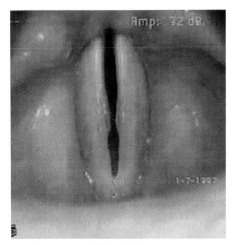

Figure 4.1.

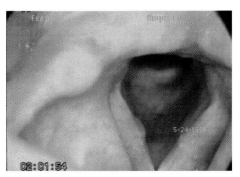

Figure 4.2.

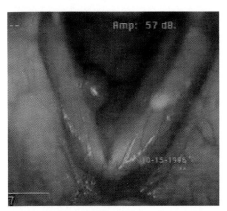

Figure 4.3.

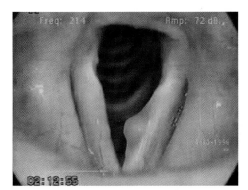

Figure 4.4.

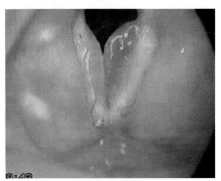

Figure 4.5.

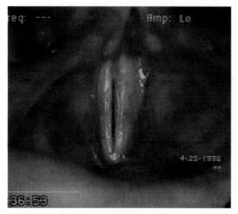

Figure 4.6.

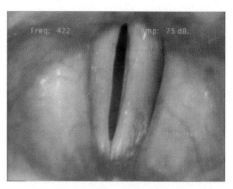

Figure 4.7.

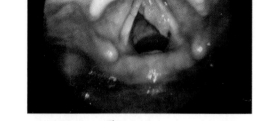

Figure 6.1.

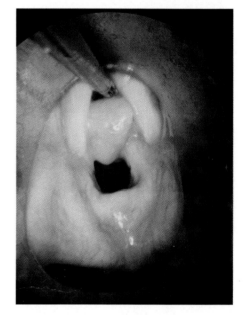

Figure 6.2.

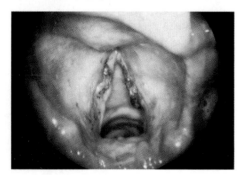

Figure 6.3.

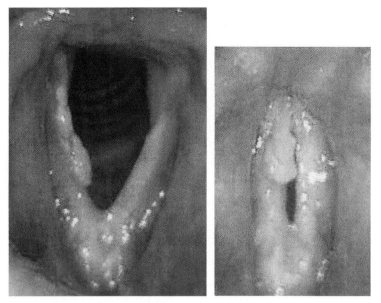

Figure 6.4.

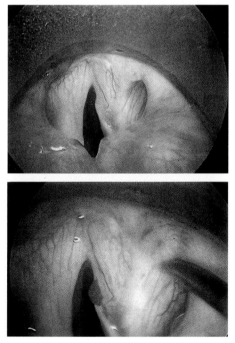

Figure 6.5.

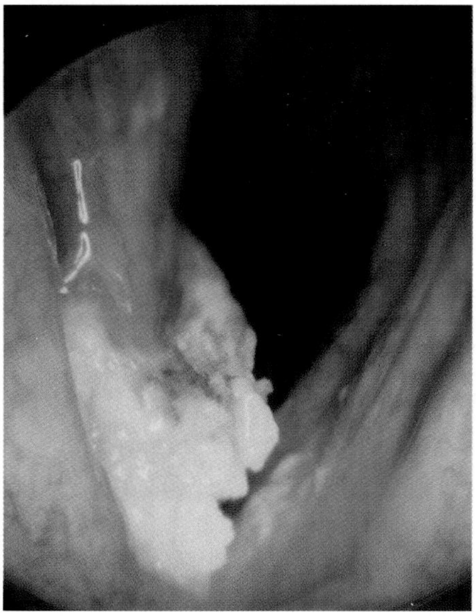

Figure 6.6.

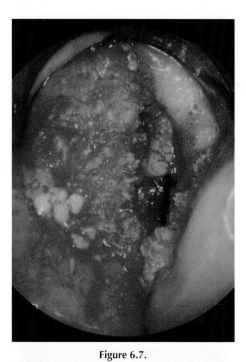

Figure 6.7.

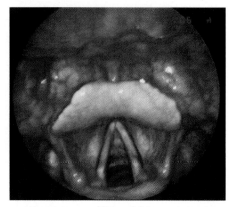

Figure 8.2.

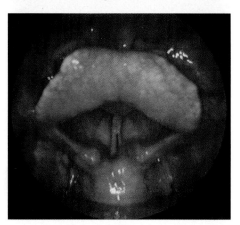

Figure 8.3.

Understanding Voice Problems

A Physiological Perspective for Diagnosis and Treatment

THIRD EDITION

Understanding Voice Problems

A Physiological Perspective for Diagnosis and Treatment

THIRD EDITION

Raymond H. Colton, Ph.D.
Professor and Chair, Department of Communication Sciences and
 Disorders
Syracuse University, Syracuse, New York
Professor Emeritus, Department of Otolaryngology and Communication
 Sciences
Upstate Medical University, Syracuse, New York

Janina K. Casper, Ph.D.
Professor Emeritus, Department of Otolaryngology and Communication
 Sciences
Upstate Medical University, Syracuse, New York

Rebecca Leonard, Ph.D.
Adjunct Professor, Department of Otolaryngology/HNS
University of California, Davis, California

With Contributions From:
Susan Thibeault, Ph.D.
Assistant Professor, Division of Otolaryngology—Head and Neck
 Surgery, Department of Surgery
The University of Utah, Salt Lake City, Utah

Richard Kelley, M.D.
Assistant Professor, Department of Otolaryngology and Communication
 Sciences
Upstate Medical University, Syracuse, New York

Selected Color Photographs by Eijii Yanagisawa, M.D.

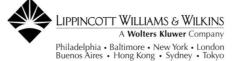

LIPPINCOTT WILLIAMS & WILKINS
A **Wolters Kluwer** Company
Philadelphia • Baltimore • New York • London
Buenos Aires • Hong Kong • Sydney • Tokyo

Acquisitions Editor: Pam Lappies
Managing Editor: Matt Hauber
Project Management: Hearthside Publishing
Marketing Manager: Mary Martin
Production Editor: Julie Montalbano
Designer: Holly McLaughlin
Compositor: TechBooks
Printer: Quebecor—Versailles

Printed in the United States of America

Library of Congress Cataloging-in-Publication Data

Colton, Raymond H.
    Understanding voice problems : a physiological perspective for diagnosis and treatment/
Raymond H. Colton, Janina Casper ; color photography by Eijii Yanagisawa.—3rd ed.
        p. ; cm.
    Includes bibliographical references and index.
    ISBN 978-0-7817-4239-9
    ISBN 0-7817-4239-0 (hardcover)
    1. Voice disorders—Pathophysiology. I. Casper, Janina K. II. Title.
    [DNLM: 1. Voice Disorders—physiopathology. 2. Voice Disorders—therapy.
        3. Larynx—physiology. 4. Voice Disorders—diagnosis.
    WV 500 C725u 2006]
    RF510.C65 2006
    616.85′5—dc22   2005007656

07 08 09
2 3 4 5 6 7 8 9 10

To David W. Brewer, M.D., our teacher, colleague, friend and a fine human being. Your dedication and contributions to the field of voice will not soon be forgotten.

Preface

There was a time when books on the topic of the voice and its disorders were few and far between. Within the last 25 years or so, we have been witness to an explosion of interest in the voice by clinicians, scientists, physicians, and singers. This multidisciplinary interest in the voice has led to a remarkable sharing of knowledge through the establishment of voice clinic teams, the publication of dedicated scholarly journals, electronic communication, and an abundance of conferences spanning not only a broad range of topics but also spanning the globe.

We are indebted to those who pioneered and pursued an interest in phonation, in how the larynx works, and in how to alter or correct its function. They persevered despite criticism by some who found these early efforts lacking in scientific stringency. We, our students, and our patients are the beneficiaries of their persistence. Nevertheless, much remains to be done. Although heartened and encouraged by the increasing numbers of scientists and clinicians, teachers, and singers interested in study of the larynx and voice production, we are dismayed by its continuing "stepchild" status in training programs for speech–language pathologists and otolaryngologists, and in singing pedagogy programs.

That, in large measure, is the reason for this book. We have been fortunate in being part of an interdisciplinary team that has studied normal and disordered phonation both clinically and experimentally for many years. Through this experience, we have evolved a philosophy and framework for the examination of laryngeal function and for clinical management of the voice-disordered patient that differed from others in its emphasis. Over the years we have presented our ideas in many lectures and courses and, if we are to judge by feedback received, have found our approach to be well received and helpful. Indeed, the team approach to voice disorders has now become the norm and is practiced in many hospitals, clinics, and other facilities where the diagnosis and treatment of voice disorders occurs.

That approach was our guide and led to the first edition of this book. We intended it to be used by students and practitioners alike in all of the specialty areas involved in the management of the voice, including otolaryngology, speech–language pathology, and coaching of the singing and dramatic voice. We intended this book to be used as a reference text by other medical specialists, such as pediatricians, family practitioners, and internists, who might be the first to come in contact with the patient with a voice disorder. We believe that the first edition broke some new ground and helped to move the study and care of the voice more firmly into the physiological domain.

The second edition of the book was also well received and is used in many of the training programs in the United States and in parts of the rest of the world. In that edition, we updated and expanded many sections to reflect then current practice and new knowledge. That same aim is reflected in this third edition. Indeed, the growth of knowledge in the field required not only updating and revising, but also the addition of entire chapters. We continue to believe that understanding voice disorders must begin with an understanding of normal phonatory physiology and acoustics. Based on such knowledge, the student, speech–language pathologist, or otolaryngologist can better understand the pathophysiology that results from traumatic voice use, pathological conditions, or neurological involvement. Because there is not a one-to-one relationship between physiology and acoustics, it is not always possible to predict specific pathological conditions or alterations in physiology on the basis of acoustics or perception alone. Thus, neither acoustic nor perceptual data are sufficient for the diagnosis and treatment of voice disorders. State-of-the-art imaging, increased knowledge of the pathophysiology together with understanding the acoustic and perceptual factors, and individual psychodynamics must all be added to the equation in determining diagnosis and planning treatment.

We are firm advocates of the differential diagnosis model and have attempted to emphasize that throughout the text. A differential diagnosis can only be carried out if it is based on knowledge. Indeed, one of the fascinations of the area of voice is the amalgamation of knowledge from various fields that must be brought to bear on the diagnostic process. The team approach is thus an ideal mechanism to support this need. The approach to management has at its core the normalization of physiology, which we believe will bring with it normalized phonation. When normalization is not a realistic goal because of structural or neuromotor constraints, the approach builds on making the most of what remains functional. The choice of therapy technique is predicated on a knowledge-based problem-solving approach, rather than on an uninformed gunshot approach. The "if it works, use it" approach may be occasionally successful but may be totally inappropriate at other times. It is important to know when to use a technique and to be able to at least speculate about why it works or fails to do so. We firmly believe that wherever possible, a technique used in voice treatment should be based on a firm theoretical basis, have solid scientific evidence when possible, and be in keeping with principles of learning. The clinician must understand the nature of the altered physiology, must take into account the psychological dynamics that may be operative, and must then be able to select an appropriate approach to rehabilitation that will address these issues. The intertwined relationship between the voice and the person is an essential component in both diagnosis and management. However, even in the patient with a psychologically based voice disorder, the deviations in the manner of voice production and voice use must be understood.

In writing this book, we have presumed that the reader will have been exposed to the study of laryngeal anatomy, physiology, neuroanatomy, and neurophysiology. Therefore, the chapters dealing with these topics appear at the end of the book and are designed to be reviews of essential concepts rather than extensive teaching chapters. Some have commented to us that these chapters would be better placed at the beginning of the book. But we prefer to emphasize the essential clinical nature of the book right from the beginning and firmly believe that the student should come to the study of voice disorders thoroughly grounded in the basic anatomy and physiology of the larynx and related structures.

We have confined ourselves to those problems having laryngeal integrity and function at their core. Thus, there is little discussion of the difficulties with voice experienced by the deaf and by those with severe hearing impairment. Although we have come to learn that there may be physiological differences in phonation between the hearing and the (congenitally) deaf, the problem usually lies primarily in the absence of acoustic input, not in abnormality of the larynx. For the same reason we have excluded discussion of the resonance problems of hyper- and hyponasality. The velopharyngeal mechanism and the anatomical structures involved in that mechanism are at the core of most aberrant resonance characteristics, rather than the phonatory mechanism. Another problem area that is absent from this book is that of the patient without a larynx. The phonatory demands of that population require the learning of an alternative mode of sound production that can no longer involve the larynx. Such problems are unique to this group and are well and thoroughly covered in other readily available publications.

The structure and philosophy of this revised edition retains much of the organization of the previous editions. A new addition is that of a third author, Dr. Rebecca Leonard, whose insight, clinical and research skills, and clear thinking have added much throughout the revised text. Chapter 1 introduces the study of the larynx, beginning with its important biological functions. The uniqueness of our human ability to speak is dependent in part on the ability of the larynx to produce the acoustic signal we call voice. The changes in that signal that accompany lifespan changes are reviewed, as is voice production. Various models of the team approach to the diagnosis and management of voice disorders are introduced. Chapter 2 is key to the philosophy of this book. We have approached the process of differential diagnosis in the manner usually experienced in the real world when the patient presents with certain symptoms. We follow the process through the steps that the practitioner must pursue in narrowing the possibilities until a diagnosis and cause are assigned. Case studies are presented as an aid to understanding the process. Our scheme rests on nine primary symptoms of disorders of voice and expands from there to the various signs—perceptual, acoustic, and physiological—that would be consistent with the symptom.

In Chapter 3, Dr. Susan Thibeault discusses current information and concepts about the microstructure of the larynx. Chapter 4 addresses traumatic use of the larynx, with a focus on the physiological effects related to specific vocal behaviors. Expanded information on stroboscopic findings is a feature of this revised text. One of the unique aspects of this book is a lengthy section in this chapter devoted to the effects of drugs on the voice. The use of over-the-counter as well as prescription drugs is extensive. Their effects on the laryngeal mucosa have been largely overlooked. There is still a paucity of experimental evidence about these effects. Voice problems associated with nervous system involvement are discussed in Chapter 5. Although voice problems in this population are extensive, the available data on the acoustic parameters of the voice or the physiological parameters of airflow and laryngeal muscle action potentials are exceedingly limited.

Chapter 6 is devoted to a discussion of voice problems associated with the organic: disease and trauma. These are areas about which the speech–language pathologist must be knowledgeable. Chapter 7 traces the development and occurrence of voice disorders in children and concludes with a more extensive treatment of the aging voice than appeared in the first two editions. The section on geriatric voice addresses some of the current problems and concerns of this growing segment of our population. An extensive section on taking the voice history introduces Chapter 8, and its length emphasizes our concern about the relatively minimal training speech–language pathologists and otolaryngologists usually receive in this critical area of communication between patient and practitioner. The remainder of the chapter is given over to descriptions and discussion of methods of laryngeal examination and testing procedures, both instrumental and noninstrumental. The information that has been generated about the larynx and its function through the use of stroboscopy has been updated and expanded. Dr. Richard Kelley, the otolaryngology member of our team, discusses phonosurgery, and the surgical management of voice problems, in Chapter 9.

The focus of Chapter 10 is vocal rehabilitation, a primary method used to alter phonatory behavior. The chapter begins with a discussion of some general concepts, principles, and guidelines that we believe are critical to the undertaking of a vocal rehabilitation program. The role of voice therapy in the treatment of disorders associated with traumatic voice use, pathological conditions, neuromotor involvement, and some unusual problems is discussed. A variety of specific treatment techniques are offered. Each is described, and a rationale for its usefulness is provided. This section contains updated information on various therapy techniques as well as patient outcomes. The outcome of our treatment for all kinds of communication disorders has received much more attention since the publication of the second edition of this book. Much more information is available to assess the effect of our treatment on a patient's everyday function and on the quality of life. Some controversial areas related to voice therapy and some unresolved issues are discussed, and the final sections of this chapter briefly address the issues of prevention and malpractice.

Chapters 11 through 13 were described earlier as reference chapters. They deal with the anatomy, physiology, and neuroanatomy and neurophysiology of the vocal mechanism, in that order. It is our intent that these chapters be referred to frequently as a differential diagnosis is pursued. Chapter 14, the final reference chapter, provides normative data against which patient data can be compared. By placing this material in a separate chapter, we have made it readily accessible for reference use. And finally, the Appendix offers a variety of forms and protocols that we have found to be useful in our assessment and examination procedures and includes a copy of the rating form proposed by the Consensus Conference on Voice Perception for rating patient voices.

We have also included a DVD containing video samples of the stroboscopic examinations of many of the patients presented in Chapter 2 and 7. We have also included a unique case presentation and examples of surgical procedures.

As much as possible, we have attempted to construct our sentences so as to avoid the use of sex-specific pronouns. When this attempt resulted in convoluted language structure that became an obstacle to understanding, we have chosen to use gender pronouns (i.e., his or her) interchangeably. The reader should be aware that despite the particular pronoun used, we are speaking of both sexes unless it is clearly stated otherwise. Furthermore, because this book is intended for a broad audience, we have adopted the use of the English alphabet rather than phonetic symbols to describe vowel sounds (such as /ee/ for the sound in "see").

We are indebted to Susan Thibeault, Ph.D. for her excellent treatment of vocal fold histology (Chapter 3) and to Richard Kelley, M.D. for his superb chapter on surgical intervention (Chapter 9). We also wish to thank again Dr. Miroru Hirano, a leader and innovator in the study of vocal fold physiology who contributed to the earlier editions of the book.

Many others have helped in diverse ways with the preparation of this book. Dr. David W. Brewer has, throughout the years, been a source of constant support and encouragement. We thank him for that and for his insightful reading and critique of much of the text. We acknowledge the help of the late Samuel Mallov, Ph.D., Professor Emeritus of Pharmacology, SUNY Health Science Center at Syracuse, who checked the accuracy of our comments about the effects of drugs on the voice. Martha Hefner, medical illustrator at the SUNY Health Science Center, along with Elinor Griep, Brian Harris, and Craig Palmer, provided splendid illustrative material, and always with a smile. We are grateful for the generosity of Eijii Yanagisawa, M.D., in sharing with us his superb photographic skills. Others have read various sections of the manuscript in preparation and have given us valuable direction. We wish to thank Peak Woo, M.D., Fran Lowry, Carol Friedenberg, the late Herbert N. Wright, and

Joanne Chilton. For this revised edition, we want to thank the many colleagues who have offered support and encouragement by adopting this textbook for use with their students and by providing us with such useful and positively reinforcing feedback.

We each have families who have been supportive and patient throughout this process. They have been deprived of attention, of our presence, and of the availability of the computer, but not of our gratitude and love.

Contents

Chapter 1

Introduction and Overview

BIOLOGICAL IMPORTANCE OF THE LARYNX

The structures that make up the larynx play a role in support of an important life-sustaining function, that of respiration. The vocal folds (both true and false), the aryepiglottic folds, and other structures within the larynx were designed to maintain and protect the airway from foreign substances. The architect of the human body realized that the respiratory system needed multiple levels of protection from foreign substances, including the harmful effects of the environment. Numerous protective mechanisms therefore exist in the respiratory tract, but the most vigorous exist in the larynx. Some are mechanical and act to close off the airway; others are expulsive and serve to force foreign substances out of the airway. All are reflexive and operate under involuntary control.

Many sensory endings within the larynx collect information about the state of the larynx and transmit this information through several reflex arcs, as well as directly, to the central nervous system. (See Chapter 13 for more detailed information.) These sensory systems exist to inform the brain about the state of the environment within the respiratory tract. Wyke (1967, 1969) and others (Bradley, 2000; Lucier, Daynes, & Sessie, 1978; Sant'Ambrogio, Mathew, Fisher, & Sant'Ambrogio, 1983; Warner, 1998) have written extensively about these reflex control mechanisms. The various levels of these reflex mechanisms within the larynx provide an elaborate system of precautions to protect the airway and maintain life. For example, sensory endings in the laryngeal lining respond to mechanical forces such as air pressure, and these sensory endings signal information about the state of these forces to higher centers. Although these reflex mechanisms speak primarily to the biological importance of the larynx, they also may be very important to consider in understanding the physiology of normal human phonation and its disorders.

Speech is an overlaid function; that is, the systems used to produce speech were developed long before humans learned to speak. These systems have evolved over eons and reflect the unique place of speech in human existence. Clear evidence of this evolution is seen in the multiplicity of the protective laryngeal reflex mechanisms. It is important to recognize that these protective "natural" acts may sometimes be the cause of a voice disorder. For example, excessive coughing, a protective act, can result in trauma to the vocal folds and cause edema, which in turn will interfere with the vibratory characteristics of the vocal folds. By the same token, rapid, random movements of the vocal folds at rest may interfere with normal vibratory motion. Central neurological dysfunction or disruption in a reflex arc may create abnormal motions, which may interfere with phonation or, indeed, threaten life.

The biological function of the larynx can never be ignored. The examiner who accidentally touches the back wall of the pharynx when performing an indirect mirror examination or rigid endoscopy can attest to the rapid reflexive motions of the pharynx and larynx that result from the "gag" reflex. The reflex or biological functions of the larynx can be subtle in their effects, however, and may not be apparent to either the untrained observer or the experienced eye. Many reflex endings are sensitive to small changes of movement or air pressure that serve to inform the central nervous system about the normal operation of the airway. The respiratory cycle itself and the activity of the nerve controlling the diaphragm may be affected by these changes. They also affect the discharge pattern of the intrinsic laryngeal muscles. The effects of these subtle changes are important to consider for an understanding of the physiology of normal voice production.

We are still young in our understanding of the physiology of the human body. Our fascination with modern instrumentation has produced a good deal of information about human voice production (Baken & Orlikoff, 2000). Nevertheless, the fundamental mechanisms of bodily function and regulation must not be ignored. Reflexes are primitive neural control subsystems. They operate at a very low level in the hierarchy of neural functioning and control large muscle actions. These mechanisms are always there, however, waiting in the wings, so to speak, to alter body function. Our awareness and appreciation of their role should be apparent to us and to our patients if we are truly to understand human voice function.

THE LARYNX AND THE VOICE

The voice is an integral part of that uniquely human attribute known as speech. The larynx and its capabilities are important in two broad areas: biological function and speech. The larynx houses the major source of sound used during speaking. The vocal folds produce a tone that becomes modified by the pharynx, palate, tongue, and lips to produce the individual sounds of speech. Voice is present for most vowels and for many of the consonants. The point at which the vocal folds begin to vibrate relative to the movement of the other articulators (i.e., lips, tongue, palate, etc.) is critical if the speaker is to produce the intended sound. The larynx must operate in close synchrony with other parts of the speech production apparatus if intelligible speech is to be produced. Although the voice is not visible to the eye during speech production, its absence or malfunction is obvious.

In addition to its role as a carrier of words, the voice also can produce music and express emotion—it acts as a mirror of the inner self. The singer with superb control of the vocal instrument brings immense pleasure to the listener. Although the singer's words may be conveying a verbal statement, the phrasing, control of pitch, and dynamic range may communicate an even stronger message. In classical singing, for example, it is the rare listener who is not enthralled by the sound of a clear and beautiful high C, sung with ease, power, and majesty. The singing of a choir or the chanting of prayers can lead to a unique religious experience.

The actor's voice, resonant and full of meaning, can add significantly to the message and the intensity of emotion. Indeed, the actor's delivery of the words can sometimes be more engrossing to the listener than the words themselves.

The voice serves as an emotional outlet. Both laughter and crying release emotion and frequently serve important cathartic functions. Shouts of joy and screams of rage or fear convey meanings that are easily recognized.

The voice reveals the inner self. It is a reflection of the personality of the individual (Rosen & Sataloff, 1997). We recognize the stereotypical driving, hard-hitting voice of the salesperson, the nasal singsong of the perpetual whiner, and the monotonous, de-energized voice of the depressed. The voice of an outgoing person may be characterized by variety in the pitch, loudness, or quality. Conversely, a monotone voice, one with little variety, may characterize the withdrawn individual or the loner who wishes not to be disturbed. Markel and his colleagues (1964, 1973) have shown that the pitch, loudness, and tempo of the voice can be used to reflect the personality of the individual and correlate well with other standardized tests of personality measurement.

The speaker's voice is used to attract as well as to repel people. A soft, soothing voice is more apt to calm an agitated person than a strident and loud voice. Conversely, a strident, loud voice may be used effectively to repel someone. We instantly use a loud, "firm" voice to dispense with a pushy salesperson or to avert a physically threatening situation.

The voice can reveal a person's physical state, as well as the physical state of the larynx. The weak or tremulous voice associated with illness is easily identified, and the voice altered by a laryngeal pathological condition is identified as abnormal.

Yes, the voice is a powerful tool that not only delivers the message but also adds to its meaning. In learning to understand the voice, it is not enough to understand its mechanical functioning. It is also necessary to recognize the important information the voice conveys about the speaker.

VOICE CHANGES IN LIFE

The voice changes dynamically, minute by minute. However, long-term changes are associated with growth and decline in life. At the major stages of life, the uses of the voice are different, as are the demands placed on it. The reasons for these differences are many and include biological maturation and the emotional and social changes that occur in the individual's life.

The Voice in Infancy and Childhood

In the first few weeks of life, the infant voice is used to express pain, pleasure, displeasure, and hunger. Crying, the major avenue of communication for the infant, is rich in its ability to communicate (Lester, 1985).

Crying reflects the beginning ability of the infant to control his or her voice (Robb, Goberman & Cacace, 1997; Robb & Goberman, 1997). It is a gross physical act that can be described as ballistic in nature. In other words, crying, once started, runs its course and stops. Little can be done to stop the crying once it has begun. As the infant grows older, he is more responsive to the environment and also gains more control of the physical apparatus used to produce the cry. Consequently, the quality of crying is seen to reflect physical and psychological growth. As the infant gains finer and finer motor control, the cry becomes increasingly controllable and much more purposeful in its use.

The next most obvious voice use change occurs as the child begins to use the voice in the production of speech sounds. Concurrently, the child is learning the sounds of his specific language. Then, the child can use the voice to express ideas and moods. At other times, the child may use the voice merely as the expression of play in itself. As the child matures, increasingly complex and sophisticated differentiation of acceptable modes of vocal behavior develops. This differentiation begins in infancy. The infant's vocal response to a caretaker's familiar voice differs from that given to an unfamiliar voice. Generally, the child's vocal response differs based on the familiarity of the voice heard. Children learn that the voice of the playground is not the voice of the classroom. Such differentiation continues through life in many subtle ways.

The voice reflects the physical development of the child. The infant possesses a larynx that is pliable and has a low level of neuromuscular coordination. It is also small, with short vocal folds. The small structure means that the pitch of the infant's voice will be high. The infant's ability to control the tension of the vocal folds is limited. Moreover, the limited ability of the infant to control the air pressure required for speech results in short bursts of sound, many of which are rather loud. As the infant grows, the ability to control vocal pitch and loudness increases (Boone, 1987). This development is reflected in the longer cries, which are lower in pitch and vary in loudness depending on the circumstances.

In summary, during infancy and childhood, the characteristics of the voice depend on the physical, cognitive, and emotional maturation of the child. The physical size of the vocal folds is a major determinant of the fundamental frequency of the child's voice. The infant, with a small larynx and short vocal folds, exhibits the highest vocal pitch, whereas the older child, whose larynx has grown, possesses a lower vocal pitch. Adult vocal pitch is not attained until puberty, when the larynx reaches its adult size.

Loudness variation is less affected by these growth changes and more affected by the level of motor control exhibited by the child. Quality variation reflects physical growth changes of the vocal folds, changes in the size and shape of the entire vocal tract, and finer control of the neuromuscular system. Differentiation of appropriate voice use characteristics depends not only on physical abilities but also on cognitive and social growth and awareness.

The Voice of the Adult

By age 18 years or perhaps younger, the voice reaches its mature or adult stage. The fundamental frequency is where it will remain for several decades. The individual has full control over the dynamic range (loudness) of the voice and can produce many variations of pitch and voice quality. These vocal abilities reflect the maturation of the anatomical and physiological systems for the support of speech (Kahane, 1982).

Although the adult voice has been attained by age 18 years, much refinement still can occur to expand vocal abilities. Indeed, vocal training for the singer or the actor most appropriately begins when this level of maturation has been reached. Pitch range can be extended, vocal control can be increased, and voice quality can be enriched.

The way the voice is used depends on the demands of the situation. These demands may include the teacher's need to instruct and maintain discipline, the minister's need to deliver a forceful sermon or to be consoling, or the salesperson's need to sell a product.

The voice is easily taken for granted. We can traumatize it with constant use and frequent misuse. We can expose it to the harmful effects of smoke and alcohol and expect it to be unaffected. Typically only when we experience difficulty talking do we cease taking it for granted and seek help. Often we have difficulty recognizing potentially traumatic habits and making the necessary changes, even when our lives are threatened.

The Aged Voice

After 65 years of age or so, the voice begins its decline, much the same way other body functions begin to decline (Beasley & Davis, 1981; Kahane, 1981; Linville, 2001). The voice, however, does not always mirror the extreme or rapid changes that may occur in the physical functioning of the body. Aged individuals in good physical condition possess voices that are similar in their characteristics to the voices of younger persons (Ramig & Ringel, 1983). Some singers can maintain their voices well into their 70s. The voice may retain the essential elements of beauty, although it may not exhibit the range or degree of vocal control that was present in younger years.

For others, however, the voice readily betrays the effects of aging. Voices that show a decline or increase in habitual vocal pitch, decreased control of loudness, or changes in voice quality may be showing signs of diminished physical status. Acoustic changes such as upward or downward frequency shifts, poorly controlled loudness, and quality changes reflect to some degree the physiological changes that occur in the larynx with increasing age.

The vocal demands of the aged adult also may be different from those of the younger adult. After retirement, the salesperson no longer must use that voice to sell a product. The retired minister no longer has to deliver that forceful sermon. The decline of bodily function is usually accompanied by reduced demand on the system. That is not to say that the voice is no longer important to the elderly. On the contrary, the voice is important, but in a different way. It retains its importance in the communication process. It is used to maintain contact with friends and relatives. For some individuals, verbal communication becomes the only way to maintain human contact and control of the environment.

PRODUCTION OF THE VOICE

To most lay people, the way in which the voice is produced is a mystery. The term *voice box* is commonly used to refer to the larynx, the voice-generating mechanism. Most people know they have one and that it is somewhere in the throat below the chin. From experience they know that when they have laryngitis, they cannot talk, or that their voices sound "funny," but few understand why those changes occur. Some people may be aware that after strenuous voice use, such as yelling at a sports event, their voices may sound hoarse. They surmise that the hoarseness has to do with "straining" the voice. Some people may even realize they can manipulate their voices in many ways, for example, raise or lower pitch, increase or decrease loudness, and change their voice quality. This is such common knowledge that it is taken for granted without thought about the workings of the mechanism that is capable of producing such changes.

Understanding phonatory physiology goes beyond knowing laryngeal anatomy and recognizing various laryngeal pathologies (Aronson, 1990; Kahane, 1982). Treatment of the voice-disordered patient demands such a knowledge base. Disturbed physiology may be a by-product of pathological conditions and may persist after the pathological condition is resolved. Conversely, disturbed physiology may be the cause of tissue changes. Whatever the treatment modality, restoration of normal function, or the closest possible approximation of it, is the goal.

The basic concepts of phonatory physiology have been understood for many years (Lieberman, 1968; Titze, 1994; van den Berg, 1958). Recent technological advances have, however, significantly increased our knowledge base (Hirano, 1981a; Kahane, 1981). The inaccessibility of the larynx, especially during the phonatory act, has hindered our ability to understand its functioning more fully. In 1855, Garcia developed the laryngeal mirror (Moore, 1937) and made it possible to visualize the larynx with the naked eye. Since then, greatly improved techniques of laryngeal visualization as well as sophisticated analyses of laryngeal acoustics and improved methods of measuring physiological events related to phonation have resulted in a greater understanding of phonatory physiology (Fritzell & Fant, 1986).

Understanding the physiology of phonation is intimately bound up with an understanding of laryngeal anatomy and neuroanatomy, as well as respiratory function. Changes in the structures, in the tissues, or in motor control, whether the result of neurological insult, trauma, congenital anomaly, lesion, or disease process, will distort normal physiology in some fairly predictable ways. This disturbed physiology will, in turn, have an effect on the acoustic characteristics of the voice. Physiology also can be altered by changes in muscular and skeletal tensions, with concomitant changes in the acoustics. Therefore, there is an interdependence and interaction among anatomy, physiology, neurology, and acoustics. It is necessary to understand this interaction to treat the voice problem effectively. Teachers of the professional voice must increase their working knowledge of the complex phonatory process.

All users of voice, as well as those who treat or train it, can benefit from an understanding of how the voice works. Simple knowledge of the effects of vocally traumatic behaviors and the need for good vocal hygiene is important to the prevention of certain types of laryngeal pathological conditions and could be potent preventive measures for reducing the incidence of vocal nodules and certain polyps. Some people, without the benefit of specific voice training, are able to use their voices in strenuous ways without encountering any vocal problems. They are the exceptions. Most people who use the voice in chronically strenuous ways are at risk for developing vocal difficulty.

Most professional voice users have had vocal training, although it is rare for such training to include more than a cursory understanding of phonatory physiology. Typically, voice coaches have been taught by other voice coaches, and techniques are passed on that are believed to produce the desired results. Little objective evidence exists that these techniques do what they are purported to do. Although some techniques appear to be spectacularly successful, others have done unwitting damage to voices.

Professional voice users need to understand the workings of their instrument to use it most effectively and maintain its health. In addition to professional singers and actors, the category of professional voice users should be expanded to include teachers, coaches, ministers, salespersons, cheerleaders, and others who use their voices extensively and perhaps strenuously in the performance of their occupations.

The growth of interest in the voice and the recognition of the need for multidisciplinary involvement in its care have resulted in increased understanding of the science underlying voice physiology among vocal coaches and singers as well. The many multidisciplinary voice conferences throughout the world attest to this and continue to disseminate information.

THE VOICE TEAM

Many professionals representing numerous disciplines or fields of study are concerned with the voice. Some are concerned with basic studies of laryngeal function, others are concerned with medical problems affecting the voice, and others are concerned with the evaluation and treatment of voice problems. Still other disciplines are focused on developing the voice to its pinnacle of performance ability. Each discipline brings its particular focus and area of expertise to bear on diagnosis, treatment, or teaching.

The internist, the family practitioner, or the pediatrician may be the first specialist to come in contact with a patient with a voice problem. These primary care physicians must be aware of the voice as a sign of health or illness. For example, persistent hoarseness is recognized among medical personnel and the public as one of the early warning signs of cancer. Other vocal symptoms if recognized can be helpful in the early diagnosis of certain disease processes. Recognition and identification of the existence of a problem is only the first step. This must be followed by appropriate treatment or referral for further evaluation or treatment.

The otolaryngologist is the most appropriate specialist for the diagnosis and treatment of medical laryngeal problems. Although a growing number of otolaryngologists specialize in the treatment of voice problems, most will be expected to treat a variety of laryngeal and other otolaryngological problems. Laryngitis, vocal fold nodules, polyps, loss of voice, or hoarseness of undetermined origin are among the problems that affect the voice and are typically identified by otolaryngologists.

As is true for otolaryngologists, many speech–language pathologists work with the voice-disordered patient, but relatively few have made this an area of specialization. The appropriately trained speech–language pathologist is the specialist who diagnoses and treats problems of phonatory function, or "vocal pathology." The mode of treatment offered by speech–language pathologists focuses on the modification of phonatory behavior. Indeed, the speech–language pathologist's broad-based understanding of behavior, whether it be the result of inappropriate voice usage, disturbed physiology, or a manifestation of underlying psychological problems, uniquely qualifies this professional to aid in the diagnostic process, as well as to provide a primary resource for nonmedical treatment.

Voice scientists have added immeasurably to our understanding of phonatory physiology and acoustics through experimental verification of hypotheses. They are not usually directly involved in either treating or teaching the voice user. However, the information available from laboratory studies of the voice can be helpful in establishing a diagnosis, validating treatment approaches (Verdolini & Titze, 1995), and in documenting change in vocal function as a result of treatment. Furthermore, much can be learned about phonatory physiology from the study of abnormal function.

Neurolaryngology, the specialized neurological approach to laryngeal function, is a fairly new and developing area of knowledge, with far-reaching clinical implications. Many movement disorders have laryngeal components that have not been well documented and are not well understood. Indeed, it is not unusual for a phonatory problem to be the first symptom of a motor disorder. A neurolaryngologist could be a valuable member of any team concerned with voice disorders.

Imaging techniques are powerful tools assisting in the diagnosis of pathological conditions. Laryngologists whose special area of expertise focuses on head and neck problems are frequently involved in initial and subsequent assessments of laryngeal abnormality. Radiologists provide further information relative to the size, location, and extent of a lesion through a variety of imaging techniques. Such information is frequently critical to diagnostic and management decisions, especially those that involve surgery. Imaging techniques such as magnetic resonance imaging (MRI) or computed tomography (CT) (Baer et al., 1987; Brooks, 1993; Leboldus et. al., 1986;

Piekarski, 1992; Stark et. al., 1984; Wippold, 2000) scan can provide additional information about the state of the larynx and the vocal tract during speaking and singing.

Patients whose voice problems are an expression of deep-rooted emotional problems may require psychotherapy (Aronson, 1990; Aronson, Peterson, & Litin, 1966; Diehl, 1960). Referral to a psychotherapist is indicated when it has been determined that the vocal problem exhibited by the patient may be an expression or symptom of significant psychiatric disability. Our understanding of the bond between voice and personality has been enhanced by the contributions of the fields of psychiatry and psychology.

Teachers and coaches of the singing and the speaking voice are interested in maximizing the individual potential of each of their students while maintaining the health and structural integrity of the vocal mechanism. Their unique knowledge of the professional voice and their deep interest in its correct use necessitates a good knowledge of vocal anatomy and physiology. This is especially true because the vocal demands on singers and actors are frequently much greater than for the average speaker. Furthermore, even subtle changes in vocal production may be critical to a performance.

The number and variety of disciplines involved in the understanding and management of the voice give testimony to the complexity of the process of phonation. Our experience in the "team approach" to understanding the voice and its disorders has led us to an appreciation of the active involvement of a variety of disciplines working together in the assessment process. The benefits of this interactive interdisciplinary team approach accrue not only to the patient, but also to the professionals involved. Each team member brings a particular perspective and knowledge base to the diagnostic process, extending by far the single examiner's expertise. For example, the otolaryngologist is highly skilled in assessment of the health or disease state of the larynx, the speech–language pathologist specializes in the phonatory function of the mechanism and the manner in which it may be disturbed by various conditions, and the singing coach recognizes problems in vocal technique that are specific to the singing voice.

The team approach may take various forms, each with its own set of advantages and disadvantages. A description of several models follows.

Model A

The patient is seen individually during the course of a few hours by various specialists who are located within the same facility or in close proximity. Typically either the otolaryngologist or the speech–language pathologist will perform a videostroboscopic laryngeal examination. The team of specialists may subsequently meet to review the videotaped examination, discuss their various findings, and agree on a treatment plan, or individual reports may be directed to the team leader, who incorporates them into a complete report with recommendations for treatment.

ADVANTAGES

The patient is seen on a single day, ensuring that all specialists are seeing the patient at the same point in the course of the problem. Each specialist has the necessary time to carry out a complete evaluation. The opportunity for interaction among team members exists if the team meets together to discuss the findings. Although it may take a few hours, this model nonetheless can be a time saver for the patient.

DISADVANTAGES

The process involves duplication of information that the patient must provide to each specialist. Team members do not have the input from other findings until after they have made their own assessments and arrived at their own plan. Even though the examinations take place within a few hours, patients do fatigue, and the voice heard by one examiner may be quite different from that heard by another. The patient is usually not present when the team meets, precluding further immediate assessment based on input from any individual specialist. For example, if the stroboscopic examination is performed by the otolaryngologist, the voice clinician may not have the opportunity to extend that examination into a phonoscopic (vocal behavior) examination, or, conversely, a voice clinician may fail to adequately examine the area for signs of disease. The alternative here is for the patient to undergo two separate examinations, the ramifications of which are obvious. Furthermore, if there is a time lag between the actual examinations and the team meeting, much can be lost through dulling of memory. If individual findings are reported to a single individual, the opportunity for invaluable interaction among specialists is lost.

Model B

The patient is seen individually by various specialists over the course of several weeks. In this type of model, individual reports are typically sent to a single individual who is the manager of the case. That individual blends all of the information and makes recommendations for treatment.

ADVANTAGES

The only plus for this model is the involvement of various disciplines rather than a single specialist who functions without the benefit of additional information.

DISADVANTAGES

This process may take some time to complete. Over that course of time, the patient's problem may undergo various changes in type, degree, and severity. Thus, each specialist may be seeing quite a different picture. There is no opportunity for true interdisciplinary interaction. It is time consuming for the patient and may prolong a problem by postponing appropriate intervention. Most of the disadvantages cited for the first model also apply here.

Model C

The patient is seen either by the laryngologist or the speech–language pathologist, and a video laryngostroboscopic examination is done. The history and tape may then be reviewed jointly by these two specialists and a diagnosis and treatment plan agreed to, or, after the tape is reviewed individually, a consensus is reached regarding diagnosis and treatment. Additional specialists may be consulted as needed.

ADVANTAGES

This model may be a time saver for all concerned—the patient has one examination, and only one specialist's time is involved in the examination. If specialists review the examination together, a degree of interdisciplinary interaction is preserved.

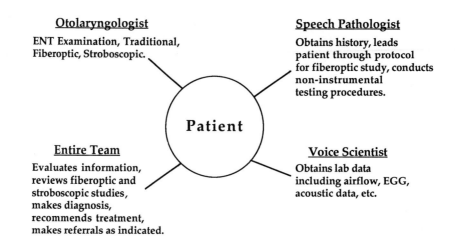

Figure 1.1. The Team Approach.

DISADVANTAGES

The patient is usually not present when the specialists meet, thus precluding the possibility of additional examination or data gathering at that time. Acoustic and other laboratory data may not be obtained at the time of the initial examination. If the specialists do not jointly review the examination tape, there is a lack of interaction. If further assessments are needed the time necessary to complete the examination becomes extended, and interaction of all involved usually becomes minimal.

Model D

The model that we find most satisfactory is one in which a number of specialists are present and interact with the patient and each other at the time of the video laryngostroboscopic/phonoscopic examination with the opportunity for further individual assessments to follow (Fig. 1.1). In our model, laboratory data (acoustic and physiological) are obtained immediately before or after the endoscopic examination. The team discusses the findings and presents the diagnosis and treatment plan to the patient, with full opportunity for questions to be raised and answered. Patients have the opportunity to view the laryngeal imaging study, and, with staff direction, they are able to observe laryngeal or vocal pathological conditions or other problems.

ADVANTAGES

An obvious advantage of this model is that all of those involved hear the same sample of voice and observe the larynx at the same time. Each specialist has the opportunity to ask questions during the history taking and to request that a specific phonatory task or non-phonatory gesture be elicited during the examination. For example, the speech–language pathologist may wish to assess laryngeal function through the use of both the rigid and the flexible endoscopes to appreciate aspects of phonatory physiology or to engage in preliminary treatment probing. There is an opportunity for immediate discussion of the case, and, because the patient is still present, further examination is possible if it seems warranted. Diagnosis and treatment plan are formulated by the team and discussed with the patient. The interdisciplinary interaction is extremely valuable.

The history and findings are clearly recalled by all without reliance on memory over time.

DISADVANTAGES

The number of people present (three or more) can sometimes be overwhelming to patients if they have not been prepared to expect this. The history can only address major areas and may not uncover more subtle or underlying problems that are not appropriately discussed in the presence of the full team. Often such problems, if present, emerge when the patient begins an individual treatment protocol. At that time, the individual practitioners attain a better understanding of the patient and can more appropriately explore other issues.

Although we are committed to Model D of the team approach, we recognize that it is not a universal mode of operation. Otolaryngologists often see patients with voice problems in their offices and refer to a speech–language pathologist only those patients they believe are appropriate candidates for voice therapy. Those referrals frequently may be based on indirect mirror examinations, with minimal information provided to the speech–language pathologist. ASHA (1993) guidelines and Preferred Practice Patterns make it clear that all patients with voice disorders must have a laryngological examination before the initiation of voice therapy.

When referrals for voice therapy fail to provide adequate information on which to base a therapy approach, it is incumbent on the speech–language pathologist to request additional information. That can be accomplished in a variety of ways. Professional protocol requires that additional information be sought from the referring physician. If the speech–language pathologist is appropriately trained in phonatory function assessment and has access to videostroboscopic equipment, such an examination is appropriately carried out. If neither of these avenues provides the necessary information, patients can be directed to a voice laboratory or other resource where additional information or a second opinion may be obtained.

SUMMARY

The larynx serves essential reflexive biological functions that protect the airway and maintain life. These basic functions determine the limits of voice and may occasionally affect its function. The larynx also provides the acoustic signal for speech, that uniquely human capability. Singing, dramatic exposition, laughing, and crying fulfill additional human needs through the voice. The voice reflects individual identity, personality, and life stage. An understanding of phonatory physiology, as well as of those factors that may disturb it, is necessary for all professionals involved in the care of the voice and for all professional voice users. Assessment of the voice-disordered patient is enhanced by input from various disciplines through a team approach.

Chapter 2

Differential Diagnosis of Voice Problems

In this chapter, and throughout this book, we use the term *diagnosis* in two distinct ways. In the first sense, it refers to the process one should engage in when attempting to determine the nature of a problem. That process involves examination and observation, a problem-solving approach. However, in the second sense, the word *diagnosis* refers to the decision that is the end product of the diagnostic process.

The diagnostic process can be likened to solving a puzzle. Each piece of the puzzle must be examined from many perspectives. Each piece is only a part of the total picture. As a piece is found, it is placed into the puzzle, until the picture is complete. As often happens, one or more pieces may be missing. In those instances, more time is required to search for the missing pieces. In the process of diagnosis of voice disorders, there also may be missing pieces. The solution may not be apparent, and ongoing examination of all relevant information must continue.

Analysis of voice problems involves the examination of many individual components. These components include the statement of the problem, the symptoms, and the history or related information, as well as a set of signs observed or measured by the examiners. The examination of these components may involve a variety of procedures, including the following:

1. Interview
2. Examination of medical records
3. Rating of auditory perceptual characteristics
4. Measurement of acoustic, aerodynamic, vibratory, and muscle action events
5. Examination of the laryngeal structures and their function
6. Evaluation of other bodily functions and systems as deemed appropriate
7. Experimental therapy, or treatment probing, in which attempts are made to manipulate the patient's vocal behavior

The successful completion of the diagnostic process requires a solid base of information. Diagnosis of voice disorders requires a thorough understanding of laryngeal anatomy and physiology. Research on all phases of the voice is proceeding at a very rapid pace, and exciting and significant information is being reported about how the voice works and the structures and mechanisms that are needed to maintain this function. A fundamental understanding of phonatory physiology is essential so that rational hypotheses can be formulated about the voice problem and the conditions accompanying it. Moreover, the clinician must be able to formulate hypotheses concerning the expected changes in physiology based on analysis of perceptual and acoustic information. The clinician must be aware of and sensitive to the relationship between personality and voice. Knowledge about the various pathological conditions and how they affect phonation is, of course, essential.

The diagnostic process is differential. That is, it is necessary to consider all the possible causes of a problem and to proceed through them all as if each is the real cause until proved otherwise. The differential aspect of the diagnostic process involves consideration of the basic question, what specific problem or problems might comprise these component parts? The available information relative to the patient is then matched against each of these hypotheses in the search for a match, a good fit.

The process of differential diagnosis begins anew with each patient. In the clinical setting, patients present with a complaint or perhaps even several complaints. The challenge for the diagnostician is to track down all of the pieces of data essential to an understanding of the physiology, to the making of a diagnosis, and perhaps to knowledge about cause.

WHAT IS ETIOLOGY?

Etiology is defined by Webster's Third New International Dictionary as "a science or doctrine of causation or of the demonstration of causes." Symptoms and signs describe various components of the problem, providing part of the raw data necessary for determination of the cause. The first step in the treatment of any medical problem is determination of its cause, its etiology. Recognition of the correct cause is essential for proper treatment. It is not only unwise but also potentially dangerous to treat a problem for which a well-considered etiology has not been established. An incorrect etiology may result in improper treatment, lack of needed treatment, or, at the very worst, may compromise a patient's life. For example, laryngitis is a common cause of hoarseness and is treated not only by otolaryngologists but also by pediatricians, family physicians, and internists. In many cases, laryngitis is caused by an upper respiratory infection and is appropriately treated with medication. However, hoarseness may be a sign of many other pathological laryngeal conditions, including malignant lesions, and as such should be evaluated with all possible causes in mind. In our experience, some patients have followed a protracted and unsuccessful course of medical treatment only to have subsequent examination show the presence of a vocal fold lesion as the cause of the hoarseness.

Assigning an etiology is not always easy. It is possible for a condition to be unobservable and to escape careful and thorough examination. A condition also may persist when the original cause of the problem is no longer present. For example, an untrained singer may have developed vocal nodules while engaged in strenuous voice use and abuse for a period of several months. The behaviors that led to the pathological condition may no longer be present, but the resultant tissue changes persist. It is important to be aware of antecedent conditions that may be responsible for the present problem.

SYMPTOMS AND SIGNS

The words "signs and symptoms" are used frequently in medical literature (Brewer, 1975). What do they mean, and how can the distinction between them help the diagnostic process?

What Is a Symptom?

A symptom is a complaint. It is what the patient reports about the problem and its characteristics. Symptoms may be described in various ways and are not always clearly stated. The patient may complain of sensations associated with phonation, such as pain along the side of the neck or soreness in the throat region after prolonged conversation. Other complaints may refer to perceptual characteristics of the voice, such as hoarseness, scratchiness, or perhaps a wobbly voice. Some symptoms can be verified; some cannot. For example, you cannot "feel" the patient's pain or record it. However, the report of pain is a very important symptom and can be a potent factor in directing the clinician's thinking about a problem. Other feelings (e.g., dry throat, scratchy throat, etc.) also may be difficult to verify. Symptoms, verifiable or not, have reality for the patient and must be given serious consideration by the speech–language pathologist and the otolaryngologist.

What Is a Sign?

Signs are characteristics of the voice that can be observed or tested. For example, hoarseness may be the patient's complaint, but it is also a sign that can be observed and measured independently. Signs represent an inventory of vocal characteristics based on examination, observation, and measurement.

Signs Versus Symptoms: Why the Distinction?

Despite the fact that patients' symptoms have reality for them, they do not tell the full story. Sometimes they can be misleading, they are frequently underreported, and they may not be the most salient and significant vocal characteristics present in the voice. Thus, symptoms may provide only part of the picture of the patient's vocal difficulty.

Signs provide more objective information. Because each sign is not unique, there may be redundancy in the data. For example, hoarseness may include the following acoustic signs: low fundamental frequency, reduced variability of fundamental frequency, increased frequency perturbation, increased spectral noise, and a large s/z ratio. (See "Acoustic Signs" later in this chapter for a more complete discussion.) A little redundancy is probably good because it may help the clinician assess the reliability of the patient reports. The lack of consistent reporting of redundant signs may alert the clinician to probe more deeply into the patient's history. Which of these component signs are significant is sometimes difficult to determine, and it is not always possible to record all of them in a single patient. However, knowing how one relates to another and to the underlying pathophysiology will assist the speech–language pathologist and the otolaryngologist in properly interpreting the sign and evaluating its significance.

This section presents the major symptoms and signs of voice problems. In the next three sections, we discuss perceptual, acoustic, and physiological signs. Finally, each of the symptoms discussed in this section is presented in greater detail, with a listing of the major perceptual, acoustic, and physiological signs, as well as potential causes that might produce the symptoms and signs. The emphasis throughout this chapter is on the process of discovering and interrelating the perceptual, acoustic, and physiological signs to the underlying pathological condition or pathophysiological condition and eventually to the cause of the problem.

MAJOR SYMPTOMS OF VOICE PROBLEMS

In our experience, patients with voice problems tend to present nine major symptoms. Not included in this list are symptoms reflective of a problem with resonance caused by incompetent velopharyngeal closure. These have been traditionally considered voice problems, but they are not phonatory problems. There may be some other minor symptoms or different classification schemes, but we believe that these nine primary symptoms are basic. It is important to recognize that symptoms do not usually occur singly but more often appear in combination.

The nine symptoms shown in Table 2.1 are as follows:

1. Hoarseness: This symptom reflects aperiodic vibration of the vocal folds. Some patients will use the term *hoarse* to refer to this symptom, whereas others might use terms such as *raspy* or *rough* voice.
2. Vocal fatigue: Patients complain of feeling tired after prolonged talking and often state that continued talking requires a great deal of effort. Moreover, they may report occasional raspiness or hoarseness, which tends to be most apparent at the end of a working day.
3. Breathy voice: Patients sometimes complain that they are unable to say complete sentences without running out of air and needing to replenish the air supply to continue talking. They further report having difficulty being heard, especially in noisy situations. They also may complain of a dry throat. We usually label the voice as *breathy*, although patients will not always use this term.
4. Reduced pitch range: This symptom is usually associated with singers who complain that they are experiencing difficulty producing notes that had previously presented no problem. Typically these are the notes that occur at the upper end of their singing range, although some singers have difficulty in the transitional area of their frequency range, for example, in moving from one register to another. They also may complain of tiredness and soreness in the throat area.

Table 2.1. Nine Primary Symptoms of Voice Problems

Hoarseness
Vocal fatigue
Breathy voice
Reduced phonation range
Aphonia
Pitch breaks or inappropriately high pitch
Strain/struggle with voice
Tremor
Pain and other physical sensations

5. Aphonia: Aphonia means absence of voice. The patient speaks in a whisper and may sometimes complain of a variety of symptoms, including dryness in the throat, soreness, and a great deal of effort in attempting to speak.

6. Pitch breaks or inappropriately high pitch: A patient may complain of periodic squeakiness and of voice cracks. The voice seems out of control, and the patient reports never knowing what sound will come out. Therefore, we have labeled this symptom as pitch breaks, although it is also possible to describe it as the inappropriate use of high pitch or puberphonia. Often this symptom is reported by a male adolescent who uses an inappropriately high pitch as the habitual voice rather than the more typical lower-pitched post pubertal male voice.

7. Strain/struggle voice: These patients report that it is difficult to talk. This may include inability to get voicing started or to maintain voice. They report that it is a strain to talk; they experience a great deal of tension while speaking and become fatigued because of the effort involved.

8. Tremor: Patients may complain that the voice is wobbly or shaky. They are unable to voluntarily produce a steady sustained sound. This shaky voice is usually very regular and consistent.

9. Pain and other physical sensations: Patient reports about pain vary. Some report pain on both sides of the neck lateral to the larynx; others localize the pain to a specific unilateral area or to mid-larynx, and a few report pain radiating into the upper chest. In some patients this may be the only symptom, although that is very rare. Other physical sensations reported by patients include feelings of a lump in the throat, feelings of strain or tension, or the sensation of dryness. Sometimes, the patient's main concern is a frequent cough.

These nine symptoms are the most common in our experience, and the terms used are those patients have used themselves in discussing their problem or are descriptive of their reporting. Patients may report several symptoms, but usually the symptom mentioned first or emphasized should be considered the primary symptom and probably will relate most directly to the eventual etiology of the vocal problem.

MAJOR SIGNS OF VOICE PROBLEMS

Perceptual Signs

Perceptual signs of voice problems are the characteristics of an individual's voice that are perceived by the listener/observer. Although they are often considered subjective, they have psychological reality and may be assessed objectively and compared across listeners (see Chapter 8 for methods of scaling perceptions). Clinically, the perceptual signs—the clinician's perception of voice characteristics—paired with the history serve as initial guideposts in the process of differential diagnosis.

Many adjectives have been used to describe voice qualities (Aronson, 1990; Colton & Estill, 1981; Perkins, 1971). The list of perceptual signs to be presented in this chapter encompasses a variety of perceptual characteristics that serve to focus our attention on clinically useful voice characteristics. Some of these characteristics have reasonably clear, well-defined, measurable acoustic correlates, and others do not. For example, we are not able to differentiate hoarseness and roughness acoustically. Both hoarseness

Table 2.2. Perceptual Signs of Voice Problems

Pitch
    Monopitch (reduced pitch variability)
    Inappropriate pitch
    Pitch breaks
    Reduced pitch range

Loudness
    Monoloudness (reduced loudness variability)
    Loudness variation (soft, loud, or uncontrolled)
    Reduced loudness range

Quality
    Hoarse or rough
    Breathy
    Tension
    Tremor
    Strain/struggle
    Sudden interruption of voicing
    Diplophonia

Other Behaviors
    Stridor
    Excessive throat clearing

Aphonia
    Consistent
    Episodic

and roughness have increased perturbation and a noisy spectrum. As another example, tension can be observed by a clinician, but its measurement becomes problematic. Indeed, we would be hard put to specify the exact loci of vocal tension, its acoustic parameters, and how to measure it.

Perceptions by their very nature are hard to describe verbally. They are subjective and individual, being influenced by personal preference, experience, and culture. In the following discussion of perceptual signs of voice (Table 2.2), we have grouped them within the broad areas of pitch, loudness, quality, non-phonatory behavior, and aphonia (absence of phonation). The definitions of the terms are worded so as to provide meaningful guidelines without undue restriction on individual experience.

PITCH

Pitch is the perceptual correlate of fundamental frequency.

Monopitch

This term refers to a voice that lacks variation of pitch during speech. There is a marked absence of inflectional variation and in some instances inability to voluntarily vary pitch. Monopitch can be one of many signs characteristic of neurological impairments that may affect the voice. It also may simply be a reflection of an individual's personality or, more significantly, of psychiatric disability.

Inappropriate Pitch

This refers to the voice that is judged to exceed the range of acceptable pitch for age or sex, being either too low or too high. Norms for fundamental frequency (the acoustic correlate of pitch) are available for age and sex (see "Acoustic Signs" later in this chapter). The high-pitched voice of a young child is perceived to be inappropriate when produced by an adult, and vice versa. Similarly, the pitch range for an adult female voice does not generally extend as low as might be acceptable in an adult male. The perception of voice pitch and the subsequent judgment of the acceptability of that pitch, based solely on perception, can be fraught with danger. Research has shown (Plomp, 1976; Wolfe & Ratusnik, 1988) that other characteristics of voice quality can affect our perception of pitch. Thus, although the hoarse voice of a person with a vocal lesion may be perceived to be lower than acceptable, actual measurement of the fundamental frequency may fail to corroborate that perception (Shipp & Huntington, 1965). The pitch of a voice is related to the size of the larynx and its structures. A vocal pitch higher than expected may reflect underdevelopment or immaturity of the larynx based on endocrinological factors or perhaps a congenital anomaly. Vocal pitch also may be excessively low because of endocrinological factors such as hypothyroidism or the use of male hormone by women. Vocal pitch also may be too high or too low based on individual preferences or habit.

Pitch Breaks

Unexpected and uncontrolled sudden shifts of pitch in either an upward or downward direction are readily perceived even by the untrained and unsophisticated listener. They are frequently associated with the changing voice of the adolescent male and are usually a temporary stage that resolves with time. Occasionally pitch breaks persist beyond the expected laryngeal growth period. Pitch breaks, however, also may occur as a result of a laryngeal pathological condition or as an accompaniment to conditions that involve some loss of neural control of phonation.

Reduced Pitch Range

Sometimes, a patient may complain about a reduction in pitch range, usually at the high end of the range, and an inability to produce these pitches without excessive strain or at all. Very rarely do patients complain about loss of the low end of their range.

LOUDNESS

Loudness is the perceptual correlate of intensity.

Monoloudness

This refers to voice that lacks variation in loudness level. The use of increased loudness for emphasis is absent, and there may be an inability to voluntarily vary loudness. In this category, the perception does not attend to the actual level of loudness being used but rather to the variability of the level during speaking. Monoloudness may be (a) an indication of neurological impairment in which the ability to voluntarily control and vary loudness may be lost; (b) a reflection of psychiatric disability; or (c) a habit associated with personality.

Loudness Variation

When variations in loudness are extreme, either too soft to be heard easily in average conversational settings or excessively loud for the setting, they are perceived as a sign of a problem. Although norms are available for dynamic range (the softest to the loudest sound a person is able to produce; see "Acoustic Signs" later in this chapter), appropriate loudness levels are dependent on the specific speaking situation. Unpredictable and uncontrolled variation of loudness level, explosive to fading, constitutes another sign of loudness variability that is beyond accepted norms. Voices that are too soft or too loud may be a reflection of auditory dysfunction, of personality, or of habit. A habitually loud speaker may have grown up in a large and noisy family in which excessive loudness was the norm, or may have had to speak loudly to be heard by a hearing-impaired relative. The inability to control vocal loudness also may be attributable to the loss of neural control of the phonatory mechanism or to problems affecting the respiratory mechanism. Variations in vocal loudness, from explosive to almost aphonic, also may be a reflection of psychological problems.

Reduced Loudness Range

Reduction in a patient's loudness range usually involves a loss of the ability to produce loud sounds. Many times, reduced phonational range and reduced loudness range occur in the same patient.

QUALITY

Hoarse or Rough

These words are descriptors of a voice quality that is noticeably aberrant in its lack of clarity, its increased noisiness, and its discordance. Although hoarseness/roughness may be the primary perceptual characteristic of an abnormal voice, its perception may be paired with other characteristics such as breathiness, tension, or strain. The degree of hoarseness/roughness in the voice is related to the acoustic correlates of perturbation (see later discussion under "Perturbation") and to the noisiness of the spectrum (see later under "Signal-to-Noise"). Pathological conditions that affect the vibratory behavior of the vocal folds will usually result in some degree of perceived hoarseness/roughness.

Breathy

This designation refers to the perception of audible air escape during phonation. The voice lacks clarity of tone and is usually reduced in loudness. A breathy voice quality is related to the amount of airflow produced. Norms for airflow measures are available (see Chapter 14), and its measurement can verify the perception of breathiness. Excessive airflow through the glottis is usually a reflection of inadequate glottal closure. Inability to fully adduct the vocal folds during phonation may be the result of peripheral neurological problems, of central neurological impairment, of the presence of a lesion that interferes with closure, or of improper use.

Tension

Tension in the voice suggests to the listener a "hard edge" to the voice, combined with hard glottal attacks and sometimes observable muscular tension in the external neck. Tension is a perception that is difficult to verify through measurement. Assumptions can be made about the dynamics of vocal tension, such as increased tension of certain muscle groups, but we do not have adequate data to determine the most salient muscle groups nor the amount of tension that is acceptable in the normal voice. In many instances, tension seems to be related to "hyperfunctional" usage patterns. However, it also may be a reflection of compensatory behavior in the presence of some laryngeal pathological condition or neurological disability.

Tremor

This sign may be described as regularly rhythmic variations in pitch and loudness of the voice that are not under voluntary control. The voice is perceived as unsteady, "wobbly," or quavering. Tremor is a perception that can be verified through measurement. Indeed, the rate of the tremor can be an important factor in determining the underlying pathological condition (see "Voice Tremor" later in this chapter). Tremor of any type is usually a reflection of a central nervous system dysfunction that results in some loss of control of the phonatory mechanism.

Strain/Struggle

The voice perceived to reflect strain/struggle behavior suggests difficulty in initiating phonation and struggle to maintain phonation. As speech is produced, there is the perception of inability to control voicing as it fades in and out. Actual voice stoppages may occur. Physical correlates of these perceptions, such as voice onset time, silence, and variations of fundamental frequency and sound pressure level (SPL), are accessible to objective measurement. However, the perception of the strain and struggle behavior is qualitatively unique and is not well expressed by the various objective measurements. The precise cause of this vocal difficulty is still unclear, but most voice specialists believe that it is a manifestation of a laryngeal dystonia. Some experts continue to believe that, in a certain percentage of these patients, the cause is psychological.

Sudden Interruption of Voicing

A sudden unexpected drop in loudness and an equally unexpected change in voice quality to breathy voice is a very noticeable perceptual sign. The breathy voice may last only a fraction of a second and may occur repeatedly within an utterance, alternating with essentially normal voicing. This perceptual sign of an abnormal voice may be the result of sudden, unexpected, and involuntary abduction of the vocal folds, or delayed adduction when making the transition from unvoiced to voiced phonemes (Ludlow, 1995), the cause of which is usually neurological dysfunction. Again, these perceived voice characteristics (e.g., loudness variability, airflow changes) are accessible to objective measurement.

Diplophonia

This word literally means "double voice." It is said to be present when two distinct pitches are perceived simultaneously during phonation. Theoretically this occurs when the vocal folds are under differing degrees of tension or mass and each vibrates at a different frequency. No consistent pattern of the perception of diplophonia as a consequence of a given pathological condition appears to exist.

OTHER BEHAVIORS

Stridor

The term *stridor* refers to noisy breathing, involuntary sound that accompanies inspiration, expiration, or both, and it is indicative of a narrowing of the airway at a certain point. Although the pitch or quality of the stridulous sound is taken by some to be diagnostic (Cotton & Richardson, 1981), the judgments of these factors appear to be based entirely on perception. Although the frequency and intensity of stridor could be measured, we know of no such measurements. The presence of stridor is always an abnormal finding and one with potentially serious implications, because it is a reflection of blockage of the airway.

Excessive Throat Clearing

A frequent accompaniment to a variety of voice disorders, excessive throat clearing probably represents an attempt by the patient to clear excess mucus from the vocal folds, or it may be a response to the sensation of "something in the throat." It is a natural behavior but is considered a perceptual sign of disordered voice when it occurs frequently and consistently.

APHONIA

Consistent

This is an absence of voicing, usually perceived as whispering, that is constantly present. Aphonia may be the result of bilateral vocal fold paralysis, in which the vocal folds are unable to adduct, or a result of central nervous system dysfunction, or it may be a psychogenic problem.

Episodic

Episodic aphonia may take a number of forms. A patient may exhibit unpredictable, involuntary aphonic breaks in voice production that last for only a fraction of a second. Another patient may experience aphonic periods lasting minutes, hours, or even days. Yet another patient may experience a gradual fading of voice to the aphonic state, particularly with increased physical fatigue. Momentary involuntary aphonic breaks are not uncommon during the speech of patients with laryngeal pathological conditions. Episodic aphonia may be observed in patients with central neurological dysfunction of the flaccid type, as noted in myasthenia gravis. However, episodic aphonia may be psychologically based.

Acoustic Signs

Voice is produced by movements of the vocal folds interrupting the egressive airstream. The movements of the folds are controlled by the biomechanical characteristics of the folds themselves, the magnitude of the air pressure beneath the folds, and their neural control. Pathological conditions may affect these movements by interfering with any of these variables.

Vocal fold movement results in periodic interruption of the airstream at rates appropriate for the perception of sound. Acoustics is the study of sound, and voice acoustics can provide important information about vocal fold movement. However, acoustics is one stage removed from the movements of the vocal folds. Although acoustic signs are, at best, imperfect mirrors of the underlying vocal fold physiology, there is a great deal of correspondence between the physiology and acoustics, and much can be inferred about the physiology based on acoustic analysis. Moreover, acoustic parameters are probably the easiest to record and to analyze objectively. Many acoustic parameters of the speaking voice can be measured by various instruments, such as the Visi-Pitch (Kay Elemetrics, Lincoln Park, NJ) or one of several computer programs such as Computerized Speech Lab (CSL) (STR, Victoria, BC/Kay Elemetrics, Lincoln Park,

Table 2.3. Acoustic Signs of Voice Problems

Fundamental Frequency
    Mean or average speaking fundamental frequency
    Frequency variability
    Phonation range
    Perturbation

Amplitude
    Average overall sound pressure level (SPL)
    Amplitude variability
    Dynamic range
    Perturbation

Signal-to-Noise Ratio (Harmonics-to-Noise Ratio)

Vocal Rise or Fall Time

Voice Tremor

Phonation Time

Voice Stoppages

Frequency Breaks

Normal Acoustics

NJ), CSpeech (CSpeech, Bend, OR), Dr Speech (Tiger DRS, Seattle, WA), EZVoice (Internet Soft Solutions, Scarborough, ON), or SuperScope II (for the Mac) (Superscope Technologies, Batavia, IL).

Many acoustic signs may be associated with any given pathological condition (Table 2.3). Some are unique and others redundant. For example, jitter (variations of period from one pitch period to the next, also known as frequency perturbation) and noise spectrum may reflect the basic aperiodicity of the vibrating vocal folds. Jitter may be easier to measure and therefore have greater clinical utility. All acoustic signs reflect some aspect of the underlying pathological condition of interest, however.

FUNDAMENTAL FREQUENCY

The frequency of vibration of the vocal folds is often referred to as fundamental frequency (F_o). This acoustic characteristic is usually defined as average fundamental frequency or, in the instance of spontaneous speech or reading, speaking fundamental frequency. Also of interest is the variability of fundamental frequency, usually expressed as the standard deviation of frequency and sometimes labeled the pitch sigma. The range of frequencies that can be produced by the voice also may be of interest and is called phonational range. Finally, there is considerable interest in the short-term stability of the vocal folds. This stability (or lack thereof) is reflected in the measure termed frequency perturbation.

Mean Fundamental Frequency

Considerable normative data exist on fundamental frequency during speech for males and females of all ages (Baken & Orlikoff, 2000). Males should produce average fundamental frequencies during conversational speech between 100 and 150 Hz, whereas

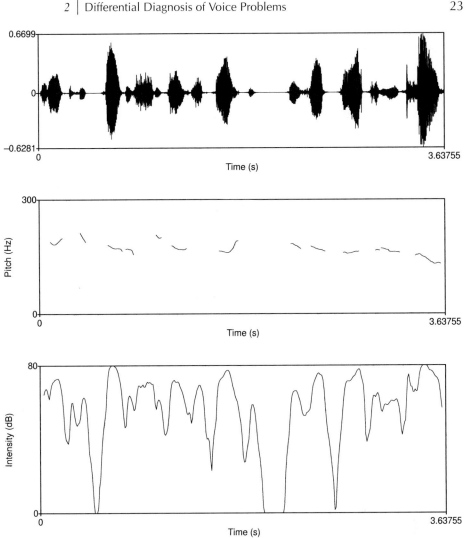

Figure 2.1. Example of an analysis of fundamental frequency and sound pressure levels in a sentence produced by a normal female speaker. The upper panel shows the waveform of the sentence. The middle panel shows a plot of fundamental frequency. The gaps in the plot indicate no measurable fundamental frequency. The lower panel is a plot of the envelope of the waveform to show the variation of SPL. The analysis and the plots were made with the Praat, Ver 3.9.34, written by Paul Boersma & David Weeninkn ©1992–2001.

females should produce fundamental frequencies between 180 and 250 Hz (Hollien, Dew, & Phillips, 1971). The middle panel of Figure 2.1 shows an example of fundamental frequency as a function of time for a sentence produced by a normal female speaker. The speaking fundamental frequency was 197.97 Hz. Pathological conditions may affect the vibrating frequency, with the result that males or females will produce either too high a frequency or too low a frequency. By too high or too low, we mean frequencies that lie outside the range expected for normal phonation.

Pitch should not be confused with frequency. Pitch is the psychological feature of the voice, whereas frequency is the physical feature. It is possible to perceive a voice as having excessively low pitch without an excessively low fundamental frequency (Wolfe & Ratusnik, 1988).

Frequency Variability

The standard deviation of fundamental frequency (or pitch sigma) reflects frequency variability for a reasonably large time segment or passage. During speech, both fundamental frequency and intensity vary depending on the sounds, the words uttered, and the intent of the message. Computing the standard deviation of frequency during a sentence or paragraph will provide an estimate of this longer-term variability. In Figure 2.1, the standard deviation of fundamental frequency for the sentence of the normal speaker was 27.97 Hz. In the literature, the standard deviation of fundamental frequency is usually expressed in semitones and labeled the pitch sigma. The pitch sigma of this production was 3.19 semitones FL. As a general guideline, normal speakers should be expected to exhibit pitch sigmas between 2 and 4 semitones for both males and females (Baken, 1987; Linville & Fisher, 1985; Mysak & Hanley, 1959; Stoicheff, 1981). Patients are sometimes unable to produce normal variability. This acoustic measure would presumably be related to the perceptual features of monopitch, although little research has been reported on the relationship between fundamental frequency variability and the perception of monopitch.

Phonational Range

Phonational range refers to the range of frequencies that a person can produce. Normal young adults should be able to produce a phonational range of approximately three octaves, with singers' ranges slightly higher than those of nonsingers (Baken & Orlikoff, 2000; Colton & Hollien, 1972). Phonational range decreases with age (Linville, 1987).

Perturbation

Perturbation refers to the irregularity of vibration of the vocal folds and is often referred to as vocal jitter or vocal shimmer. If the irregularity is in the time of vibration, it is called jitter. If the irregularity is in the amplitude of vibration, it is called shimmer. Vocal jitter is a variation of glottal period or frequency perturbation or the change of frequency from one successive period to the next (Casper, 1983; Horii, 1979, 1980, 1982). Normal speakers have a small amount of perturbation, which may represent variation in vocal fold mass, tension, muscle activity, or neural activity (Baer, 1979; Pinto & Titze, 1990). An example of perturbation in a normal speaker's sustained vowel production is shown in Figure 2.2. The average jitter is expressed as a percentage of the average fundamental frequency and is 1.57%. Chapter 14 summarizes some of the data on normal perturbation.

When pathological conditions affect the vocal folds, their vibrations will show increased aperiodicity (Hecker & Kreul, 1971; Koike, 1967b; Lieberman, 1963). Many possible pathological conditions can affect vibration, including but not limited to growths on the vocal folds, changes in the mucosa, variations in the composition of the vocal folds, variations in muscle function, and variations in the motor control of the muscles controlling the vibration. Thus, perturbation may not be useful for differentiating among causes but may reflect the extent or severity of a pathological condition (Colton, Reed, Sagerman, & Chung, 1982).

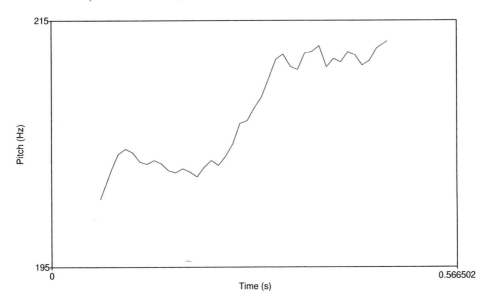

Figure 2.2. Fundamental frequency of a short segment of a sustained vowel produced by a female speaker.

AMPLITUDE

Several acoustic variables reflect the amplitude or strength of the tone produced by the vocal folds. Many are expressed in decibels. Overall, SPL refers to the average sound pressure level of an utterance (sustained vowel, spontaneous sentence, or paragraph). Amplitude standard deviation is simply a measure of amplitude variability, whereas dynamic range reflects the range of vocal amplitudes an individual can produce. Finally, amplitude perturbation reflects the short-term variation of amplitude from one glottal period to the next.

Overall SPL

The average overall SPL in decibels provides an indication of the strength of the vocal fold vibration. If a person speaks softly, the overall SPL will be low. Conversely, if a person speaks loudly, the overall SPL will be high. Everyday conversational speech may exhibit SPLs between 70 and 80 dB (Baken, 1987). SPLs as a function of time for a normal male speaker's production of a simple sentence are shown in Figure 2.1 (lower panel). The mean SPL was 60.6 dB.

Amplitude Variability

During speech or a reading passage, the amplitude of speaking will vary depending on the sounds spoken and the message. Variability of amplitude during speech would be expressed as a standard deviation. The standard deviation of SPL for the normal speaker in Figure 2.1 was 18.33 dB.

Dynamic Range

This is the range of vocal intensities that a person can produce. Normal speakers should be able to produce minimum intensities of approximately 50 dB and maximum intensities of approximately 115 dB; intensities for males are slightly higher than for females (Coleman, Mabis, & Hinson, 1977). Figure 2.3 presents the mean dynamic

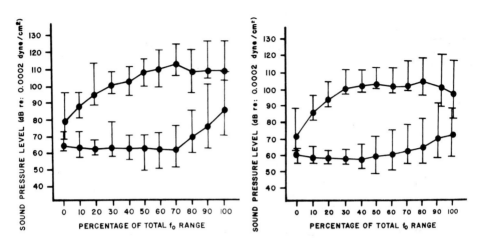

Figure 2.3. The left panel presents the average and range for 10 male subjects, whereas the right panel presents the average and range for 12 female subjects. Each subject produced a sustained vowel at 10% increments of their fundamental frequency ranges and at minimum and maximum SPL.

ranges as a function of fundamental frequency for the normal subjects in the Coleman, Mabis, and Hinson study. Note how the SPLs at the extremes of the fundamental frequency range are much smaller than the dynamic ranges at the mid frequencies.

Perturbation

As was the case for fundamental frequency, the amplitude of the vocal fold tone may vary from one cycle to the next. This characteristic is called amplitude perturbation or shimmer. Growths on the vocal folds or poor neural control of the vocal folds would be expected to affect the stability of the vocal folds during vibration. Therefore, shimmer should reflect the kind and degree of pathological condition that a speaker might exhibit. Chapter 14 summarizes some of the available data on shimmer for normal speakers.

SIGNAL-TO-NOISE RATIO

Noise is random, aperiodic energy in the voice. It may occur throughout the entire frequency range of the voice, or it may be located in certain frequency bands. Normal voices have low levels of noise, whereas abnormal voices show greater noise levels (Emanuel & Sansone, 1969; Fujiu, Hibi, & Hirano, 1988; Hanson & Emanuel, 1979; Isshiki, Kitajima, Kojima, & Harita, 1978; Kitajima, 1981; Newman & Emanuel, 1991; Wolfe & Steinfatt, 1987; Yanagihara, 1967a; Yumoto, Gould, & Baer, 1982; Yumoto, Sasaki, & Okamura, 1984). Two general approaches have been developed for the analysis of noise components in voice.

The first, reported by Yanagihara (1967b), uses spectrograms to classify voices, using the level of noise near the second formants of several vowels. As such, the system is qualitative although based on objective data. It may not provide data that might differentiate subtle differences among patients, differences that might assist in diagnosis.

The second approach analyzes the level of noise directly. An example of this approach is the harmonics-to-noise ratio, a variant of signal-to-noise ratio (Yumoto, 1987; Yumoto, Gould, & Baer, 1982; Yumoto, Sasaki, & Okamura, 1984). Harmonics-to-noise ratios greater than 1.0 mean that the harmonic energy was greater than the noise energy. Normal speakers are expected to have harmonics-to-noise ratios much greater than 1.

Noise may be generated in two ways. First, there may be a noise source at or near the vocal folds (e.g., air rushing against the open vocal fold). Second, greater aperiodicity of vibration may show up as greater noise in the spectrum (Klingholz & Martin, 1985). Most procedures for the measurement of noise would not be able to distinguish between these two sources. Nevertheless, increased noise levels are associated with problems that affect the vibrating frequency of the vocal folds or create additional, unwanted sources of sound at the level of the vocal folds.

VOCAL RISE OR FALL TIME

The ability of the vocal folds to start tone production quickly or to stop phonation quickly may be impaired by pathological conditions. The time it takes to produce a tone of full amplitude is referred to as rise time. The time it takes for the vocal folds to stop producing a tone is called fall time. Rise time is also associated with vocal attack. It has been shown that some pathological conditions will affect the time it takes the vocal folds to attain their maximum displacement from their most closed position (Koike, 1967a). Pathological conditions affecting the neural control of laryngeal muscles would theoretically be expected to have a pronounced effect on the rise or fall time of glottal amplitude, although little work has been reported on these relationships.

VOICE TREMOR

Tremor refers to a regular variation in the fundamental frequency or amplitude of the voice (Aronson, Brown, Litin, & Pearson, 1968a; Izdebski & Dedo, 1979; Ludlow, Bassich, Connor, & Coulter, 1986). As a patient attempts to sustain a tone at a constant frequency, there is a slow variation of frequency around the desired constant frequency. Usually, this variation is between 3 and 5 Hz above or below the mean fundamental frequency, although it could be higher or lower than these limits. Tremor also may be exhibited by slow variation in the amplitude of the voice signal. Tremor is usually associated with variations in muscle activity levels or the control of the muscles used in phonation. As such it is usually associated with central nervous system dysfunction and not with impaired peripheral motor control or vocal fold pathological conditions.

Figure 2.4 presents an example of tremor on a sustained vowel. Note the slow oscillations of SPL during the production. Measuring the distance between the peaks of the SPL oscillations would yield the tremor rate, which in this example was approximately 5 Hz.

PHONATION TIME

Maximum phonation time refers to the maximum time a subject can sustain a tone on one breath. As a rule of thumb, one would expect normal adult male subjects to produce a vowel for approximately 20 seconds; adult female subjects, approximately 15 seconds; and children, approximately 10 seconds (Kent, Kent, & Rosenbek, 1987). However, these values may vary considerably between people and among age groups. Phonation time may vary as a function of trials. With proper instruction and practice, as few as three trials may be sufficient (Bless & Hirano, 1982; Sawashima, 1966). Short maximum phonation times reflect inefficiency of the phonatory or respiratory system.

Another measure of phonation time is what is referred to as the s/z ratio (Boone & McFarlane, 1988; Eckel & Boone, 1981), or the maximum sustained phonation time

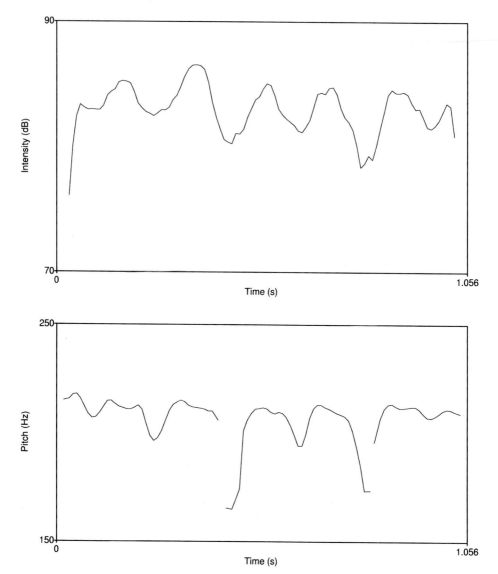

Figure 2.4. Example of tremor in a voice. The upper panel shows the amplitude variation of this sustained vowel produced by a female with essential voice tremor. The lower panel shows the corresponding trace of fundamental frequency.

of /s/ divided by the maximum sustained phonation time of /z/. A normal speaker would be expected to sustain both the voiceless /s/ and the voiced /z/ for approximately equal durations, resulting in a ratio of 1. However, in the presence of a disturbance of vocal fold vibratory behavior or ability to close the glottis, the duration of sustained voicing for /z/ would be expected to suffer. The resulting s/z ratio becomes increasingly larger as the discrepancy between sustained productions of these sounds (z shorter than s) becomes greater. For a group of normal subjects, Eckel and Boone (1981) reported average s/z ratios between 0.4 and 2. Based on the results of their statistical tests between normal and pathological speakers, they suggest that any s/z ratio greater than 1.4 may indicate a vocal pathological condition. S/z ratios for children were similar (Shearer, 1983; Tait, Michel, & Carpenter, 1980; Weinberg, Bosma, Shanks, & DeMyer, 1968).

VOICE STOPPAGES

Normal speech consists of phonation, noises, and silences. The latter are usually brief. When silences become longer than normally expected or appear unexpectedly during phonation, they call attention to themselves, disrupt intelligibility, and are considered abnormal. In some disorders, the voice may suddenly stop for a brief period and then revert to its previous level. These interruptions would be observable in the spectrum of the sound.

FREQUENCY BREAKS

Frequency breaks refer to sudden shifts of fundamental frequency either upward or downward. One would expect that these would be related to the perceptual pitch breaks often reported in the literature in the speech of patients with certain vocal pathological conditions.

NORMAL ACOUSTICS

Finally, it is possible that a patient with a phonatory problem will exhibit acoustic features typical of a normal voice. In other cases, the differences between a normal and abnormal voice may be so subtle that they are not manifest in these acoustic signs.

Measurable Physiological Signs

The physiological signs that may be affected by pathological conditions include aerodynamic features (airflow and pressure), vibratory behavior (contact area, waveform shape), and muscle activity (as recorded by electromyography). These are summarized in Table 2.4.

Table 2.4. Measurable Physiological Signs of Voice Problems

Aerodynamics
- Airflows (increased, decreased, variable)
- Air pressures (increased, decreased, variable)

Vibratory Behaviors
- Aberrant glottal pulse shape
- Slowed opening and closing phases of vocal folds
- Inadequate or excessive closed times
- Irregularity or asymmetry of vocal fold motion
- Mucosal wave changes

Muscle Activity
- Absent, reduced, or excessive levels
- Involuntary rhythmic variations of level
- Sudden, unexpected bursts of activity
- Slow rise or fall in amplitude
- Diminution of level with sustained phonation
- Imbalance of paired muscle activity

AERODYNAMIC MEASUREMENTS

Airflow

During normal speech, airflow may range between 50 and 200 mL/sec, with males producing higher flows than females (Hirano, 1981b). Usually, the measurement of airflow represents airflow rates computed over 1 to 5 seconds of phonation and therefore represent many hundreds of glottal cycles. It is possible to measure the peak flow that occurs during an individual vibratory cycle. If possible, peak flow measures should be differentiated from the steady airflow rates that occur during speech. The steady airflow rates for speakers with various vocal fold pathological conditions are greater than those for normal speakers. Normal speakers exhibit a small amount of airflow when the vocal folds adduct, whereas speakers with a vocal pathological condition may produce larger than normal airflows during the closed phase of the vocal folds. If closure of the vocal folds is compromised by a lesion or by poor muscular or neural control, airflow rates will be greater than normal.

Air Pressure

The magnitude of air pressure beneath the vocal folds is important in producing vibration and determining the intensity of the sound. Typical pressures beneath the vocal folds (subglottal air pressure, lung pressure, or alveolar pressure) range from approximately 0.3 to 2.0 kPa[1], depending on the loudness of the sound. Pressures between 0.2 and 0.9 kPa would be expected for conversational speech levels (Brodie, Colton, & Swisher, 1988; Holmberg, Hillman, & Perkell, 1988; Shipp & McGlone, 1971). Higher than normal levels may indicate either excessive lung pressures or inefficient valving of the vocal folds.

Variability of airflow or pressure may be important to measure in persons with vocal pathological conditions. Excessive variation could be associated with poor motor control of the vocal folds or of the respiratory system.

Phonation Threshold Pressure

Phonation threshold pressure is the minimum pressure required to initiate vocal fold vibration (Titze, 1992b). It is dependent on the pitch of the phonation and determined by the degree of opening between the vocal folds, the thickness of the vocal folds, the velocity of the mucosal wave, and the viscosity of the tissue (Titze, 1994). It may be a very important measurement to obtain when describing the pathophysiology of phonation and appears to reflect the level of hydration of the vocal folds (Verdolini-Marston, Titze, & Druker, 1990; Verdolini, Titze & Fennell, 1994).

VIBRATORY BEHAVIOR MEASUREMENTS

Vibratory characteristics of the vocal folds are important in determining the final acoustic output of the vocal folds. Many of these characteristics have been studied by using high-speed films. Information about some of the vibratory characteristics can be obtained from stroboscopic examinations or by using indirect techniques for assessing laryngeal function. Some of the more popular systems include (a) electroglottography (EGG); (b) inverse filtering of the oral airflow waveform (flow glottogram); and (c) photoglottography (PGG).

---

[1]kPa is kilopascals, a unit of pressure measurement in the MKS (Meter-Kilogram-Second) system. 1 kPa is approximately equal to 10 cm H_2O.

During normal voice function, the shape of the airflow pulse or the shape of the area pulse is different depending on the mode of vibration[2] (Colton & Estill, 1981; Timcke, von Leden, & Moore, 1958). Similarly, the shape of the airflow pulse through the glottis is different (Rothenberg, 1981; Sundberg, 1987). In pathological conditions, the pattern of glottal opening becomes irregular and distorted (von Leden, Moore, & Timcke, 1960), as does the airflow pulse (Colton & Brewer, 1985). Thus, analysis of glottal area from high-speed films or airflow waveform shape can help to describe the vibratory characteristics of voice-disordered patients.

MUSCLE ACTIVITY MEASUREMENTS

Pathological conditions may affect the muscles that control vocal function directly by affecting peripheral function or indirectly by affecting the central nervous system. Clinically, muscle function can be assessed by observing the movements of the structures themselves (i.e., vibration of the vocal folds) or by recording the electrical activity of the muscles (electromyography [EMG]). Faaborg-Andersen (1957, 1964; Faaborg-Andersen & Sonninen, 1960; Faaborg-Andersen & Vennard, 1964) was among the first to use EMG in the analysis of muscle function in the larynx. Many studies since that initial work have been concerned with various muscles of the larynx in healthy subjects as well as in subjects with voice disorders. EMG is an invasive technique and should be performed only by those skilled in its application. EMG cannot and should not be performed on every patient (Basmajian, 1979). For a few patients, however, EMG can be a valuable technique to assess laryngeal function (Faaborg-Andersen, 1957; Lindestad & Persson, 1994; Parnes, 1988; Parnes & Satya-Murti, 1985).

When a muscle is activated for a task, an EMG recording will show a fairly rapid rise in the amplitude of the signal, followed by a consistent level of activity. When muscle activity ceases, the recording will show a fairly rapid fall in amplitude to a low level of baseline activity adequate to maintain the tonus of the muscle (Basmajian, 1979; Kotby & Haugen, 1970). Pathological conditions may severely reduce or increase the background levels as well as the muscle levels during contraction (Kotby & Haugen, 1970; Sawashima, Sato, Funasaka, & Totsuk, 1958). Muscles may be slow to become activated and slow to turn off, or a sudden unexpected burst of muscle activity may be superimposed on steady activity during muscle contraction, or muscles may show normal levels of activity when first contracted but with continued contraction, diminishing levels. There also may be differences of level between pairs of muscles controlling the vocal folds, suggesting a difference of activity between the two muscles (Hiroto, Hirano, & Tomita, 1968). Normal EMG levels, onsets, and offsets will be found in those patients whose laryngeal pathological condition does not affect muscles or their neural control.

Observable Physiological Signs

STROBOSCOPIC OBSERVATIONS

The stroboscope has become increasingly popular in the diagnosis and treatment of voice problems. Recent models are relatively easy to use and provide sharp imaging (Elias et al., 1997; Faure & Muller, 1992; Hertegard & Gauffin, 1995; Hirano, 1981b;

---

[2] The vocal folds may produce different modes of phonation depending on the characteristics of the mucosa, tension in the epithelium and muscle, and other inherent physical characteristics of the tissue. See Titze (1994), pp. 97–100, for more information.

Table 2.5. Observable Physiological Signs of Voice Problems—Stroboscopic

Degree of glottal closure
Phase closure
Vertical level
Amplitude of vibration
Mucosal wave
Vibratory behavior
Phase symmetry
Periodicity

Hirano, Feder, & Bless, 1983; Kitzing, 1985; Poburka, 1999; Shohet et al., 1996; Tsunoda et al, 1997; Woo, 1996).

The stroboscope flashes a light at a rate equal to or approximating the vibrating rate of the vocal folds (Alberti, 1978; Kitzing, 1985). If the flash rate is equal to the vibrating rate of the vocal folds, they appear to stand still because they are illuminated at the same phase of each (or same point within each) vibratory cycle. If the rate is slightly different from the vibration rate of the vocal folds, they are illuminated at different phases of their vibratory cycle. The effect is a slowing of the vibratory motion of the vocal folds, permitting observation of vibratory details.

The strobe must measure the fundamental frequency of the vocal folds to function. This measure is available to determine the regularity of vocal fold vibration.

The stroboscopic signs of laryngeal pathological conditions are obtained from the recordings of the strobe images (Fex, 1970; Kallen, 1932). Their recognition, like many of the signs previously discussed, depends on the knowledge and skill of the examiner. The signs listed in Table 2.5 are based on those presented by Bless (unpublished technical manual, B&K Stroboscope Course), Hirano (1981b; Hirano & Bless, 1993), and our own experiences with stroboscopy.

Glottal Closure

The extent and configuration of glottal closure can be described based on the stroboscopic images. The terms most commonly used to describe glottal closure include: complete closure, posterior chink, anterior chink, bowed, hourglass configuration, irregular closure, and incomplete closure.

Phase Closure

This parameter refers to the relative amounts of time that vocal folds are open and closed during a phonatory cycle. (Be aware that the stroboscopic image is not a representation of cycle-by-cycle behavior, but rather is a composite of a number of cycles; therefore, the use of the term *phonatory cycle* in discussing stroboscopic observations is not entirely accurate. With that understanding, however, it is convenient to use the term in a stroboscopic context.) In a whisper or in aphonic speech, the vocal folds would be predominantly open, whereas in vocal hyperfunction the closed phase might predominate. The gauge for normal is an equal distribution of open to closed time.

Vertical Level

The vocal folds should be on the same vertical level so that as they approximate they appear to be at the same height. In cases of trauma, paralysis, or other neurological involvement, this may not always be true. One fold may appear to lie consistently at a level lower than the other. Because the examiner is looking at the vocal folds from above, and the view is only two-dimensional, it is not always possible to assess their vertical level.

Amplitude of Vibration

This parameter refers to the extent of horizontal excursion of the vocal folds as they open and close during phonation. This parameter is greatly affected by the loudness of phonation, becoming greater as loudness increases. At modal pitch and loudness, the expected amount of movement from the midline should approximate one third the visible width of the vocal fold. The movement of each vocal fold is rated individually. Differences in movement between the two folds may be diagnostically useful information.

Mucosal Wave

The mucosal wave is a rippling motion that can be observed as it travels mediolaterally across the superior surface of the vocal folds. It is a reflection of the complex structure and behavior of the vocal folds. It is most easily seen at low or middle pitches and usually disappears at high pitch. Normally the mucosal wave travels smoothly across the visible width of the vocal fold but can be limited by pathological conditions, scarring, or stiffness. In some instances the wave may appear to be larger than normal. This can occur in the presence of highly fluid-filled polypoid degeneration. This parameter is rated separately for each vocal fold.

Vibratory Behavior

This refers to the presence or the absence of vibratory behavior in the entire vocal fold. The extent of vibratory behavior may vary from normal to partially absent to totally absent. Once again, each vocal fold is rated independently.

Phase Symmetry

During phonation, the vocal folds should appear to move as mirror images of each other. As both folds open in phase they separate in unison and then approach each other and close in unison. That action is referred to as phase symmetry. Variations in this movement can be observed when the voice is disordered. For example, the vocal folds may appear to follow one another with one fold closing (moving toward the midline) as the opposite fold opens (moves away from the midline). This behavior may be constant or it may be intermittently present.

Periodicity

Periodicity is an estimate of the regularity of vibration of the vocal folds. Judgments of periodicity may be made in a number of ways. Through observation it is possible to subjectively judge whether the movement of the two vocal folds appears to be regular and periodic. It is most apparent when the strobe is placed in manual mode and the time at which the strobe light flashes is adjusted to show what appears to be a stopped frame. That is, the flashes are set to occur at the same point within each vibratory cycle. Normal vibration filmed in this manner will show a stopped frame with some small amount of movement because of the natural jitter in all voices. Fluctuation and variation of the fundamental frequency often can be observed on screen in the readout of that measure, or it can be observed as slow or rapid variations in the apparent motion of the vocal folds.

Table 2.6. Observable Physiological Signs of Voice Problems—Laryngoscopic

Vocal fold approximation
Vocal fold movement
Tissue changes
Pyriform changes
Anteroposterior laryngeal dimensions
Ventricular folds
Anatomical malformations and congenital anomalies
Vocal fold lengthening
Vertical laryngeal position
Involuntary laryngeal activity
Phonatory apraxia
Normal-appearing larynx

LARYNGOSCOPIC SIGNS

In this section, we describe those physiological signs that can be observed by using a variety of visualization techniques without the stroboscopic feature. These techniques include indirect mirror examination, flexible nasendoscopy, examination with a rigid oral endoscope, direct laryngoscopy under anesthesia, and ultra-high-speed photography. Table 2.6 summarizes the observations that can help to establish a diagnosis. The ability to make these observations may vary with the visualization technique used.

Vocal Fold Approximation

Variations of vocal fold approximation may include (a) incomplete closure along the length of the one or both vocal folds; (b) bowing of the vocal folds, seen as a central gap; and (c) lack of approximation of the vocal processes, resulting in a posterior chink. These behaviors also may be seen in video laryngostroboscopic recordings.

Vocal Fold Movement

Adductory or abductory movement of one or both vocal folds may be reduced or absent because of a variety of conditions. The vocal folds may (a) not adduct (move to the midline); (b) not abduct (move away from the midline); or (c) adduct excessively or abduct involuntarily and at inappropriate times during phonation. It is, of course, not possible to see the vibratory movements of the vocal folds with continuous light endoscopy.

Tissue Changes

A host of changes can affect the vocal fold mucosa or deeper tissue layers of the true vocal folds. These include edema, inflammation, and benign, malignant, or premalignant lesions. Each has a characteristic appearance or site of occurrence (see Chapter 3).

Pyriform Changes

The opening of the pyriform sinuses usually increases with adductory movement of the vocal folds. Lack of aperture variation of the pyriform sinus cavity is usually a sign of laryngeal paralysis and is a significant sign to note when attempting to differentiate between paralysis and arytenoid ankylosis or dislocation (Brewer & Gould, 1974).

Anteroposterior Laryngeal Dimensions

During phonation of the sustained /ee/ vowel, the distance between the epiglottis and arytenoids (anteroposterior dimension) is sufficient to allow visualization of the full length of the vocal folds in most normal speakers, particularly if the vowel is produced at a high pitch. However, in some persons, the epiglottis and arytenoids can be seen to approach each other during phonation, thereby shortening this anteroposterior dimension and obscuring visualization of the vocal folds. The extent of the visualization will depend on the phonatory conditions produced by the patient (i.e., pitch, loudness, and vowel). Marked compression of the arytenoids and epiglottis also can be observed in hyperfunctional voice production.

Ventricular Folds

The ventricular folds are located superior and lateral to the true vocal folds, and there is variation in the degree of their movement. During phonation they are usually seen to maintain their position relative to the edge of the true vocal folds. However, sometimes they appear to move toward the midline, obscuring all or part of the true vocal folds (Freud, 1962). They may even approximate each other during phonation. In some cases, false fold activity may represent a compensation for impaired true folds. For example, if a true fold is paralyzed, the false fold on the involved side may attempt to approximate the midline during phonation.

Anatomical Malformations and Congenital Anomalies

Structures may be malformed as the result of a congenital anatomical deformity (Ferguson, 1970; Ward, 1973; Cohen, 1985) or as the result of abnormal growth and development. Laryngomalacia, a softness or abnormal flaccidity of the laryngeal cartilages, is the most common congenital laryngeal anomaly and may resolve by 1 to 2 years of age (Cotton & Richardson, 1981; Hollinger & Brown, 1967). This condition shows a characteristic movement pattern of the larynx involving a downward and anterior displacement and a bowing of the aryepiglottic folds during inspiration. Other congenital problems include (a) subglottal stenosis, a thickening of subglottal tissues that may be sufficient to obstruct the airway; (b) vocal fold paralysis, often a temporary condition lasting approximately 4 weeks (Hollinger & Brown, 1967); and (c) laryngeal web, a band of tissue (which may vary in extent) joining the two vocal folds usually at the anterior commissure.

Vocal Fold Lengthening

Vocal fold lengthening is usually observed as vocal pitch is raised. This is seen fiberoptically as a lengthening of the distance between the arytenoid cartilages and the epiglottis as the vocal folds elongate. In some persons, the elevation of pitch does not produce this effect.

Vertical Laryngeal Position

The larynx is able to move in the vertical dimension. This can be visualized in laryngoscopic examination as a rising of the larynx as pitch is raised and a descent below resting level as pitch is lowered. Degree of movement varies among individuals and between trained and untrained singers (Shipp, 1975; Shipp & Izdebski, 1975). For further discussion on vertical laryngeal position, please see Chapter 4, "High Laryngeal Position."

Involuntary Laryngeal Activity

Rhythmic involuntary movement of laryngeal structures in the resting state, in the absence of phonation, is often seen accompanying neurologically based disorders (Parnes, Lavarato, & Myers, 1978). Another common observation is the movement of the arytenoids toward the midline. In voluntary effort closure, a medial squeezing and "closing down" of the entire larynx occurs. On occasion, such a movement occurs involuntarily and is described as hyperadduction. The normal larynx, when viewed at rest, maintains a relatively static posture with a fully open glottis. In some individuals, random, arrhythmic movement of various structures may be observed.

Phonatory Apraxia

Phonatory apraxia is an inability to produce phonation volitionally. Although seemingly normal movement of the vocal folds and other laryngeal structures may be observed during swallow and reflexive activities, it is absent when the person is asked to phonate voluntarily (Aronson, 1990).

Normal-Appearing Larynx

Despite the perception of a vocal abnormality, the larynx may appear to be normal in structure and function.

INTERRELATIONSHIPS OF PERCEPTUAL, PERCEPTUAL, ACOUSTIC, AND PHYSIOLOGICAL SIGNS

The signs of voice problems are not independent of one another. That is, interrelationships occur among the physiological, acoustic, and perceptual signs. Simply stated, movements of the vocal folds (physiology) create pressure disturbances in the air (acoustics) that are received by the ear and processed in the nervous system (perception).

A change in the structure of the vocal folds (e.g., a lesion, a tissue change) or a change in their manner of use (e.g., excess tension, inadequate energy) will affect the acoustic signal produced, which in turn will alter the perception of the voice. For example, a mass on the vocal folds may interfere with their closure. Consequently, air will continue to flow during that part of the vibratory cycle in which the vocal folds should be completely closed. This disturbed physiology will create a weak acoustic disturbance. Furthermore, because of the constant flow of air through a small glottal opening, an increase of noise level may occur. The weaker acoustic signal in combination with noise from the air striking the vocal folds will create the perception of breathiness.

As another example, the fundamental vibrating rate of the vocal folds is determined by their mass, length, and tension. If there is a mass on the vocal folds (e.g., a polyp or nodule), the basic vibrating rate will be altered. Vocal folds with a large mass would vibrate at a lower rate, producing a lower fundamental frequency and the perception of a lower pitch (Isshiki, Tanabe, Ishizaka, & Board, 1977). Masses on both vocal folds that are asymmetrical in size will each vibrate at a different rate, producing greater aperiodicity of vibration and increased frequency and amplitude perturbation. Greater perturbation usually is associated with the perception of greater roughness or hoarseness in the voice.

Many signs are redundant and provide the same kinds of information but perhaps in a different way. For example, it is often the case that jitter, shimmer, and signal-to-noise ratios are highly correlated because they reflect the instability of the vocal folds and any noise that they may create. This redundancy is probably good for two reasons: (a) multiple similar but not identical observations of the same effect (i.e., instability) help to confirm the effect; and (b) should it not be possible to measure one of the variables, another can be used to assess the effect of interest.

Signs cannot be viewed in a vacuum. Signs interrelate within a domain (physiology, acoustics, or perception) and across these domains. Patterns of signs accompany different voice problems and, when considered in combination with laboratory tests, physical examination, and the patient's history, assist in the accurate diagnosis of the voice disorder.

DIFFERENTIAL DIAGNOSIS OF VOICE PROBLEMS DEMONSTRATED IN NINE CASE STUDIES

In the previous sections, we have defined the terminology used to describe the symptoms and signs of voice disorders. In the following sections, each of the nine symptoms is explored in further detail in the manner of the differential diagnosis process, using case studies. The first case is presented and followed by a discussion of the process of differential diagnosis as it applies to that case. For each of the other cases, we present only the case study, with questions designed to guide the reader's thinking. Tables providing those signs that are consistent with each major symptom are also provided throughout the text. Please keep in mind that an individual patient would not necessarily present with all of the signs listed in the tables.

Hoarseness

G.N. is a 46-year-old woman referred for a consultation because of hoarseness. The patient reported that this voice quality had existed for about 2 years, and she was concerned about the possibility of cancer. Apparently, there was a family history of cancer including throat cancer. She had previously seen an otolaryngologist, who suggested a diagnosis of vocal fold nodules.

> Q. MOST ENT PHYSICIANS WILL PERFORM AN INDIRECT MIRROR EXAMINATION ON VOICE PATIENTS. WHAT WOULD YOU EXPECT TO SEE ON AN INDIRECT EXAMINATION OF THE VOCAL FOLDS IN A PATIENT WITH VOCAL FOLD NODULES?

G.N. also reported soreness in the neck area after speaking, and sometimes this pain began in the neck region and spread down to her chest.

> Q. IS SUCH A COMPLAINT CONSISTENT WITH A DIAGNOSIS OF NODULES AND IF SO, WHY?

G.N. had been referred to a speech–language pathologist (SLP) before being seen by us and received voice therapy with no significant results. She reported to us that during the therapy, when little progress was being noted, the SLP had told her that if she were a more forgiving person she could expect more progress.

> Q. DO YOU THINK PERSONALITY CHARACTERISTICS AFFECT PROGRESS IN THERAPY, AND IF SO, WHAT MIGHT THOSE BE?

G.N. works with handicapped children and uses her voice considerably during the day. She denies throat clearing, is a smoker, and drinks 3 to 4 cups of coffee a day.

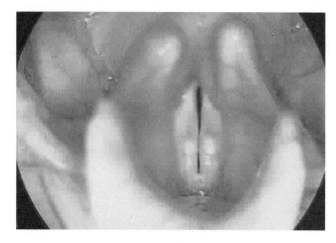

Figure 2.5. Patient G.N. Pretreatment.

Q. MOST PEOPLE ARE FAMILIAR WITH THE EFFECTS OF SMOKING ON THE BODY, BUT WHAT IS THE POTENTIAL SIGNIFICANCE OF DRINKING 3 TO 4 CUPS OF COFFEE DURING THE DAY?

G.N.'s general ENT examination of mouth, nose, and ears was negative; however, the laryngostroboscopic examination (Fig. 2.5) showed bilateral mid-membranous lesions with decreased mucosal wave at the lesion sites and prominent blood vessels leading to both lesion masses.

Q. IS THERE ANY SIGNIFICANCE TO THE DECREASED MUCOSAL WAVE AROUND THE MASSES? DOES THE PRESENCE OF A PROMINENT BLOOD VESSEL LEADING TO A LESION SUGGEST ANY DIAGNOSIS?

Bilateral vocal fold cysts were diagnosed. Voice therapy is not usually very effective with cysts. However, G.N. did participate in a preoperative visit with our SLP for counseling about the surgery and education on vocal fold anatomy and physiology. Numerous suggestions were given to facilitate a successful surgical outcome. Needless to say, she was also counseled by our otolaryngologist to reduce or eliminate her smoking.

Approximately 3 months after this initial examination, G.N. underwent surgery for removal of the two vocal fold masses. On follow-up examination approximately 1 week later, her voice was dysphonic, strained, and breathy. She reported that it required considerable effort to phonate. Approximately 2 weeks after surgery, G.N. was seen again and noted a problem initiating voice production. During the examination, she produced a very severely dysphonic voice, essentially aphonic. The strobe examination showed that although both vocal folds were mobile, closure was incomplete. Mucosal wave was significantly reduced, and there was mild erythema of both folds. Both vocal folds appeared to be stiff, probably as a consequence of surgery.

G.N. was seen again approximately 2 months after surgery. She had returned to work and was talking approximately 6 hours per day. Her voice was still hoarse and soft. She reported some strain in her neck but denied any significant vocal fatigue. The strobe examination showed bilateral vocal fold scarring, most likely the combined result of surgical removal of the cysts and vocal overuse too soon in the postoperative period. She was referred to our SLP for further voice therapy to help increase vocal fold vibratory behavior and achieve a more flexible voice.

Q. WHAT KIND OF THERAPY MIGHT HELP ACHIEVE THESE GOALS?

The patient in this case was referred to the speech–language pathologist with a stated diagnosis, vocal nodules, made by an otolaryngologist. The primary symptom expressed by the patient, hoarseness, was consistent with that diagnosis. Table 2.7 shows the perceptual signs that may accompany the symptom of hoarseness. A number of these signs were noted in this case during the initial voice evaluation, for example, hoarse voice quality, increased breathiness, episodic aphonia, excessive throat clearing, and increased tension.

Table 2.7. Signs That May Be Associated With the Symptom of Hoarse Voice

Typical Complaint: "My voice is hoarse or groggy. People think I have laryngitis."

Perceptual Signs
    Hoarseness/roughness
    Breathiness
    Laryngeal tension
    Inappropriate pitch
    Excessive throat clearing
    Episodic aphonia
    Pitch breaks

Acoustic Signs
    Restricted phonation range
    Restricted dynamic range
    Excessive spectral noise
    Greater jitter
    Greater shimmer
    Reduced maximum phonation time and high s/z ratios
    Reduced fundamental frequency variability

Observable Physiological Signs—Laryngoscopic
    Anteroposterior shortening
        Functional
    Increased ventricular fold activity
        Functional
        Compensatory
            Paralysis
            Fixed cord
            Inadequate closure
    Tissue change
        Nodules
        Polyps
        Carcinoma
        Papilloma
        Leukoplakia
        Edema
        Cyst

Continued.

Table 2.7. (continued)

Color change
   Burns
      Heat
      Chemical
   Other vocal fold lesions
Variations of vocal fold approximation
   Posterior chink
      Functional
   Bowing
      Reduced muscle tonus
   Keyhole
      Aged voice
   Incomplete anteroposterior approximation
      Paralysis
      Functional
      Ankylosis
      Dislocation
Anatomical malformation
   Congenital
   Malacia
   Stenosis
   Web
Trauma
   Blunt
   Penetrating
   Surgery
Normal larynx
   Functional
      Psychogenic
      Misuse
   Neurological
   Minor or hidden tissue change

Measurable Physiological Signs
   Aerodynamics
      Increased flow
      Increased air pressure
   Vibratory
      Aberrant glottal pulse shape
      Irregularity or asymmetry of vocal fold motion
      Mucosal wave changes
   Muscle activity
      Higher than normal levels
      Imbalance of paired muscle activity
      Normal activity

Table 2.7 lists those acoustic signs that would be consistent with the symptom and the perceptual signs. In other words, our ears hear certain vocal characteristics, some of which are accessible to measurement, thereby providing an independent corroboration of our perception. We would therefore expect to find a certain degree of match between the perceptual and the acoustic signs. In this case, we find reduced phonational range, a significant s/z ratio, and reduced phonation time.

Let us examine these factors a little more closely. Remember that hoarseness was given as a perceptual sign. A lesion, such as a nodule, on the vibratory edge of the vocal fold mucosa will disrupt vibratory behavior by adding mass at a specific location on the vocal fold. Addition of the same amount of mass distributed along the entire length of the vocal fold would most likely reduce fundamental frequency. In the case of a nodule, the extra mass loads down the vocal fold and affects its periodicity. Stiffness of the vocal fold cover is also increased because of the biomechanical characteristics of the nodule. This disruption results in a disturbance of the periodicity of the signal, creating a noisy signal that is perceived as hoarseness. The increased mass and stiffness of the folds also interferes with their ability to stretch and vibrate at a more rapid rate; therefore, pitch elevation is affected, and phonational range is decreased.

The s/z ratio is based on the theory that vocal fold vibration sufficient to produce phonation (i.e., /z/) can be maintained for a period equal to the time that airflow can be maintained without vocal fold activity (i.e., /s/). When a lesion is present on the vocal folds, there is incomplete glottal closure or very brief contact, resulting in a loss of air and a reduction in the ability to sustain phonation. The resulting s/z ratio becomes significantly greater than 1.4, which is reported to be the upper end of the normal range (Eckel & Boone, 1981). Similarly, the maximum time that phonation can be sustained is reduced. When air leakage during phonation is of a sufficient degree, there will be a perception of breathiness.

Excessive throat clearing is a common observation in patients who have vocal nodules or other lesions. These patients report the sensation that something is in the way of their being able to talk and that they must first attempt to dislodge it by clearing the throat, often quite strenuously. Unfortunately, this leads in a cyclical fashion to increased vocal trauma, which results in an exacerbation of the symptoms, which leads to an increased feeling of the need to clear the throat, and so on.

When a vocal fold lesion is present and maximum phonation time is reduced, it is not unexpected to find momentary episodes of absence of voicing. This occurs because the patient is unaccustomed to the reduction in the ability to sustain phonation or because there was insufficient effort, air pressure, or vocal fold approximation to compensate for the extra demands placed on the system by the presence of the lesion.

We would expect that breathiness would be reflected in greater than expected airflow during phonation. Indeed, when this patient was seen for further examination, one of the physiological aerodynamic signs (see Table 2.7) was increased flow. The glottal pulse shape was aberrant, revealing the poor glottal closure.

Stroboscopic examination, which was helpful in making the diagnosis of a vocal fold cyst, indicated reduced mucosal wave in the area of the cyst (see Table 2.5) and prominent vessels leading into the lesions. The laryngoscopic signs noted on fiberoptic laryngoscopic examination showed some tissue change, which appeared as a lesion on the superior surface of the vocal fold mucosa at a midway point along its length (see Table 2.6).

During the differential diagnosis process, the pieces must fit together. The process can work from a starting point of the patient's complaint, or it can work backward, as it were, from a previously arrived-at diagnosis. It is typical for speech–language pathologists to be in the position of having patients referred with a stated diagnosis. In certain cases, however, the observations and perceptions of the speech–language pathologist and information about the acoustic and physiological signs do not seem to be consistent with the diagnosis. Further examination is often warranted in such cases. On other occasions, as typified by the case of G.N., the symptoms and signs may be consistent with the diagnosis, yet the patient's treatment course suggests the need for further exploration of the case. It is especially important to recognize that, in the case of G.N., all the perceptual, acoustic, and physiological signs could have been consistent with the original diagnosis. The stroboscopic and laryngoscopic signs were the determining factors in making the diagnosis, and the suspicion of the speech–language pathologist, based on sudden and unexpected worsening of a condition, was the catalyst for reexamination of the original diagnosis.

Although some case history material was provided in the description of G.N., that part of the diagnostic process has been only briefly considered in this chapter. We do not mean to suggest that it is not an essential part of the process. Indeed, a thorough case history is essential and will be fully covered in Chapter 6.

We explore the other primary symptoms of voice problems and the differential diagnosis process in the remainder of this chapter. Each symptom is accompanied by a case study that typifies the symptom. However, we do not explain each case in the same amount of detail provided for G.N. Consult the tables for listings of all the various signs that we believe to be consistent with the symptom. Following the process should lead the reader to an understanding of the interrelatedness of the various factors, that is, perception, acoustics, and physiology, and the need for complete evaluation. In turn, this understanding should help to eliminate the cookbook approach to voice problems and replace it with the ability to follow the process of differential diagnosis in a thoughtful and reasoned manner.

Vocal Fatigue

J.S. is a. 55-year-old man who has sung professionally most of his adult life, primarily in clubs and on cruise ships. Several years ago, he began to experience difficulty with his voice. He described his symptoms at that time as an inability to increase vocal intensity without voice "breaks," and poor quality and control in the high part of his pitch range. Initially, he was able to compensate for these problems by manipulating his material, for example, shifting to a lower singing key and adjusting the amplitude of his accompaniment so that he did not have to "force" his voice. However, over the last year he began to experience vocal fatigue during performances. The frequency and severity of these incidents eventually caused him to suspend his singing career. In the interim, he has had other employment but continues to experience symptoms of vocal fatigue and difficulty increasing vocal intensity. He is not a smoker. He described no injuries to his neck and no surgical procedures that required intubation or affected the head or neck. At the time of this evaluation, he was taking medications for symptoms of gastroesophageal reflux.

> Q. WHAT TYPES OF VOCAL AND LARYNGEAL PATHOLOGICAL
> CONDITIONS MIGHT ACCOUNT FOR THE SPECIFIC CONTEXTS
> OF J.S.'S DYSPHONIA, I.E., DIFFICULTY WITH QUALITY AND
> CONTROL OF HIGH PITCHES AND INABILITY TO GENERATE
> INCREASES IN VOCAL INTENSITY?

J.S.'s speaking voice at the time of this evaluation was pleasant and judged to be within normal limits in quality. Phonatory function testing showed a fundamental frequency

Table 2.8. Signs That May Be Associated With the Symptom of Vocal Fatigue

Typical Complaint: "My voice gives out at the end of the day."

Perceptual Signs
    Monopitch
    Tension
    Breathiness
    Hoarseness

Acoustic Signs
    Restricted phonation range
    Reduced variability of fundamental frequency
    Normal acoustics

Observable Physiological Signs—Laryngoscopic
    Variations of vocal fold approximation
        Functional
    Tissue change
        Color
        Nodule
    Change of laryngeal position
        Muscle tension
    Normal-appearing larynx
        Neurological
        Myasthenia gravis

Measurable Physiological Signs
    Aerodynamic
        Increased airflow
    Vibratory
        Inadequate closed time
    Muscle activity
        Muscle imbalance
        Excessive levels
        Variation of level

range of 23 semitones and a fundamental frequency average of 102 Hz. Maximum phonation duration on a vowel sustained at comfortable pitch and loudness levels was 20 seconds. Mean and peak flows for a briefly sustained vowel were within normal limits but were elevated on a long sustained vowel and on a rapid syllable repetition task. Glottal resistance estimates for the same syllable repetition task were at the low end of normal for these measures. Measures of cycle-by-cycle variability in the voice (i.e., jitter, shimmer, harmonic-to-noise ratio) were within normal limits.

Laryngeal imaging with rigid endoscopy and stroboscopy showed both true vocal folds to be within normal limits in color. Mobility of both folds on abduction and adduction also appeared within normal limits. At rest, the left fold appeared somewhat thinner than the right. Under stroboscopic filming, a sulcus (or vergeture) was apparent on the left fold (Fig. 2.6). The cause of these furrows, or grooves, along the vibratory edge of the fold are not completely understood, but they may be related to cysts that rupture and produce scarring. The affected portion of the fold's vibratory margin is typically thin and stiff. At comfortable fundamental frequencies and intensities,

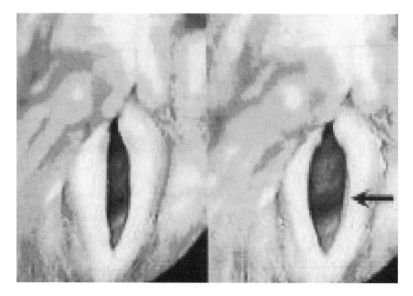

Figure 2.6. 55-year-old man, professional singer, complaining of poor quality at high F_{o}s, inability to generate loud vocal intensities, and vocal fatigue during performances. Note sulcus/vergeture on left true vocal fold.

glottal closure during phonation appeared complete (Fig. 2.7). However, glottal closure during vibratory cycles produced at high fundamental frequencies and elevated vocal intensities was incomplete (see Figs. 2.6 and 2.7).

Q. DO THE SYMPTOMS AND PHONATORY FUNCTION DATA APPEAR CONSISTENT WITH EACH OTHER? DO THE OBSERVATIONS FROM LARYNGEAL IMAGING SEEM TO ACCOUNT FOR BOTH THE SYMPTOMS AND THE PHONATORY FUNCTION FINDINGS?

The impression of the Voice Team was that the abnormality of the left fold could account for the patient's symptoms. That is, increases in vocal intensity require increases in subglottal pressure, and an accompanying increase in resistance in the true vocal folds. In J.S., the apparent inability of the left fold to increase resistance and maintain closure during vibratory cycles appeared consistent with his complaint of poor ability to increase vocal intensity, and also could explain the elevated airflows and reduced maximum phonation times noted on phonatory function testing. Similarly, the patient's description of poor quality and loss of control at fundamental frequencies high in his range could be explained by the glottic incompetence (persistent glottal gap during vibratory cycles) noted on laryngeal imaging for elevated fundamental frequencies. The team felt, furthermore, that the pathological condition described, and its consequences for voice production, were consistent with the patient's complaint of vocal fatigue, in particular, during vocal performances.

J.S. had previously undergone voice therapy, and although he reported learning a great deal about voice production and vocal hygiene, the treatment had not resolved his dysphonia. When symptoms necessitate, the treatment for this condition is typically surgical and may involve an attempt to alter the tissue at the site of the pathological condition, or a medialization or augmentation procedure of the involved fold to allow

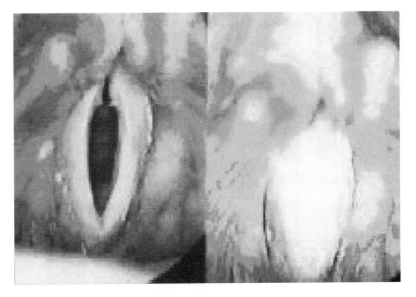

Figure 2.7. Opening and maximum closing during vibration at comfortable fundamental frequency and intensity. Note closure is complete (and voice quality good).

better contact between the true vocal folds during phonation. These options are now being considered for J.S.

Breathy

M.T., a 58-year-old woman, was referred to the Voice Clinic with a diagnosis of bowing of the true vocal folds and marked dysphonia. M.T. has been an elementary school teacher for over 30 years. She reported episodes of hoarseness during this time, perhaps

---

Table 2.9. Signs That May Be Associated With the Symptom of Breathy Voice

Typical Complaint: "My voice is weak. I run out of air. People can't hear me."

Perceptual Signs
  Breathiness
  Little loudness variation
  Hoarse/rough
  Episodic aphonia

Acoustic Signs
  Restricted phonation range
  Restricted dynamic range
  Reduced sustained phonation time
  Increased s/z ratio
  Excessive spectral noise
  Increased perturbation
  Increased shimmer

Continued.

Table 2.9. (continued)

Observable Physiological Signs—Laryngoscopic
  Variation of vocal fold approximation
    Incomplete a-p approximation (most prevalent)
      Paralysis (adductor)
      Functional
      Ankylosis
      Dislocation
      Neurological
      ALS
      Parkinson's
      Myasthenia gravis
    Posterior chink
      Functional
    Bowing
      Aging
      Reduced muscle tonus
  Lack of movement of one or both vocal folds
    Paralysis
    Ankylosis
    Dislocation
    Carcinoma
  Lack of change in appearance of pyriform sinuses
    Paralysis
  Anatomic malformation
    Congenital
    Laryngomalacia
    Trauma
      Blunt
      Penetrating
      Surgery
    Tissue change
      Burns
        Heat
        Chemical

Measurable Physiological Signs
  Aerodynamic
    Increased airflow
    Increased air pressure
  Vibratory
    Aberrant glottal pulse shape
    Inadequate closed time
    Irregularity and asymmetry of vocal
      fold motion
    Mucosal wave changes
  Muscle activity
    Absent or reduced levels
    Imbalance of paired muscle activity

2 to 3 times per year, but never so severe that she had been unable to teach. Approximately 3 months ago, she experienced symptoms of laryngitis and became extremely hoarse and breathy. The use of amplification in her classroom reportedly did not help significantly, and she described near complete loss of her voice by mid-day. Though some improvement was noted with periods of voice rest, her dysphonia did not resolve. For the last 10 weeks, she has been unable to teach and is performing administrative duties. Her medical history was not significant for factors that may have produced her dysphonia. She did not smoke, and she denied symptoms associated with gastroesophageal reflux.

Q. WHY ARE SMOKING AND REFLUX HISTORIES IMPORTANT TO KNOW IN PATIENTS? WHAT ARE THE POSSIBLE EFFECTS OF THESE CONDITIONS ON VOCAL FOLD TISSUES AND VOICE? WHAT CONDITIONS MIGHT PRODUCE THE SYMPTOMS M.T. DESCRIBES?

Perceptual signs noted at the initial evaluation included moderate breathiness and vocal strain. By the end of most breath groups, voice was aphonic. Phonatory function testing showed fundamental frequency range reduced and speaking fundamental frequency within normal limits. Maximum phonation time on a vowel sustained at comfortable fundamental frequency and intensity was 12 seconds. Mean airflow for a briefly sustained vowel produced at comfortable fundamental frequency and intensity was within normal limits. However, on a syllable repetition task produced at 80 dB, airflows were markedly elevated. Pitch perturbation, i.e., jitter, was consistently over 3% on 5 repetitions of a vowel sustained at comfortable fundamental frequency and intensity.

Laryngeal imaging with rigid endoscopy and stroboscopy showed both true vocal folds within normal limits in color and symmetrically mobile on abduction and adduction. On phonation, a persistent glottic gap during vibratory cycles was observed. The impression was that this was produced by granulation tissue, in particular, on the right posterior true vocal fold (Fig. 2.8). Early contact at this site appeared to frequently preclude complete closure of the folds. The situation was more marked with increasing vocal intensity. At soft voice, closure was more complete. Under stroboscopic imaging, mucosal wave characteristics appeared within normal limits in amplitude and symmetry.

The clinician may be wondering whether "glottic incompetence" of the type described is synonymous with the term "bowing." In our experience, bowing is more often used to characterize thinness and atrophy of the vocal folds sometimes associated with aging, or perhaps to changes in muscle tension associated with certain neurogenic conditions. The Voice Team did not feel that M.T. demonstrated bowing of this type. Certainly, however, the effects of the early posterior closure produced glottic incompetence and voicing similar to what can be observed in patients who have bowing of the true vocal folds.

Q. WHAT FACTORS MIGHT HAVE CONTRIBUTED TO THE GRANULATION TISSUE NOTED?

Based on these findings, M.T. was placed on strict voice conservation and a reflux protocol. She was advised to avoid vocal fatigue, loud talking, and talking other than in one-on-one situations. It was also recommended that she return to the Clinic for voice therapy. One goal of therapy would be to attempt to change vocal and vocal fold behavior in a manner that minimized contact pressures at the site of the pathological condition.

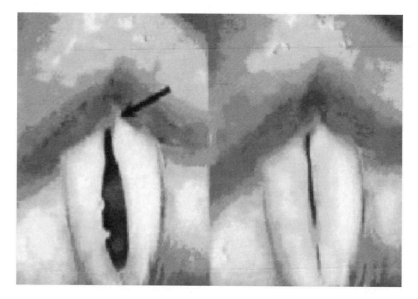

Figure 2.8. 58-year-old woman, elementary school teacher, with complaint of progressive hoarseness and vocal fatigue over last 2 years. Note apparent granulation tissue at arrow that interferes with closure of true vocal folds during voicing. At right, folds are shown at maximum closure during phonation at comfortable F0 and I0 levels. Voice quality is breathy.

Q. WHAT VOICE THERAPY STRATEGIES CAN YOU THINK OF THAT MIGHT HAVE THIS EFFECT?

In Figure 2.9, M.T.'s vocal folds are shown 2 months after her initial evaluation. The posterior granulation tissue has resolved to some extent, and closed phases of vibration appear appropriate. Interestingly, airflow values obtained at this time were substantially below normal, which may have reflected the patient's attempts to conserve air in the face

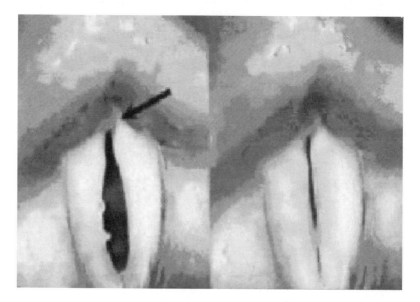

Figure 2.9. Some improvement is noted 6 weeks later after reflux precautions and strict voice conservation.

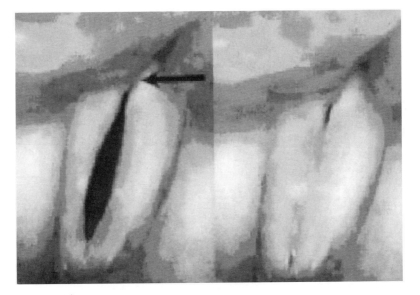

Figure 2.10. Additional improvement is noted after voice therapy. Frame at right shows good closure between the vocal folds (and good voice quality) at comfortable F0 and I0.

of glottal gapping. Thus, a second goal of therapy was to normalize airflow and achieve a better balance between respiratory and phonatory behavior. These objectives were successfully achieved, and a sample of the patient's voice post-treatment is presented in an audio sample on the companion DVD. In Figure 2.10, additional improvement in vocal fold closure is noted after voice therapy, although a small amount of residual pathological condition is still present.

> Q. WHAT TREATMENT STRATEGIES CAN YOU THINK OF THAT MIGHT ADDRESS THE ISSUE OF ACHIEVING BALANCE BETWEEN RESPIRATORY AND PHONATORY COMPONENTS OF VOICE PRODUCTION?

Reduced Pitch Range

M.D. is a 46-year-old woman referred by another ENT because of a persistent voice problem. She is a professional singer who has sung locally in the community for over 20 years. She also does much of the scheduling for the band for which she sings and notes that this activity requires considerable telephone work. M.D. reports that she has lost the top of her range in recent months and is hoarse when speaking. She also describes having reflux in the past but does not believe she has any symptoms currently.

> Q. WHAT WOULD BE THE EFFECT OF REFLUX ON THE LARYNX AND VOCAL FOLDS? WHY SHOULD THE ENT CAREFULLY EVALUATE REFLUX SYMPTOMS?

Previous ENT examinations have indicated a mild vocal fold edema and a right hemorrhagic lesion. Topical steroids were tried with little positive result. She was treated for reflux with little improvement of her voice. At this time, no behavioral modifications or changes in the voice were instituted.

Table 2.10. Signs That May Be Associated With the Symptom of Reduced
Phonation Range

Typical Complaint: "I am not able to produce the high notes of my range during singing."

Perceptual Signs
  Tension
  Pitch breaks
  Normal-sounding voice

Acoustic Signs
  Restricted phonational range
  Restricted dynamic range

Observable Physiological Signs—Laryngoscopic
  Tissue change of vocal folds
    Nodule
    Color
  Normal-appearing larynx
    Functional
      Misuse
      Improper vocal technique
    Minor or hidden tissue change

Measurable Physiological Signs
  Muscle
    Excessive levels
    Normal physiology

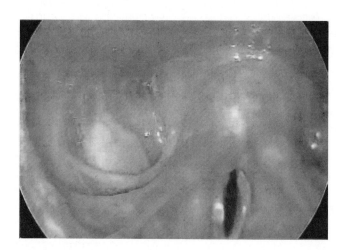

Figure 2.11. Patient M.D. Initial visit.

A rigid strobe examination was attempted; however, because of her gag reflex, it was abandoned in favor of a flexible examination (Fig. 2.11). Bilateral vocal fold edema was found along with interarytenoid erythema. The right vocal fold had a superior surface hemorrhagic lesion.

In addition to continuing M.D.'s antireflux medication, voice therapy was also recommended. Surgery was considered but not recommended at this time because of concerns that the patient would not follow prescribed vocal rest and proper postoperative rehabilitation. M.D. was seen for one session of voice therapy and counseled about proper voice hygiene, including water intake, and conservative voice use, i.e., restrictions on amount and type of talking. Vocal exercises also were recommended. A second therapy session focused on using soft glides and a more relaxed mode of phonation.

M.D. was seen again and reported that she was unable to continue voice therapy because it was not covered by insurance. At this time, she continued to have difficulty with her speaking voice and described "pushing through" her singing performances. She stated that she was doing considerable talking on the phone, and although she had successfully managed to sing for the past few months, a much more demanding schedule was forthcoming, and she was concerned about her voice.

The endoscopic strobe examination showed a slight posterior chink, erythema, and slight stiffness of the right vocal fold. Our ENT was concerned that when she started singing again, the voice would worsen. He suggested that she continue voice therapy and start lessons with a singing coach to improve her technique. She was offered exploratory microlaryngoscopy to better determine the problem, but she declined. She has not followed through with any surgery, nor has she continued her voice therapy sessions.

Aphonia

J.F., a 16-year-old girl, presented to our Voice Clinic accompanied by her mother. J.F. is a junior in high school and lives with her mother and two younger brothers. The parents have been separated for 5 years, and the father lives in another state. J.F. was essentially aphonic, and the mother reported that this has been the situation for the past 3 months. J.F. was able to whisper, and we obtained the history from her in that mode. She reported the onset of the problem after a sinus infection when she was able to produce sound only at a very high pitch. Her voice continued to worsen until only the whisper was left. Although no strain was noted during the whispering, J.F. claimed that her throat often hurt and that it was a strain to even produce a whisper. She denied any prior episodes of voice difficulty, although she has had sinus infections previously. In addition to this problem, J.F. reports TMJ (temporomandibular joint) problems and inability to fully open her mouth that began suddenly with facial spasms while she was lifting weights. She has been treated for this problem for the past year and a half with physical therapy, some surgical intervention—the details of which she was unable to provide—and muscle relaxant drugs. She claims that these treatments have resulted in minimal improvement.

> Q. WHAT ARE SOME POSSIBLE CAUSES OF APHONIA? WHICH OF THOSE DO YOU THINK COULD EXPLAIN THIS GIRL'S APHONIA?

Throughout the history taking and the examination, J.F.'s mother appeared very anxious and concerned, although J.F.'s affect seemed quite unconcerned. Video fiberoptic laryngeal examination was performed, using both rigid and flexible scopes.

Table 2.11. Signs That May Be Associated With the Symptom of Aphonia

Typical Complaint: "I lost my voice" or "My voice is gone."

Perceptual Signs
    Breathiness
    Consistent aphonia

Acoustic Signs
    Excessive spectral noise

Observable Physiological Signs—Laryngoscopic
    Variations in vocal fold approximation
    Incomplete vocal fold approximation
    Bilateral adductor paralysis
    Lack of movement of vocal folds
    Phonatory apraxia
    CNS lesion

Measurable Physiological Signs
    Aerodynamics
        Increased airflow
        Increased air pressure
    Vibratory
        Not applicable
    Muscle activity
        Unknown

Q. GIVEN THE APHONIA, OF WHAT VALUE DO YOU THINK A STROBOSCOPIC EXAMINATION WOULD BE AND WHY? WHAT WOULD YOU ANTICIPATE THE POSITION OF THE VOCAL FOLDS WOULD BE DURING PHONATION FOR THE VARIOUS POSSIBLE CAUSES YOU CONSIDERED ABOVE?

The examination showed normal laryngeal structure and function except during speech.

In carrying out nonvocal acts such as swallowing and whistling, the vocal folds were noted to ab/adduct normally. During whispered phonation, the vocal folds remained apart. When asked to produce sounds such as a cough, clearing the throat, producing a high pitch, etc., J.F.'s response was always delayed and tentative at first but nothing more than the whisper was ever produced.

Q. WHAT DIAGNOSIS/DIAGNOSES WOULD YOU BE CONSIDERING AT THIS TIME?

J.F. was referred for voice therapy and was subsequently seen for six sessions. We were using a working diagnosis of aphonia of psychogenic origin. The patient could best be described as a very resistant patient and very guarded. Despite the use of a variety of techniques and gentle but pointed probing, J.F. continued to deny any problems and stated that everything in her life was fine. She remained totally aphonic for the first two sessions.

Q. WHAT THERAPY TECHNIQUES WOULD YOU ATTEMPT WITH THIS PATIENT?

During the third session, the clinician indicated to J.F. that this therapy approach seemed not to be meeting with any success and might therefore need to be terminated. Quite suddenly her voice began to improve, but in very gradual steps. By the sixth session, entirely normal voice was restored, but J.F. had never provided any verbalized insight into any areas of concern. The clinician strongly recommended to J.F., to the mother, and to the referring physician that, despite the return of voice, issues had not been resolved for which counseling should be sought.

Pitch Breaks or Falsetto

V.P. is a 16-year-old boy with a history of voice problems beginning in the seventh grade. He was initially treated for reflux by his family physician without any change in his voice. A CT scan of the neck indicated no abnormalities. He was seen twice a week for 5 weeks by an SLP elsewhere with no improvement in his voice.

Table 2.12. Signs That May Be Associated With the Symptoms of Pitch Breaks or Inappropriately High Pitch

---

Typical Complaint: "My voice sounds squeaky."

Perceptual Signs
   Inappropriate pitch level
   Pitch breaks

Acoustic Signs
   Higher than expected speaking fundamental frequency
   Rapid shifts of fundamental frequency
   Restricted phonation range
   Restricted dynamic range
   Reduced maximum phonation time

Observable Physiological Signs—Laryngoscopic
   Normal-appearing larynx
      Functional
   Anatomical malformations
      Hormone imbalance
      Web

Measurable Physiological Signs
   Aerodynamics
      Decreased airflow
   Vibratory
      Inadequate closed times
      Mucosal wave changes
   Muscle activity
      Excessive levels

Q. WHAT WAS THE PURPOSE OF THE CT SCAN OF THE NECK?

Q. WHAT PERCEPTUAL SIGNS OF THE VOICE WOULD YOU WANT INFORMATION ON?

V.P. described his voice problem as consisting of pitch breaks and unsteadiness. He feels that his voice is unpredictable. He admits to being a quiet and shy person. He does play tennis and does well academically. During the interview, he was dysphonic with numerous pitch breaks and difficulty sustaining a low modal pitch.

V.P. was examined stroboscopically using a flexible endoscope, and no abnormalities were noted in the larynx or vocal folds. A diagnosis of puberphonia was made, and V.P. was referred to the SLP team member for voice therapy. Interestingly, his mother accompanied V.P. to the diagnostic session and remarked that she was not concerned about his voice. Later in the session, she stated that the new, deep voice that V.P. had demonstrated was not his voice.

During the first and only therapy session, an appropriate pitch and smooth phonation could be elicited in a number of ways. The remainder of the session was spent in establishing this lower pitch and smoothness of pitch, incorporating it into conversational speech. V.P. seemed accepting of this new sound, although he is a young man who reveals little emotion. Discussion of the problem and of the "new" sound was pursued, and again V.P.'s responses, although relatively minimal, demonstrated a willingness to use this new voice. He was willing to use the voice when his father returned to the room. The SLP did not believe that further therapy was necessary because V.P. seemed comfortable with the new sound and was using it consistently for much of the session. V.P. was asked to be in touch with us by phone so that we could ascertain that the change was adopted. He was urged to contact us if there were any setbacks.

Strain/Struggle

M.V. is a 48-year-old obese woman who reported difficulty with her voice for many years. She stated that her speech is very effortful and unpredictable, and at times she cannot produce any sound. She also complained of TMJ discomfort. She is a nonsmoker and denies use of alcohol or recreational drugs. She claims to be in fairly good health with the exception of the above complaints. Perceptually her speech was marked by frequent voice stoppages, some of which were prolonged. During these prolonged stoppages, facial grimacing was noted as she appeared to be struggling to produce voice. She also demonstrated aphonic episodes, especially at the end of sentences. She was unable to sustain a vowel in a smooth, unbroken voice quality for more than 2 seconds.

Q. ARE THESE SYMPTOMS CONSISTENT WITH A DIAGNOSIS OF SPASMODIC DYSPHONIA (SD)?

Q. WHAT OTHER DIAGNOSES WOULD BE PART OF YOUR DIFFERENTIAL DIAGNOSTIC LIST?

Videolaryngoscopic examination was performed by using a flexible fiberscope in the continuous light condition. The patient's symptoms were more severe during this examination than they had been during conversation. The image was marked by much strain, with the vocal folds remaining in the closed vibratory phase most of the time. Once again, no smooth, uninterrupted sustained phonations were elicited.

Table 2.13. Signs That May Be Associated With the Symptom of Strain/Struggle

Typical Complaint: "My voice just stops. I can't get anything out."

Perceptual Signs
    Strain/struggle voice
    Tension
    Sudden interruption of voicing
    Loudness variation (uncontrolled)
    Tremor

Acoustic Signs
    Unexpected voice stoppages
    Spectral interruptions
    Reduced sustained phonation time

Observable Physiological Signs—Laryngoscopic
    Effort closure of the larynx
        Spasmodic dysphonia
        Myoclonus
        Hyperkinetic dysarthria
        Mixed dysarthria (ALS)
        Functional
    Anteroposterior shortening of the vocal folds
        Spasmodic dysphonia
        Functional
    Rhythmic movement of laryngeal structures
        Spasmodic dysphonia
    ALS
        Essential tremor
        Myoclonus
    Arrhythmic movements of laryngeal structures
        Spasmodic dysphonia

Measurable Physiological Signs
    Aerodynamic
        Decreased airflow
        Increased air pressure
    Vibratory
        Excessive closed times
        Aberrant glottal pulse shape
    Muscle activity
        Excessive levels
        Sudden, unexpected bursts of activity
        Involuntary rhythmic variations of level
        Slow rise or fall of signal amplitude

Q. DOES THIS INFORMATION CONFIRM THE DIAGNOSIS OF SPASMODIC DYSPHONIA? WHY WAS A FLEXIBLE FIBERSCOPE USED RATHER THAN THE RIGID SCOPE? WHY WAS THE CONTINUOUS LIGHT CONDITION USED? (YOU MAY WISH TO RETURN TO THE LAST TWO QUESTIONS WHEN YOU HAVE LEARNED MORE ABOUT VARIOUS EXAMINATION TECHNIQUES.)

The examiners thought that more information was needed at this time to assist in making a diagnosis. Therefore, the patient was referred to a neurologist for EMG examination to determine whether there was evidence of excessive muscle action potentials

Q. WHICH MUSCLES DO YOU THINK MIGHT SHOW SUCH EXCESS ACTIVITY IN SD?

Q. THE NEUROLOGIST'S REPORT INDICATED THAT THE PATIENT'S EXAMINATION WAS NORMAL AND FAILED TO SHOW ANY EXCESSIVE MUSCLE ACTION POTENTIALS. WHAT DOES THIS INFORMATION MEAN TO YOU REGARDING YOUR DIAGNOSIS THUS FAR?

Further diagnostic information seemed to be needed. Therefore, the patient was referred for diagnostic voice therapy. She was seen for three sessions of such therapy over a 3-week period. Her symptoms remained the same, and at no time were we able to elicit significantly smoother voice quality despite the trial of numerous techniques.

Q. WHAT DOES THE TERM "DIAGNOSTIC VOICE THERAPY" SUGGEST TO YOU? (THINK ABOUT SOME VOICE THERAPY TECHNIQUES YOU MIGHT TRY WITH THIS PATIENT.)

It was decided at this time to move forward with the diagnosis of adductor SD, despite the fact that we continued to believe that there might be an overlaid component of muscle tension dysphonia. This was explained to the patient, and treatment with botulinum toxin (Botox) was recommended. The patient subsequently received Botox injections into the thyroarytenoid muscles bilaterally. Her posttreatment course was typical of patients with SD. Her voice quality was markedly improved by this treatment, and she has continued to receive these injections every 3 to 4 months on average.

Tremor

M.L. is a 74-year-old woman who was referred because of problems with her voice for the past few years. Her husband agreed that her voice was problematic and further stated that her head bobbed occasionally. The patient reported that she had experienced some spasms in her voice, but she does not believe that her speech is effortful.

Q. WHAT COULD THE OBSERVATION MADE BY HER HUSBAND ABOUT THE HEAD BOBBING MEAN?

The ENT examination showed an elderly but alert woman with no evidence of tremor in the arms and hands. However, head oscillations were noted. All cranial nerves were tested and were intact.

A flexible stroboscopic examination showed rhythmic oscillations of the larynx, especially on the production of a sustained /ah/ and /ee/. In Figure 2.12, note the variation of position of the arytenoids and vocal folds from one image to the next.

Table 2.14. Signs That May Be Associated With the Symptom of Tremor

Typical Complaint: "My voice wobbles. My voice is unsteady."

Perceptual Signs
  Tremor
  Monopitch
  Monoloudness
  Loudness variations/uncontrolled

Acoustic Signs
  Voice tremor
  Restricted phonation range
  Restricted dynamic range
  Less variability of
      Fundamental frequency
      Intensity
  Slow rise or fall in signal amplitude

Observable Physiological Signs—Laryngoscopic
  Rhythmic movements of laryngeal structures
      Essential voice tremor

Measurable Physiological Signs
  Aerodynamics
      Periodic variations of airflow
  Vibratory
      Aberrant glottal pulse shape
  Muscle activity
      Involuntary rhythmic variations of level

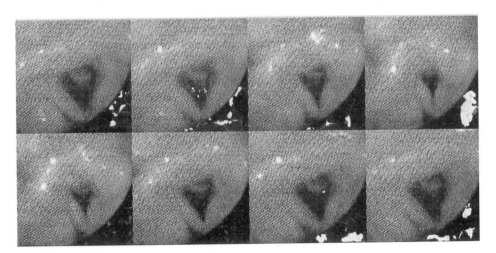

Figure 2.12. Patient M.L. Initial visit. This figure is a sequence of frames as the patient breathed quietly. Note the changes of position of the vocal folds indicating movement of the vocal folds and arytenoids during breathing when the vocal folds should remain open.

These images were taken from a segment of the examination in which the patient was not phonating and was presumably at rest. There was periodic movement of the arytenoids and vocal folds during this time. The companion video clip on the DVD shows these rhythmic oscillations during the first part of the examination. A diagnosis of vocal tremor was made. Options discussed with the patient included referral to a neurologist, medications, Botox, or no treatment.

> Q. WHAT KINDS OF MEDICATIONS HAVE BEEN USED TO TREAT TREMOR AND HAS SUCH TREATMENT BEEN SUCCESSFUL? BOTOX TEMPORARILY PARALYZES THE MUSCLES OF THE LARYNX. HOW MIGHT THIS BE EXPECTED TO HELP IN THE TREMOR THAT IS A CENTRAL NEUROLOGICAL PROBLEM?

M.L. decided to have the Botox injection. Two units of the drug were injected into the thyroarytenoid on each side. She was then seen for voice therapy 5 days after the injection and noted to have a breathy voice.

> Q. WHY WOULD THIS PATIENT BE REFERRED TO A VOICE THERAPIST WITH THIS DIAGNOSIS?

The severity of the tremor appeared to have been reduced compared with the pre-injection examination. The nature of the voice therapy was discussed with the patient, and techniques were suggested to prolong the benefit of the injection. These techniques included (a) reduction of loudness—do not try to push the voice; (b) increase speaking rate; (c) speak in shorter phrases; and (d) allow the natural breathiness that occurs because of the Botox to prevail and continue a more breathy, confidential voice.

Approximately 4 months after her first injection, M.L. was seen again for another Botox injection. She reported that she had prolonged breathiness for several weeks after the first injection. The effects of the tremor were becoming more marked over the last few weeks. Because of her rather long period of breathiness after the last injection, it was decided to reduce the amount of Botox from 2 to 1.5 units, again on both sides. Two weeks after the injection, M.L. reported that she had been breathy for about a week and had a little trouble swallowing. The voice sounded strong and much smoother than before the injection.

Pain and Other Physical Sensations

As noted in the initial discussion of this section, symptoms are reported by patients in a variety of ways. Thus, rather than a single case presentation representative of a single symptom category, we present a number of patients who report specific types of pain or sensations and relate that sensory information to the underlying pathophysiology.

J.F. reports having a severe cough for several weeks. After resolution of the cough, he noted residual slight hoarseness that did not abate. He also complained of slight soreness and burning in a localized area on the left neck near the posterior aspect of the larynx. He was found to have a contact granuloma over the left vocal process slightly superior to the vocal fold. This lesion was surgically removed but recurred and required two additional surgeries. The granuloma recurred yet again. Each time the soreness recurred and was always localized to the same spot. According to the patient's report, the pain was exacerbated by phonation.

Q. WHY WOULD PAIN BE PRESENT AND WHAT COULD BE HAPPENING DURING PHONATION TO INCREASE THAT PAIN?

A 24-hour pH probe study had ruled out gastroesophageal reflux as a contributing factor. J.F. was referred for a course of voice therapy when a video laryngostroboscopic study showed a consistent pattern of approximation of the arytenoids occurring before closure of the vocal folds. This pattern could be described as a "toeing in" of the arytenoid cartilages.

Voice therapy was directed at changing this closure pattern and reducing the force of the contact. The granuloma reduced in size, and the symptom of pain was eliminated.

Q. WHAT COULD ACCOUNT FOR THE RESISTANCE OF THIS GRANULOMA TO TREATMENT?

A CT scan showed the probable answer. The left arytenoid was found to be entirely calcified. Thus, the thin mucosal cover overlying a hard and "nongiving" calcified cartilage was unable to absorb the impact forces of arytenoid closure. Although this is not a typical case, it again focuses attention on the need for thorough and ongoing assessment.

L.D. is a 26-year-old woman who has been singing with various local rock groups for approximately 10 years. Until this past year she had never experienced more than fleeting hoarseness that never lasted more than 2 days and rarely occurred. This year she has noticed increasingly frequent episodes of hoarseness that have now culminated in a constant degree of hoarseness that does not go away. Although her singing voice was affected, others seemed not to be aware of it. She was aware that she had to work harder to produce voice, that she was changing musical arrangements to avoid the upper range (which was especially difficult), and that she was exhausted by the end of a set. She finally sought medical attention because she began to experience pain and soreness that radiated from the neck down to her upper chest. It was the pain that frightened her into recognizing that she had a problem.

Q. IN THIS CASE, WHAT SPECIFICALLY DO YOU THINK COULD BE CREATING PAIN OR SORENESS? WHY WOULD THAT SORENESS BE IN THE AREAS DESCRIBED?

L.D. was found to have vocal fold nodules, and a course of voice therapy was prescribed. After two sessions of voice therapy directed at eliminating traumatic vocal behavior, restricting the amount of talking, and using a very soft breathy voice when it was necessary to talk, L.D. reported that the pain was gone. Voice therapy was continued for another six sessions, with eventual resolution of the nodules. L.D. had no further complaint of pain.

Q. WOULD THIS BE CONSISTENT WITH YOUR RESPONSES TO THE QUESTION ABOVE?

A 35-year-old minister, R.S., complained of vocal fatigue and of soreness on both sides of the neck lateral to the larynx. This soreness was especially intense as he was giving sermons. Laryngovideostroboscopy with a rigid oral endoscope was performed and, on sustained vowel productions, revealed healthy vocal folds with good vibratory behavior, normal mucosal wave, normal amplitude, good closure, and good phase symmetry. Very slight inflammation of the larynx was observed.

Table 2.15. Summary of Peceptual, Acoustic, and Physiological Signs That May Accompany the Nine Major Voice Systems

Symptom

Perceptual Sign	Hoarse	Vocal Fatigue	Breathy Voice	Reduced Phonational Range	Aphonia	Pitch Breaks, Inappropriately High Pitch	Strain/Struggle Voice	Tremor	Pain and Other Physical Sensations
Monopitch		X							
Monoloudness	X	X						X	
Hoarseness	X	X	X						X
Breathiness	X	X	X						X
Tension				X			X	X	X
Tremor							X	X	
Strain/struggle	X						X	X	
Inappropriate pitch			X		X				
Loudness variation							X	X	
Stridor	X								
Throat clearing	X	X	X		X			X	X
Aphonia—constant	X		X						
Aphonia—episodic	X			X		X	X		
Pitch breaks						X			
Sudden interruptions					X			X	
Normal									

Symptom

Acoustic Sign	Hoarse	Vocal Fatigue	Breathy Voice	Reduced Phonational Range	Aphonia	Pitch Breaks, Inappropriately High Pitch	Strain/Struggle Voice	Tremor	Pain and Other Physical Sensations
Mean frequency	X	X				X			
variability		X						X	
perturbation	X								
shifts						X			

Table (rotated on page). *Symptom* columns across; acoustic measures and laryngoscopic signs down.

	Hoarse	Vocal Fatigue	Breathy Voice	Reduced Phonational Range	Aphonia	Pitch Breaks, Inappropriately High Pitch	Strain/Struggle Voice	Tremor	Pain and Other Physical Sensations
					Symptom				
Phonational range	X		X	X		X		X	
Mean intensity	X	X	X	X				X	
variability	X	X						X	
perturbation	X	X	X						
dynamic range	X	X	X	X		X		X	
Spectrum									
noise	X		X		X				
harmonic energy	X	X	X						
interruptions							X		
Phonation time									
maximum	X	X	X				X	X	
s/z ratio	X	X	X				X		
Unexpected pauses							X		
Tremor	X							X	
Normal	X		X						
Observable Physiologic Sign—Laryngoscopic									
Variation of VF approximation	X				X				X
Vocal fold movement			X		X		X		
Tissue changes	X	X	X	X					
Pyriform sinuses			X						
AP laryngeal dimension	X	X			X			X	
Ventricular fold activity		X	X		X		X		X
Anatomical malformation	X					X			X
Vocal fold length	X				X				
Vertical laryngeal position	X	X			X				
Rhythmic movements	X						X	X	

Continued.

61

Table 2.15. (continued)

Columns grouped under the heading **Symptom**: Hoarse, Vocal Fatigue, Breathy Voice, Reduced Phonational Range, Aphonia, Pitch Breaks Inappropriately High Pitch, Strain/Struggle Voice, Tremor, Pain and Other Physical Sensations.

Hoarse	Vocal Fatigue	Breathy Voice	Reduced Phonational Range	Aphonia	Pitch Breaks, Inappropriately High Pitch	Strain/Struggle Voice	Tremor	Pain and Other Physical Sensations	Observable Physiologic Sign—Laryngoscopic
						X		X	Effort closure
						X			Arrhythmic movemets
			X	X	X				Phonatory apraxia
X	X								Normal

Hoarse	Vocal Fatigue	Breathy Voice	Reduced Phonational Range	Aphonia	Pitch Breaks, Inappropriately High Pitch	Strain/Struggle Voice	Tremor	Pain and Other Physical Sensations	Measurable Physiological Sign
X	X	X		X	X	X	X		Airflow
X	X	X		X		X			Air pressure
X		X				X	X		Glottal pulse shape
	X		X						Open/closed phases
X		X							Vibratory behavior
									Muscle
X	X	X	X		X	X		X	levels
X	X					X	X		rate changes
						X			bursts
									onset/offset
						X			level decay
X	X	X							paired muscle activity
X			X						Normal

Q. WHAT OTHER TYPE OF EXAMINATION MIGHT YOU WANT AND WHY?

We thought that use of the flexible nasendoscope might allow the patient to provide a sample of the speech he uses when he gives a sermon, thereby allowing us to visualize phonatory behavior in that mode. What we observed did not come as a total surprise. Marked anteroposterior squeezing was noted, and the entire larynx moved superiorly as he began phonation.

Q. DO THESE OBSERVATIONS HELP TO EXPLAIN THE NATURE AND LOCATION OF THE PAIN AND VOCAL FATIGUE OF WHICH THE PATIENT COMPLAINED? HOW AND WHY?

SUMMARY

In this chapter, a basic approach to the diagnosis of voice problems is presented. The approach, based on the medical model of differential diagnosis, carefully considers the patient's symptoms (complaints) and relates them to the signs of the patient's voice problem. There are four categories of signs: perceptual, acoustic, measurable physiological, and observable physiological.

Nine primary symptoms are presented: hoarseness, vocal fatigue, breathiness, loss of range, aphonia, pitch breaks, strain/struggle, tremor, and pain. These are defined and discussed within the context of case studies of individual patients.

Signs can be observed and tested independently of the patient's report. The major perceptual signs associated with voice problems include those related to pitch, loudness, and quality, as well as aphonia and non-phonatory signs. Acoustic signs include reduced phonation and dynamic range, higher or lower fundamental frequency, perturbation, low or high intensity, and spectral noise. Measurable physiological signs include reduced or excessive airflow and pressure, aberrant airflow or electroglottographic waveform, reduced or excessive muscle activity, and unusual muscle activity. Observable physiological signs are those stroboscopic signs that include mucosal wave, level of folds, symmetry of vocal folds, and amplitude of vocal fold motion. Laryngoscopic signs include tissue change, vocal fold approximation, anteroposterior approximation, movement of the vocal folds, and anatomic malformations. Table 2.15 presents a summary of the relationships between symptoms and signs discussed in this chapter.

Case studies have been presented to illustrate the symptoms of a voice problem and the signs associated with each symptom. The process by which the symptoms and signs are considered in the making of the diagnosis of a voice problem is emphasized in this chapter. The diagnosis of a voice problem is an ongoing, dynamic process. It is incumbent on those who work with patients with voice disorders to continue to ask questions about the nature of the problem and the treatment approach.

Chapter 3

Morphology of Vocal Fold Mucosa: Histology to Genomics

Voice is created as a consequence of vibration of the vocal folds. The quality of voice production is dependent on the uniquely layered ultrastructure of the vocal folds, which is defined by its cellular and extracellular matrices (ECM). Pathological changes of the vocal fold ECM alter vocal quality secondary to loss of normal vibratory function and alteration of tissue viscosity and thereby create mild to debilitating levels of dysphonia. Select characteristics of the layered structure have been documented for normal and pathological states, but methodologies have been limited to histological and immunohistological analyses. Little has been completed using cellular, molecular, or genetic techniques such as gene expression analysis (i.e., polymerase chain reaction or northern analysis) and protein synthesis analysis (i.e., Western blot or enzyme-linked immunosorbent assay [ELISA]). Significant unanswered questions concerning the ECM and its effect on vocal fold vibration remain. However, recent advances in protein and genetic engineering have allowed for expansion of our knowledge of the ECM, particularly regarding its role in providing homeostasis between the cellular elements and the surrounding stromal matrix.

This chapter begins with an introduction to ECM biology, followed by a section on characteristics of the ECM specific to the vocal fold lamina propria. When dyshomeostasis between the cellular and stromal matrix occurs, pathological vocal fold ECM ensues. The final section contains descriptions of benign vocal fold lesions detailed by characteristics of their ECM.

THE EXTRACELLULAR MATRIX (ECM)

The ECM is formed of connective tissue, which is composed of cells and an organized meshwork of macromolecules. Various kinds of connective tissue exist, which differ in the types and amounts of cells and macromolecules present in their ECM. Variations in the relative amounts of the different types of matrix macromolecules and the way they are organized in the ECM give rise to a variety of structures. At one time, the ECM was thought to solely provide structure and support for tissue. Today's conventional wisdom suggests that the ECM not only provides support but also provides homeostasis between the cell and its surroundings.

The ECM is a molecular complex composed mainly of fibrillar proteins (fibrous and interstitial), proteoglycans, and glycosaminoglycans (GAG). The fibrous matrix macromolecules are secreted largely by fibroblasts (Martins-Green 1997). Molecules and amount present vary with tissue type and at different stages of development in a single tissue type.

Fibrillar proteins are frequently broken down into two functional types: structural (collagen and elastin) and mainly adhesive (fibronectin and laminin). Collagens account for 25% of total mammalian protein mass; currently 19 subtypes of collagen are known (Ehrlich, 2000). After being secreted into the ECM, the collagen molecules assemble collagen fibrils, which can aggregate into large bundles referred to as collagen fibers. Collagen provides strength to tissue. Elastin is made of a highly hydrophobic (water-fearing) protein that when secreted into the ECM becomes highly linked with other elastin proteins. Elastin is responsible for the tissue's ability to recoil after stretch. Fibronectin, a glycoprotein (sugar molecular with a protein attached), has multiple forms. It is secreted into the blood by the liver. Fibronectin contains multiple binding sites for collagen, heparin, fibrillin, integrins, and cell surface receptors. It participates in such varied biological activities as inflammation, malignant metastasis, and thrombosis. Laminin is known to bind to collagen type IV, heparin, and cell surface receptors (Alberts, 1999). Laminin and fibronectin are responsible for organizing of the ECM and cell binding in the ECM in differing tissue types.

GAGs are unbranched chains composed of repeating sugar units (Alberts, 1999). GAGs are negatively charged and strongly hydrophilic or "water loving." They tend to adopt an expansive conformation and attract large amounts of sodium, which causes large amounts of water to be absorbed by the tissue. This allows the tissue to be able to withstand large compressive forces. Hyaluronan is the simplest of GAGs; it consists of a regular repeating sequence of sugar units. It has been suggested that hyaluronan functions in resisting compressive forces, wound repair and lubrication (Alberts, 1999; Balazs & Larsen, 2000; Chan & Titze, 1999).

Proteoglycans are composed of GAGs that are also attached to a protein. They are a diverse group. Proteoglycans are believed to play a major role in signaling between cells and serve to regulate the activity of other proteins. A family of small proteoglycans includes decorin, biglycan, fibromodulin, and lumican. Decorin has been found to inhibit collagen formation and modify the structure of collagen. Fibromodulin has also been shown to regulate the formation of collagen. Biglycan and lumican have unknown roles.

ECM regulation is the process by which old proteins are broken down and new proteins are made. Under normal physiological conditions, the maintenance of the proteins is tightly controlled through a balance between synthesis and degradation. Any changes in this balance can alter normal tissue architecture, impair tissue function, and change the mechanical support for tissues. Net degradation or net synthesis of the ECM is most often associated with pathological conditions. For example, benign vocal fold lesions are thought to be a result of either net degradation or net synthesis of the ECM.

Matrix metalloproteinases (MMPs) are a family of molecules that break down specific ECM components. MMPs are made and secreted by the connective tissue and are known to be important in both normal remodeling and in the early destruction on the ECM occurring in many diseases (Murphy & Docherty, 1992). Twenty MMPs have been identified, each acting against a specific protein. The major natural inhibitors of MMPs are the tissue inhibitors of MMPs (TIMPs) (Alberts, 1999). TIMPs are complex glycoproteins that work to prevent matrix degradation by the MMPs. There are two types of TIMPs in humans, TIMP-I and TIMP-II. We know that ECM regulation is a tightly controlled process. It is dependent not only on total amount of secreted proteins, but also on activation and inhibition of MMPs by TIMPs.

VOCAL FOLD ECM BIOLOGY

The lamina propria of the vocal folds is connective tissue made up of ECM. All of the components and characteristics of the ECM described in the previous section are pertinent to the vocal fold lamina propria. Table 3.1 summarizes ECM components known to be in the vocal folds. The dynamic interactions between proteins, proteoglycans, and glycoproteins provide a balanced environment for normal vocal fold development. In general, fibrous proteins provide structural maintenance, whereas the interstitial proteins may affect the mechanical properties of the vocal fold through changes in tissue viscosity, fluid content thickness of lamina propria layers and even collagen fiber population density and size. If disequilibrium occurs in the levels of components of the lamina propria (LP), pathological vocal fold conditions arise.

Hirano (Hirano, 1974; Hirano & Kakita, 1985) was the first to provide a detailed description of the morphological structure of the human vocal folds. Histologically, the human vocal fold has been divided into three distinct layers: epithelium, lamina

Table 3.1. Vocal Fold Lamina Propria Extracellular Matrix Fibrous and Interstitial Proteins Function and Location in the Lamina Propria

ECM Constituent	Function	Localization in Normal Lamina Propria
Collagen	Provides strength to lamina propria (Gray, Titze, Alipour, & Hammond 2000).	Density increases across superficial layer of lamina propria to deep layer of lamina propria (Gray et al., 2000).
Elastin	Provides stretch and recoil of the lamina propria (Gray et al., 2000).	Highest density in middle layer of lamina propria (Gray et al., 2000).
Hyaluronic Acid	Effects tissue viscosity, tissue flow, tissue osmosis, tissue dampening (Laurent, Laurent, & Fraser, 1995). Attracts water.	Found throughout the vocal fold with the highest density in the ILLP (Butler et al., 2001).
Decorin	Promotes lateral association of collagen fibrils to form fibers and fiber bundles in the ECM. Binds to fibronectin (Iozzo, 1997).	Found throughout lamina propria. Highest density is in the superficial layer of the lamina propria (Gray et al., 1999).
Fibronectin	Induces cell migration and ECM synthesis. May be involved in the development of fibrosis (Ehrlich, 2000).	Found throughout the lamina propria, including the BMZ (Gray et al., 1999).
Fibromodulin	Plays role in collagen fibrillogenesis (Ignotz, 1986).	Found in the intermediate and deep layers of the lamina propria (Gray et al., 1999).

propria, and muscle. The more superficial tissue was termed the cover and the deeper tissue named the body. The cover–body theory of phonation (Hirano & Kakita, 1985) suggests that superficial and medial tissues slide and move over the more rigid body tissue. This theory necessitates that histologically the superficial and medial tissues allow freedom of movement whereas the deeper tissues are more tightly bound. This is indeed what occurs ultrastructurally.

Epithelium

The epithelium of the vocal fold (medial edge) is composed of stratified squamous cells. This is adjacent to ciliated pseudostratified epithelium of the posterior glottis, ventricular folds, and trachea and stratified columnar epithelium of the epiglottis. Work by Fisher, Telser, Phillips, and Yeates (Fisher, Telser, Phillips, & Yeates, 2001) has demonstrated the presence of sodium potassium adenosine triphosphatase channels in the vocal fold epithelium. These channels are important for water movement in and out of the vocal fold, providing an intrinsic mechanism for vocal fold hydration. As an additional protective mechanism, a mucociliary blanket, i.e., a layer of mucus, which serves to prevent dehydration of the underlying epidermis, covers the epidermis.

Lamina Propria

The lamina propria has been categorized into three layers based on histological composition. The three middle vocal fold layers are superficial (SLLP), intermediate (ILLP) and deep (DLLP) lamina propria. This is illustrated in Figure 3.1. ECM is the major

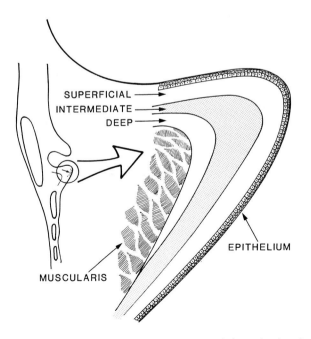

Figure 3.1. A schematic of the five layers of the vocal fold—the epithelium, the three layers of the lamina propria (superficial, intermediate, and deep), and the thyroarytenoid muscle.

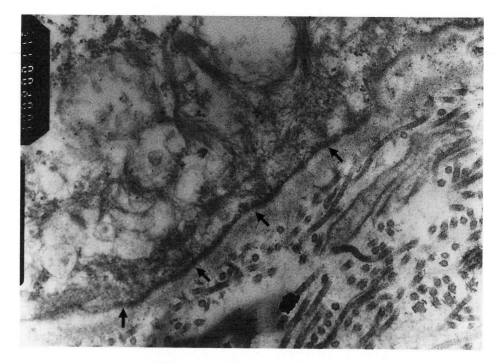

Figure 3.2. A normal vocal fold basement membrane zone (specialized ECM) taken with transmission electron microscopy. The arrows indicate the thickened region separating the superficial lamina propria from the epithelial cells.

constituent of superficial, intermediate, and deep layers of the lamina propria. The innermost vocal fold layer is the thyroarytenoid muscle.

The basement membrane zone (BMZ), a specialized ECM, divides and secures the epithelium to the SLLP. This zone can be broken down into the lamina lucida and the lamina densa. Anchoring filaments (made of collagen type IV and fibronectin) secure the lamina lucida to the lamina densa. Anchoring fibers (collagen VII) loop between the lamina densa and SLLP. Figure 3.2 shows the electron microscopic photograph of the BMZ of normal vocal folds. The number of anchoring fibers in the BMZ appears to vary depending on the location in the vocal fold, with the density appearing greatest in the midmembranous fold area. Gray et al. (Gray, Pignatari, & Harding, 1994) have speculated that these anchor fibers may provide increased structural integrity for this delicate tissue transition and interface, particularly in regions of high shear and stress. Additionally, the population density of anchoring fibers may be genetically determined. Briggaman & Wheeler (Briggaman & Wheeler, 1975) determined that the average person may have between 80 to 120 anchoring fibers per unit area of BMZ (in skin), whereas someone who has the recessive gene that does not create as many anchoring fibers may have only 40 to 60 anchoring fibers per unit area. Persons who are homozygous for the recessive gene will have few or no anchoring fibers. Given Gray et al.'s (Gray et al., 1994) speculation, there may be a specific genetic predisposition for vocal lesions in areas of high shear and stress. This speculation has not been tested.

The SLLP is a pliable, flexible region also known as Reinke's space. Generally, the SLLP is made up of loose fibrous elements, and it is the loose nature of the fibrous elements that gives this layer the ability to move liberally during voicing.

Hammond et al. (Hammond, Zhou, Hammond, Pawlak, & Gray, 1997) found relatively small amounts of mature elastin and collagen (types I, II, and III) and hyaluronic acid (HA) in the SLLP. They report that the elastin in the SLLP is present in nonfibrillar forms—elaunin and oxytalan, which are not verified using the common EVG elastin stain. Decorin, fibronectin, macrophages, and myofibrils were described by Pawlak et al. (Pawlak, Hammond, Hammond, & Gray, 1996) and Catten et al. (Catten, Gray, Hammond, Zhou, & Hammond, 1998), using immunocytochemical techniques, in the SLLP. Macrophages and myofibrils are cells that are present when there is inflammation and cell repair occurring. Their presence suggests constant tissue injury and repair in the SLLP. Interestingly, minimal macrophages and myofibrils are found elsewhere in the LP. Decorin's role in reducing fibrosis and scarring after injury is well documented in the dermal literature (Sayani, Dodd, Nedelec, Shen, Ghahary, Tredget, & Scott, 2000). Its high concentration in the SLLP may be a reason surgical procedures limited to this area rarely involve scar formation. Fibronectin has many roles, including structural, adhesive, and reparative, indicating that it may be necessary for the assembly and maintenance of other proteins and cells of the LP ECM (Hirschi, Gray, & Thibeault, 2002).

The ECM constituents observed in the SLLP differ from those seen in the ILLP and DLLP. Overall, a concomitant increase occurs in the presence of fibrous and interstitial proteins in the ILLP and DLLP. The ILLP and DLLP make up the vocal ligament. The increased presence of fibrous and interstitial proteins in this area of the LP is suggestive of the body's requirements to enhance tissue ligament performance for specific vocal needs. The ILLP is marked with a distinct elevation in the relative amount of elastin (Hirano, 1981) and collagen, and this continues through the DLLP (Hammond, Gray, & Butler, 2000). Fibromodulin and fibronectin are present in both layers. The GAG HA is present at its highest concentration in the ILLP (Gray, Titze, Chan, & Hammond, 1999), particularly in the infrafold area of the ILLP. Speculatively, the presence of HA in the ILLP may provide bulk and thickness to the vocal folds, indirectly affecting vocal fold pliability (Ward, Thibeault, & Gray, 2002). There is a direct relationship between pliability and thickness in vocal fold vibration (Yumoto, Katata, & Kurokawa, 1993).

A schematic representation of the major ECM constituents is presented in Figure 3.3.

Age and Gender Differences in the Lamina Propria

Little has been published assessing age and gender differences in the ECM constituents of the LP. In newborns, the entire LP is uniform in structure, resembling the SLLP (Hirano, 1981). Fibroblast density is highest in newborns, with a decrease as one ages (Hirano, 1981).

Gender-related differences and age differences have been reported for collagen (Hammond et al., 2000). Infants have significantly less collagen than adults, and males have greater amounts of collagen than females. The difference in the amount of collagen across the layers of the LP was minimal across ages and gender, with more collagen present in the DLLP.

No gender differences have been reported for elastin, but there are age-related differences. Sato and Hirano (Sato & Hirano, 1997) and Hirano, Kurita, and Sakaguchi (Hirano, Kurita, & Sakaguchi, 1989) found less elastin with age, whereas Hammond et al. (Hammond, Gray, Butler, Zhou, & Hammond, 1998) found increases in elastin

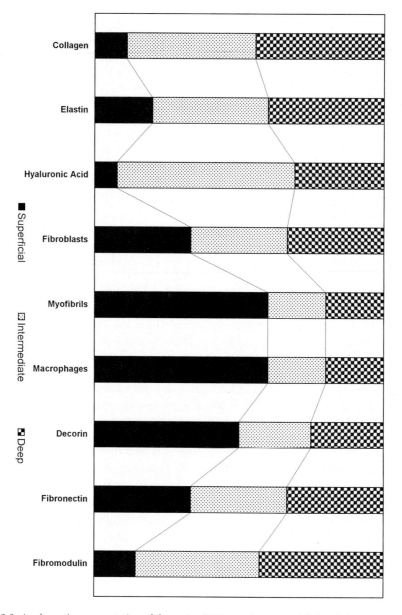

Figure 3.3. A schematic representation of the major ECM constituents and their relative proportion distribution across the three layers of the lamina propria. Relative amounts should not be compared across constituents, only across layers for each individual constituent.

with age, with a subsequent thinning of the SLLP secondary to infiltration from the middle layer protein or atrophy. The disparate findings between these two research groups may be explained by the methodology used. Hammond et al. (1998) used a quantitative image analysis system and fewer samples. Sato and Hirano (1997) and Hirano, Kurita, and Sakaguchi (1989) used a qualitative visual assessment on more vocal fold specimens. Gray et al. (2000) suggest that the dissimilar elastin findings may be explained by possible racial variations in the specimens.

Gender differences have been found in regard to HA (Butler, Hammond, & Gray, 2001). Males have significantly more HA than women (3:1 male:female). When controlling for age, a sex difference was found in the concentration of HA across the depth of the LP. Females have less HA in the SLLP and more HA in the DLLP than males. Because HA is known to influence the biomechanics of voice production and voice quality by affecting tissue viscosity, thickness, and hydration, less HA in the SLLP may imply less protection from vibratory trauma and overuse. This may explain in part why more females than males suffer from phonotrauma (Butler et al., 2001).

BIOLOGY OF BENIGN VOCAL FOLD LESIONS

The increasing density of the layers of the vocal fold dissects it into two functional biomechanical layers—the body and the cover. The body is composed primarily of muscle, whereas the cover is the LP. The shape (determined by the ECM) and tension of the cover determine the vibratory characteristics of the folds and subsequent vocal quality. The shape and tension may be modified by benign lesions, which arise from the cover and change the biomechanics and thus the voice source. The composition of the ECM of the LP is altered in benign lesions. This change in ECM composition directly influences tissue viscosity, which can lead to higher phonation threshold pressure necessary for voice production (Titze, 1992). As technology progresses, more details regarding the genetic and molecular cellular activity responsible for causing these changes is revealed. As the molecular ultrastructure is defined for pathological states, a better understanding of how these alterations subsequently affect the vibratory characteristics of the vocal folds can be determined. Table 3.2 summarizes the molecular ultrastructure of common benign laryngeal lesions.

Vocal Fold Nodules

Vocal nodules are regarded as a result of vocal fold abuse, and changes in the BMZ have been demonstrated. Thickening of the BMZ (Gray et al., 1994) and increased fibronectin (Courey, Shohet, Scott, & Ossoff, 1996), which may represent tearing forces and subsequent wound repair in the subepithelium, have been reported. Figure 3.4 compares a normal vocal fold BMZ with the BMZ of a vocal fold with nodules. It is easy to see the increased thickening of the BMZ in the presence of vocal fold nodules. Kotby et al. (Kotby, Nassar, Seif, Helal, & Saleh, 1988) further report nodular lesions with gaps at the intercellular junctions, disruption and duplication of the BMZ, and collagen fiber dispositions. Gray et al. (Gray, Hammond, & Hanson, 1995) have proposed that the disorganized BMZ (particularly injury to the anchoring fibers) may leave the vocal fold in a predisposed state for repetitious injury, and the fibronectin deposition may lead to increased stiffening of that part of the membranous fold.

Vocal Fold Polyps

Histological analyses of vocal fold polyps and comparison with normal vocal fold LP structure have found less fibronectin deposition, more vascular injury (thrombosis), fibrin and iron deposition (Courey et al., 1996; Dikkers & Nikkels, 1995) in the presence of vocal fold polyps. Analysis of protein levels with Western blot showed decreased collagen levels and increased fibronectin levels in five polyps (Thibeault, Gray, Li, Ford, Smith, & Davis, 2002). Increased fibronectin may be responsible for the

Table 3.2. Extracellular Matrix Characterizations of Benign Vocal Fold Lesions

Vocal Fold Lesion	Histopathology	Genomic Pathology
Nodules	Abnormal BMZ with altered anchoring fibers Increased fibronectin Increased collagen	Not reported to date
Polyps	Fibrin Iron deposition Decreased fibronectin Thin BMZ	Altered gene levels for epithelial genes involved in BMZ organization Increased fibronectin protein Decreased collagen protein
Cysts	Lined with columnar or squamous epithelium Thickened BMZ	Not reported to date
Reinke's Edema	Hemorrhage Fibrin Edematous lakes Thickened BMZ	Decreased messenger RNA levels for fibronectin Increased messenger RNA levels for decorin
Granuloma	Focal ulceration Desquamating epithelium Edematous lamina propria Inflammatory cells Neutrophils	Altered gene levels for genes involved in wound healing and inflammation
Scar	Conflicting reports of collagen levels depending on age of scar Conflicting reports of procollagen levels depending on age of scar Increased fibronectin Decreased elastin Decreased HA Decreased decorin Decreased fibromodulin	Not reported to date
Sulcus Vocalis	Epithelial thinning Loss of layered lamina propria, Inflammation	Not reported to date

decreased mucosal wave observed with videostroboscopy preoperatively in these five patients.

The state of the BMZ in vocal fold polyps is unknown. Thibeault et al. (Thibeault, Hirschi, & Gray, 2002), using microarray genetic analysis to measure gene expression levels in one vocal fold polyp, report abnormal levels for genes that are involved in epithelial differentiation and BMZ formation. Loire et al. (Loire, Bouchayer, Cornut, & Bastian, 1988), Kotby, Nassar, Seif, Helal, and Saleh (1988), and Courey, Shohet, Scott, and Ossoff (1996) report atrophy of the epithelium of VP with a thin BMZ and an intact BMZ, respectively, in their histological samples.

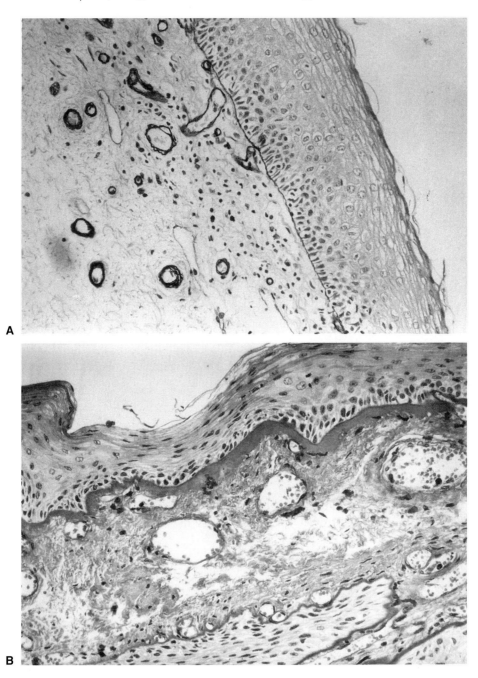

A

B

Figure 3.4. **A.** A light microscope image of a normal vocal fold with a normal basement membrane zone. **B.** A light microscope image of a vocal fold polyp with thickened basement membrane zone.

Vocal Fold Cysts

Vocal fold cysts can be lined with columnar or squamous epithelium (Shvero, Koren, Hadar, Yaniv, Sandbank, & Feinmesser, 2000), with a BMZ thickness that is between that of polyps and nodules indicating some degree of BMZ injury (Courey et al., 1996).

Reinke's Edema

Reinke's edema is manifested by edema of the SLLP, and Dikker and Nikkels (1995) have described hemorrhage, fibrin, edematous lakes, and thickening of the BMZ. Genomic messenger RNA levels were measured in four Reinke's edema samples—decreased gene expression levels for fibronectin and increased decorin levels were reported (Thibeault et al., 2002). Increased decorin levels in the SLLP may be present as an active reparative process.

Vocal Fold Granuloma

Histological structural analysis of granulomas show defined ulceration, with desquamating epithelium and lamina propria that is swollen and marked with infiltration by chronic inflammatory cells and neutrophils (Shin, Watanabe, Oda, Umezaki, & Nahm, 1994). Genomic microarray analysis for messenger RNA levels (Thibeault et al., 2002) report altered gene levels for inflammatory and wound healing genes. This indicates that granulomas are an injury. This would be consistent with the literature that suggests that granulomas are a result of vocal abuse or gastroesophageal reflux. Both cause injury to the larynx.

Vocal Fold Scarring

Vocal fold scarring causes significant changes in the physical properties of vocal fold tissue, altering the body–cover relationship and inhibiting propagation of normal mucosal wave. Histological characterization of fibrous and interstitial proteins of the LP in vocal fold scarring has been used in animal models. Differing results have been reported depending on animal model and healing time. Young scar tissue (2 months) (Rousseau, Hirano, Welham, Thibeault, Bless, & Ford, 2002; Thibeault, Gray, Bless, Chan, & Ford, 2002), ultrastructurally, has been defined by no change or a decrease in collagen levels, with markedly increased procollagen levels (precursor to collagen) and fibronectin with decreased HA, elastin levels, decorin, and fibromodulin (Thibeault, Bless, & Gray, 2002). More chronic scar formation (6 months) is characterized by increased collagen, decreased procollagen, and decreased elastin (Rousseau et al., 2002). The relationship between the tissue stiffness observed in vocal fold scar and fibrous and interstitial proteins does not seem to be straightforward and requires further investigation.

Sulcus Vocalis

Sulcus vocalis has been described as an indentation, groove, or furrow along the medial edge of the vocal fold, with varying thickness, involving differing layers of the LP, depending on the severity of the sulcus. The lesion may only involve the epithelium or it may involve several or all of the layers of the LP up to and including the thyroarytenoid muscle. Histopathological findings include epithelial thinning and loss of the

LP cellular layered structure with minimal inflammatory response (Ford, Inagi, Khidr, Bless, & Gilchrist, 1996).

SUMMARY

Vocal fold biology is intricate. Normal vibratory function is dependent on the complex interactions within the ECM. An understanding of the normal layered structure of the vocal folds is necessary for all clinicians. Knowledge of the pathological changes that occur with the presence of a vocal fold lesion provides a better understanding of changes that are seen concomitantly in vocal fold vibratory patterns and perceived in voice quality. We have a basic understanding of the vocal fold structure. This is an exciting and rich area for research. With the use of more advanced molecular and genetic techniques, our knowledge of vocal fold biology and genetic implications for voice disorders is expected to expand rapidly over the next decade.

Chapter 4

Phonotrauma: Its Effects on Phonatory Physiology

The term *phonotrauma* was proposed by Verdolini (1999) as a more appropriate and less punitive term than the traditionally used "vocal abuse" terminology. Although we agree with Verdolini's arguments in this matter, and accept the use of the term *phonotrauma* as an umbrella term, there are still times, it seems to us, when the nature of phonatory behavior is best described by the word *abusive*, that is, the behavior abuses (or traumatizes, if you prefer) the tissues of the vocal folds sufficiently to cause a change in the voice. We caution voice clinicians, however, to explain their use of terminology to patients in ways that do not "blame the victim." Another term that we find useful is "misuse of the voice," which is described later in this chapter.

Phonotrauma refers to vocal behaviors that are thought to contribute to the development of voice problems. Some of these behaviors are considered sufficiently damaging and abusive of the vocal fold tissues to affect the voice, whereas others simply represent the misuse of the voice. The behaviors are thought to contribute to the laryngeal tissue changes that result in the formation of benign lesions such as nodules, polyps, and cysts or contact ulcers. Other behaviors, or the extent to which they are present, may be thought of as mechanisms of misuse. Such behaviors may or may not result in laryngeal tissue changes. What vocal behaviors produce trauma to the voice? How much trauma can laryngeal tissues tolerate? How do patterns of phonotrauma evolve, and what maintains them? How does phonotrauma create voice problems? These questions must be asked, and surprisingly few answers are available. In this chapter, we discuss the current state of knowledge about phonotrauma, including both abuse and misuse categories.

MISUSE

Misuse suggests voice production behaviors that distort the normal propensity of the phonatory mechanism to work effectively and efficiently. An efficient system produces its best results with a minimum of effort. A car engine whose various components are in top working condition so that its operation is smooth and uses the least energy to perform its work is said to be operating efficiently. Similarly, a phonatory system in which the individual components are healthy and the coordination and interaction with all of its supporting parts and systems is in tune produces voice in an efficient manner.

Table 4.1. Characteristics of Vocal Behaviors Categorized as Misuse

A. *Increased Tension or Strain*
   1. Hard glottal attack
   2. High laryngeal position
   3. Anteroposterior laryngeal squeezing

B. *Inappropriate Pitch Level*
   1. Puberphonia
   2. Persistent glottal fry
   3. Lack of pitch variability

C. *Excessive Talking*

D. *Ventricular Phonation*

E. *Aphonia and Dysphonia of Psychological Origin*

Smooth operation of the voice may be altered in a number of ways. Each of us can voluntarily produce voice in a variety of manners, some of them efficient, some inefficient. Those who work with disordered voices should be able to produce inefficient as well as efficient voice to better understand how various changes in voice production can be made. For example, take a breath, and as you begin to speak tighten your chest to the point of almost holding your breath. Without taking another breath, try to count to 10. How does it feel to talk like that? Where do you feel the tensions? How did it change the sound of your voice? As another example, try to squeeze your larynx tightly and speak in a hoarse voice. Think about how that feels and what you have done to change the sound of your voice. As a final experiment, pick a pitch about two tones above your present pitch level and try to converse, and then do this at a pitch about two tones lower than your comfort level. Has your larynx height changed? What does it feel like to try to do this? What does it do to your breathing, your degree of tension, your inflection patterns?

All of these activities could be categorized as vocal misuse, yet all are within the ability of each of us to produce. In Table 4.1, we have identified some of the behaviors that, when used habitually, constitute misuse. Each of these is discussed in the following sections.

Increased Tension or Strain

Descriptions of what is meant by increased vocal tension abound but frequently lack specificity. The judgment of vocal tension is most frequently made on a subjective basis. The subjectivity may be the reporting by the patient of the sensation of tension, or sometimes even pain, accompanying speaking, or it may be the judgment of the voice clinician based on auditory or visual observations. There are few objective methods of documenting tension, and there are none that can be put to routine clinical use to provide measurement of specific muscle tensions. Biofeedback using externally placed electrodes has been attempted, but it is not at all clear what specific muscles are being tapped, nor is there sufficient information available to identify which muscles are the most significant in assessment of vocal tension.

In cases of vocal misuse, the laryngological examination may be negative for the presence of lesions but with perhaps a suggestion of increased redness or slight swelling of the vocal folds. In some cases, it is noted that a strand of mucus forms and reforms between the vocal folds at the nodal point, a sign thought by some to be an early indication of, or tendency toward, nodule formation. We have found flexible fiberoptic examinations to be of significant help in identifying patterns of excessive laryngeal tension in some patients. The specific, observable signs of that tension are hard glottal attack, high laryngeal position, and excessive medial compression.

In any discussion of behaviors thought to constitute vocal or laryngal "misuse," it is important to note that the normal larynx is capable of a wide range of behaviors. For example, when the larynx is protecting vocal folds, it is usual to see ventricular folds; approximation of the arytenoid cartilages with the epiglottis by the arytenoids, or medial compression; squeezing of the false supraglottal structures so as to obscure visualization of the laryngeal inlet and true vocal folds. In fact, these gestures are necessary and critical to safe swallowing. Similarly, such behaviors may sometimes reflect a strategy for achieving a certain vocal output, for example, anteroposterior approximation of the arytenoids and epiglottis during loud voice production. Our understanding of normal laryngeal behavior is in fact not complete, and we need to be careful in characterizing any isolated behavior as hyperfunctional or abusive. However, when we observe behaviors that appear to require excessive effort or more work to produce voice, and when these behaviors appear to contribute to our perception of the speaker's voice as dysphonic, then it is reasonable to think of them as constituting "misuse"—anteroposterior laryngeal squeezing and excessive medial compression, for example.

A number of authors have discussed behaviors that may fall into this category (Koufman & Blalock, 1991; Morrison & Rammage, 1993; Rosen & Murry, 2000).

HARD GLOTTAL ATTACK

The hard glottal attack or glottal coup is a term that describes a manner of initiating vowels, usually characterized by rapid and complete adduction of the vocal folds before the initiation of phonation. This adducted state, which may be accompanied by considerable muscle tension, requires that subglottal pressure be increased to overcome vocal fold resistance and initiate phonation. The characteristic sound of a hard glottal attack is an abrupt, explosive, and hard-edged onset of phonation. This form of voice initiation is often visible fiberoptically, especially when subjects are asked to produce isolated vowel sounds (Casper, Colton, Brewer, & Woo, 1989). It appears to be produced in at least two ways. In one method, medial compression of the vocal folds is observed almost simultaneously with the onset of phonation. The second variation is characterized by prephonatory laryngeal constriction in which the ventricular folds approach each other, as do the arytenoids and the epiglottis, obscuring visualization of the true vocal folds. As phonation is initiated, there is a reduction in the forced adduction and a sudden springing open of the larynx as the true vocal folds become visible. Again, it is important to interpret such behaviors with caution. We have observed occasional evidence of this hard glottal attack in speakers who were judged to have normal voices and who were not experiencing any voice problems. It is a behavior that may occur on occasion in most speakers. In some instances, the behavior may be a reaction to the examination procedure and the tensions associated with it. Whether this particular behavior is identified as evidence of misuse must depend in part on the degree of its presence and the circumstances under which it is observed. In general, when the hard glottal attack is present to a significant degree, it is but one of several behaviors that give evidence of increased tension and strain.

HIGH LARYNGEAL POSITION

Vertical laryngeal height has been the subject of some study and controversy. It has been reported that untrained singers show greater laryngeal elevation with increased pitch level than do trained singers (Shipp, 1987; Shipp & Izdebski, 1975). There are different schools of thought among singers, singing coaches, and voice scientists relative to the benefits of maintaining a low laryngeal position. Many believe that raising laryngeal height with elevation of pitch is improper singing technique and detrimental to the voice (Sundberg & Askenfelt, 1983). However, more recently, Sundberg reported that an X-ray study of two well-trained female singers showed an increase in vertical laryngeal height with an increase in pitch, in what he described as a "very elegant" and "well-trained" behavior (Shipp, Guinn, Sundberg, & Titze, 1987). Varying laryngeal position may be useful and raising the larynx during singing may not be misuse. Many differences between singing and speaking make suggesting that a particular behavior in one activity is the same or has the same effect in the other activity difficult. Raising the larynx results in (a) a shortening of the vocal tract, with a subsequent raising of all formant frequencies; (b) a stiffening of vocal fold tissues that alters the vibratory pattern and increases fundamental frequency; and (c) an increased tendency for tight vocal fold closure. This tight adduction is a desirable and essential part of the swallowing process wherein the larynx elevates and a tight valving maneuver ensues, thereby protecting the lower airway. In speaking, it is not variability of laryngeal height that is suggestive of excessive tension but rather a speaker's tendency to consistently speak with the larynx in an elevated position. Shipp et al. (Shipp, Guinn, Sundberg, & Titze, 1987) believe that the human body seems naturally to do that which is easiest to do, and it seems to optimize itself for a given task. Furthermore, they suggest that the speaker who constantly maintains a low laryngeal posture may be using more energy in doing so than the speaker who allows the mechanism to move freely.

Vocal tension is characterized by increased tension in both the intrinsic and extrinsic laryngeal muscles. However, we are not yet able to isolate the contributions of each muscle group to voice problems associated with misuse. Indeed, the system as a whole is so interactive that when excessive tensions exist in one muscle, they will probably occur also in some other muscles. Thus, although laryngeal height is primarily controlled by extrinsic laryngeal muscle activity, we cannot attribute a voice disorder to that condition alone and must recognize the total physiological disturbance. A high laryngeal position may be related to excessive tension in both extrinsic and intrinsic muscle groups. Sundberg and Askenfelt (1983) stated that "the muscles used for raising the larynx also may affect the way in which the vocal folds vibrate" (p. 307), which underscores the relationship between larynx height and the voice source. Shipp (1987) also addressed this relationship and reported that increased stiffening of the vocal fold margin results from the upward stretch of tissues created by laryngeal height elevation.

It is not unusual for patients with this particular pattern of hyperfunction to report sensations of pain or soreness in the neck lateral to the larynx, sometimes radiating upward or downward. These patients also report that their voices tend to become worse with increased use and that by the end of the workday they feel it takes too much effort to talk.

ANTEROPOSTERIOR LARYNGEAL SQUEEZING

In the endoscopic laryngeal examination of voice-disordered patients, we have often observed (usually in the absence of observable pathological conditions) a "squeezing" of the larynx in which the epiglottis and the arytenoids approach each other during phonation. A similar but not identical movement is typical in the production of the low back vowels (e.g., /ah/), when the tongue position dictates a posterior movement of the epiglottis. That movement is a natural one in which none of the "squeezing" elements is present. During production of the vowels /ee/ and /oo/, the epiglottis is normally expected to be pulled somewhat anteriorly and superiorly, making the vocal folds fully visible. This does not occur in patients with this "squeezed" larynx. These patients, even in the production of the /ee/ and /oo/ vowels, as well as other stimulus materials heavily loaded with these vowels, demonstrate anteroposterior "squeezing" behavior to the extent that visualization of the true vocal folds along their full length is often obscured. Another vocal maneuver that is normally expected to "open" the larynx when it is being viewed endoscopically is pitch elevation. However, persons who tend to habitually use very tight laryngeal posture with anteroposterior shortening maintain that closed posture even as they raise pitch. In fact, they often encounter difficulty in raising pitch and may exhibit a reduced phonational range. We believe that this vocal behavior is an indication of disturbed phonatory physiology, probably caused by excess strain and tension.

Inappropriate Pitch Level

A common concept in the voice literature is that of optimum pitch. Clinicians are instructed that the use of a too high or too low habitual pitch level is a frequent cause of voice disorders. Much therapy time is spent in identifying what is purported to be an individual's optimum pitch, and therapy is then directed toward teaching the patient to use that pitch. We have difficulty with this approach for a number of reasons.

If the fundamental frequency of a person's voice is altered by a pathological condition, for example, it seems to us that attempts to "measure" an optimum pitch are immediately flawed. The most common methodology espoused for obtaining the so-called optimum pitch is described by Fairbanks (1960) and involves obtaining a measure of phonational range. Recall, however, that phonational range is often reduced in the presence of certain laryngeal pathological conditions and voice disorders. Despite the apparently widespread use of the concept of optimum pitch, no data demonstrate or document its validity or its therapeutic efficacy. (See Chapter 10 for further discussion of this topic.) The physiological approach to voice disorders, based on an understanding of vocal fold physiology and acoustics, suggests that a disturbance of physiology caused by mass lesions, manner of use, or abnormal motor control will result in acoustic changes. Thus, an inappropriate pitch level, if indeed it is present, may well be a sign of a problem rather than the cause of the problem. Attention needs to be paid to the underlying cause of the problem, and when the physiology is normalized or improved, then the pitch level of the voice will also improve or normalize. Indeed, it is quite possible for a person to speak at a totally appropriate pitch level and yet do so in an abusive way.

Judgments of the pitch of a voice can be made subjectively, but those perceptions should always be checked against objective measurement of fundamental frequency. Perception of pitch levels can be quite erroneous, especially in the presence of hoarseness or excess noise energy in the voice. Objective measurement of fundamental frequency rather than casual judgments of pitch may be made easily by using methods described in Chapter 8 and should always be done before any judgments about the acceptability of this parameter are considered. However, in a very rough voice, even measurements of fundamental frequency should be suspect because of the difficulty in obtaining reliable and accurate estimates of the period of vibration.

Inappropriate pitch is typically the hallmark of puberphonia, persistent glottal fry, and lack of pitch variability. Recognize, however, that inappropriate pitch may be only one sign of an underlying problem.

PUBERPHONIA

This category is referred to in the literature by a number of names: adolescent falsetto, pubescent falsetto, incomplete mutation, and mutational falsetto, to name a few. We have chosen to use the term *puberphonia* (not as the most desirable, but as the least objectionable) because it suggests the developmental stage at which this problem is encountered (puberty) and tells us that it involves the voice (phone). Rather than add yet another term, we prefer to describe the nature of the problem.

Puberphonia refers most simply to the persistence of a high-pitched voice beyond the age at which voice change is expected to have occurred. This is primarily a male problem. Although some women continue to have very high-pitched and childlike voices into their adult years, there is little stigma attached to this situation, for two reasons: First, the lowering of the fundamental frequency in women (3–4 semitones) as a result of laryngeal growth is not as marked as for men (one octave); second, women are expected to have higher-pitched voices. Thus, the presence of a high-pitched voice in a woman is not always perceived to be as unusual or inappropriate as in a man. That is not to deny, however, that a childlike voice can be inappropriate, can jeopardize a woman's employment status, and can negatively affect how she is perceived.

In cases of puberphonia, it is important that a determination be made first as to whether an organic abnormality is present. The adequacy of laryngeal growth must be assessed, and potential endocrinological problems must be ruled out. The laryngeal examination and the history may provide sufficient information regarding these concerns. The vocal symptoms include not only the inappropriately high-pitched voice but also often hoarseness and some degree of breathiness. The voice tends to sound unstable and uncertain, and the patient's reporting often confirms that perception: "It sounds funny, and I never know what it is going to sound like" is a commonly heard self-description of the voice problem. Pitch breaks also may be heard. Although the onset of the problem is, by definition, during the adolescent growth spurt and the emergence of secondary sex characteristics, it may persist for a considerable length of time before any treatment is sought.

Psychosocial factors, such as difficulty with male identification or with the acceptance of emerging adulthood, have been frequently cited as the primary causative factors. Our experience, however, suggests that, if present, these factors are not overwhelming in their expression. It seems quite logical to us that a certain percentage of young boys may have fairly traumatic voice change experiences not only in the psychological sense but also in the physical sense.

Pitch breaks may be frequent and extreme, and the lack of control over the voice may be pronounced. Feelings of embarrassment result and are aggravated by a lack of understanding of what is happening. An understandable reaction to such feelings might be an attempt to hold on to the voice that is known (the child voice) and to attain control of what otherwise seems to be an uncontrollable behavior. In many cases, when asked if they have another voice, young men with this problem will answer in the affirmative. In some, we have observed a profound sense of relief when this admission has been made and reassurance has been provided about the normalcy of the "hidden" voice. Indeed, for many, little additional treatment has been necessary beyond providing a period of practice in using the new voice, coupled with encouragement and guidance. In others, the process of "releasing" the adult voice (see Chapter 10) is usually very effective in producing a more typical adult voice within a short period. We are not aware, through either personal experience or perusal of the literature, of post-therapy failures wherein there is a regression to the high-pitched voice. We also have not been impressed that the young men who have presented with this problem in our clinic have had difficulty with male identification. Indeed, we would not describe the sound of their voices as ever having been effeminate. The characteristics of an effeminate voice comprise speech mannerisms and suprasegmental differences that go well beyond just the presence of a higher than expected pitch level. We believe that the theory of the domineering mother figure and the weak father figure as the primary underlying cause for the maintenance of the inappropriately high pitch level has not been validated, and we do not believe it to be true.

We have recently become aware of several cases of "falsetto-like" voice in the female. These voices exhibit instability similar to that described for the puberphonic male with frequent pitch breaks and elevated fundamental frequency. The underlying cause and the pathophysiology in these cases has not been well explored, but they appear to differ from other psychogenically based voice problems in that the voice has not undergone a recent change. It has been consistently present for many years, with no recall of it ever having sounded different. In the cases we have encountered, eliciting and establishing a more appropriate pitch level and vocal stability has been accomplished fairly readily through voice therapy.

PERSISTENT GLOTTAL FRY

Glottal fry, vocal fry, or pulse register is described as one of the three normal voice registers, the other two being loft (falsetto) and modal. These registers are characterized by a change in the mechanical mode of vibration (Fairbanks, 1960), and there is usually some overlap in the frequency of phonation between adjacent registers. Daniloff, Shuckers, and Feth (1980) state that the physiologically complex larynx "can vibrate in three (or more) relatively different ways, giving rise to airflow modulation that yields acoustically and perceptually distinct vocal quality" (p. 209). Glottal fry is the register lowest in fundamental frequency and the least flexible. The vocal folds are noted to close quickly, and the closed phase of the vibratory cycle is very long relative to the length of the entire period (Hollien, Moore, Wendahl, & Michel, 1966). Moore and von Leden (1958) described the occasional occurrence of two open phases during one vibratory cycle. Zemlin (1988) reported that the closed phase occupies approximately 90% of the cycle. In describing the characteristics of glottal fry as seen in high-speed motion pictures, he observed tightly approximated vocal folds whose free edges, however, appeared flaccid. Zemlin further noted that air seemed to "bubble up" between the folds near the junction of the anterior two thirds of the glottis. Glottal fry is produced with much lower airflows than the other registers (Murry, 1971), and air is released in irregularly timed bursts. Pulsated voice, according to Perkins (1983), allows the production of only very low fundamental frequencies, with a decay of energy in every glottal cycle. Glottal fry has a very characteristic sound, which has been described variously as similar to the popping of corn, the imitated sound of a motor boat engine, or a creaky voice. The vibratory pattern is so slow that individual vibrations of the vocal folds are heard. The amplitude of vocal fry sound is very low.

Although glottal fry is a normal mode of vibration, its consistent and habitual use is atypical and may be considered misuse of the voice. It is difficult to produce glottal fry with adequate volume for many speaking situations. A person using this mode of phonation will show increased tension when attempting to increase vocal loudness. The lack of flexibility of pulse register makes it difficult to achieve variation of fundamental frequency and results in monotonic voice. Complaint of a sense of vocal fatigue and a constant awareness of vibration even below the larynx are typically heard from speakers who habitually use glottal fry.

LACK OF PITCH VARIABILITY

Some individuals speak in a monotone, with barely perceptible variations in fundamental frequency, as corroborated by acoustic analysis. A monotonic voice may be a sign of neurological dysfunction affecting the ability to control pitch, a reflection of psychological depression, or it may be a habitual pattern that is a sign of misuse. We have been impressed with the presence of this problem in untrained speakers who lecture or frequently address large groups. They do not know how to modulate their pitch level for maximum communication effectiveness. In this type of pattern, the phonatory mechanism establishes a "set" that rarely varies. This set includes a certain configuration of the vocal folds, with the adductory and contact forces occurring with the same strength and in the same area over and over again. This behavior fails to take advantage of the flexibility of the phonatory mechanism and tends to become fatiguing. It is not unusual to find that persons with this pattern allow their voices to drift into vocal fry at the end of utterances. The delivery usually is perceived as lacking in energy, vitality, and interest.

Excessive Talking

Each larynx has a physiological limit that varies not only from person to person but also intraindividually, as influenced by numerous factors. A healthy, well-rested, well-nourished, emotionally stable individual may encounter no vocal difficulties despite heavy voice use demands. However, should that same person be physically exhausted, eating poorly, and perhaps taking some medication, the same amount of demand on the larynx, or even less, may result in phonatory problems. Factors of individual selectivity are involved in determining the physical tolerance limits of body structures and systems. Therefore, it is not possible to predict whether excessive talking per se will result in a problem or, if a problem does result, how severe the impairment will be.

Excessive talking may result in vocal fatigue. The voice quality may be reported to become slightly rough or hoarse, the voice may sound weak, and the person may report that talking requires effort. Frequently, those who have such complaints in the presence of a chronic pattern of excessive voice use report that a night's rest or a weekend with fewer vocal demands may temporarily restore the voice to normal but that the symptoms recur with the next period of excessive voice use. Patterns of misuse do not always occur as single, isolated behaviors. The excessive talker may also engage in other patterns of vocal misuse or abuse. Thus, a distinction should be made between amount of talking and manner of talking (i.e., is it just a lot of talking or is it a lot of talking in an excessively loud or tense voice?).

Ventricular Phonation

The diagnosis of ventricular phonation is usually made when laryngological examination shows greater than expected movement of the ventricular folds toward the midline. Visualization of the true vocal folds is often largely obscured by the compression of the ventricular folds, particularly in indirect mirror examination. Use of the flexible fiberoptic laryngoscope often permits visualization of some part of the true vocal folds or of their adductory and abductory movements. Stroboscopic examination can document whether actual ventricular fold vibration is present.

Ventricular fold phonation has been described as being low in pitch, very hoarse in quality, rattling, rumbling, cracking, reduced in intensity, and diplophonic (Aronson, 1990; Case, 1984). However, acoustic data to support these perceptual descriptors are not available. The pathophysiology of ventricular phonation is not well understood (see Chapter 10 for further discussion). We have observed it as a manifestation of a psychogenic dysphonia (Brewer & McCall, 1974), as a compensatory behavior in the absence of adequate vocal fold movement (Woo, Casper, Brewer, & Colton, 1995), as one component in a pattern of hyperfunction, and as an unexplained phenomenon. Other studies have reported use of the false folds related to a variety of conditions affecting the true vocal folds (Von Doersten et al., 1992) Furthermore, in a study of normal nonsymptomatic speakers, Casper, Brewer, and Colton (1987a) observed much variability in the degree of medial movement of the ventricular folds accompanying adduction of the true vocal folds.

Therapeutically, we have found ventricular phonation to be reversible when its cause is psychological or when it is a manifestation of hyperfunction. Its use as compensatory behavior may well be very functional, allowing the individual to produce the best voice of which he is capable. In such instances, it is an appropriate behavior requiring neither change nor elimination unless improved function of the vocal folds can be restored. When the cause is unclear, or when it is a true compensatory behavior, we have found this increased ventricular fold activity to be very resistant to change through behavioral therapy.

When excess medial compression of the ventricular folds is present in the absence of laryngeal pathological conditions, and when a voice problem seemingly related to this ventricular fold activity is present, ventricular phonation may be considered vocal misuse.

Aphonia and Dysphonia of Psychological Origin

No single way exists to characterize the patterns of misuse of the phonatory mechanism exhibited by persons whose voice problems are psychogenically based. In our experience, we have encountered a wide diversity of patterns, including (a) total aphonia in which even the voiceless consonants were inaudible and the vocal folds were maintained in an abducted posture; (b) dysphonia in which the laryngeal mechanism was held in a tension equal to that of very forceful effort closure, with episodic bursts of explosive vocalization alternating with extreme hoarseness; (c) dysphonia in which the ventricular folds appeared to adduct; and (d) dysphonia so variable that it encompassed normal voicing, aphonia, hoarseness, and very strained phonation, all within two or three sentences. In all of these instances, when the physiology was normalized, so too was the voice. Therapeutic approaches to achieve normalization are discussed in Chapter 10.

DIFFERENTIATING MISUSE FROM PHONOTRAUMA

Before discussing phonotrauma, it is appropriate to return to some of the questions posed in the first paragraph of this chapter. We have thus far discussed the vocal behaviors that we believe constitute misuse. However, the line between misuse and trauma is very thin, and perhaps rather than there being a division between the two, the behaviors might be thought of as existing along a continuum. Bear in mind, however, that a continuum is only a scale. It is usually thought to represent lesser or greater degrees of a behavior (in this case), but it does not necessarily imply progression of a behavior or disorder along the continuum. Thus, a pattern of misuse such as puberphonia can remain misuse and may not necessarily develop into a problem of greater severity. We are unable to predict whether or when misuse may become abuse and lead to tissue change. It is logical to assume that excessive talking, for example, might at some point result in actual tissue changes. Indeed, many patients with lesions such as nodules or polyps admit to being incessant talkers. However, we all know nonstop talkers who never develop a voice problem. Certainly there are individual selectivity factors operating about which we know little.

How patterns of misuse evolve is often difficult to determine or track down. One of the most frequently asked questions we have encountered clinically, and often a difficult one to answer, is the patient's incredulous wonderment about how it is possible, after several decades of presumably talking correctly, to no longer be doing so. We have no prospective information about this and therefore can only theorize retrospectively, using the information provided by patient recall. There are inherent dangers in doing this because most people are usually unaware of their speaking patterns until they encounter difficulty. To speak, to produce voice, is so innately human that very little conscious effort or thought is involved. Furthermore, memory is often flawed. The tendency to date the onset of a problem to a coincident event or one closely related in time is sometimes very useful, but it also may be totally misleading.

The most common antecedents to vocal misuse that seem to have validity include periods of increased personal tension or of greater than usual demands on the voice. A change in employment that requires new demands, including greater vocal demands, is one such example. Patients frequently report an episode of what they describe as laryngitis as the precipitating event. This laryngitis is reported to have been but one symptom of a more extensive upper respiratory infection, or it may have been an isolated symptom. Whereas other symptoms resolve, the altered voice persists. Some patients recall periods of voice difficulty in the past that they ascribed to laryngitis and that had always resolved spontaneously within a short time. On occasion they may report that these episodes had become increasingly frequent and that each one had taken longer to resolve. Because producing voice is such a "natural" phenomenon, and because sensory feedback from the larynx is so limited, it is possible to change phonatory behavior with little awareness of having done so. In the presence of laryngitis, whether caused by infection or by vocal fold edema resulting from misuse, adjustments in phonatory behavior need to be made to produce any voice. It is conceivable that these changes may go unrecognized and persist after the precipitating condition has resolved or may

Table 4.2. Abusive Behaviors

A. Excessive, prolonged loudness
B. Strained and excessive use during period of swelling, inflammation, or other tissue changes
C. Excessive coughing and throat clearing
D. The screamer and noise maker
E. Sports and exercise enthusiast
   1. Observer
   2. Participant

contribute to maintaining the condition. One other factor that is often neglected must be considered. That is, we are not the same person from moment to moment or day to day. Our bodies are constantly changing and reacting to nutritional status, to drug intake, to effects of age, to environmental factors, to emotional state. A behavior that may have been present for many years and tolerated by the body may, because of some of these factors, become intolerable and create what appears to be a sudden change in body function. It is also possible that the body reaches a threshold of tolerance for a certain behavior, the effects of which may have been minimal but cumulative. The changes may have been so gradual as to have gone unnoticed until the cumulative effect surpassed threshold level.

PHONOTRAUMA

Recognizing the fine distinction between misuse and trauma and the possibility of misuse becoming traumatic behaviors that we categorize as trauma tend to be harsher than those previously described, with a greater likelihood of causing trauma to the laryngeal mucosa. Table 4.2 presents vocal behaviors that we categorize as being abusive of the mechanism.

Excessive, Prolonged Loudness

In this category, speakers who traumatize voice, we would include persons who have habituated patterns of excessively loud voice use, those who spend much time talking above high levels of environmental noise, teachers who have come to depend on loudness as a means of capturing and maintaining attention and discipline, cheerleaders, aerobics instructors, some ministers, sports coaches, and untrained or poorly trained singers, speakers, or actors whose activity requires loud voice usage, often in environments not conducive to good voice production.

The mechanism for loudness requires the creation of increased resistance of the laryngeal valve until an appropriate level of air pressure is produced and released. The vocal folds must be adducted strongly to create the increased medial compression required for this valving capability. Awareness of this mechanism explains the traumatic nature of excessive or prolonged loudness. The laryngeal mucosa, especially along the glottal edge, may become irritated, inflamed, and swollen. This may result in altered mass and affect the stiffness of the cover of the vocal folds. Vibratory behavior is changed and reflected in the sound of the voice. Continued use of the voice in this harsh manner may lead to further tissue changes, resulting in organized local lesions at the point of the greatest force of contact of the vocal folds, that is, the midpoint of the vibratory portion of the vocal folds. (In more generalized pathological conditions, a greater extent of the vocal folds may be affected.) The ability to fully adduct the vocal folds may be altered by mass lesions, and this will change the sound of the voice. Leakage of air through an incompletely closed glottis is heard as noise and adds a breathy component to the voice. As changes in phonatory function occur, there is a natural tendency on the part of the speaker to make compensatory adjustments. However, these attempts often constitute further trauma and can result in greater tissue damage.

Daniloff et al. (1980) have pointed out that untrained speakers and singers have difficulty changing vocal parameters (e.g., pitch, loudness) independently of one another. Thus, as loudness is increased, the increased air pressure produces faster vocal fold vibration, resulting in an elevation of pitch. This may put additional strain on the mechanism.

Strained and Excessive Use During Periods of Swelling, Inflammation, or Other Tissue Changes

In the previous section, we mentioned the negative effect of continued use of excessive and prolonged loudness after such behavior had already resulted in irritation of the vocal fold mucosa. At other times similar caveats must be recognized. Edema of the vocal folds may result from infection, allergic reaction, or noxious environmental agents. Other conditions, such as chronic sinusitis with purulent drainage and gastroesophageal reflux, may serve to irritate, swell, and inflame the mucosa. Excessive drying of the tissues, resulting from the use of certain drugs (discussed later in this chapter), extreme dryness of heated buildings (caused by inadequate humidification or the use of wood-burning stoves for heating), excessive use of alcohol, or reduced function of mucous glands can also increase the vulnerability of the mucosa. The chances of creating further damage to the vocal folds are increased if traumatic vocal behaviors occur in the presence of any of these conditions. Tissues that are not in their healthiest and strongest condition are unable to withstand added stress. Often a patient may report that a voice problem seemed to begin with an episode of laryngitis, but that normal voice did not return after the infection had cleared. Persons who rely heavily on voice use are often the most likely to engage in traumatic behavior by continuing to use their voices during periods of laryngeal irritation. They tend to strain and exert greater than usual effort to produce as much voice as possible, and in so doing increase the trauma. They also may produce other tissue changes that persist after the infection has cleared.

Excessive Coughing and Throat Clearing

All of us cough and clear our throats. Coughing may be in response to a local irritation or to infection and serves a life-sustaining purpose in guarding the airway against the entry of foreign objects. The cough reflex evokes a blast of air at high pressure as a mechanism for expelling anything that has attempted to pass through the larynx. It is also the reaction to irritation of the mucosa of the vocal fold edge. The sensation of needing to clear the throat may result from momentary collection of mucus on the vocal folds that interferes with phonation. For some people, certain foods may create a reaction of increased mucus secretions (dairy foods seem to be the most common culprits) and an increased need to clear the throat. An allergic reaction of irritation and swelling of the vocal fold mucosa also can result in the need to cough or clear the throat. During upper respiratory infections or other illnesses, or as a reaction to drugs or treatment such as radiation therapy, the mucus tends to thicken and become tenacious.

The sensation aroused seems to make clearing the throat necessary. Inadequate laryngeal lubrication may result from drug effects, from emotional reactions such as stage fright, from excessive smoking or drinking, or from poorly functioning mucus glands.

A chronic cough is one that persists for longer than 3 weeks. Fourteen percent to 23% of adults who do not smoke are reported to have a persistent cough (Wynder, Lemon, & Mantel, 1965). Smokers have a greater incidence of coughing. Chronic cough, usually dry and unproductive, can result from irritation of the mucosa caused by smoking, secondary to reflux of stomach contents in patients with gastroesophageal reflux disease (GERD) (Deveney, Benner, & Cohen, 1993; Gaynor, 1991; Koufman, 1991; Olson, 1991; Wilson, Pryde, Cecilia, & Macintyre, 1989) (see Chapter 6 for more complete discussion of this topic), postnasal drip, asthma, chronic bronchitis, and some medicines.

Occasional coughing and throat clearing are not of concern. When these behaviors become excessive or habitual, they can be abusive. The entire larynx and supraglottal structures are involved in a cough. High-speed films of coughing behavior show wide glottal opening first, followed by firm and protracted glottal closure during which large lung pressures build up, and ending in a complex expulsive phase (von Leden & Isshiki, 1965). The vocal folds and supraglottal structures, including the posterior pharyngeal wall, are all involved in that final vibratory phase and show periodic undulations of a violent nature. Very vigorous laryngeal activity also has been described during throat clearing (Timcke, von Leden, & Moore, 1959). An understanding of the "violent" nature of these behaviors makes it clear that both excessive coughing and habitual throat clearing can be damaging to the sensitive laryngeal mucosa.

An inventory of traumatic behaviors frequently indicates habitual throat clearing as one such behavior. The pattern can be so habituated that it is at an involuntary level, and the patient's general level of awareness of it is limited. Most patients who exhibit this behavior report sensations of something in the throat that they feel they must dislodge to begin to speak. A habitual, hacking cough and frequent throat clearing are recognized hallmarks of the cigarette smoker and occur in response to the mucosal irritation caused by the noxious agents and the heat of the inhaled substances. They also may be symptomatic of an allergic reaction or other laryngeal irritation.

The Screamer and Noise Maker

Some young children are the prime exhibitors of these behaviors. They tend to be aggressive youngsters who talk a lot, habitually using loud voice in most situations, and engaging in much yelling and screaming in interactions with family and friends, be it in anger or in play (Barker & Wilson, 1967; Toohill, 1975; Wilson & Lamb, 1973). Parents frequently report that a child has been a "screamer" since infancy, being perhaps the only one in the family to be so categorized. On other occasions the report implicates other family members who also tend to be "loud" in their vocal behavior. Because of factors of individual selectivity coupled with amount and degree of excessive screaming, a child may begin to exhibit a voice problem. Vocal nodules are often referred to as "screamer's nodes" because of their frequent occurrence in association with excessive screaming and yelling behavior.

Another manifestation of abuse of the voice most frequently noted in young children is that of using the voice to make a variety of sound effects. Not all such behavior need be abusive; however, many of the sounds typically produced by these children tend to involve strained vocalizations. Some children take special delight in producing the most unusual sounds they can devise. Others tend to supply all of the sound effects during play, not only for themselves but also for their friends.

Many more boys are implicated in screaming and noise making than girls. The incidence of vocal nodules is similarly greater for boys than girls (Coyle et al., 2001; Moore, 1986; Senturia & Wilson, 1968). Aronson (1990) assigns the "abnormal speaking behavior" of these youngsters to personality or emotional factors. Barker and Wilson (1967) studied the amount and type of voice use in the classroom of children with hoarse voices and compared them with a group of children with normal voices. They noted that those with hoarseness produced almost three times as many vocalizations within a 2-hour period as those with normal voices. These dysphonic children were also observed to be more behaviorally active during unstructured classroom time than the control group of children. A further finding of interest was that 65% of the hoarse children came from families in which there was much intrafamily conflict, whereas only 35% of the non-dysphonic children had such a family background.

Sports and Exercise Enthusiast

OBSERVER

Prime demonstrations of vocal phonotrauma may be seen at many sporting or political events. The roar of the crowd is made up of many individual roars. In concert with the crowd noise, it becomes difficult to monitor the loudness of an individual voice. In the heat of the moment, and in keeping with socially accepted behavior, the louder the scream or yell, the better. These loud yells are usually produced with great tension and with elevated pitch, which adds to the degree of tension under which the laryngeal mechanism is held. This behavior and its results are so commonly known that lay people talk about screaming until the voice is gone. Indeed, even Shakespeare commented on this phenomenon in Henry IV with the exclamation, "For my voice, I have lost it with halloing and singing of anthems."

The delicate vocal fold mucosa becomes edematous and irritated in response to this abuse, thereby increasing the mass of the folds and interfering with their vibratory behavior. The severity of the vocal symptoms will be related to the extent of this irritation and the tissue reaction to it. However, return to normal or slightly reduced vocal use plus a good night's rest will usually suffice to restore the vocal folds to their normal condition. Should the person continue to use the voice abusively, or place greater demands on it than the weakened mucosa can withstand, however, further deterioration of both the condition of the mucosa and the dysphonia may occur.

PARTICIPANT

A number of sports or fitness exercises by their very nature may set the stage for vocal trauma. Whenever it becomes necessary to build intrathoracic pressure, the laryngeal valve is involved, and effort closure of the glottis often results. Producing voice under this condition is very stressful. When lifting weights, for example, it is necessary for the person to build and maintain lung pressure as ballast against which the weight may be lifted. This is a reflexive behavior when attempting to lift any heavy weight. Weightlifters often produce grunting sounds during the actual lift. It is not difficult to recognize the abusive nature of phonation produced with the larynx and vocal folds in tight adduction and with increased subglottal pressure present. Similar effort closure of the glottis occurs accompanying a tennis serve or a golf drive.

In other types of sports, it is often necessary for team members to yell to one another above the noise of the spectators. Aerobics instructors who not only participate in the routine but also verbally cue the class above the sound level of the music are a new group of voice abusers to encounter problems. Persons who use motorized sports equipment such as snowmobiles and talk above the noise of the engines also may find themselves having repeated episodes of dysphonia.

When dealing with vocal misuse or phonotrauma, it is essential to pursue an exhaustive history of voice use. Patients do not readily identify behaviors other than the obvious ones, such as screaming, excessive talking, and loud singing. It is necessary for the clinician to explore the full range of potentially traumatic vocal behaviors. Although we have attempted to highlight many such behaviors, our listing is probably not all inclusive. Each voice clinician will be able to add to it from personal experience.

DAMAGING EFFECTS OF DRUGS ON THE VOICE

This section of the chapter will deal with the known and potential effects of drugs on the voice. Although the taking of drugs does not come under the category of a vocal behavior, the effects of drugs can be potentially damaging to the mucosa and disruptive to phonation. For these reasons, we have chosen to place this material in this chapter.

Research on the effects of various drugs on the laryngeal mucosa and laryngeal physiology is almost nonexistent. Therefore, in discussing the effects of drugs on voice, we are talking about expected effects based on an understanding of drug action and laryngeal anatomy and physiology. The following summary is based on the work of pharmacologist F. Gene Martin (1983, 1984, 1988), who presents five basic pharmacological principles to keep in mind when discussing the general effects of drugs:

1. Biological response variability: There is wide biological variability in individual response to drugs, based on a large variety of factors, including age, body composition, kidney function, genetic inheritance, biochemistry, stress level, disease, drug/drug interaction, and nutritional status. Responses may differ both quantitatively and qualitatively.

2. The placebo effect: The expectation of an effect may influence the type and degree of effect obtained. This is a poorly understood but generally accepted phenomenon.

3. Dose–response relationship: The intensity of the effect of a drug is usually expected to be proportional to the dose administered or taken; that is, the larger the dose, the greater the effect, proportionally. However, the dose–response relationships of most drugs form sigmoid-shaped curves rather than straight lines when their effects are plotted against dosage. Such curves indicate that the intensity of a drug increases gradually at first, then rapidly, and then gradually again, eventually reaching a ceiling or plateau level as the dose is increased incrementally (stepwise). Increasing the dose after the ceiling effect has been obtained produces no further enhancement of effect and may only produce undesirable

toxic side effects. Allergic reactions to drugs may appear with any dose, no matter how small, and the intensity of allergic effects is not related to the magnitude of the dose.

4. Multiple effects of a single drug: Drugs may have a multiplicity of effects. Those that are not the specifically intended effect are usually referred to as side effects. These are the effects that most frequently have ramifications for voice production.

5. Drug efficacy versus drug dosage: The efficacy of a drug is of more concern than its potency. Thus, if drug A produces a desired level of response at a lower dose than drug B does, it does not necessarily mean that drug A is better than B. Drug A may, in fact, be worse, if even at its lower dose it produces more undesirable side effects than drug B. It matters little to the patient whether the pill swallowed contains 5 mg or 200 mg of a drug. What matters is the production of an adequate therapeutic effect and the absence of unacceptable side effects with a given reasonable dose.

To those basic principles an additional caution should be included concerning the geriatric population. Elderly people may respond differently, quantitatively or qualitatively, than younger persons do to the same dose of the same drug. This difference in response is caused by the loss, reduction, or alteration of certain body structures and functions with aging, as, for example, a reduced ability to metabolize or absorb certain drugs. Furthermore, many drugs are combinations of several agents, each of which may have an effect on the voice. It is important for the consumer to be aware of these combinations and their possible effects. The voice-related effects of drugs may be classified in the following seven categories: (a) coordination and proprioception; (b) airflow; (c) fluid balance; (d) secretions of the upper respiratory tract; (e) structure of the vocal folds; (f) irritation of vocal fold mucosa; and (i) miscellaneous. The various classes of drugs and their effects are shown in Tables 4.3 and 4.4.

Table 4.3. Drug Classes and Their Laryngeal Effects

Drug Type	Coordination and Proprioception	Airflow	Fluid Balance	Secretions of the Upper Tract	Structure of the Vocal Folds	Irritation of the Vocal Fold Mucosa
CNS stimulants	X					
CNS depressants	X					
Anesthetics	X					
Bronchial dilators and constrictors		X				
Diuretics and decongestants			X			
Corticosteroids			X			
Drying agents				X		
Wetting agents				X		
Androgens					X	
Lower esophageal sphincter effects						X

Table 4.4. Some Common Drugs and Their Possible Voice Side Effects

Drug Group	Brand Name	Manufacturer	Generic Name	Effect on Voice
Antiasthmatic	Azmacort	Rhône-Poulenc	Triamcinolone	Patients using inhaled steroids sometimes experience significant voice changes (including complete loss of voice). The onset of symptoms and severity of symptoms is highly variable among patients. Studies show that discontinuation of inhaled steroids restores the voice in dysphonic patients, but symptoms may not resolve immediately.
Anticoagulant	Coumadin Warfarin	Dupont Barr	Warfarin	Vocal performers, particularly, should be cautious about using medications that decrease platelet function during periods of strenuous voicing demands, due to an increased possibility of vocal fold hemorrhage.
Antidepressant	Paxil	Glaxo-SmithKline	Paroxetine	Paxil and Zoloft may have a drying effect on the body, including vocal fold tissues, which can lead to hoarseness, soreness, voice changes, or laryngitis. Additionally, dry vocal tissues may be more prone to injuries such as nodules.
	Zoloft	Pfizer	Sertraline	
Antihistamine	Allegra Zyrtec Zantac	Aventis Pfizer Glaxo-SmithKline	Fexofenadine Cetirizine Ranitidine	Antihistamines have a drying effect on mucous membranes that may cause hoarseness, sore throat, voice changes, or laryngitis. In addition to irritation, dry vocal folds may be more prone to injuries such as nodules.
Antihyper-lipidemic	Mevacor Zocor	Merck	Lovastatin Simvastatin	No effects on voice or speech mechanisms have been reported.

Continued.

Table 4.4. (continued)

Drug Group	Brand Name	Manufacturer	Generic Name	Effect on Voice
Cardiovascular	Zestoretic	AstraZeneca	Lisinopril/ HCTZ	Two adverse reactions are possible: (1) excessive coughing has been associated with the use of ACE inhibitors, which in turn may lead to hoarseness and possible vocal tissue damage; and (2) the diuretic component may have a drying effect on mucous membrane.
Hormone	Necon 1/35	Watson Lab	Norethindrone	The use of oral contraceptives has not been shown to significantly affect female voices.
Diuretic	Lasix Bumex Demadex	Aventis Roche	Furosemide Bumetanide Torsemide	Diuretics have a drying effect on mucous membranes, including those used for speaking and singing. Hoarseness, sore throat, voice changes, or laryngitis are possible symptoms. In addition to irritation effects, dry vocal folds may be more prone to injuries.
Nonsteroidal antiinflam-matory	Naproxen Ibuprofen	Various	Naproxen Ibuprofen	Vocal performers, particularly, should be cautious about using medications that decrease platelet function during periods of strenuous voicing demands, due to an increased possibility of vocal fold hemorrhage.
Steroid decongestant	Flonase Flovent Nasonex Rhinocort	Glaxo-SmithKline Schering AstraZeneca	Fluticasone Fluticasone Mometasone Budesonide	Throat irritation and dryness, cough, hoarseness, and voice changes are all possible adverse reactions.

Material excerpted from www.ncvs.org/ncvs/info/vocol/rx.html.

Coordination and Proprioception

Any agent that is stimulating or depressing to the central nervous system has the potential to affect coordination, including the fine motor control of phonatory behavior. Central nervous system stimulants include amphetamines, dextroamphetamine sulfate (Dexedrine; GlaxoSmithKline, Research Triangle Park, NC), cocaine, caffeine, and phenylpropanolamine (PPA), the active agent in over-the-counter diet aids. Stimulants are used primarily as recreational drugs and appetite depressants. Their adverse effects may include nervousness and tremor and difficulty in performing acts requiring well-controlled coordination. For example, the shaky or tremulous voice of a person who is highly agitated results from a breakdown of the ability to control fine aspects of voice production. Central nervous system depressants include alcohol, barbiturates, tranquilizers such as diazepam (Valium, Roche Pharmaceuticals, Nutley, NJ) and chlordiazepoxide hydrochloride (Librium, Roche), and chloral hydrate. They are used primarily as antianxiety agents and produce a sedating effect that in high enough doses may have a negative influence on muscle coordination. For example, slurred and slowed speech are well-recognized hallmarks of the person who has had too much to drink.

Diazepam (Valium) is often prescribed for patients with a variety of voice disorders. However, administration of diazepam is usually unproductive of any beneficial change in voice production or in the alleviation of voice symptoms. In a study of the effect of diazepam on respiratory and laryngeal muscle activation, Ludlow, Schulz, and Naunton (1988) reported strong inter-individual respiratory and phonatory effects, which may be age related. Laryngeal activation (as at the onset of phonation) decreased in their older subjects, whereas it increased in their younger subjects. The authors cautioned that use of diazepam as a treatment for spastic dysphonia or other movement disorders affecting the voice may, in some individuals, result in a worsening of symptoms. Furthermore, they called attention to the not uncommon administration of diazepam or other such medications to subjects in studies of laryngeal muscle activity during speech, suggesting that this practice may significantly alter the results of such studies. Another group of drugs that affect the central nervous system are those that produce an anesthetic effect. Local anesthetics such as benzocaine (Americaine, Celltech), lidocaine (Xylocaine), procaine hydrochloride (Novocain), or phenol may be the primary ingredients in over-the-counter lozenges and sprays used to treat a sore throat. These agents are capable of blocking nerve impulse conduction and reducing pain sensation. Pain serves as an alarm system, indicating the presence of a problem somewhere in the body. The usual response to throat or laryngeal pain is to reduce voice usage. Reduction of pain by the use of these analgesic agents masks the presence of the problem, and the individual may then be prone to overstressing voice use. Leonard and Ringel (1979) reported some changes in laryngeal behavior after the dripping of a local anesthetic onto the vocal folds.

Airflow

Drugs that either dilate or constrict the bronchioles will affect the movement of pulmonary air through the larynx. Bronchodilators, such as albuterol (Proventil, Ventolin), metaproterenol sulfate (Alupent), and others are used primarily as antiasthma agents. Negative side effects may be nervousness and tremor. Bronchoconstrictors potentially have a more adverse effect on voice production. The mechanism most often used to cause bronchoconstriction pharmacologically is an allergic reaction. The effects may vary from very mild discomfort and wheezing to a significant, even life-threatening effect on respiratory function. Many environmental irritants, such as dust, pollen, and molds, produce similar effects in individuals with sensitivity to these environmental factors.

Fluid Balance

Fluid balance in the mucosa of the vocal folds may have a very significant and direct effect on voice production. Many drugs, either as a consequence of their primary intended effect or as their side effect, work in such a way as to reduce edema either systemically or in a more localized manner. Diuretics, which reduce the formation of edema, are commonly used in the treatment of high blood pressure and heart or kidney failure. Perhaps the most widely used group of agents with the effect of reducing edema are the decongestants, many of which are sold as over-the-counter preparations in tablet, capsule, or liquid form or as topical sprays (e.g., oxymetazoline hydrochloride [Afrin], pseudoephedrine hydrochloride [Sudafed, etc.]). These are used in the treatment of the symptoms of cold, cough, allergy, or sinus problems.

Vocal fold edema, under most circumstances, is the result of protein-bound water (Lawrence, 1987; Sataloff, 1987a) and will not be responsive to diuretic agents. Corticosteroids, often used as drying agents in the treatment of vocal fold edema in performers after vocally abusive episodes, affect protein-bound water directly. Although they are often effective, they offer only a palliative, not a curative, effect. A patient may be using a diuretic agent for a number of reasons not directly related to vocal fold edema. In such instances, the danger of reducing the normally desirable fluid level in the laryngeal mucosa must be kept in mind. Long-term use of decongestants may cause a rebound effect wherein, as the vasoconstrictive effects of the drug wear off, there is a return of the edema and congestion to a greater degree than was previously present. As a result, a vicious cycle may be established in which the patient must continue to take the decongestant in an attempt to counteract the side effect that is being caused by the drug itself. The long-term effects of vasoconstriction and the adverse effects from the loss of adequate fluid balance include a reduction in blood flow to the mucosa; loss of electrolytes with concomitant decrease of potassium level, leading to a decrease in energy and a sedating effect; increased nervousness and tremor; and potential damage to the mucous membranes. Edema formation in reaction to drugs occurs primarily in the form of an allergic response. Agents that cause an allergic reaction in a patient may have more than a single effect. Whereas bronchoconstriction may be one effect, edema of the mucosa may occur simultaneously. Edema of the laryngeal mucosa also may occur in response to vocal abuse, trauma, infection, and environmental allergens.

Corticosteroid inhalants are used in the treatment of asthma. Their effect on voice is not entirely clear. Williams, Baghat, DeStableforth, Shenoi, and Skinner (1983) reported dysphonia and bilateral vocal fold bowing in patients using an inhaled corticosteroid. The vocal fold bowing appeared to be related to the dose and potency of the drug used and was believed to represent a local steroid myopathy. The bowing and concomitant dysphonia were reversed in all patients after cessation of use of the steroid inhalant. Watkin and Ewanowski (1979) reported that prolonged administration of aerosol-delivered triamcinolone acetonide (Kenalog), a drug used by chronic asthmatics, results in significantly altered vocal tract functioning and an elevation of fundamental frequency of approximately 20 Hz. They reported that changes were evident after 1 year of use, with a cumulative effect described after 2 years.

Secretions of the Upper Respiratory Tract

According to Martin (1983, 1984, 1988), exposure to agents that affect upper respiratory tract secretions occurs with great frequency. Many drugs act as drying agents by causing a reduction in secretions of the salivary and mucus glands. Furthermore, Martin states, a major portion of our lives "is spent in buildings with very low humidity, and we are continuously breathing air with moisture levels similar to that of the Sahara" (Martin, 1988; McClean, 1987; Stoicheff, Giampi, Passi, & Fredrickson, 1983). A vicious cycle ensues in which breathing dry air results in dryness and irritation of the mucosa, which leads to coughing, which serves to further irritate and dry the mucosa.

Among the drugs creating a drying effect, the most common are the antihistamines used in the treatment of allergy, cold, cough, sinus, motion sickness, and insomnia. Drugs functioning as antispasmodic agents (e.g., atropine, scopolamine, diphenoxylate hydrochloride [Lomotil], etc.) used in the treatment of diarrhea also create a reduction in glandular secretions. The action of antitussive drugs such as codeine and dextromethorphan hydrobromide (Benylin DM), used in cough remedies, is drying, and a side effect is sedation. Antipsychotic agents such as chlorpromazine hydrochloride (Thorazine) and haloperidol (Haldol) and antidepressant agents such as amitriptyline (Elavil) and lithium carbonate (Lithane, Lithobid) cause drying and sedation. The last group of drying agents is the antihypertensive drugs used in the treatment of high blood pressure, such as methyldopa (Aldomet), reserpine (Sandril, Serpasil), and captopril (Capoten).

The most effective wetting agent is water, abundantly available and easily consumed. Ambient humidity may be voluntarily controlled, as may the amount of water consumed. Expectorants, used in the treatment of cough, are agents that increase secretions. However, many of these products contain other drugs that have the opposite effect. Guaifenesin (Robitussin, Glycotuss) is the most commonly used expectorant drug and can be obtained as the only drug in a product. Saliva substitutes (e.g., dibasic sodium phosphate [Moi-stir], sodium carboxymethylcellulose [Salivart], etc.) have recently become available and appear to be very helpful as wetting agents. They are used primarily by persons who have salivary gland pathological conditions but can be used effectively to combat the dry mouth caused by the use of drying agents and also by pre-performance anxiety. Thompson (1995) has suggested that the efficacy of wetting agents has not been proved, and perhaps the most beneficial effect may be the increased water intake required while taking this medication.

Changes in Structure of the Vocal Folds

The androgens, which are structurally related to the male hormone testosterone, change the actual structure of the vocal folds. They are used in the treatment of hormonal imbalance (frequently in postmenopausal women), in sexual reassignment from female to male, and by body builders seeking to increase muscle mass. Androgens cause an increase in the mass of the vocal folds, which, of course, results in a change in the voice, referred to as the virilization of the voice. Once this change has occurred, it is irreversible (Damste, 1967). A synthetic androgen, danazol androgen (Danocrine), is commonly used in the treatment of benign fibrocystic breast disease, although a side effect of voice change occurs in approximately 10% of the patients treated. It is not yet clear whether these voice changes are reversible (Martin, 1988). These agents can be used effectively to lower fundamental frequency of the voice in individuals who have undertaken sexual reassignment from female to male.

Irritation of Vocal Fold Mucosa

Laryngeal tissue (as well as esophageal and pharyngeal) is susceptible to irritation and damage caused by the acidic contents of gastric juices that reflux into the hypopharynx in gastroesophageal reflux disease (GERD). Lower esophageal sphincter (LES) pressure has been reported to be decreased by the following drugs: atropine, dopamine, smoking, calcium blockers, sedatives/tranquilizers, nitrates, theophylline, and adrenergic drugs (Gaynor, 1991). Because a decrease in the tightness of the LES is implicated in the pathophysiology of GERD, it is logical to assume that use of any of these drugs may predispose an individual to GERD. Caffeine, fat, alcohol, and highly spiced foods are also believed to reduce LES pressures. (See Chapter 6 for more information on GERD.)

Miscellaneous

Martin (1983, 1984, 1988) notes additional agents that are thought by some to have an effect on voice production and on performance, although they do not specifically fit any of the previous categories. These include ototoxic drugs, herbal teas, aspirin, beta blockers, and tobacco and other smoked or inhaled drugs.

HEARING

A number of drug groups are known to be potentially ototoxic. Some of these are aminoglycoside antibiotics, such as amikacin sulfate (Amikin) and tobramycin sulfate (Nebcin), which are used intravenously in life-threatening disease states. Certain diuretics, referred to as "loop" or "high ceiling" diuretics, such as furosemide (Lasix) or bumetanide (Bumex), used in the treatment of heart failure and high blood pressure, also have the potential to create hearing loss. Some drugs used in chemotherapy for cancer are also suspected to have ototoxic side effects, and their use should be monitored closely. Obviously the loss of hearing will not have a direct effect on laryngeal anatomy. However, laryngeal physiology may be indirectly affected in the profoundly and congenitally hearing impaired, and in those who have acquired hearing impairment of a severe degree, and perhaps not an immediate effect on laryngeal physiology. Indirectly, however, this loss of hearing may affect vocal production, and it is likely that vocal physiology may be altered over time. When vocal loudness considerations are a component of a voice disorder, auditory acuity must be taken into account.

HERBS AND ALTERNATIVE THERAPIES

An estimated that 42% to 57% of the population of the United States have used some form of alternative medical therapies including the ingestion of various herbs and other organic material (Fisher & Veronneau, 2000). Furthermore, approximately 1 in 5 individuals who take a prescribed medication also use herbal substances. The problem is that many individuals do not inform their physicians that they are taking the herbal supplements. Serious negative interactions have been known to occur between prescribed medications and herbal materials. Moreover, herbs may have an undesirable side effect, and some have been reported to produce serious health problems and even death. For many herbal preparations, the claimed benefit has not yet been substantiated.

The lay person's view of herbs is that they are natural substances and therefore cannot cause any harm. That may be true when taken in moderation and recommended by a reliable source. Unfortunately, herbal preparations are not regulated by the FDA and are considered food supplements. Thus, there are no regulations regarding the purity or even the accurate labeling of these substances.

Herbal substances may have adverse effects. Some documented adverse effects include hallucinogenic actions, sedative, or cardiovascular reactions (Fisherft & Veronnneau, 2000). Surow and Lovetri (2000) have described most of the adverse reactions to alternative medical therapies. These possible reactions to commonly used herbal preparations are shown in Table 4.5. Some of these adverse reactions are dose related or could be caused by impure or undocumented additional substances in the herbal preparation. How does one know which herbs are good and which are not? How does one know where to purchase these herbs with a reasonable assurance about their purity and content? The web site of B&K Prescription Shop, a seller of herbs and supplements, has some good tips for the wary consumer (www.bkrx.com/tips.htm). Check this page for a complete list of tips. The best advice is to be wary of any advertising claims of the efficacy of herbal supplements, buy from a reputable (and large) manufacturer, look for standardized products, consult with your physician especially if you are taking any medications, and be wary of fad products. Singers should be even more careful about these preparations because they may have subtle effects on the body and perhaps the voice. However, there have been few, if any, scientific studies of reported effects on the voice of taking herbal substances. (See Table 4.5.)

Table 4.5. Commonly Used Herbs, Their Claimed Benefit and Possible Adverse Effects

Product	Claimed Use(s)	Adverse Effects
Echinacea (E. Purpurea)	Immune stimulant generally used for colds, sore throat, and flu. Used for treatment and prophylaxis	Possible allergies
Garlic (Allium sativum)	Lowers cholesterol and blood pressure	May cause GI irritation
Ginger (Zingiber officinale)	Helps prevent motion sickness, morning sickness	GI upset in large doses
Ginkgo (Ginkgo biloba)	Improves memory, circulation, helps treat depression, Impotence	Minor GI disturbances
Ginseng (Panax ginseng)	Reduces stress, improves stamina, Adaptogen	Nervousness and excitation first few days of taking
Saw palmetto (Serenoa repens)	Benign prostatic hyperplasia	Very few. Headache reported.
St. John's wort (Hypericum perforatum)	Mild to moderate depression	Avoid use with other antidepressants. May cause photo-sensitivity.

Based on table presented at www.bkrx.com/herbs.htm.

ASPIRIN

Aspirin has anticoagulant properties that are not usually of consequence to the average voice user unless that individual has a bleeding disorder or is taking another anticoagulant medication. Because the professional voice user is called on to use the voice strenuously, the risk of vocal fold hemorrhage may be somewhat greater than for the average speaker. Such risk may be further increased, and particularly so if that person is taking aspirin or any preparations containing acetylsalicylic acid.

BETA BLOCKERS

During times of stress and fear, the adrenal glands release the chemicals epinephrine and norepinephrine. The increased level of these chemicals results in rapid heartbeat, tremor, elevated blood pressure, sweaty palms, dry mouth, respiratory tension, nausea, and an urge to urinate. These are also the well-known symptoms of the phenomenon known as stage fright. Beta blockers, of which propranolol (Inderal) is the most common, act to block the effect of epinephrine on glands, smooth muscles, and the heart, thereby reducing the symptoms described above. Whether the reduction of symptoms produces enhanced performance has not been determined. Instrument musicians have been reported to demonstrate improved performance and a lessening of subjective stage fright symptoms with the use of beta blockers (Brantigan, Brantigan, & Joseph, 1982; James, Pearson, Griffith, & Newburg, 1977; Liden & Gottfries, 1974). Evidence of their effectiveness in singers is less conclusive. Gates and Montalbo (1987) suggest that low-dose (20 mg) beta blockade had no significant effect on singers' performance. In an earlier study, Gates, Saegert, Wilson, Johnson, Shepard, and Hearne (1985) reported a deleterious effect on singing quality with the administration of beta blocker in high doses (40–80 mg). There does not appear to be strong evidence that beta blockers significantly enhance performance. Indeed, some have suggested that heightened pre-performance anxiety serves a useful purpose in that it lends a degree of intensity and excitement to the performance that might be lost if beta blockers were used. Data to support this contention or its corollary are not yet available.

TOBACCO AND OTHER SMOKED OR INHALED DRUGS

We should not leave this section on the effect of drugs on the voice without some direct mention of tobacco, marijuana, and other drugs that are smoked or inhaled. There is very convincing evidence (Burch, 1981; Hammond, 1966; Kahn, 1966; Wynder, Covey, Mabuchi, & Muchinski, 1976; Wynder & Stellman, 1977) that smoking cigarettes is closely related to laryngeal cancer. The vast majority of individuals who present with laryngeal carcinoma have a history of heavy smoking. Precancerous conditions such as leukoplakia and hyperkeratosis are also closely linked to smoking. Some smokers present with very boggy, polypoid vocal folds (Reinke's edema), a condition that is benign but usually results in significant dysphonia and can be severe enough to compromise the airway. Redness and generalized irritation of the mucosa of the upper respiratory tract and the larynx are often present in persons who use tobacco, marijuana, and other inhaled substances. The harmful effects of inhaling environmental smoke has been documented (U.S. Department of Health and Human Services, 1986). Lung cancer and emphysema are also known to be directly related to smoking. When the respiratory system is compromised, there is a direct effect on voice production. Thus, even in the absence of an actual laryngeal pathological condition, the effects of smoking on lung function are sufficient to produce a broad effect on phonation.

VOCAL PATHOLOGIES SECONDARY TO PHONOTRAUMA

In this section, we discuss pathological conditions that are thought to be caused by or contributed to by vocally traumatic behaviors. These conditions are nodules, polyps, cysts, edema, chronic laryngitis, and sulcus vocalis. However, as noted above, phonotrauma may not be the only cause of some of these pathological conditions. Indeed, in some cases, the exact cause is still in question. All of the pathological conditions do appear to have an abusive component even if it may not be the primary cause.

Throughout this section, we report some of the data that we have collected on a large sample of patients with benign lesions (Colton et al, 1997). In this project, we analyzed various acoustic and aerodynamic variables before treatment and at selected intervals after treatment. We also studied the patients' own perceptions of their disability and rated the degree of dysphonia. These patients were treated with medical, surgical, or voice therapy, depending on the specific diagnosis and presenting symptoms. Specific results are presented in the appropriate sections that follow.

Nodules

PRIMARY VOICE SYMPTOM: HOARSENESS

Description and Etiology

Nodules are localized benign growths on the vocal folds that are usually thought to be the result of vocal abuse. They are a reaction of the tissue to the constant stress induced by frequent, hard oppositional movement of the vocal folds. In the initial stages of the formation of a nodule, the trauma causes localized edema on the vocal fold edge. Early or acute nodules are fairly soft and pliable; they may be reddish and are mostly vascular and edematous. The remainder of the vocal fold also may be edematous, and the entire larynx may be slightly inflamed. In this early stage, the nodule may be evident only on one side and may be easily mistaken for a polyp. With continued trauma, the tissue undergoes hyalinization and fibrosis and becomes firm. Chronic or "older" nodules are usually hard, white, thick, and fibrosed. Arnold (1962, 1980) reported that at this chronic stage of nodule development, the epithelium may show hypertrophy, horny or very rough surfaces, and a change in the type of cells present. Chronic nodules are usually bilateral and not always entirely symmetrical. Figure 4.1 is an illustration of a pair of vocal nodules.

Some controversy exists about the distinction between nodules and polyps. A polyp is a projecting mass with a central core of fibrous tissue of greater density than the lamina propria and covered by a normal or slightly hyperplastic epithelium (in contrast to nodules). Clinically, there are times when the distinction between the two lesion types is very clear and other times when the difference is minimal. Histologically, the distinction between nodules and polyps is not much clearer. Fitz-Hugh, Smith, and Chiong (1958) reviewed the histological findings of 300 consecutive cases of benign tumors of the vocal folds. They commented on the difficulty of distinguishing among nodules, polyps, and polypoid degeneration. Many nodules were classified as polyps and vice versa, on review. They eventually concluded that a nodule was a trauma-related lesion consisting of a local nodular or polypoid degeneration of the lamina propria. They state that a polyp has its origin in the subepithelial (or Reinke's) space. From the perspective of the voice clinician, both types of pathological condition frequently respond to conservative treatment, particularly in their acute or early stages.

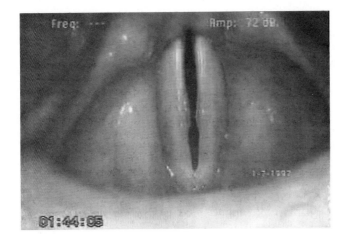

Figure 4.1. A vocal fold nodule. See color plate.

Gray and his colleagues (1987) have described some of the histological changes that occur as a result of extended phonation, and the changes that occur in nodules of the vocal folds. Hyperphonation results in several changes to the vocal fold epidermis, including (a) damage to the microvilli; (b) creation of a cobblestone appearance along the surface; and (c) damage to the surface and underlying cells (Gray, Titze, & Lusk, 1987). Nodules appear to result from damage to the basement membrane zone (BMZ), an area connecting the outer epidermis to the lamina propria. Trauma produces a disorganization of the BMZ that reduces the strength of the attachment of the epidermis to the lamina propria.

Nodules occur more frequently in adult women and young, pre-pubescent male children. In their retrospective study of 1,158 patients with voice disorders seen in two ear, nose, and throat (ENT) offices in Ohio over 3 years, Coyle, Weinrich, and Stemple (2001) reported that approximately 10% of patients had vocal fold nodules. Of the total number of patients reviewed, 12.5% of women had vocal nodules, whereas 6.6% of men had vocal nodules. Most of the patients with nodules were between the ages of 25 and 44 years. Although this study had a large number of patients, one should interpret their results with caution for two reasons. First, the study only reports the prevalence of voice problems for two medical practices in one midwestern state. Second, the study is retrospective with the lack of controls one might wish in a study such as this.

Luchsinger and Arnold (1965) considered general physical constitution, personality, and local laryngeal signs to be important predisposing conditions for nodules (or polyps). Allergies or thyroid imbalances may contribute to precipitating factors; tobacco and alcohol use may be aggravating factors.

In adults, nodules occur most frequently in women between the ages of 20 and 50 years. In children, nodules occur predominantly in boys from 3 to 6 years of age. The children are typically reported to be prone to excessive loud talking and screaming.

Perceptual Signs and Symptoms

Hoarseness and breathiness are the major perceptual signs of nodules. Some individuals complain of soreness or pain in the neck lateral to the larynx that may radiate upward to the ear or downward to the upper chest. Some have the sensation of something in the "throat" that they need to try to clear. Difficulty in producing pitches in the upper third of the range is a complaint especially true for singers. The degree of hoarseness or breathiness present may be related to the size and firmness of the nodules and may vary from slight to moderately severe.

Acoustic Signs

The acoustic characteristics of a patient with vocal fold nodules will depend on a number of factors, including the severity of the dysphonia. Depending on the size of the nodule, a patient may have a mild, moderate degree of dysphonia. In some cases, a patient may be perceived to have a normal voice even though a vocal nodule can be seen on videostroboscopy. In our study of 35 adult female patients with vocal fold nodules (Colton et al.,1997), we found that most of our patients were perceived as only mildly dysphonic, a factor that should be kept in mind when evaluating the results of our acoustic studies.

Acoustically, a patient with nodules exhibits increased frequency and amplitude perturbation (jitter and shimmer) with a fundamental frequency within the normal range. Davis (1981) reported pitch perturbation quotient (PPQ) values of 2.61% and 1.87% for two patients with nodules, compared with a PPQ of 0.42% for normal speakers. Others have reported similar greater than normal frequency perturbation measurements in the presence of nodules. Our group of 35 female patients with nodules had an average jitter of 0.32% and average shimmer of 2.72%. Takahashi and Koike (1975) reported a mean relative average perturbation (RAP, see section in Chapter 2 on frequency perturbation) of 0.0084, whereas Ludlow, Coulter, and Gentges (1983) reported a mean jitter of 9.26 microseconds, compared with a normal value of 5 microseconds. Davis also reported an amplitude perturbation quotient (APQ) of 9.07% and 15.33% for the nodule cases, compared with a normal APQ of 6.14%.

Phonational range may be markedly reduced in these patients, especially at the upper end. Our group of 35 patients had a mean phonational range of 24 semitones FL, a value slightly less than would be expected for normal female speakers. The magnitude of the reduction in phonational range appeared to depend on the severity of the dysphonia. For example, patients perceived to be normal or only slightly dysphonic had an average phonational range of approximately 28 semitones, whereas patients perceived to be moderately dysphonic had an average phonational range of 21 semitones. The single patient perceived as "very dysphonic" had a phonational range of slightly more than 7 semitones.

The patient also may show a reduced dynamic range, with marked inability to produce high sound pressure levels. Our patients showed an approximately 27dB range at a single comfortable pitch, a value somewhat lower than others have reported (Coleman, Mabis, & Hinson, 1977). Again, patients with more severe dysphonia tended to have smaller dynamic ranges.

Eckel and Boone (1981) reported an average s/z ratio of 1.65 for their group of 28 patients with nodules and polyps. Normal subjects produced an s/z ratio of 0.99. Spectrum analysis of a patient's phonation typically shows evidence of noise in the spectrum (Arnold & Emanuel, 1979; Yanagihara, 1967b), the degree of which depends on lesion size and severity of the accompanying hoarseness. Interestingly, nodules seem to produce little effect on fundamental frequency of phonation (Murry, 1978).

Measurable Physiological Signs

Airflow in a patient with nodules may be equal to or slightly higher than normal (Iwata, Esaki, Iwami, & Mimura, 1976; Iwata, von Leden, & Williams, 1972). Tanaka and Gould (1985) reported a mean value of 275 mL/sec in their two patients with nodules. Normal male subjects produce flows of approximately 125 mL/sec. Woo, Colton, and Shangold (1987) reported a mean flow rate of 265 mL/sec for their combined polyp and nodule group, collapsed across 14 male and 18 female subjects. In their study, normal speakers produced a mean flow rate of 144 mL/sec. The magnitude of the increase of airflow rates appears to depend on the severity of the lesion (Shigemori, 1977). Lung pressures also may be high because of the tendency for an individual to increase the driving force to overcome incomplete glottal closure (Tanaka & Gould, 1985). However, in our sample of 35 females with nodules, we found some elevation of pressure (6.41 cm H_2O) versus as compared with normal (Colton et al., 1997). Our patient group showed some elevation of leakage airflow and slightly elevated peak airflows, the magnitude of which depended on the severity of dysphonia. Electroglottograms show decreased closing times of the vocal folds and an irregular pattern. Normal electromyogram levels would be expected, although it is possible for these to be elevated if the patient shows excessive laryngeal tension.

Observable Physiological Signs

Laryngoscopy. Nodules typically have been described as benign lesions located at the junction of the anterior third and posterior two thirds of the vocal folds. There the forces encountered during vibration are the largest (Luchsinger & Arnold, 1965). The posterior one third of the vocal fold (i.e., the vocal process) is composed of stiff cartilage that does not vibrate. The remaining two thirds of the vocal folds vibrate, and it is at the midpoint of this vibrating portion that the contact forces will be the greatest. However, in a recent study of 24 patients with vocal nodules, Casper, Colton, Brewer, Kelley, Woo, and Griffin (1995) reported that one third of those patients were found to have nodules located at mid-cord. Laryngoscopically, there may be evidence of incomplete closure of the vocal folds, especially in the area surrounding the nodules, or a large posterior chink. Some edema of the folds is not uncommon, and there is increased vascularity.

Stroboscopy. According to Kitzing (1985), the vocal folds will show normal symmetry and periodicity but reduced amplitudes and mucosal waves at the nodule site and reduced glottal closure. In view of the greater frequency perturbation found in patients with vocal nodules (as reported in "Acoustic Signs," above), Kitzing's finding of normal periodicity is questionable. A small nodule may have a minimal effect on the vibratory frequency of the vocal folds. Hirano and Bless (1993) report absence of the mucosal wave in the nodule area when the mass is firm, but find it present and unchanged when the nodule is edematous and soft. In our study of stroboscopic signs in a group of 30 female patients with nodules (Colton, Woo, Brewer, Griffin, & Casper, 1995), the amplitude of the vocal fold movement was slightly reduced. Glottal closure had traditionally been described as having an hourglass appearance. Using frame-by-frame analysis procedures in which even a single frame of vocal fold closure results in a "complete closure" rating (Colton et al, 1995), approximately 47% of our patients with nodules exhibited an posterior chink closure pattern, whereas 32% showed an hourglass closure pattern. Eighteen percent of the patients showed complete closure. When viewed as a gestalt (rather than frame-by-frame), the "appearance" of both hourglass closure and posterior chink ratings would be more predominant. In another study (Casper et al, 1995), we found that approximately half of the nodules identified could be described as being pinpoint in shape, with the remainder described as broad based.

Pathophysiology

A nodule will increase the mass of the cover of the vocal fold. The stiffness of the cover will be increased by a hard and firm nodule and decreased or unchanged by a soft and pliable one (Hirano, 1981a; Hirano & Bless, 1993). The mechanical properties of the transition layers and the muscle may not be affected by the nodule. However, Gray's recent work on the BMZ (Gray, 1991; Gray, Hirano, & Sato, 1993; Gray, Pignatari, & Harding, 1994) suggests the BMZ area as the possible site of some damage. Because the mechanical properties of the cover are very important in determining the vibratory characteristics of the vocal folds, a nodule may have a pronounced effect on the mechanics of vibration. The extra mass along the medial edge of the vibrating vocal folds results in increased aperiodicity of vibration, greater frequency perturbation, and greater hoarseness. Depending on the size of the nodule, glottal closure also will be affected. Incomplete closure (such as occurs in the hourglass configuration) permits increased air escape, resulting in the perception of breathiness.

Polyps

PRIMARY VOICE SYMPTOM: HOARSENESS

Description and Etiology

A polyp may take a number of forms that may affect voice differentially and require different interventions, and the subsequent effects and treatment may also vary. If the polyp is localized, it may show up as pedunculated (attached to the vocal fold only by a slim stalk of tissue) or it may be sessile (closely adhering to mucosa). Another variant is that of hemorrhagic polyp, which has the appearance of a blood blister. If the lesion is diffuse, it may cover half to two thirds of the entire length of one or both vocal folds. These lesions are usually referred to as polypoid degeneration or Reinke's edema and are discussed in a separate section. The distinction between polyp and polypoid degeneration is sometimes confusing. According to Lowenthal (1958), the pathological conditions are very similar in that they are localized or diffuse inflammatory tumors involving the space of Reinke. Histologically, both types are also very similar.

Polyps are thought to result from a period of vocal abuse, although they can occur as the result of a single traumatic incident, such as yelling at a basketball game. The latter tend to be hemorrhagic polyps with sudden onset of hoarseness. Luchsinger and Arnold (1965) considered polyps and nodules to have the same cause and to differ only in degree. According to Jackson (1941), a polyp is larger and more vascular, edematous, and inflammatory than a nodule, which is described as an organized mass of tissue (Fig. 4.2).

Polyps are usually predominantly unilateral, although sometimes a small polyp can be found on the contralateral side. This apparent contralateral polyp may, in reality, be a lesion created by the contact with the unilateral polyp during phonation. Although polyps usually occur on the free margin of the vocal folds, they also may be found on the superior surface of the folds as well as in the subglottis. In the latter case, there may be little or no alteration in the voice. Polyps also may involve almost the entire length of the vocal fold (Fig. 4.3).

It is easy to see how acute nodules can be mistaken for polyps. Polyps usually occur in Reinke's space (the superficial layer of the lamina propria) and may consist of dilated blood vessels, fibrotic tissue, and small hemorrhages.

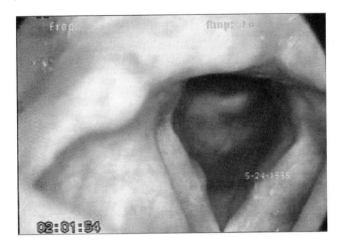

Figure 4.2. A single vocal fold polyp. See color plate.

Polyps constituted approximately 7.7% of the patients seen in ENT practices reported by Coyle et al. (2001). A little more than 5% of these patients were female and slightly less than 2.5% were male. We studied 25 patients with vocal fold polyps (Colton et al., 1997). Eighteen of these patients were female, with a mean age of 48 years. The remainder were males with a mean age of 44 years. Because of missing data, the reports about the acoustic, aerodynamic, and stroboscopic data that follow in the appropriate sections are based on 23 subjects (15 females, 7 males).

Perceptual Signs and Symptoms

Typical perceptual signs of a polyp include hoarseness, roughness, or breathiness. In addition, the patient may report the sensation of something in the throat.

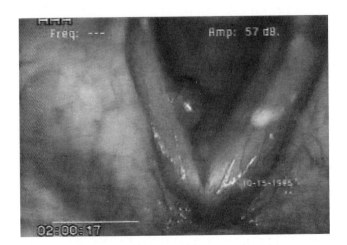

Figure 4.3. Larger hemorrhagic polyp in the middle of the vocal fold. See color plate.

In our polyp patient group, 35% of the women and 17% of men exhibited a "moderate" severity of dysphonia. The next most frequent category was "very severe" (22% women; 4.35% men). Thus, the polyp group exhibited a greater severity of dysphonia than did the nodule group discussed in the last section.

Acoustic Signs

The acoustic features created by a polyp are very similar to those of a nodule. Increased jitter and shimmer would be expected, depending on the location of the polyp. Davis (1981) reported a PPQ of 0.60% and an APQ of 11.68% for his one patient with a polyp. Normal PPQ is 0.42%, and APQ is 6.14%. We found jitter scores that ranged from 0.27% to 1.83%, the latter for a group of female subjects with a "moderate" severity rating. Reduced phonational and dynamic ranges, as well as increased spectral noise, also would be anticipated acoustic characteristics. We found a significant reduction of phonational range for both male and female patients with vocal fold polyps. Please note that the "slight" dysphonia category for both sexes and the "very" dysphonic category for males had each included only one patient. Our data for dynamic ranges showed little difference between patients with polyps and normal speakers.

Measurable Physiological Signs

Increased airflow may be present if the polyp interferes with complete glottal closure, but available data regarding this matter are somewhat variable. In one report, 18 patients with polyps had an average airflow rate of 162 mL/sec (Iwata, von Leden, & Williams, 1972), whereas in another report, Iwata et al. (Iwata, Esaki, Iwami, & Mimura, 1976) reported an average airflow rate of 253 mL/sec for 29 male patients and 247 mL/sec for 19 female patients with unilateral polyps. In the same study, patients with bilateral polyps had airflow rates of 256 mL/sec (8 males) and 359 mL/sec (8 females). For their seven patients with polyps, Tanaka and Gould (1985) reported a mean flow rate of 223.71 mL/sec. Woo, Colton, and Shangold. (1987) reported a mean flow rate of 265 mL/sec for their combined polyp and nodule group, collapsed across 14 male and 18 female subjects. In the Woo et al. study, normal speakers produced a mean flow rate of 144 mL/sec. We found significantly greater alternating airflow rates for our group of 23 patients but no differences in leakage airflow. Subglottal or lung pressure also appears to increase because of attempts to produce phonation in the presence of a leaky glottis (Tanaka & Gould, 1985). Our patient group had subglottal air pressures within normal limits, but the average open quotients were markedly reduced as compared with the normal group. Electroglottograms tend to suggest decreased closing times of the vocal folds and irregular patterns. Muscle action potentials would again be expected to be normal, unless the patient showed excessive laryngeal tension.

Observable Physiological Signs

Laryngoscopy.   Polyps can be visualized with standard continuous light laryngoscopy, using a mirror or flexible endoscope. They typically appear as rather large masses on one vocal fold, sometimes with a very broad base, sometimes attached to a stalk. Most times they appear somewhat translucent, although on occasion they may be red and apparently blood-filled.

Stroboscopy.   Stroboscopically, asymmetry of motion of the vocal folds and increased aperiodicity are noted. Polyps tend to show distinct phase differences between the two folds, especially if the lesions are grossly different in size or if the lesion is unilateral. The vibratory amplitude of the vocal folds is reduced, but the effect of the polyp on mucosal waves, especially in the vicinity of the polyp, may vary from being decreased or absent (as in the case of a hemorrhagic polyp) to being increased (as in large sessile polyps) to being normal (as in a pedunculated polyp). Glottal closure also may be affected (Hirano, Feder, & Bless, 1983; Kitzing, 1985). In our study of 24 patients with polyps (Colton, Woo, Brewer, Griffin, & Casper, 1995), the most common closure pattern was irregular. Aperiodicity of vocal fold movement may be increased, although in our study (Colton et al., 1995), the most frequent periodicity category rating was regular. In some instances, the polyp lags in movement behind the vocal fold proper and thus appears as a "coupled" movement. Our study further revealed that the amplitude of vocal fold movement in patients with polyps was moderately decreased, especially for the affected fold. Vibration of the affected vocal fold was also altered by presence of the lesion (Colton, Woo, Brewer, Griffin, & Casper, 1995); i.e., there was little or no mucosal wave, especially over the site of the lesion.

Pathophysiology

A polyp will increase the mass of the cover of the vocal folds. If the polyp is soft, edematous, and pliable, the stiffness of the cover will be decreased (Hirano, 1981a). However, if bleeding, hyaline degeneration, or other histological changes are present, stiffness of the cover may be increased (see Chapter 3). The mechanical properties of the transition layers and the muscle should not be affected. As described in the case of nodules, the mechanical properties of the cover will determine the vibratory characteristics of the vocal folds. The extra mass at the midpoint of the vibrating vocal folds results in increased aperiodicity of vibration, greater frequency perturbation, and greater hoarseness. However, if the polyp is pedunculated, the effects on vibration are likely to be minimal, because the mass of the polyp does not affect the cover directly. Depending on the size of the polyp, glottal closure may be affected. If excessive air can escape through the closed glottis, breathiness will be perceived.

Intracordal Cysts

PRIMARY VOICE SYMPTOM: HOARSENESS

Description and Etiology

Intracordal cysts appear as small spheres on the margins of the vocal folds (Fig. 4.4) and sometimes on the superior surface. They may be mistaken for early nodules, because small nodule-like growths may appear on one cord but not the other. Cysts are predominantly unilateral and often can be mistaken for early nodules or polyps. Cysts also may occur in association with vocal nodules (Monday, 1983).

Intracordal or retention cysts may be caused by blockage of a glandular duct in which there is retention of mucus (Cornut & Bouchayer, 1989; Monday, 1983). Typically the cyst is lined with glandular epithelium, may appear to have a slightly yellowish color, and does not drain spontaneously. Because there is no way for the mucus to escape, a cyst may, with time, grow larger. Another type of cyst, usually smaller than a retention cyst, is the epidermoid cyst. Epidermoid cysts, another variant of the vocal folds, have

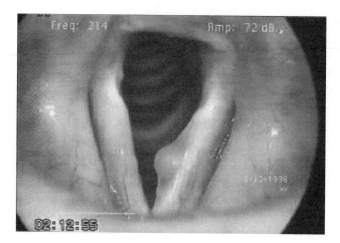

Figure 4.4. Intracordal cyst. See color plate.

a strong similarity to epidermal cysts of the skin. Cornut and Bouchayer (1989) make a clear distinction between epidermoid and retention.

In most patients with intracordal cysts, making the differential diagnosis is difficult. The presence of a dilated blood vessel leading almost directly to the cyst may be one differentiating sign. Pseudocysts are yet another variant. They are easily mistaken for polyps or nodules because they appear in the same area. They tend to be unilateral and have a translucent appearance. They occur most frequently in young adult women (Bouchayer, Cornut, Witzig, Loire, Roch, & Bastian, 1985; Monday, 1983). Cysts often occur in professional voice users. The cause of cysts is not entirely clear, but it is thought that vocal trauma may be a contributory factor that starts the process of cyst development.

Perceptual Signs and Symptoms

Typical signs of a cyst include hoarseness and a lowered pitch. The patient may report a "tired" voice.

Our sample of cyst patients consisted of 3 men and 9 women. The most frequent dysphonia severity rating was "moderate." One patient had missing data; therefore, the data presented in the following sections were pooled across severity ratings from 11 patients.

Acoustic Signs

The female patients in our sample of patients with vocal fold intracordal retention cysts exhibited a significantly lower than normal value for phonational range. No other differences were statistically significant. This was the only acoustic measure that reached significance.

It is also possible that different types of cysts may produce differing acoustic signs.

Measurable Physiological Signs

Again, there are few physiological data available regarding patients with cysts. However, higher than normal average airflows might be expected if glottal closure is incomplete and as a result of elevated offset flows and higher than normal peak flows. The closing phase of the vocal folds, as seen in an electroglottogram, also may be slower than normal.

Observable Physiological Signs

Laryngoscopy. Identification of a cyst can be very difficult. Bouchayer et al. (1985) reported that in only 10% of their cases was a cyst obvious on initial examination. However, the appearance of fullness of the vocal fold and dilated capillaries raised the suspicion of a cyst in 55% of cases. Endoscopically, cysts are sometimes highlighted by a persistent light reflection from the slightly raised area of the cyst. The tell-tale sign noted above, of a dilated and prominent blood vessel, can further be described as a vessel that flows laterally or irregularly across the fold and appears to terminate at the site of the cyst.

Stroboscopy. Stroboscopy has been found to be very helpful in the diagnosis of a cyst because there is an absence of mucosal wave in the area over the cyst, and the typically round shape of the lesion is very visible. Other signs include greater aperiodicity and reduced glottal closure (Kitzing, 1985). In our sample of 12 patients with cysts, 42% had an hourglass closure pattern, 33% a posterior chink pattern, and 25% had complete closure. We have also noted that the vibration of the two folds was often asymmetric, especially over the area of the cyst (Colton, Woo, Brewer, Griffin, & Casper, 1995). Amplitude of the affected side, in particular, was decreased in our patient sample.

Pathophysiology

A cyst originates in the superficial layer of the lamina propria (Hirano, 1981a). As the encapsulated lesion grows, it increases the distance between the cover and the lamina propria but usually does not extend into the layers. A cyst increases the mass and stiffness of the cover, whereas the transition layers and the body are unaffected.

Edema

PRIMARY VOICE SYMPTOM: HOARSENESS

Description and Etiology

Although edema refers to the buildup of fluid that occurs primarily in the superficial vocal folds, all edema does not have the same appearance or cause as in the layers of the lamina propria. The outermost layer includes Reinke's space, which comprises loose, pliable fibers. When it occurs in the first layer of the lamina propria, fluid collects at this site, and it is referred to as Reinke's edema because Reinke's space occurs in this layer (Fig. 4.5). Other names used to refer to this condition are diffuse polyposis or polypoid degeneration. Some apparent swelling of the vocal folds, especially when localized, also may be a sign of a cyst. The lesions are seen bilaterally but are usually asymmetrical in size.

Edema is a natural reaction of tissue to trauma and misuse. It may result from misuse or excessive use of the voice or as a concomitant result of infection or inflammation. Persons taking certain drugs may have edema as a side effect. Edema is often a component of an allergic reaction. When the vocal folds are involved, they appear edematous but tend to be pale. In addition to vocal abuse, chronic Reinke's edema is most often associated with smoking. It appears to occur more frequently in women,

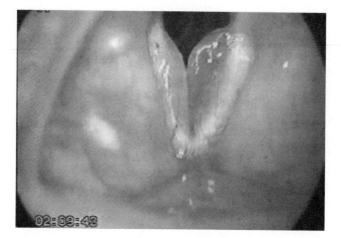

Figure 4.5. Reinke's edema. See color plate.

especially if they are long-term smokers (Bastian, 1986; Nielsen, Hojslet, & Karlsmose, 1986).

Perceptual Signs and Symptoms

Typical symptoms of edema include a lower than normal pitch level and hoarseness. If the Reinke's edema is particularly severe, the patient may complain of shortness of breath because the edematous vocal folds may partially block the airway. In some other cases of edema (not polypoid), patients complain of loss of pitch range and increased effort required to produce voice. Thirteen patients in our group had edema. Twelve of the 13 were female, and, therefore, we only report our data for the female patients.

Acoustic Signs

The fundamental frequency of phonation is lower than that expected for the sex and age of the patient. Bennett, Bishop, and Lumpkin (1987) reported a mean fundamental frequency of 108 Hz for their group of 29 females with Reinke's edema, and 91 Hz for their six male patients. In our sample of 12 patients, the fundamental frequency was lower than normal but the difference failed to reach significance. Jitter and shimmer on the vowel /ah/ were also within normal limits but significantly greater on the vowel /oo/. The only acoustic variable that was significantly lower than normal was dynamic range.

Measurable Physiological Signs

Electromyographic recordings also may show no abnormalities. Our patients showed a significantly greater mean flow rate than normal. Pressures and vocal efficiency measures were within normal limits.

Observable Physiological Signs

Laryngoscopy. In Reinke's edema, the vocal folds have the appearance of enlarged, fluid-filled, boggy structures. They do not appear firm or solid. The edema usually involves most of the full length of the vocal folds bilaterally. In some respects,

Reinke's edema gives the appearance of broad-based polyps occupying the full length of the vocal fold. Vocal folds also may be seen to be edematous, but without the boggy appearance of Reinke's. In such cases, they have a firmer, rounded appearance, rather than flat with a rounded, superior surface along the full length of the folds.

Stroboscopy. Stroboscopic features of Reinke's edema are expected to show greater than normal excursion of the mucosal wave and complete glottal closure. In our published study of four patients with Reinke's edema (Colton, Woo, Brewer, Griffin, & Casper, 1995), the mucosal wave was slightly decreased but glottal closure was complete. In our larger sample of 12 patients, a complete closure pattern was again most frequent, but there were more ratings of moderately decreased and severely decreased mucosal wave. Amplitude of vibration of the vocal folds was also moderately decreased. We have found that the vibration of the two folds was often symmetrical. In superior surface edema, the stroboscopic appearance may be quite different. The vocal folds may appear to be stiffened with reduction of both amplitude of vibration and mucosal wave.

Pathophysiology

Edema affects the superficial layer of the lamina propria. The mass of the cover is increased. However, stiffness of the cover may depend on the specific nature of the lesion. Bennett, Bishop, and Lumpkin (1987) suggested that Reinke's edema disturbs the elasticity of the cover, resulting in decreased stiffness. Such a reduction in stiffness would allow for greater amplitudes of vibration. The transition layers and body are not affected in Reinke's edema. The increase in bulk and reduction of stiffness would contribute to a lowered fundamental frequency of vibration.

Laryngitis

A number of inflammatory conditions are referred to as laryngitis. One is reflux laryngitis, thought to be caused by reflux of the stomach contents. This condition is discussed in a later chapter. Another kind of laryngitis, acute laryngitis, is due to an upper respiratory infection, either bacterial or viral in nature. The third form is caused by phonotrauma and can be either acute or chronic. The following discussion focuses on this last type of noninfectious laryngitis.

In their study of 1,158 patients, Coyle et al. (2001) reported that laryngitis was one of the fifth most frequently occurring pathological conditions that occurred in their identified population. Patients with laryngitis of any form were not included in our study of benign lesions.

PRIMARY VOICE SYMPTOM: HOARSENESS

Description and Etiology

Laryngitis is an inflammation of the vocal folds and larynx. It may result from exposure to noxious agents (tobacco, alcohol, drugs), acidic gastric contents (GERD), environmental agents (allergens, dust), or phonotrauma. Laryngitis also may be the result of upper respiratory infections, which have a generalized effect on the mucosa of the respiratory tract, including the larynx (Fig. 4.6). The problem may be acute or chronic. Acute laryngitis resulting from bacterial or viral infection requires medical attention and is not directly related to phonotrauma. However, it does affect voice production

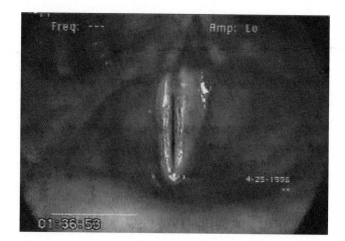

Figure 4.6. Acute laryngitis. See color plate.

and indirectly may be aggravated by vocal excesses, as is described later. Chronic abuse can lead to chronic laryngitis with persistent inflammation and perhaps a thickening and drying of the vocal folds. Laryngitis may lead to tissue changes, such as nodules, polyps, or hypertrophy of the laryngeal epithelium.

Perceptual Signs and Symptoms

The symptoms of laryngitis include marked roughness or hoarseness of the voice with accompanying sensations of discomfort and dryness in the throat. When secondary to infection, the hoarseness may persist for some time after the infection has been controlled. Continued heavy use of the voice during this time may contribute to exacerbate the laryngitis and contribute to the continued hoarseness. The pitch level of the voice may appear to be either higher or lower than normal, and it will be difficult to speak in a loud voice.

Acoustic Signs

Greater than normal frequency and amplitude perturbation would be expected. Takahashi and Koike (1975) found a mean relative average perturbation (RAP) of 0.0069 and 0.0078 in their two female patients with chronic laryngitis. Their nine normal subjects had a mean RAP of 0.00582. Takahashi and Koike (1975) reported a mean fundamental frequency level of 103 Hz for one of their female patients with chronic laryngitis, and 284 Hz for the other. Thus, fundamental frequency may be either elevated or reduced. Fundamental frequency may be related to the severity of the cordal involvement and thus may be either elevated or reduced. One would also expect that phonational range would be reduced (Shipp & Huntington, 1965). Maximum sustainable intensities may be much lower than normal. Finally, there should be greater than normal spectral noise in the voice.

Measurable Physiological Signs

When laryngitis is present, airflow and air pressures may be elevated, especially if there is incomplete glottal closure. However, average airflows appear to be within normal limits (Hirano, 1981b; Hollien, 1975; McGlone, Richmond, & Bosma, 1966). Based on our experience, vibratory airflows show increased variability from one cycle to the next, and there may be greater than normal offset and peak airflows. Woo et al. (1987) reported a mean flow rate of 222 mL/sec for their combined acute, chronic, and post-radiation laryngitis group, collapsed across 7 male and 11 female subjects. (Normal speakers produced a mean flow rate of 144 mL/sec.) The electroglottographic signal may show marked variability from one cycle to the next, although closure times may be normal.

Electromyographic levels would be expected to be normal or slightly elevated.

Observable Physiological Signs

Laryngoscopy. Laryngitic larynges in the acute stages show a marked redness; small, dilated blood vessels may be visible on the inflamed folds. Chronic laryngitis may not be marked by inflammation, but rather by thickened and dry epithelium.

Stroboscopy. The vocal folds may show increased asymmetry and aperiodicity, with reduced mucosal waves and reduced amplitude. We have noted a jerk-like movement of the mucosal wave, in which the wave appears to travel along part of the surface at one speed, then changes its speed for the remainder of its travel. The movement also may be called biphasic (Woo, personal communication, 1988). There is a stiff, jerky quality to this movement.

Pathophysiology

Laryngitis affects the cover of the vocal folds by increasing its stiffness, but may have little effect on the mass of the vocal folds.

Other Comments

Chronic laryngitis, if allowed to continue untreated, may result in serious complications, including laryngitis sicca, which is characterized by marked atrophy of the mucosa of the larynx. The major abnormality is the lack of vocal fold lubrication because of the reduction in or absence of glandular secretions. The vocal folds become dry and sticky, and a chronic cough may be present as the system attempts to remove the thick secretions that gather adherent to the vocal folds tissues. On occasion, laryngeal crusting may result, requiring surgical removal.

Other forms of laryngitis result from diphtheria, tuberculosis, and syphilis, all of which are extremely rare. Another special form of laryngitis is acute epiglottitis, in which the inflammatory changes affect the mucosa of the epiglottis. Epiglottitis may be life threatening if the epiglottis becomes sufficiently enlarged to result in airway obstruction. Emergency treatment may be required. Antibiotics may be used to control the infection, or steroids may be used to reduce the inflammation (Sataloff, 1987a).

Sulcus Vocalis

Sulcus vocalis did not appear in the list of pathological conditions seen in the two ENT practices in Ohio reported by Coyle et al, 2001. We only had 4 patients with sulcus vocalis in our study of patients with benign lesions of the vocal folds.

PRIMARY VOICE SYMPTOM: HOARSENESS

Description and Etiology

Sulcus vocalis refers to a condition in which a furrow along the upper medial edge of the vocal folds is observed. Bastian (1986) describes it as an "epithelial-lined furrow or pocket whose lips parallel the free edge of the cords" (p. 1974). In a cross-section of the vocal folds, the furrow appears as a pocketed ledge on the medial surface of the vocal folds (Fig. 4.7). The longitudinal extent of the furrow is variable, as is its depth. If very deep, it seems to divide the vocal fold in half. According to Arnold (1980), sulcus vocalis may be associated with other laryngeal or oral asymmetries. Ford et al. (1996) described 3 different types of sulci and their differential effects on the lamina propria.

The cause of sulcus vocalis is uncertain, although Bastian (1986) attributes it to vocal misuse and abuse. Luchsinger and Arnold (1965) in their review of the literature summarized the possible causative factors as being congenital, developmental, or traumatic. Bouchayer et al. (1985) argued for a congenital cause. The disorder is rather rare, at least in Europe and the United States (Luchsinger & Arnold, 1965); it may be more prevalent in Japan (Hirano, 1981b). According to Hirano and Bless (1993), sulcus vocalis is either congenital or the result of repeated chronic inflammatory processes.

Perceptual Signs and Symptoms

Symptoms include a breathy, hoarse voice quality that apparently is caused by incomplete closure of the vocal folds and disturbed vibratory behavior. Hirano et al., 1990, reported that 64% of their patient sample of 126 with sulcus vocalis had a mild breathiness. Lindestad and Hertegard (1994) estimated that the pitch was higher than normal in 72% of their sulcus patients.

Acoustic Signs

Hirano et al. (1990) reported jitter (PPQ) and shimmer (APQ) within normal limits for their sample of 126 patients. Normalized noise energy was also within normal limits. Maximum phonation time was only slightly shorter (18.1 seconds) than normal.

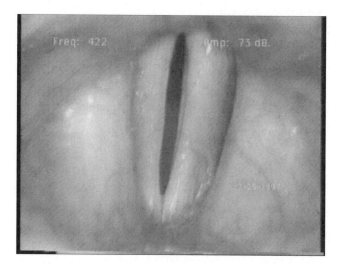

Figure 4.7. Vergeture (sulcus). See color plate.

Phonational ranges were 22.7 semitones for unilateral sulci and 19.4 semitones for bilateral sulci, a value lower than would be expected.

Measurable Physiological Signs

Airflows may be slightly elevated (Shigemori, 1977), although Hirano et al. (1990) reported a mean flow rate of 148 mL/sec for patients with unilateral lesions and 195 mL/sec for patients with bilateral lesions. These values are slightly higher than the mean flow rates for normal speakers (see Chapter 14) but are probably within normal limits. We found that in our 4 patients, mean flows and peak flows of our patients were greater than would be expected. Leakage flow was within normal limits.

Electroglottographic recordings may show increased perturbation, with the possibility of short closed times.

Observable Physiological Signs

Laryngoscopy. Laryngoscopically, a sulcus will be seen as a depression or line along the upper medial edge of the vocal fold. The depression may be variable in length from partial to the entire length of the vocal fold and may vary in depth from shallow to very deep. Sulci may be either unilateral or bilateral.

Stroboscopy. Hirano at al. (1990) reported an incomplete glottal closure pattern in 69 of their 126 patients with sulcus vocalis in combination with slightly decreased amplitude of vibration and a slightly decreased mucosal wave. Lindestad and Hertegard (1994) reported a spindle-shaped glottal closure pattern as most frequent in their sample of 47 patients with a sulcus. Of these patients, 79% also had a diminished mucosal wave. Forty-nine percent of the patients with bilateral lesions had slightly decreased amplitude of vibration, whereas only 21% of the patients with a unilateral lesion showed a decrease. In cases of unilateral sulcus, a mucosal wave usually can be seen across the superior surface of the uninvolved vocal fold, but it may be diminished in amplitude (Lindestad & Hertegard, 1994).

Pathophysiology

The sulcus is located in the superficial layer of the lamina propria, which decreases the mass of the cover but may increase its stiffness. The body and the transition layers are normal.

Bouchayer and Cornut (1984) have identified a variant of sulcus that they term vergeture. Lindestard and Hertegard (1994) describe a vergeture as an adhesive type of lesion wherein the epithelium attaches directly to the underlying muscle through the division produced by the sulcus. They use the term *sulcus vocalis* to refer to a pocket-like appearance of the mucosa. Distinguishing these two forms of a sulcus may be difficult, especially without the use of a stroboscope, and may only become clear during microscopic laryngeal surgery.

SUMMARY

Phonotrauma is a recently proposed term that is meant to cover the broad category of vocal behaviors that may cause phonatory or laryngeal tissue changes. Such behaviors may include voice misuse and behaviors that are damaging to the vocal fold tissues. The goal of this chapter is to sensitize the practitioner to the many forms that misuse and abuse of the phonatory mechanism may take. As defined here, the primary misuses of the voice include hard glottal attack, elevated laryngeal posture, anteroposterior squeezing, and inappropriate pitch level. Traumatic behaviors include excessive coughing and throat clearing, yelling, shouting, cheerleading-type activities, and prolonged loud talking. These behaviors may result in mechanical trauma to the vocal folds or vocal processes. Continued trauma may result in the production of tissue changes that will alter the vibratory characteristics of the vocal folds, which in turn results in hoarseness or roughness in the voice. In some cases, the tissue alteration will prevent complete glottal closure and result in the production of breathy phonation. An understanding of these behaviors will allow the clinician to help patients make a thorough inventory of their own behaviors.

The goal of this chapter's section on drugs is to increase awareness of the potential phonatory effect of a vast array of pharmaceuticals, many of which are frequently considered to be quite benign, especially if they are of the over-the-counter variety. There are certainly many overriding reasons why drugs must be used in the treatment of various conditions, even if some degree of voice change may occur. However, the practitioner who works with the voice patient must be aware of the effects various drugs may have on voice or on mucosal tissues. This can be particularly critical for the professional voice user.

In the last section, a variety of specific tissue changes associated with vocal misuse and phonotrauma have been reviewed, including vocal nodules, polyps, cysts, edema, laryngitis, and sulcus vocalis. Although some of these conditions may be caused by

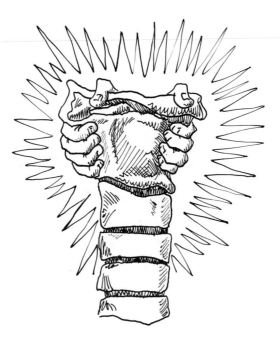

Figure 4.8. Phonotrauma.

infection, viral agents, external trauma, congenital disposition, or disease, phono-trauma is often considered to be directly or indirectly involved as either a precip-itating or exacerbating factor. Recognition of the contribution of phonotrauma to these conditions is necessary to arrive at a treatment protocol that will be effec-tive in reducing or eliminating these damaging vocal behaviors, restoring the voice to the best quality attainable, with the least trauma and expense to the patient (Fig. 4.8).

Chapter 5

Voice Problems Associated With Nervous System Involvement

ROLE OF THE NERVOUS SYSTEM

The nervous system is that portion of the body concerned with the control of body functions. Viewed as a unit, it is responsible for the total control of all systems in the body, even self-regulating systems that are capable of carrying out their own functions. The smaller units of the body's organizational system (cells, tissues, and organs) function only within their own little world and in an environment that must be controlled. It is the responsibility of the nervous system to create this environment by regulating systems that provide for the proper nourishment, temperature regulation, gas exchange, and by-product disposal necessary for all the component parts to work effectively.

Coordination of function is another aspect of the control exerted by the nervous system. One system must work at the proper time if another system is to function properly. Within a system, the various parts must perform their tasks at the proper times for the final output of the system to be meaningful and productive. The necessity for coordination is even more apparent in the production of skilled motor acts involving the various striated muscles of the body. Simple walking is an example of a highly skilled motor act involving the properly timed contraction and relaxation of various muscles for its smooth action.

The nervous system is divided into two major parts: the central nervous system (CNS) and the peripheral nervous system (PNS). The CNS is that portion residing within the cranial cavity or skull and vertebral column. The peripheral nervous system (PNS) resides throughout the body outside of the cranium. The CNS is responsible for the initiation and coordination of function, whereas the PNS carries the instructions of the CNS to the various organs and muscles of the body.

The nervous system also may be divided into two components, according to whether information is conducted to the CNS (afferent) or from the CNS (efferent). Indeed, information from muscles, organs, and tissues is needed by the CNS for proper control to be maintained. Information from the outside world via the several senses is also used by the CNS to make it possible for the body to exist in the hostile world. Without the nervous system, the body cannot live. With a damaged nervous system, the body cannot function "normally" in its environment.

GENERAL CHARACTERISTICS OF NERVOUS SYSTEM DYSFUNCTION

The nervous system may malfunction because of disease, abnormal growths, accidents, or trauma. The nature of the malfunction will depend on where the problem occurs. In some cases there will be difficulty in initiating an action or activity, whereas in others the activity will begin without difficulty but control of it may be impaired. In still other cases, incoming information will be distorted or nonexistent, so that the nervous system will not have the proper information for the control of motor or organ activity appropriate for the task at hand.

The CNS is responsible for initiating skilled motor acts that involve the starting and stopping of motor activity. Walking is a good example of an activity that must be initiated and terminated. Most internal body functions are ongoing; that is, once started, they continue or else the body will to cease to function (e.g., blood flow, respiration, temperature regulation). Other internal body functions are episodic and may be stopped and started (e.g., digestion, hormone production). Speech itself is a very good example of an act that is constantly started and stopped even during its execution. There are centers and cells within the CNS that have this function of starting an act. If damaged, the initiation of the act may not take place or will be delayed, uncertain, or otherwise impaired.

The CNS also coordinates function. There are many examples of the need for coordination of body systems, the act of walking being just one. Speech is also a highly coordinated event involving coordination within and among bodily systems (e.g., phonation, respiration, articulation). Damage to the CNS may affect control of coordinated function.

Lower brain centers, including the spinal cord, maintain a measure of control, albeit local, on muscles and systems. For example, muscles must be maintained in a state of readiness for action. Muscle tone reflects this state of readiness. Muscles show steady levels of electrical activity even when they are not being used for a motor act. This state of readiness is often regulated and maintained by lower neuron systems. The CNS exerts its control by inhibiting the activity of the lower centers, so that they do not get out of control. Damage to the CNS can result in the disruption of this inhibition and the production of unnecessary or unwanted movements.

Finally, incoming sensory information is critical for the control process. The CNS must know when the right foot has touched the floor to command the left leg to rise and move the left foot forward. Otherwise the walker will fall flat on his face or cease moving. The CNS relies on visual information to properly control the hand and arm in reaching for the glass of water on the kitchen table. Deprived of sensory information, the organism will not know about the environment and its potential effects. Incoming sensory information need not be entirely external. Internal sensory information is also critical for neural control. Examples of internal sensory information include joint kinesthetics, position sense, pain, pressure, and temperature. Kinesthetic feedback from joints and muscles must be available if skilled movements are to be possible. The job of the CNS is to receive and integrate information and prepare a proper plan for dealing with it.

ROLE OF THE NERVOUS SYSTEM IN PHONATION AND SPEECH

Speech is a complex, fine motor act that involves several diverse systems or parts of systems for its execution. The respiratory system, basically designed for the exchange of gases for use by the tissues of the body, is also used for speech, with contributions from the digestive system, primarily the mouth, jaw, and teeth. Speech requires the use of the respiratory system mechanically, that is, for the generation and control of the airflows and pressures needed for speaking. Thus, the control of the respiratory system for life support and the control of the respiratory system for speaking are quite different. The nervous system must provide the control appropriate to the task at hand. Furthermore, during speech, there must be a high level of coordination among the chest wall, the abdominal mechanical system, the larynx and pharynx, and the lips, tongue, teeth, and mandible so that all function at the proper time and for the length of time necessary for the production of the individual sounds. During the act of speaking, the system receives information about the state of its structures and muscles via both kinesthetic and acoustic feedback. Thus, the auditory system is yet another important system that must enter into the control exercised by the nervous system.

Disease, malformation, or injury will affect the control capabilities of the nervous system. The manifestation of nervous system damage will vary depending on where the lesion occurs. If the lesion occurs at the cortex, many components of speech may be affected, including the ability to use language, to initiate speech, to produce muscle movements necessary to produce intelligible speech or control muscle movements, or to receive information from the body systems about where they are and what they have done. The symptoms and signs that the patient presents are critical to the proper diagnosis of the problem and identification of the source of the problem.

In this book, we are interested in the effects of nervous system damage on the control of phonation. Although the system remains complex, a finite set of brain sites and pathways have been shown to be important for the control of phonation. Lesions will produce specific symptoms that will help the diagnostician identify the site of lesion. Some of the possible problems affecting phonation and their possible locations in the nervous system are discussed by Barlow, Netsell, and Hunker (1986). They note that in the lateral precentral cortex, a convergence of pathways from other parts of the brain appears to be the site of the final common pathway through the brain to the periphery. Lesions at this site would be expected to result in complete loss of phonation, because input from the higher control centers will have been lost. Furthermore, lesions in this area and other adjacent areas also would be expected to produce loss of function in other muscles concerned with speech. Consequently, such lesions will be expected to produce aphonia or dysphonia, dysarthria, and perhaps even aphasia. Lesions in the anterior cingulate cortex are also reported to produce akinetic mutism in humans (Barlow, Netsell, & Hunker, 1986). In monkeys this area seems to be critical for the control of conditional, learned vocalization. Lesions in other areas of the brain (e.g., basal ganglia, periaqueductal gray) produce a disruption in phonation characterized by breathiness, roughness, tremor, or complete disruption of vocalization. Lesions in the cerebellum result in ataxic dysarthria and changes in the velocity of lip and jaw movements and would presumably affect the speed of movements of structures in the larynx. Larson, Sutton, and Lindeman (1978) concluded that the cerebellum is very important in the control of pitch and loudness of phonation but is not required for the initiation of phonation.

One way to consider the neurological problems that affect phonation would recognize the levels of organization within the nervous system, as discussed previously. The following is such a scheme, proposed by Ward, Hanson, and Berci (1981). It is both simple and effective as an aid in understanding how a specific lesion or syndrome may affect phonation.

1. Afferent sensory, autonomic
    Sympathetic Nervous System: prepares body for stressful situations, producing a fight-or-flight type of response
    Parasympathetic Nervous System: restores body to normal after excitement and acts to calm the system

2. Efferent motor
    Upper motor neuron (cortex and pyramidal tracts)
    Extrapyramidal (reticular substance)
    Cerebellar
    Nuclear (lower motor neurons)

ORGANIZATION OF THE NERVOUS SYSTEM AND VOICE PATHOLOGY

The following section is a brief review of the major systems involved in phonation. More complete information about the nervous system can be found in Chapter 13. Ward et al. (1981) discuss the role of the afferent or sensory system in the control of phonation. Our discussion here concentrates on the efferent or motor system involved in the control of phonation.

In the cortex, area 4 of the precentral gyrus is very important in the control of vocalization. Neurons from this and other areas of the cortex converge to form the corticobulbar tracts. These tracts pass through the internal capsule and cerebral peduncle and eventually constitute what is known as the pyramidal tracts (Fig 5.1). At the upper part of the medulla, many fibers cross over (decussate) to the opposite side and continue down to the nucleus ambiguus in the brainstem. As discussed in Chapter 13, the nucleus ambiguus houses the motor nuclei for the 9th, 10th, and 11th cranial nerves. Thus, lesions anywhere along this pathway may involve the precentral cortex, the corticobulbar tracts, the internal capsule or the cerebral peduncles, the medulla, the brainstem, or the nucleus ambiguus itself, causing differential effects on phonation.

The extrapyramidal system (Fig 5.2) consists of the reticular substance, corpus striatum (with the caudate and lenticular nuclei), and the basal ganglia (specifically the globus pallidus and the substantia nigra) (Ward, Hanson, & Berci, 1981). Lesions here affect the coordination of laryngeal function. Athetoid movements are characteristic of patients with lesions in these areas. Degeneration of the basal ganglia and the reticular substance produce the symptoms typical of parkinsonism (see later section on parkinsonism for a more complete discussion of this disease). The Shy-Drager syndrome, in which there is progressive abductor paralysis of the larynx, is thought to be a disease affecting the extrapyramidal system, as well as the motor nuclei of the vagus (see later section on Shy-Drager syndrome for a more complete discussion of this disease).

Lesions in the cerebellum affect the coordination of motor function and result in slurred speech and problems with coordination of the various speech systems, as well as nonspeech symptoms, such as ataxia, nystagmus, and gait problems. The voice may

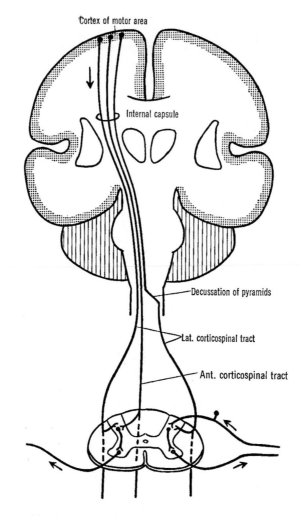

Figure 5.1. Schematic of the direct (pyramidal) motor pathway. (From Gardner, E., Fundamentals of Neurology. Philadelphia: WB Saunders Co, 1963.)

exhibit a breathy quality, or it may exhibit spastic behavior. In the Arnold-Chiari malformation, for example, the vocal folds may typically demonstrate involuntary abduction (see later section on Arnold-Chiari malformation for a more complete discussion).

Lower motor neuron problems occur in the brainstem and medulla. Many syndromes result from lesions in the medulla and voice will be affected, as will the functioning of the palate, pharynx, tongue, face, and other body parts. Lesions in the nucleus ambiguus may produce classic symptoms of a combined paralysis of the superior and recurrent laryngeal nerves, resulting in flaccid vocal folds. Such lesions, depending on their extent, also may affect the palate and pharynx.

Finally, there can be an interruption of control in the peripheral nerves supplying the larynx itself. Such a disturbance can result from lesions or injury to the superior laryngeal nerve, the recurrent laryngeal nerve, or both. Furthermore, the lesions may be either unilateral or bilateral. Again, the specific symptoms presented by the patient will help to determine the proper diagnosis and locus of the problem.

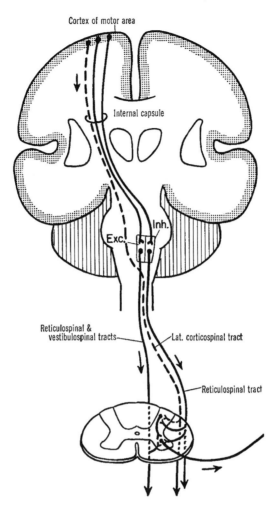

Figure 5.2. Schematic of the indirect (extrapyramidal) motor pathway. (From Gardner, E., Fundamentals of Neurology. Philadelphia: WB Saunders Co, 1963.)

In some voice problems, neurological involvement is suspected but cannot be determined with certainty. Some of these problems may involve diffuse areas of the brain, and no specific single site of lesion can be determined. In other instances, the cause is unknown or described as idiopathic in nature. However, "unknown" or "idiopathic" is not a diagnosis. It should signify a temporary condition during which further data are gathered in the search for the diagnosis. A more precise diagnosis may result from additional testing, but occasionally the simple passage of time reveals additional symptoms that help to refine the diagnosis. In some cases, a more specific diagnosis may remain undetermined or unknown.

In the following discussion about specific neurological problems that affect the voice, a primary vocal symptom will be stated. In most cases, this refers to the most frequently reported symptom for that disease, as reported by Aronson, Brown, Litin, and Pearson (1968b). In some cases, other studies were used to identify the primary vocal symptom. There usually are additional voice symptoms associated with each neurological problem. These are discussed for each disease in the section entitled "Perceptual Voice Signs and Symptoms."

CLASSIFICATION OF NEUROLOGICAL VOICE DISORDERS BASED ON PHONATORY DYSFUNCTION

Ramig and Scherer (1992) have proposed an organizational scheme that focuses on the phonatory dysfunction affected by the disorder and emphasizes the general form of treatment for it. In this way, the speech–language pathologist (SLP) is provided an over-all framework within which to direct treatment. Three general categories of phonatory dysfunction may be affected by neurological disorders. These are (a) adduction problems; (b) stability problems; and (c) coordination problems (Ramig & Scherer, 1992; Smith & Ramig, 1995). The authors recognize that a given neurological problem may affect one or more of the three areas. The overall organizational framework is shown in Table 5.1.

Table 5.1. Classification of Neurological Disorders of Voice Based on Phonatory Dysfunction

Classification	Neurological Disorder
I. Adduction or Abduction Problems	
A. Hypoadduction	Myasthenia gravis
	Parkinsonism
	Peripheral nerve paresis/paralysis
	Shy-Drager
	Supranuclear palsy
B. Hyperadduction	Adductor SD
	Huntington's disease
	Pseudobulbar palsy
C. Malabduction	
II. Phonatory Stability	
A. Short-term (jitter & shimmer)	Most neurological disorders
B. Long-term (tremor)	Essential tremor
	Parkinsonism
	ALS
III. Phonatory Incoordination/ Voiced-Voiceless Distinction	Abductor SD
IV. Mixed Disorders	Cerebellar ataxia
	Multiple sclerosis
V. Miscellaneous Disorders	Tourette syndrome
	Other miscellaneous disorders (see Table 5.5)

Adapted from Table 14-2, Smith and Ramig, 1995.

ADDUCTION OR ABDUCTION PROBLEMS

HYPOADDUCTION

Myasthenia Gravis

PRIMARY VOICE SYMPTOM: BREATHINESS

Description and Etiology

"Myasthenia gravis is a chronic autoimmune neuromuscular disease characterized by degrees of weakness of the skeletal (voluntary) muscles of the body (NINDS Myasthenia Gravis Information Page, http://www.ninds.nih.gov). Patients with myasthenia gravis show a characteristic weakening of the striated muscles and a prolonged return of function after activation. Muscles innervated by cranial nerves seem most susceptible to this disease. The disease is relatively rare, with an incidence of 2 to 10 per 100,000 (Garfinkle & Kimmelman, 1982). It tends to affect the sexes differentially in terms of incidence and age of onset. It occurs twice as often in women and much earlier than in men. Onset for women is reported in the 3rd decade of life, whereas in men it is during the 6th decade (Garfinkle & Kimmelman, 1982).

Patients with myasthenia gravis tend to show bulbar symptoms, with the earliest and most common being ptosis or drooping of the eyelids (Grob, 1961). Other symptoms include diplopia, weakness of the legs, fatigue, dysphagia, dysphonia, and blurred vision. All patients will not exhibit all symptoms. Furthermore, these symptoms are not unique to myasthenia gravis but are encountered in other disease states. The symptom of diplopia, for example, can be associated with infection, glioma of the brainstem, multiple sclerosis, toxicity, aneurysms, tumors, and trauma (Baker, 1958). Paralysis or muscle weakness also can be a sign of poliomyelitis or brainstem glioma in children. In adults, paralysis can be a sign of poliomyelitis, Guillain-Barré syndrome, brainstem glioma, cerebellopontine angle tumor, cerebral artery occlusion, amyotrophic lateral sclerosis, and pseudobulbar palsy or tumor (Tucker & Lavertu, 1992; Stuart, 1965). Carpenter, McDonald, and Howard (1979) emphasized the need for differential diagnosis among myasthenia gravis, amyotrophic lateral sclerosis, and multiple sclerosis. The unique features of myasthenia gravis are fatigability, fluctuation of function, and restoration of function after rest. These features do not occur in amyotrophic lateral sclerosis or multiple sclerosis. The voice symptoms of myasthenia gravis, because of their variability, have been mistaken for aphonia of psychological origin (Ball & Lloyd, 1971).

Some myasthenia gravis patients may present with voice or speech dysfunction as their initial symptom. Wolski (1967) reported a case of myasthenia gravis in which nasality was the initial presenting symptom. Colton and Brewer (1985) and Levine, Hatlali, and Zaggy (1985) each reported cases diagnosed as myasthenia gravis that presented unusual fiberoptic laryngoscopic findings.

In myasthenia gravis, the body's autoimmune system produces antibodies that block, alter, or destroy receptors for acetylcholine. Several tests are used in the diagnosis of myasthenia gravis. A special blood test detects immune molecules or acetylcholine receptor antibodies. A Tensilon test may be used to test for this disease. A positive response to the injection of Tensilon results in improved muscle strength and tone. Slight to moderate improvements should be interpreted with caution, because similar improvement has been noted in patients with brainstem lesions, oculomotor palsy, diabetic abducens paresis, and even in some normal subjects. The treatment of myasthenia gravis is primarily pharmacological, with occasional necessity for excision of the thymus gland.

Perceptual Voice Signs and Symptoms

The primary symptom of myasthenia gravis is the general fatigability of muscle function in the head, neck, tongue, pharynx, and larynx. Voice signs include hoarseness, breathy voice, and vocal weakness (Carpenter, McDonald, & Howard, 1979). In one study, 60% of myasthenia gravis patients presented voice symptoms (Rontal, Rontal, Leuchter, & Rolnick, 1978). The following voice characteristics were reported in ratings of 11 patients with myasthenia gravis: hypernasality, nasal emission, inspiratory voice, dysphonia, intermittent aphonia, and aspirate voice (Maxwell & Locke, 1969). Interestingly, these symptoms were completely eliminated with pharmacological treatment.

A more recent study (Mao et al., 2001) of 40 patients reported that 65% of the group exhibited hoarseness; 52.5% exhibited vocal fatigue; 30%, difficulty with pitch variation; and 20% had a breathy voice. Five or fewer patents had other symptoms.

Acoustic Signs

Few studies have been reported about the acoustic characteristics of voice in patients with myasthenia gravis. In a study of 11 women and 1 man with myasthenia gravis, average fundamental frequency of speech was found to be very similar to normal expectations in both medicated and unmedicated states (Maxwell & Locke, 1969).

Rontal et al. (1978) presented spectrographic evidence of aperiodicity and high-frequency noise in the speech of patients with myasthenia gravis.

Walker (1997) described a case of a patient whose major acoustic characteristics of the disease was a slow, steady reduction of fundamental frequency during a sustained vowel. He referred to this characteristic as the "sinking pitch sign."

Mao et al. (2001) reported lower than normal values of speaking fundamental frequency compared with age-matched and sex-matched controls (154.3 Hz vs. 172 Hz). Maximum phonation time was also reduced (16.8 seconds vs. 27.4 seconds). Shimmer, however, appeared to be within normal limits.

Measurable Physiological Signs

Electromyographic studies have shown a characteristic decrement of activity with repetitive stimulation (Warren, Gutmann, & Cody, 1977). We have studied the airflow and electroglottogram characteristics of a patient with myasthenia gravis. The data are shown in Figure 5.3. Note the extremely long opening phase of the airflow waveform cycles with a rather slow closing phase (but faster than the opening phase). The electroglottogram waveform seems to mirror these slow opening and closing phases of the vocal folds. The airflow/slope ratio (ratio of the closing slope to the opening slope) and the electroglottogram closing time were significantly greater than for normal subjects.

Mao et al. (2001) reported a significantly greater mean airflow rate for their sample of 40 patients (294.5 mL/sec vs. 111.5 mL/sec for normal control group).

Observable Physiological Signs

The characteristic sign seen in laryngoscopic evaluations is sluggishness of vocal fold abduction. Continued phonation by a patient with myasthenia gravis over time may show increasing weakness of arytenoid and vocal fold motion. Normal movement will return, however, with sufficient rest.

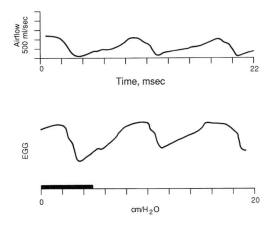

Figure 5.3. Inverse filtered airflow and electroglottogram (EGG) waveforms for a 65-year-old woman with myasthenia gravis. Note the extremely long opening phase of the vocal folds and the slow closing phase. The electroglottogram waveform mirrors these slow variations of vibration. Lung pressure was within normal limits.

There is one report of the stroboscopic signs associated with myasthenia gravis (Maeo at al., 2001) in which 92.5% of the patents exhibited what is termed mobility deficits either unilaterally or bilaterally. These deficits included mucosal wave decrements and asymmetries in phase closure and amplitude.

Pathophysiology

Muscle weakness will be expected to affect the patient's ability to raise the vocal pitch and produce a loud voice. However, these changes may occur only when the mechanism has fatigued after phonation over time. The inability to maintain the proper tension in the vocal folds will result in increased aperiodicity and the inability to maintain good glottal closure. These conditions will produce roughness or hoarseness and breathiness in the voice. Drugs can help relieve some of the symptoms of myasthenia gravis. Neostigmine and pyridostigmine (Mestinon, Valeant Pharmaceuticals, Costa Mesa, CA) are often prescribed. Immunosuppressive drugs are often used. In some cases, a thymectomy is performed. Plasmapheresis also may bring improvement (Sanders & Scopetta, 1994).

Parkinsonism

PRIMARY VOICE SYMPTOMS: MONOPITCH AND REDUCED LOUDNESS

Description and Etiology

Parkinson's disease (PD) is a progressive, degenerative disease of the CNS affecting the basal ganglia, specifically the substantia nigra, resulting in depletion of dopamine. There is also a decrease of dopamine in the caudate nucleus and the putamen. The disease results in rigidity, resting tremor, and reduced range of movement in the limbs, neck, and head. The general characteristic of PD is a slowness of movement and loss of automatic movements, referred to as bradykinesia (Brin, Fahn, Blitzer, Ramig, & Stewart, 1992). Bradykinesia also encompasses the masked facies or absence of facial expression, decreased eye blinking, decreased spontaneous swallowing, and difficulty in initiating movement on command that are features of PD. The amplitude of voluntary movement as well as postural and righting reflexes are impaired (Hoehn & Yahr, 1967). All movements may be affected. The muscles are not paralyzed but rather are hypokinetic and lack the dynamic aspects of movement. Respiratory movements also are affected, producing a shallow and irregular respiratory cycle sometimes at twice the normal frequency (Ramig & Gould, 1986). Patients may have a limited vital capacity and inspiratory capacity. These respiratory deficits may contribute to the patient's ability to produce speech of normal loudness and utterance length. Laryngeal muscle involvement also contributes to the difficulty in initiating phonation, producing adequate loudness, and varying pitch.

Although the cause of any particular case of PD is usually unknown, several causes have been hypothesized or been directly linked to the disease. Some cases of PD have been traced to a disease called encephalitis lethargica, which occurred in small epidemics in the 1920s. The last reported cases of this disease were in the 1940s (Duvoisin, 1976). With the recognition of post-encephalitic parkinsonism, the concept of multiple causes for the disease became understood. Other possible causes include an undetermined slow-growing virus, head trauma, toxic buildup, drugs, vascular trauma, or carbon monoxide poisoning (Darley, Aronson, & Brown, 1975). Iatrogenic PD is caused by antipsychotic phenothiazine drugs. It is usually reversible by withdrawal of the drug or sometimes by reduction in dosage.

Patients with Parkinson's disease may be classified into several distinct groups. The first, often referred to as idiopathic Parkinson's disease (IPD), displays the classic symptoms of this disease. Parkinson plus syndrome (PPS) involves multiple symptom atrophy. One of these syndromes is called Shy-Drager and is discussed separately. The speech and voice deficits in PPS are usually more severe, and they deteriorate faster than in patients with IPD. Other possible groups include post-encephalic parkinsonism, iatrogenic parkinsonism, juvenile parkinsonism, and secondary or symptomatic parkinsonism (Duvoisin, 1976).

Parkinson's patients can be staged according to the severity of the symptoms as discussed by Hoehn and Yahr (1967). The scale used is arbitrary but is based on the level of clinical disability observed. The stages and their definition are displayed in Table 5.2. According to the data presented by Hoehn and Yahr, staging tends to be correlated with the duration of the illness ($r = 0.97$). Other rating systems also have been proposed to assess the physical status and limitations and daily living problems that might be encountered (Martínez-Martín & Bermejo-Pareja, 1988). Speech and voice disorders are present in 75% of persons with PD, and virtually 100% will develop

Table 5.2. Stages of Degree of Severity for Patients With Parkinson's Disease

Stage	Description
I	Unilateral involvement only
II	Bilateral or midline involvement
III	Impaired righting reflexes (unsteadiness in turning or sudden change from a standing position)
IV	Severely disabling disease; patient can walk or stand but is otherwise incapacitated
V	Patient confined to bed or wheelchair

From Hoehn and Yahr, 1967.

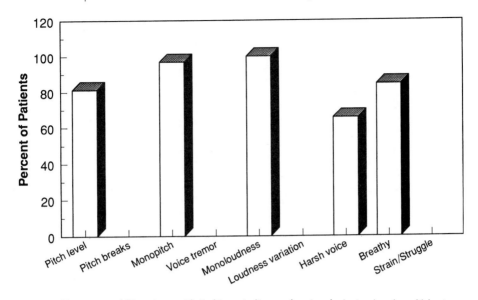

Figure 5.4. Percentage of 32 patients with Parkinson's disease showing deviant voice signs. Voice tremor was rated during contextual speech.

problems in these areas as the disease progresses into the more debilitating stages (Oxtoby, 1982; Streifler & Hofman, 1984).

Perceptual Voice Signs and Symptoms

The most frequently rated voice dimensions, as reported by Aronson et al. (1968b) (Fig. 5.4), were monopitch, excessively low pitch, and harshness. According to Aronson et al. (1968b), variability of loudness is reduced, but rate of speech is highly variable, sometimes with fast bursts and at other times a slow rate. The reduced variability of vocal loudness, pitch, and rate are thought to be the consequence of muscle rigidity and hypokinesia. Speech production is also affected by slurring and phoneme misarticulations, again associated directly with the physical symptoms described.

In a study of 200 patients with Parkinson's disease, Logemann, Fisher, Boches, and Blonsky (1978) found that 87% showed some laryngeal dysfunction and that 45% had laryngeal dysfunction as the only symptom. The specific voice signs these authors reported were breathiness (15%), roughness (29%), hoarseness (45%), and tremulousness (13.5%). Ramig (1995) reports that reduced vocal loudness is a classic speech symptom along with those noted previously. This vocal loudness reduction may be one of the first signs of PD (Aronson, 1985).

Acoustic Signs

Numerous acoustic characteristics of the voices of individuals with PD have been studied with mixed results (Aronson et al, 1968a; Canter, 1963; Canter, 1965; Kent et al., 1994; King et al., 1994; Logemann et al., 1978; Ludlow et al., 1983; Ramig et al., 1988; Ramig et al., 1990; Zwirner et al., 1991). The conflicting results of many of these studies probably had to do with the nature of the subject pool and differences in methodology and analysis procedures (Table 5.3).

Available acoustic data suggest that in patients with Parkinson's disease, the mean fundamental frequency is similar to that of normal speakers, but the variability of

Table 5.3. Some Acoustic Characteristics of Patients With Parkinson's Disease

Measure	Ludlow et al., 1983	Ramig et al., 1989	Zwirner et al., 1991	Kent et al., 1994
Avg Fund Freq (Hz)	163.9	128	120	140.7
SD FF	34.5	16	21	22
N	7[a]	8	12	22
Jitter (%)				
Average		1.26		
SD		1.05		
Jitter (ms)				
Mean			0.1	0.17
SD				0.17
Jitter ratio				
Mean	7.21			
SD	2.97			
Shimmer				
Mean		5.18	6	5.42
SD		3.43	6.6	3.2
Signal-to-Noise Ratios				
Mean		14.75	17.5	18.85
SD		2.97	4.5	4.64

[a] *Includes 4 males and 3 females.*

fundamental frequency within a speech segment is increased, probably reflecting loss of control of the motor act. Jitter and shimmer are also increased, whereas the signal-to-noise ratio is slightly decreased.

Measurable Physiological Signs

Aerodynamic. Jiang et al. (1999) reported some aerodynamic measurements made on 24 patients with stage 4 severity of Parkinson disease and 17 normal speakers of equivalent age. Mean subglottal air pressures were significantly higher in the Parkinson group compared with the normal control group. Airflow rates were not significantly different between the two groups. Laryngeal resistance was also significantly higher in the Parkinsonism group. Lin, Jiang, Hone, and Hanson (1998) found that the Parkinson group (n = 15) had significantly greater speed quotients (SQ) than their control group (n = 15) as obtained from photoglottographic recordings. They observed that the opening time of the vocal folds was longer in the patient group, which they interpreted to reflect increased rigidity of laryngeal muscles. Speed quotient may be a good measurement to make in patients suspected of PD.

Patients with PD appear to produce higher resting and background activity in the interarytenoid and posterior cricoarytenoid muscles (Guidi, Bannister, & Gibson, 1981). Lip muscles also show greater resting and background activity levels, and the degree of activity seems to be related to the side of the body most affected by the disease (Leanderson, Meyerson, & Persson, 1972). Luschei et al. (1999) reported significantly lower firing rates of the thyroarytenoid muscle in their Parkinson groups compared with a young control group. However, the firing rates were not much different for their elderly male group, suggesting that any change of firing rate of this muscle may be more attributable to aging than to the effects of the disease.

Observable Physiological Signs

Laryngoscopy.   Cisler (1927) reported diminished vocal fold movement, and Schilling (1925) described a rigor of the vocal folds. Darley et al. (1969b) reported no abnormal laryngoscopic signs. The most extensive description of laryngoscopic signs in PD patients was reported by Hanson, Gerratt, and Ward (1984). They studied 32 patients, of whom 30 had abnormal laryngoscopic signs. The most prominent sign was bowed vocal folds, and the vocal folds appeared to vibrate with greater amplitude. In 26 patients, varying degrees of laryngeal asymmetry were observed. Many patients showed a characteristic pattern consisting of a more posterior position of the vocal process, a more posterior and lateral position of the apex of the arytenoid, and a more contracted ventricular fold than seen in normal speakers. These signs were associated with the side of the body affected by the disease. Many patients also showed overclosure of the vocal folds, and 5 of the 32 exhibited an extreme degree of supraglottal constriction.

Stroboscopy.   There have been two reports on the stroboscopic signs of Parkinson's disease (Perez, Ramig, Smith, & Dromey, 1994; Smith, Ramig, Dromey, Perez, & Samandari, 1994). Smith et al. (1994) studied 22 patients with IPD. Both flexible and rigid endoscopes were used to view and record the laryngeal images as the patients produced a sustained /ee/. The images were visually rated by four experienced raters on glottal closure configuration, degree of glottal incompetence, and laryngeal hyperfunction. The results of the glottal closure configuration ratings are shown in Figure 5.5. The severity of glottal incompetence was in the mild range. As a group, the patients showed mild false fold and anterior–posterior approximation. Interestingly, although Hanson et al. (1984) found that the overwhelming majority of their patients had a bowed vocal fold configuration, Smith et al. reported that approximately 50% of

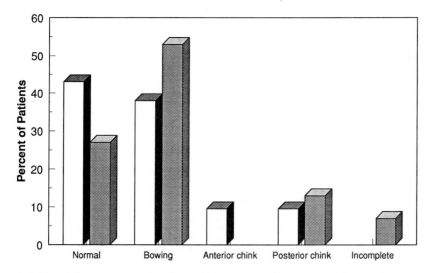

Figure 5.5. Glottal closure patterns of patients with Parkinson's disease as rated from stroboscopic video images. Open bars show data collected from flexible scope recordings, whereas filled bars show data collected from rigid scope recordings.

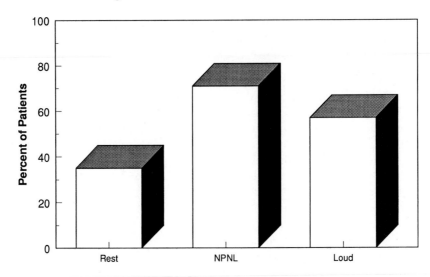

Figure 5.6. Incidence of tremor in structures of the larynx at rest and during phonation at conditions of normal pitch and normal loudness (NPNL) and loud voice among 22 patients with Parkinson's disease.

their patients exhibited such a pattern. The exact percentage depended on the type of scope used to make the recording, i.e., flexible or rigid.

Perez et al. (1994) rated tremor, phase closure, symmetry, amplitude of vocal fold lateral excursion, and excursion of the mucosal wave in 22 patients with IPD. Most of the patients (53%) exhibited tremor on at least one of the three experimental conditions. The incidence of tremor in each experimental condition is shown in Figure 5.6.

The incidence of abnormal strobe findings is shown in Figure 5.7. Many patients showed abnormal phase closure and phase symmetry, probably because of the hypotonic characteristics of Parkinson's patients.

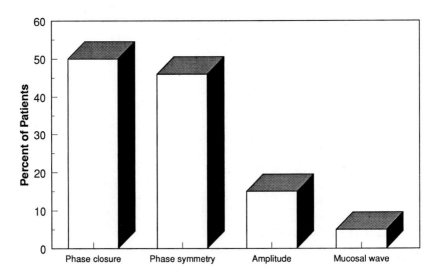

Figure 5.7. Percentage of 22 patients with Parkinson's disease showing abnormal strobe signs during phonation at normal loudness and normal pitch.

In spite of tremor, the stroboscopic signs of patients with PD can be rated successfully. These patients may show a variety of closure configurations, including bowing, anterior chinks, posterior chinks, and incomplete. Some may show a normal closure pattern. The severity of closure probably depends on the degree of severity of the disease, but in the early stages, one might expect mild symptoms, symptoms that might be correlated with the weak intensity voice often heard in these patients.

Pathophysiology

Muscle rigidity and squeezing of structures within the larynx may produce a symptom of strain/struggle in the voice. Unequal tensions in the vocal folds, as noted by Hanson et al. (1984), would be expected to produce aperiodicity, resulting in hoarseness or roughness in the voice. In more advanced stages of the disease process, patients often have much difficulty with chewing and swallowing. Management of saliva and drooling also are problematic. The typical characteristics of PD are mirrored in speech and voice production. Difficulty in initiating movement is seen in initiating speech attempts as it is in initiating walking. Muscle rigidity and hypokinesia are seen in the reduced range of motion of the speech mechanism, which results in reduced loudness (rigidity of respiratory and laryngeal muscles), monotone (rigidity of laryngeal muscles), and imprecise articulation (rigidity of all oral articulators). Tremor may be heard in the voice as well as seen in the extremities.

Shy-Drager Syndrome

PRIMARY VOICE SYMPTOM: HOARSENESS

Description and Etiology

Shy-Drager syndrome is a variant of Parkinson's disease, sometimes referred to as Parkinson's plus. It is a disease of later middle age and affects men more often than women. The major characteristic of Shy-Drager is generalized autonomic nervous system failure. It is considered one of the degenerative neurological disorders that is characterized by multiple system atrophy, not all of which include autonomic nervous system dysfunction. The initial symptoms are postural hypotension (decrease of blood pressure when the patient stands), impotence, and sphincter problems. In their study of 12 patients with Shy-Drager syndrome, Hanson, Ludlow, and Bassich (1983) reported symptoms of weakness of the accessory muscles of respiration, respiratory obstruction, limited movement of the soft palate, and dysphagia. They suggest that these symptoms are indicative of extrapyramidal, pyramidal, and bulbar involvement.

Shy-Drager syndrome was first described in two cases by Shy and Drager (1960). In one case, they were able to examine the brain after the patient's death and reported changes in the spinal cord, autonomic ganglia, and medulla (i.e., marked changes in the inferior olives) and a reduced number of Purkinje cells in the cerebellum, as well as extensive changes in the substantia nigra and the caudate nucleus of the basal ganglia.

Williams, Hanson, and Calne (1979) reported on 12 cases of Shy-Drager syndrome in which eight had moderate to severe bilateral abductor paresis or paralysis of the vocal folds. Two patients, on initial examination, showed a unilateral paresis, but these patients eventually developed bilateral paralysis as the disease progressed. They concluded that the combination of vocal fold paralysis and respiratory difficulties in some of their patients may be consistent with a lesion in the nucleus ambiguus and the retrofacial nucleus. Denervation of the posterior cricoarytenoid muscle, the muscle primarily

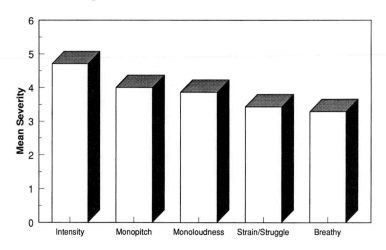

Figure 5.8. Rated severity of voice signs in 7 patients with Shy-Drager syndrome.

responsible for vocal fold abduction, has been reported in Shy-Drager patients who had bilateral abductor vocal fold paralysis (Guidi, Bannister, & Gibson, 1981).

Linebaugh (1979) reviewed 35 patients with Shy-Drager syndrome who presented with a dysarthria. He identified three major types of dysarthria: ataxic, hypokinetic, and mixed. Fifteen of the 35 presented with ataxic dysarthria, which involves the cerebellum and affects the accuracy, force, range, and timing of speech movements; 11 exhibited a hypokinetic dysarthria in which the extrapyramidal system was affected, resulting in muscular rigidity; and 9 showed a mixed dysarthria involving combinations of the extrapyramidal, cerebellar, and pyramidal systems. Linebaugh presented examples of patients with these various types and commented on how careful listening can help to distinguish among them.

Perceptual Voice Signs and Symptoms

The most complete description and study of the speech signs and symptoms of Shy-Drager syndrome was presented by Hanson, Ludlow, and Bassich (1983). They rated the speech of 12 Shy-Drager syndrome patients, using scales reported previously by Darley et al. (1969a). Shy-Drager syndrome patients were rated most severe on scales of rate of speaking (variable rate and rate[1]). The mean ratings on five voice scales are shown in Figure 5.8. The format of this figure is different from that of Figures 5.4 and 5.5. Hanson, Ludlow, and Bassich (1983) did not report the proportion of patients with aberrant ratings on the scales used, probably because of the small number of patients. Rather, the mean ratings were reported using a seven-point scale, in which 1 means normal and 7 means very severe. Other speech scales on which these patients were rated as severe included intensity (this scale may relate to the overall level of voice), imprecise consonants, reduced stress, monopitch, and monoloudness. These authors performed a discriminant analysis of these ratings to determine whether they could separate groups of Shy-Drager syndrome patients from idiopathic Parkinson patients who exhibit some of the same symptoms and from a group of normal subjects. Three scales did a very

---

[1]Variable rate was defined as a rate of speaking that alternates between slow and fast. Rate was defined as a rate of speaking that is abnormally slow or abnormally rapid.

good job of distinguishing among these groups—strain/struggle, glottal fry (a low-pitch, popping sound), and monopitch. Shy-Drager patients were rated higher on impaired function on the scales of strain/struggle and glottal fry than the PD patients but lower (less impaired) on monopitch. Perceptual speech scales may be useful in distinguishing the Shy-Drager syndrome from IPD and normal speakers.

Acoustic Signs

Various indices of perturbation were reported by Ludlow and her colleagues (1983) for a group of seven patients with Shy-Drager, four male and three female. Measurements included perturbation (in msec), DLT (perturbation after removal of fundamental frequency due to linear trend), a diplophonia ratio, fundamental frequency, and duration of phonation. As a group, the Shy-Drager patients had a mean F_0 of 160.3 Hz, compared with an f0 of 127.6 Hz for age- and sex-matched controls; the difference was statistically significant, suggesting perhaps greater vocal fold tension or muscle rigidity.[2] There were no statistically significant differences between the Shy-Drager and normal controls on any measure of frequency perturbation. The data provided some evidence of diplophonia, at least for two of the subjects.[2] Although not statistically significant, the patients' diplophonia ratio was somewhat higher (1.418) than that of the normal controls (1.046).

Measurable Physiological Signs

In a study of activity in the laryngeal muscles, Guidi et al. (1981) reported that all five of their Shy-Drager patients showed denervation of the posterior cricoarytenoid muscle, and two of the five showed fibrillation potentials in the interarytenoid muscle. Histological studies have shown marked atrophy of the posterior cricoarytenoid muscle (Bannister, Gibson, Michaels, & Oppenheimer, 1981). Interestingly, there was little evidence of cell losses in the nucleus ambiguus, suggesting a possible biochemical abnormality (Ludlow, Coulter, & Gentges, 1983). These electromyographic characteristics were very different from the muscle activity recorded in patients with IPD.

Observable Physiological Signs

The primary laryngoscopic sign seen in Shy-Drager syndrome is bilateral abductor vocal fold paresis. Hanson, Ludlow, and Bassich (1983) reported that 11 of their 12 patients presented moderate to severe abductor paresis (also reported by Williams, Hanson, & Calne, 1979). Longridge (1987) reported a case of Shy-Drager with bilateral vocal fold paralysis but did not specify whether it was of the adductor or abductor type.

We know of no studies in which the stroboscopic signs of patients with Shy-Drager syndrome have been reported.

Pathophysiology

Shy-Drager syndrome is a disease involving the pyramidal, extrapyramidal, and cerebellar systems. It also may involve atrophy of neurons in the brainstem and part of the spinal cord (Bannister & Oppenheimer, 1972). It affects the control and coordination of speech and voice. Lesions that affect the upper motor neurons will result in the

---

[2]This finding is somewhat strange because the group included males and females: it is well known that male fundamental frequencies are much lower than female fundamental frequencies. The statistical results may be accurate if the authors tested only the differences of fundamental frequency between the patient groups and their age- and sex-matched controls.

loss of muscle coordination. Lesions in the cerebellum also affect muscle coordination, whereas lesions in the medulla and brainstem affect the motor nuclei of the muscles serving the larynx, producing problems of muscle tone and function. Interestingly, the disease affects the neurons that control abductory function and not adductory function. The hyperadduction that results in strain/struggle in speech is produced by lesions higher in the brain. In many respects the disease is similar to IPD, but with its own unique features. The outlook for patients with Shy-Drager syndrome is bleak, with few surviving more than 5 or 10 years (Thomas & Schirger, 1970). The course of the disease is a steady increase in neuromuscular impairment that will eventually affect the respiratory muscles and compromise respiratory function.

Lesions of the Peripheral Nerves

PRIMARY VOICE SYMPTOM: BREATHINESS

Description and Etiology

Lesions that affect the vagus nerve somewhere along its course from the base of the skull to the larynx will result in a paresis (weakness) or paralysis of muscles in the larynx. These peripheral lesions of the vagus are the most common cause of vocal fold paralysis. The intrinsic laryngeal muscles affected will depend on the exact location of the lesion. Recall that a branch of the superior laryngeal nerve (SLN) of the vagus controls the cricothyroid muscles, whereas the recurrent laryngeal nerve (RLN) controls the remaining muscles of the larynx. The SLN branches off from the vagus high in the neck. The RLN branches off somewhat below the SLN. A paralysis of all the muscles suggests that the lesion is high in the neck or in the brainstem itself. Lesions affecting only the RLN will be much lower in the neck or as far down as the thorax.

Lesions of the SLN or RLN may affect the position of the vocal folds. In RLN paralysis, the lesion may be unilateral or bilateral and may be of the adductor or abductor type, depending on the muscles affected. In the instance of a unilateral adductor paralysis, the affected vocal fold will not be actively moved toward the midline when phonation commences. When the glottis cannot be completely closed, the quality of the voice produced will be weak and breathy. In bilateral adductor paralysis, neither vocal fold will be capable of moving to the midline, thus making phonation impossible. Furthermore, the ability to swallow will be severely compromised, with aspiration being a life-threatening sequelae. The position of the paralyzed vocal folds, that is, how far apart they are, will depend partly on whether the SLN is affected. The SLN innervates the cricothyroid muscle, which when contracted tends to contribute to adduction of the vocal folds, in addition to tensing them to create a rise of vocal pitch. Some of the symptoms associated with SLN paralysis are vocal fatigue, hoarseness, and loss of vocal range (Dursun et al., 1996). Paralysis of this muscle in addition to muscles controlled by the RLN will further reduce the adductory forces of the vocal folds, thereby increasing their distance from each other over what it might be with an RLN lesion alone. Other factors, such as degree of fibrosis of the affected fold, tension of the conus elasticus, and freedom of joint movement, also may affect the final position of the vocal folds after paralysis of the RLN or SLN (Ballenger, 1985).

Lesions also may affect the abductory function of the vocal folds, which opens the airway for inspiration. Such lesions affect the recurrent laryngeal nerve and specifically the posterior cricoarytenoid muscle, which may produce unilateral or bilateral abductory paralysis. Bilateral abductor paralysis in which the vocal folds remain in an adducted posture causes serious respiratory problems (dyspnea), for which most patients will require a tracheotomy or excision of some portion of one or both vocal folds, thereby sacrificing phonation.

Unilateral vocal fold paralysis is much more common than bilateral paralysis. In a recent study, Benninger, Gillen, and Altman (1998) reported that 79.8% of their cases were unilateral, whereas the remainder were bilateral. In their cases of unilateral paralysis, the left vocal fold was involved much more than the right side (62.5% vs. 37.5%). The more extended and circuitous route followed by the left recurrent laryngeal nerve is thought to be a factor in its vulnerability.

The cause of vocal fold paralysis is varied and, as mentioned previously, can include lesions in the brainstem itself. These high vagal lesions (from the nodose ganglion up) will affect all laryngeal muscles, as well as muscles supplied by other cranial nerves. The lesions include tumors at the base of the skull, carcinoma of the nasopharynx, or trauma. A listing of some of the lesions in this area that could affect the larynx is shown in Table 5.4.

The possible causes of low vagal lesions are even more numerous. Neuritis is a frequent cause and occurs with upper respiratory infection, infectious mononucleosis,

Table 5.4. Miscellaneous Medulla Syndromes Affecting the Vocal Folds

Name	Effect	Etiology
Wallenberg's	Paralysis of half of larynx, pharynx, palate, loss of sensation to the face, vestibular dysfunction, ataxia, Horner's syndrome	Infarction of posterior inferior cerebellar artery
Babinski-Nageotte	Similar to Wallenberg's, including paralysis of tongue, loss of position and vibratory sense	Similar to Wallenberg's, plus involvement of medial bulbar area
Cestan-Chenais	Similar to Babinski-Nageotte, except little or no involvement proximal to nucleus ambiguus	Infarction of vertebral artery below the posterior inferior cerebellar artery
Avellis'	Causes laryngeal, pharyngeal, and palatal paralysis with dysphonia and dysphagia	Vascular or inflammatory lesion in medulla; lesion in nucleus ambiguus of vagus, plus cranial part of spinal accessory
Hughlings-Jackson	Results in ipsilateral paralysis of the soft palate, pharynx, larynx, tongue, and sternocleidomastoid muscles	Intramedullary lesion or a lesion high in the lateral pharyngeal space; affects vagus, spinal accessory, and hypoglossal nerves
Schmidt's	Ipsilateral paralysis of soft palate, pharynx, larynx, sternomastoid, and trapezius muscles	Vascular lesion in caudal part of medulla
Mackenzie	Unilateral paralysis of soft palate, pharynx, larynx, and tongue	Vascular lesion in medulla
Bonnier's	General weakness	Lesion in Deiters' nucleus or associated vestibular tracts

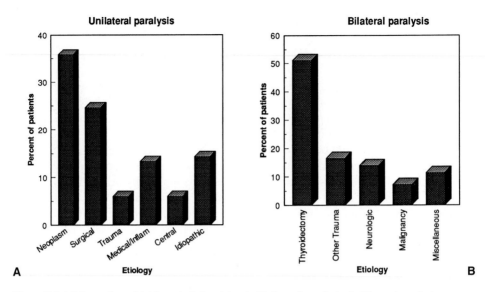

Figure 5.9. Etiology of vocal fold paralysis in adults. **A.** Unilateral paralysis. **B.** Bilateral paralysis.

sarcoidosis, and infections of the parapharyngeal spaces (Ballenger, 1985). Neoplasms in the neck, bronchi, and chest may invade and affect the nerve. Mechanical stretching or compression of the nerve also may result in paralysis of the laryngeal musculature. Among the most common causes are nonlaryngeal malignancies (primarily pulmonary), acute external trauma to the neck, surgery, and idiopathic causes (Ballenger, 1985; Tucker, 1980). The percentages for causes for both unilateral and bilateral paralysis as detailed in Benninger et al (1988) are shown in Figure 5.9. The discussion has centered on acquired paralyses. However, 10% of all congenital lesions are reported to be laryngeal paralysis (Gereau SA, LeBlanc EM, & Rubin RJ, 1995). The diagnosis may not be made immediately, because the symptoms are often nonspecific. Indeed, most congenital unilateral paralyses recover spontaneously, although the percentage is smaller in bilateral paralyses (deGaudemar, Roudaire, Francois, & Marcy,1996). Congenital bilateral paralysis occurs more frequently than unilateral and is usually secondary to CNS problems or other congenital abnormalities (Gereau et al., 1995). Daya et al. (2000) reported on their analysis of 102 cases of children with vocal fold paralysis. The group was divided about equally between unilateral and bilateral paralysis. Presenting symptoms of paralysis in children include stridor, abnormal cry, feeding difficulty, and cyanosis (Figure 5.10 Panel A). Iatrogenic causes were found more often in the unilateral paralysis group, whereas idiopathic causes were found more often in the bilateral group (see Figure 5.10 Panel B).

Some of the causes of SLN paralysis are neuritis, trauma, and iatrogenic. Dursun et al. (1996) reported that 93.6% of their cases with SLN paralysis were caused by a viral infection before the onset of the paralysis.

Perceptual Voice Signs and Symptoms

The most common perceptual symptoms of acquired unilateral paralysis are breathiness and hoarseness. Occasionally diplophonia may be present. Bilateral paralysis of the adductor type will cause severe breathiness or aphonia, but near-normal voice may be present in the abductor type. An additional perceptual sign of bilateral abductor

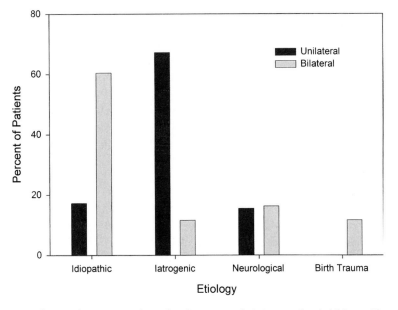

Figure 5.10. Etiology and symptoms of peripheral nerve paralysis in a study of children with unilateral paralysis (n = 53) and with bilateral paralysis (n = 49).

paralysis is inspiratory stridor that results from the passage of ingressive air over approximated vocal folds that are incapable of opening. The most common perceptual sign of congenital unilateral paralysis is a weak cry. In bilateral paralysis, stridor may be present in addition to weak cry. Vocal fatigue, hoarseness, and loss of vocal range are the most common symptoms of SLN paralysis (Dursun et al., 1996).

Acoustic Signs

No data have been published on acoustic signs in congenital paralysis, or in either abductor or adductor bilateral paralysis. Thus, the following comments apply only to acquired unilateral adductor vocal fold paralyses. We theorize that the aphonia or severe aperiodicity of voice in the presence of bilateral adductor paralysis would make acoustic analysis invalid.

Acoustically, increased aperiodicity (jitter and shimmer), a reduced pitch range, reduced variability of pitch, higher noise levels, and a reduced vocal intensity range are found. Murry (1978) reported the fundamental frequency characteristics of 20 patients with unilateral paralysis of the vocal folds as they read a standard reading passage. The patient group had a mean fundamental frequency of 127 Hz, whereas a group of 20 normal speakers had a mean fundamental frequency of 121.9 Hz. This difference was not statistically significant. The variability of fundamental frequency (pitch sigma) between the two groups of subjects was also not significant.

Davis (1981) reported pitch perturbation quotient (PPQ), or jitter, and amplitude perturbation quotient (APQ), or shimmer, values for two patients with unilateral paralysis of the vocal folds. The average PPQ was 9.165% for the patients versus 0.42% for a group of 10 normal speakers. The APQ was 12.96% for the patient group and 6.14% for the 10 normal speakers. It is difficult to generalize about these findings based on only two subjects, but they appear to be in the direction hypothesized. That is, patients with unilateral paralysis will show greater frequency and amplitude perturbation than speakers with normally functioning vocal folds.

Kim, Kakita, and Hirano (1982) carried out spectrographic analysis of some acoustic characteristics of the voices of 10 persons with unilateral RLN paralysis. They were unable to obtain accurate measures of fundamental frequency, probably because of the large amount of aperiodicity in the voice. The only difference between the patient and the normal group on amplitude variation and extent (a rough analog of shimmer) occurred between males. Other differences measured in these spectrograms included higher harmonic energy in the patient group, as well as greater noise energy. These latter features may correlate with the greater breathiness and noise levels that are present in many patients with unilateral recurrent nerve paralysis.

Measurable Physiological Signs

There have been several investigations concerned with the measurement of average airflow during the speech of patients with acquired unilateral vocal fold paralysis. Hirano (1981a) summarized several of these studies, noting that the mean flow rates in paralysis are much higher than normal, although they range from a low of 35 mL/sec to a high of 1,150 mL/sec (see Table 3.3, p. 30, in Hirano, 1981a). Normal-speaking men produce rates of approximately 110 mL/sec; women, approximately 94 mL/sec (Koike & Hirano, 1968). Yanagihara and von Leden (1967) reported a mean flow rate of 442.2 mL/sec for their 10 patients with unilateral paralysis, whereas Iwata et al. reported a mean flow of 353 mL/sec for their group of 19 unilateral paralysis patients. Hirano, Koike, and von Leden (1968) reported a mean flow rate of 312.8 mL/sec for their 10 patients with bilateral paralysis. Thus, it would appear that higher mean flow rates occur in unilateral paralysis than in bilateral paralysis.

Based on their analysis of EGG waveforms of paralysis patients, Hanson, Gerrat, Karin, and Berke (1988) were able to differentiate among four causes of unilateral vocal fold paralysis. Vagal lesions produced an open quotient that was much smaller than the other causes studied (Fig. 5.11). Measures of speed quotient showed greater variation

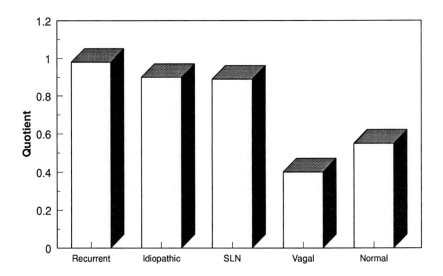

Figure 5.11. Open quotient measurements of four forms of unilateral vocal fold paralysis compared with a group of normal control subjects.

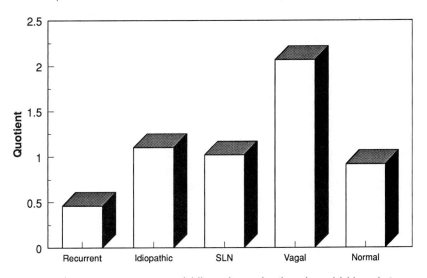

Figure 5.12. Speed quotient measurements of different forms of unilateral vocal fold paralysis compared with a group of normal control subjects.

among the four causes studied (Fig. 5.12). Perhaps measurements such as these and others yet to be tried could be used to differentiate the type of cause responsible for paralysis of a vocal fold.

We have recorded the inverse filtered airflow characteristics and electroglottograms of several patients with unilateral paralysis. One patient is shown in Figure 5.13. Note the high levels of offset flow (from baseline to lowest point on the airflow waveform), which were much greater than for the normal subjects. The airflow waveform is

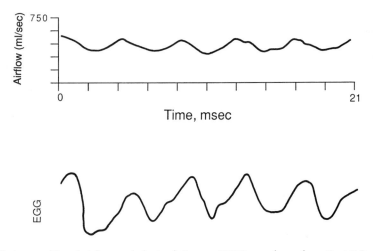

Figure 5.13. Inverse filtered airflow and electroglottogram (EGG) waveforms for patient K.B., a woman with a congenital unilateral vocal fold paralysis. Note the large airflow offset, indicative of a large leak through the vocal folds. The electroglottogram also exhibits unusual waveforms with marked change from one cycle to the next. Because of technical problems, we were unable to record the lung pressure used with this phonation.

variable, perhaps indicative of the greater aperiodicity of the vocal folds. This increased aperiodicity is also evident in the electroglottographic trace shown below the airflow trace.

Kuroki (1969) studied the subglottal pressures produced by patients with unilateral and bilateral recurrent nerve paralysis. Most patients with unilateral paralysis produced higher than normal subglottal pressures (normal, approximately 6–8 cm H_2O), and two bilateral paralysis patients showed much higher than normal subglottal pressures. This might be expected in view of the air loss during phonation and the natural tendency for the speaker to attempt to compensate for this loss with greater driving pressures below the vocal folds. Conversely, patients with vocal fold paralysis may produce greater pressures (and therefore greater flows) because of their inability to achieve glottal closure during the vibratory cycle.

Electromyography (EMG) is a valuable tool for the evaluation of vocal fold immobility (Koufman et al., 2000; Sataloff et al., 2000; Woo & Arandia, 1992). It is used to determine whether a laryngeal muscle is truly paralyzed and may help to differentiate the causes of the paralysis (Sataloff et al., 2000). The EMG interference pattern represents the sum of many motor units and shows a typical triphasic pattern in normal muscle. Little or no electrical activity may be seen in paralyzed muscles or activity that shows abnormal patterns, fibrillation, or decreases recruitment of the motor fibers. In SLN paralysis, EMG will show decreases in recruitment and fibrillation potentials (Dursun et al., 1996).

Observable Physiological Signs

Laryngoscopy.   The typical laryngoscopic view in unilateral paralysis is that of one vocal fold that does not fully adduct during phonation, while the unaffected fold moves to the midline. There may be some apparent movement of the affected vocal fold caused by movements of other structures, or by contraction of the cricothyroid (assuming an intact SLN), which will tend to exert some adductory force on the vocal folds (as described earlier), or perhaps the affected fold is driven by air pressure. Movement in the pyriform sinus on the affected side may be reduced or absent (Brewer & Gould, 1974) in patients with unilateral vocal fold paralysis. Differences in the horizontal level of the two vocal folds have been reported by Isshiki and Ishikawa (1976). Approximately half of their 56 patients showed a higher level of the paralyzed vocal fold. Reasons for this level difference may include (a) the position of the arytenoid on the paralyzed side; (b) effects of the extrinsic muscles; and (c) the possibility of a paralyzed cricothyroid muscle, which would affect the tension that can be placed on the affected fold. It should be noted, however, that others have failed to find a consistent level difference (Adran, Demp, & Marland, 1954; Ballantyne & Groves, 1978; Casper, Colton, & Brewer, 1985; Lee, 1973).

Stroboscopy.   Hirano, Feder, and Bless (1983) discussed some of the stroboscopic signs seen in patients with peripheral nerve paralysis. These signs will vary depending on the severity of involvement and the type of problem, that is, superior or recurrent nerve involvement, or both. A summary of the important signs they report for unilateral adductor paralysis is presented in Table 5.5.

Kitzing (1985) reported that stroboscopic signs in vocal fold paresis include vocal fold asymmetry and aperiodicity, greater than normal vibratory amplitudes, absence of a mucosal wave, and incomplete glottal closure. These signs are consistent with the

Table 5.5. Miscellaneous Peripheral Syndromes Resulting in Laryngeal Paralysis

Name	Effect	Etiology
Collet-Sicard	Last four cranial nerves	Tumor, meningitis, or trauma to posterior cranial fossa
Vernet's	Nerves 9, 10, 11; dysphagia and dystonia	Lesion in jugular fossa
Villaret's	Like Vernet's, including sympathetic paralysis and Horner's syndrome	Lesion in retroparotid or lateral pharyngeal space
Tapia's	Ipsilateral paralysis of tongue and hypoglossal larynx	Neoplasm where hypoglossal crosses vagus and internal carotid
Gard-Gignoux	Paralysis of vocal folds, weakness of trapezius and sternomastoid muscles	11th and vagus nerves below nodose ganglion
Klinkert	Paralysis of recurrent and phrenic nerves	Lesion in root of neck or mediastinum

nature of the disease and the perceptual, acoustic, physiological, and laryngoscopic signs discussed earlier.

We have observed many of these same signs (Table 5.6). The paralyzed fold vibrates occasionally but not at the same rate nor in the same way as the unaffected fold. There is an anteroposterior (or the reverse) ripple-like motion on the affected side. We have observed a mucosal wave on the affected fold, although it is usually not as regular as the unaffected side. Amplitude of vibration of the affected fold sometimes appears to be increased. Most often, the paralyzed fold and the non-paralyzed fold produce an aperiodic motion. A variety of glottal closure patterns are observed, but most often we have observed incomplete closure (22/39 patients).

The location of the pathological condition in vocal fold paralysis is in the muscle; that is, the thyroarytenoid muscle has little or no neural control (Hirano & Bless, 1993). Glottal incompetence with a bowed fold is sometimes seen. The stiffness of the cover and the transition layers are normal. The stiffness of the body is decreased.

Sercarz and his colleagues (Sercarz, Berke, Ming, Gerratt, & Natividad, 1992) reported on stroboscopic findings in three normal speakers whose recurrent or superior laryngeal nerves were paralyzed with drugs as well as 20 patients with unilateral paralysis. Their most significant finding was the asymmetry of traveling wave motion in the

Table 5.6. Stroboscopic Signs in Laryngeal Paralysis

1. Abnormal vibration with predominant vertical movements
2. Large irregular amplitudes
3. Poor vocal fold closure
4. Affected fold seems to flutter
5. Absence of edge deflections (upward on affected fold)

paralyzed larynx. The normal fold has the fastest traveling wave; the difference of wave velocity produced a phase asymmetry of vibration.

In SLN paralysis, Dursun et al. (1996) reported increases in amplitude asymmetry, phase asymmetry, incomplete glottal closure, decreased amplitude of vibration, and decreased mucosal wave in most of their patients. They also reported a decrease in the ability of their patients to produce a glissando pitch glide.

Pathophysiology

A paralyzed vocal fold may affect adduction or abduction of the vocal folds. Voice problems are most commonly associated with unilateral adductor paralysis. In bilateral adductor paralysis, the patient may be aphonic, but the patient's primary and potentially life-threatening problem in need of urgent attention will be loss of protection of the airway and the attendant risk of aspiration. The incidence of unilateral vocal fold paralysis is much greater than that of bilateral paralysis.

One problem encountered in the diagnosis of vocal fold paralysis is whether there is a true paralysis of the fold or if the immobility of the vocal fold is caused by fixation of the arytenoid joint or a dislocated arytenoid (Rontal & Rontal, 1986). The diagnostician must carefully explore these other possibilities either indirectly by observing other structures in the larynx (e.g., the pyriform sinus) or by directly manipulating the arytenoid to test its mobility. Electromyographic (EMG) evaluation of muscle electrical activity also may assist in making the correct diagnosis. Most important of all is a complete and careful case history (Woo, Colton, Brewer, & Casper, 1991).

In unilateral paralysis, the affected fold cannot move to the midline and assist in closure of the glottis. Because of this incomplete closure, greater than normal airflows and a weak voice will be produced. The affected fold also may exhibit muscle tensions vastly different from the unaffected cord, resulting in asymmetrical tension and increased aperiodicity in the voice. This will be perceived as roughness or hoarseness. A difference in level between the two folds also may contribute to the increased aperiodicity and excessive airflow, although its precise effect remains unknown. If the superior laryngeal nerve is involved, additional problems with pitch control may be noted.

AN UNUSUAL CASE OF UNILATERAL VOCAL FOLD PARALYSIS

R.C. is a 52-year-old man who awoke one morning with pain and pronounced weakness in both arms, slightly more pronounced on the right, with impaired manual dexterity in the right hand that prevented simple acts such as eating, writing, etc. After visiting his general practitioner, he was referred to a neurologist who performed routine neurological tests and conduction velocity tests on nerves in the right arm. The diagnosis was Guillain-Barré syndrome (acute inflammatory demyelinating polyneuropathy), and R.C. was hospitalized immediately. On the day after hospitalization, R.C. developed a breathy and hoarse voice quality consistent with a unilateral vocal fold paralysis. Also, he developed mild dysphagia. A flexible fiberoptic laryngeal examination was conducted 2 days later and showed a left vocal fold paralysis.

Guillain-Barré is a neuropathy (Dowling, Blumberg, & Cook, 1987) that affects somewhere between 0.6 to 2 individuals per 100,000 population. It is the body's reaction to a virus that the person may have had up to 8 weeks before the onset of symptoms. (R.C. reported a mild upper respiratory infection approximately 2 months previous to onset and a very mild, 1-day illness roughly 5 days before onset.) The affected individual's immune system develops antibodies in reaction to the virus that begin to attack the myelin sheaths of nerves, primarily peripheral nerves. It is probably an autoimmune T cell–mediated disease (Taft, 1988). No nerve is safe, including those that control respiration, the heart, and other vital functions. The classic symptoms of Guillain-Barré begin with weakness in the legs and ascend to the trunk, arms, head, and neck. However, other variants of the disease exist, as evinced by R.C. How far the demyelinating extends and what systems are affected is unpredictable. Until quite recently, persons with this diagnosis were hospitalized so that the progression of the disease could be monitored and appropriate life-saving interventions, such as respiratory assistance, could be introduced as necessary.

R.C. was hospitalized not only to monitor the progress of the disease, but also to start him on a treatment program of plasmapheresis (Guillain-Barré Syndrome Study Group, 1985). This treatment has been found to be an effective method of interrupting the course of the disease in some patients. During the plasmapheresis treatments, each of which can take several hours, blood is continuously extracted from the body; the white and red blood cells are separated from the plasma; the plasma is discarded; and the red and white cells are mixed with human albumen and pumped back into the patient. The theory is that the antibody causing the problem attaches itself to a protein in the plasma. Removing the plasma removes the offending antibody. R.C. remained in the hospital for 8 days and completed four plasmapheresis treatments. He did not develop any additional symptoms; indeed, the dysphagia and the acute arm pain had resolved. He still had arm weakness, vocal fold paralysis, and fatigue. He was then discharged to recuperate at home for another 2 weeks. During this time, he received two additional pheresis treatments as an outpatient. He returned to work approximately 22 days after the onset of the first symptom. The vocal fold paralysis persisted for approximately 6 weeks after its onset. R.C. recovered full use of his voice and at 3 months post onset had only mild soreness in his arms, especially his right, secondary to remyelination. Seven years post diagnosis, R.C. is doing fine, with very few residual effects.

Vocal fold paralysis is a rare complication of Guillain-Barré syndrome. It appears to respond to the treatment for the disease itself, i.e., plasmapheresis. Early diagnosis and immediate treatment appear to be critical, and patients often can experience full recovery of function with time. The presentation of vocal fold paralysis must be viewed as potentially one sign of an underlying problem that may have life threatening implications. A thorough history is critical to alert the examiner to areas that need further exploration. It is essential to rule out the presence of more diffuse disease; the presence of a neck, thoracic, or lung lesion that might be impinging on the nerve (RLN); the possibility of joint ankylosis or dislocation; and possible psychogenicity.

HYPERADDUCTION

Spasmodic Dysphonia

PRIMARY VOICE SYMPTOM: STRAIN/STRUGGLE

Description and Etiology

Spasmodic dysphonia (SD), according to Ludlow (1995), is a "focal dystonia affecting laryngeal muscle control during speech" (p. 436). It has received much attention over the past 15 to 20 years, perhaps out of proportion to its incidence. It is a relatively rare voice disorder, although judging from the many reports in the literature it appears that its numbers have increased. Perhaps this is because of the availability of methods of providing some form of symptom relief or to increased awareness of and knowledge about the disorder. SD seems to occur equally in men and women (Aronson, Brown, Litin, & Pearson, 1968b), with onset most frequently in middle age, although we have seen patients as young as 20 years with a history of onset in the teens.

The nature of the onset of SD is variable. In some patients, onset is associated with a major upper respiratory infection (Aronson, Brown, Litin, & Pearson, 1968b); in others, a traumatic emotional event is identified (Aronson, 1990; Brodnitz, 1976); and in still other patients the onset is insidious, beginning as a mild hoarseness and progressing to interrupted, strained phonation. The progression of symptoms may be rapid or may take place over a number of years.

In the past, the thinking about the causes of SD had taken two major forms (Aronson, 1990; Salamy & Sessions, 1980). Some authors advocated a psychological origin (Arnold, 1959; Block, 1965; Brodnitz, 1976; Heaver, 1959; Henschen & Burton, 1978), whereas others have implicated a neurological origin (Aminoff, Dedo, & Izdebski, 1978; Aronson, Brown, Litin, & Pearson, 1968a, 1968b; Blitzer & Brin, 1992; Rabuzzi & McCall, 1972; Robe, Brumlik, & Moore, 1960; Shaefer, 1983).

One rationale for the psychological cause is that patients often report a traumatic emotional event closely associated with the awareness of the onset of symptoms. Another reason may be the difficulty in differentiating the symptoms and signs of SD from those found in certain manifestations of psychogenic or muscle tension dysphonias. Advocates of the psychological-cause theory point to some success in therapy (voice or psychiatric), or to relief of symptoms with the use of tranquilizing or neuroleptic drugs (Brodnitz, 1976), as positive evidence of the correctness of the theory. Advocates of a neurological origin suggest that these patients had perhaps been incorrectly diagnosed.

Advocates of the neurological cause of SD point to the sizable body of evidence of associated neurological signs in these patients (Aronson, Brown, Litin, & Pearson, 1968b) and to the documented existence of abnormal findings in various tests of brain function (Aminoff, Dedo, & Izdebski, 1978; Dordain & Dordain, 1972; Finitzo-Hieber, Freeman, Gerling, Dobson, & Schaeffer, 1982; Robe, Brumlik, & Moore, 1960; Shaefer, 1983). Many of these authors also point out that there has been little actual documentation of symptom relief as a result of voice therapy or in response to psychiatric treatment. Reports of successful treatment have been anecdotal (Cooper & Cooper, 1977), and, moreover, the lack of success of these treatment protocols for patients with SD has been extensively noted (Aronson, 1990).

In the late 1970s, the unilateral severing of the recurrent laryngeal nerve was introduced by Dedo (1976), who reported lasting symptom relief in these patients. Others have also reported results of this procedure (Dedo & Izdebski, 1981, 1983; Izdebski, Dedo, & Shipp, 1981). Reports of recurrence of symptoms of SD despite the permanence of the paralysis of the severed side reduced the popularity of the procedure. Simultaneously, the use of Botox injection in the treatment of SD began to receive attention (Benninger, Gardner, & Grywalski, 2001; Blitzer, Brin, Stewart, Aviv, & Fahn, 1992; Blitzer & Sulica, 2001; Boutsen et al., 2002; Brin, Blitzer & Stewart, 1998; Courey et al., 2000; Ford, Bless, & Patel, 1992; Inagi et al., 1996; Ludlow, 1990; Shaefer et al., 1992; Whurr, Nye & Lorch, 1998; Woo, Colton, Casper, & Brewer, 1992; Zwirner, Murry, Swenson, & Woodson, 1991).

Most scientists and practitioners have come to accept that SD is a problem with a neurological substrate, one of the family of dystonias. The exact locus of the dysfunction is not clear, although many point to the basal ganglia or associated structures as the most likely location (Blitzer & Brin, 1992; Izdebski, 1992; Swenson, Zwirner, Murry, & Woodson, 1992). The problem probably has many causes (Izdebski, 1992) and may be linked to other neurological disorders (Swenson, Zwirner, Murry, & Woodson, 1992). Izdebski (1992) presented a model of SD in which sudden or sustained increases of muscle activity occur, probably in response to faulty processing of afferent information about various events within the larynx such as the variation of air pressures during phonation. The symptoms are absent in vegetative tasks and in speech tasks that do not involve phonation. Thus, in a whisper, symptoms are absent or minimal because there is no variation of air pressures or vocal fold movement. Effective treatment should focus on reducing the afferent information to the central processing unit (e.g., basal ganglia) or by reducing the motor response because of faulty input processing. Section or crush of the recurrent laryngeal nerve would potentially remove sensory input as well as motor control. Injection of botulinum toxin (Botox) reduces the motor response to any faulty input. The focal nature of SD (that is, involvement of only a few muscles) suggests that specific therapeutic techniques should be most effective in obtaining symptom relief. Perhaps, this explains why the use of drugs systemically has been reported to have little lasting effect on the amelioration of the symptoms in SD.

There are two forms of SD, the adductor type, which is discussed in this section, and the abductor type, which is discussed in its own section. An individual may have a mixed form of the problem involving both adductor and abductor musculature.

Another common name for SD is spastic dysphonia. Many believe that the use of the term *spastic* is inappropriate. "Spastic" implies lesions in the corticobulbar or corticospinal (pyramidal) systems. That does not seem to be the case in this disorder. Current evidence suggests that the underlying disease state in SD affects structures in the extrapyramidal system. Aronson et al. (1968b) suggested that the term *spasmodic* would be more appropriate.

ADD

Perceptual Voice Signs and Symptoms

The most characteristic symptom (and sign) is the struggle and strain to talk in association with intermittent stoppages of voice (Aronson, 1990; Aronson, Brown, Litin, & Pearson, 1968b; Brodnitz, 1976). Associated symptoms may include hoarseness, harshness, and tremor (Fig. 5.14). Other patients present with a creaking, choked,

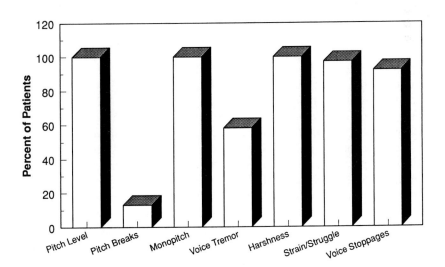

Figure 5.14. Percentage of 31 patients with SD showing voice deviations. Voice tremor was rated during contextual speech.

tense, or squeezed voice with extreme tension noted in the entire speech production system. Perceptual signs include strain/struggle, sudden interruption of voicing, tension, loudness and pitch variations, pitch breaks, and stoppages of phonation. According to Ludlow (1995), voice stoppages occur primarily in vowel productions.

Acoustic Signs

Considerable data have been reported in the literature about the various acoustic signs accompanying SD.

Fundamental Frequency. Davis, Boone, Carroll, Davenzia, and Harrison (1988) reported the average fundamental frequencies during a reading passage for 16 female and 7 male patients with adductor SD and compared these data with those of a set of control subjects. The female patients had a mean fundamental frequency of 162 Hz compared with a mean fundamental frequency of 175 Hz for the 17 female control subjects. The male patients had a mean fundamental frequency of 134 Hz compared with a mean fundamental frequency of 106 Hz for 7 male controls. These authors also reported that the SD patients had a much greater variation of fundamental frequency during the passage than the controls (21.89 semitones [ST] for females and 14.79 ST for males compared with 12.29 ST for normal females and 11.89 ST for normal males).

Fritzell, Feuer, Haglund, Knutsson, and Schiratski (1982) analyzed the distribution of fundamental frequency in the voices of four patients (three males and one female) reading a short passage. Mean fundamental frequency ranged from 111 to 238 Hz. The distribution of fundamental frequency was bimodal, with a major peak centered above 200 Hz and a minor peak centered around 150 Hz. These patients underwent section of the recurrent laryngeal nerve for relief of symptoms (see Chapter 9). Postsurgically, the fundamental frequency distribution was much lower (mean fundamental frequencies ranged from 125 to 171 Hz) and the distribution was unimodal.

Long-Term Average Spectrum. Izdebski (1984) measured the long-term average spectrum (LTAS, a spectrum computed over a sentence or paragraph) in 23 patients with adductor SD. Figure 5.15 illustrates his results. The solid line shows the spectrum of a female speaker before surgery (recurrent nerve section), and the dotted line shows the same patient after surgery. Note the high levels of high-frequency energy in the speech before surgery, but the dramatic decrease of high-frequency energy after surgery.

Fritzell et al. (1982) analyzed the LTAS in the voices of four patients reading a short passage. They reported only a slight difference of spectral shape and levels after surgery. Because there was no control group, it is not known whether the levels of energy at the higher frequencies were greater than normal. Informal comparisons of the data presented by Fritzell et al. (1982) with those presented by Hammarberg, Fritzell, Gauffin, and Sundberg (1986) for normal speakers suggests that the patient group exhibited greater than normal energy levels in the high frequencies.

Hartman, Abbs, and Vishwanat (1988) observed pronounced peaks between 4 and 7 Hz in the spectrum of sustained /ah/s produced by four patients with adductor SD. These peaks may be indicative of vocal tremor. The finding of low-frequency tremor in the frequency spectrum of these patients is of interest. Wolfe and Bacon (1976), using spectrographic analysis of a patient with adductor SD, showed a breakdown in the harmonic structure of vowels, dark areas on the spectrogram (indicating greater loudness), and sudden changes of gray levels on the spectrogram, indicating the irregular variation of voicing present in adductor SD (Fig. 5.16).

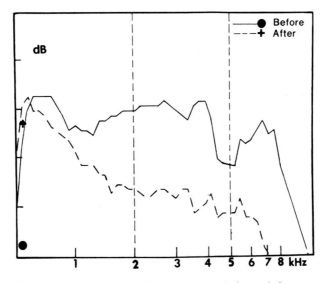

Figure 5.15. Long-time average spectra of a female patient with SD before and after recurrent nerve section.

Measurable Physiological Signs

Several studies have reported airflows and air pressures for SD patients. Hirano, Koike, and von Leden (1968) reported flows within the normal range for their eight SD patients, whereas other studies have reported low (Casper, Colton, & Brewer, 1985; Darvenzia, & Harrison, 1988; Davis, Boone, Carroll, Farmakides & Boone, 1960; Hirano, 1974, 1981b; Hollien, Dew, & Phillips, 1971; Javkin, Antonanzas-Barros, &

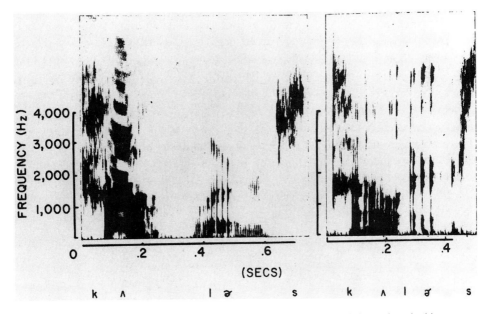

Figure 5.16. Broad-band spectrogram of a patient with abductor-type SD (left panel) and adductor-type SD (right panel). The utterance was the word "colors."

Maddieson, 1987) to very low flows (Briant, Blair, Cole, & Singer, 1983; Garrett & Healey, 1987; Hill, 1938; Hollien, 1975). In adductor SD, patients may exhibit strain during voicing, which may produce small glottal apertures through which air can flow. Low flows would be expected in this situation. We have shown very low average flow rates in patients with adductor SD (72 mL/sec) (Woo, Colton, Casper, & Brewer, 1992). Airflow rates increased after nerve section (232 mL/sec) or Botox (138 mL/sec).

Shipp, Izdebski, Schutte, and Morrissey (1988) studied subglottal air pressure magnitudes in two patients with adductor SD. They reported much higher pressures (13–14 cm H_2O) than normal (approximately 6 cm H_2O). These very high pressures are consistent with patients' reports of the increased effort required to speak. The elevated pressures in combination with the low flows suggest increased glottal resistance during voicing for patients with adductor SD.

Observable Physiological Signs

Laryngoscopy. Anatomically, the larynx appears essentially normal. However, during phonation, it is possible to observe the hyperadduction of the adductor type of SD. Hartman and Aronson (1981) reported the appearance of bowed vocal folds in 2 of 17 patients with otherwise normal-looking vocal folds. Hartman et al. (1988) reported the observations of quick adductory movements of the true vocal folds, the ventricular folds, and much of the supraglottal structures in one patient; small, irregular movements of the true vocal folds in another patient; and, in a third patient, periodic laryngospasms. In the study reported by Davis et al. (1988), most patients had normal laryngoscopic examinations, but interruption of voicing was reported to occur in seven patients because of action of the true vocal folds, in two patients tremor seemed to cause the interruption, and in four other patients the ventricular folds appeared to cause the voice stoppage. Blitzer and Brin (1992) advocate the use of flexible fiberoptic laryngoscopy to study the hyperadduction characteristics of SD.

Stroboscopy.   Few data have been reported on the vibratory characteristics of patients with SD as seen with stroboscopy. Fritzell et al. (1982) report that stroboscopy was carried out before recurrent nerve section, but no data were presented. Postsurgically, two patients showed symmetrical vocal fold vibrations, indicating a return of function to the muscle. Because patients with SD have difficulty in sustaining phonation, stroboscopic visualization of the vocal folds might be unproductive.

Pathophysiology

The pathophysiology of adductor SD is not well understood. High levels of muscle activity are seen in the thyroarytenoid muscles of some, but not all, patients with adductor SD. Muscle hypertonia or hypotonia for various groups of speakers (i.e., adductor SD, abductor SD, and normal speakers) has not been well studied or compared. The mechanism for spasmodic bursts of increased activity in specific muscles is not clear. The spasm activity of the vocal folds will have a pronounced effect on the production of sound. Excessive adductory forces will require greater than normal pressures to force the vocal folds apart during phonation. Greater air pressures will be associated with greater sound pressure levels and a more rapid opening and closing phase of the vocal folds. Rapid closing phases are associated with the production of greater energy in the higher frequencies and high-energy, high-frequency spectra. The intermittent nature of the problem will produce wide variations of spectrum and fundamental frequency unless some compensatory mechanism is employed in the attempt to maintain a steady, smooth flow of speech.

Other Considerations

In many patients with SD, other neurological signs will appear, including vocal tremor, jaw or facial jerks or tremor, hand or limb tremor, hyperreflexia, sucking reflex, torticollis, or asymmetries in the face or palate (Aronson, Brown, Litin, & Pearson, 1968b; Davis, Boone, Carroll, Darvenzia, & Harrison, 1988). The high incidence of tremor in SD patients suggests that perhaps a proportion of patients diagnosed with SD are in fact patients with essential tremor (Aronson, Brown, Litin, & Pearson, 1968a). Conversely, it is possible that in some cases SD is another manifestation of essential tremor (Aronson & Hartman, 1981; Davis, Boone, Carroll, Darvenzia, & Harrison, 1988). At the very least, the frequency of occurrence of additional neurological signs suggests that SD probably has a neurological substrate somewhere in the brain, most likely in the extrapyramidal system (Charcot, 1881).

Sharbrough, Stockard, and Aronson (1975) reported brainstem abnormalities in 7 of their 18 SD patients. They concluded that SD is "a symptom due to organic CNS disease that, in some cases, incidentally produces asymptomatic slowing of conduction within the brainstem auditory pathway" (p. 200).

Patients with SD may show abnormal auditory brainstem responses (Finitzo-Hieber, Freeman, Gerling, Dobson, & Schaeffer, 1982); that is, the capacity of the brainstem to conduct impulses is impaired. Furthermore, SD may be a disease involving multiple cranial nerves that when stressed break down and disrupt the speech system (Shaefer, 1983). Such a notion may explain why patients with SD present such variable symptoms. Blitzer and his colleagues (Blitzer & Brin, 1991, 1992; Blitzer, Brin, Fahn, & Lovelace, 1988; Blitzer, Lovelace, Brin, Fahn, & Fink, 1985; Brin, Fahn, Blitzer, Ramig, & Stewart, 1992) placed SD as a member of the family of dystonias. Dystonias are characterized by uncontrolled spasmodic muscle contractions. Dystonias may begin at any age, but many patients show either an early onset (before age 26) or late onset. They may be focal (restricted to a few muscles), segmental (involving a group of muscles), or general (involving larger areas of the body). Examples of focal dystonias are blepharospasm (involuntary eye closures), torticollis (neck twisting), and writer's cramp. Focal dystonias are apparent during the execution of a task and are not usually seen when the affected structure is at rest. Blitzer and his colleagues believe that SD is an action-induced dystonia involving the larynx. They found tremor in only 25% of their patients and question the hypothesis proposed by Aronson (Aronson & Hartman, 1981) that some SDs are a manifestation of essential tremor. The tremor is irregular and can sometimes be reduced through compensatory maneuvers (Brin, Fahn, Blitzer, Ramig, & Stewart, 1992; Folkins, 1978; Kinney, Kado, & Royner, 1972). Brin states: "Adductor SD is characterized by abnormal involuntary co-contraction of the vocalis muscle complex muscles (sic) resulting in inappropriate adduction of the vocal folds." As an action-induced, "task specific," or "functional" movement disorder, the muscles and anatomical structures are normal at rest but move inappropriately with action.

Dystonias can be induced by trauma, may have a genetic link, and show a variety of midbrain, brainstem abnormalities. Often, a psychological component may have developed in response to the dystonia and the patient's efforts to deal with the problem. SD has been very resistant to treatment. Drugs do not alleviate the symptoms in most patients; surgery of the recurrent laryngeal nerve has been shown to have limited success; speech therapy or psychotherapy do little to relieve the symptoms. Botox injection offers some relief but is not a true long-term solution to the problem.

Differentiating Spasmodic Dysphonia From Other Dysphonias

Although a number of features of SD, psychogenic dysphonia, and musculoskeletal tension (hyperfunctional) dysphonia may be similar in some respects, careful history taking, examination, and analysis of characteristics of speech production will reveal unique features of each. Patients with psychogenic problems frequently reveal a long history marked by the presence of stress; those with hyperfunctional dysphonia may report a clearly defined period of increased stresses and tensions; and the patient with SD will more frequently report increased stress since the onset of the symptoms.

The voice symptoms in the patient with psychogenic problems may be variable with return of normal voice for hours, days, or even weeks at a time; may be slightly bizarre in their presentations; show no pattern of phonemic variability; are not present in reflexive acts with associated phonation; show a consistent "phonatory set" during flexible endoscopic laryngeal examination; and often respond well to voice therapy. In contrast, patients with SD present with minimal variability and no instances of normal voice since the onset of the symptoms. The symptoms are usually in keeping with the underlying nature of the problem (not bizarre); are spasmodic, not constant, in presentation, and can be visualized to be so on laryngoscopic examination; show a pattern of phonemic variability (hyperadduction on voiced segments or difficulty in voiceless to voiced transition); have voice arrests as a very characteristic feature; and do not respond well to voice therapy. Persons with hyperfunctional dysphonia usually present with symptoms that tend to be fairly consistent; do not vary phonemically; are characterized by consistent rather than episodic vocal tension, which is visible on examination but is responsive to alteration through guided probes and suggestions; and respond well to voice therapy.

Huntington's Chorea (HC)

PRIMARY VOICE SYMPTOM: HOARSENESS

Description and Etiology

Chorea refers to a hyperkinetic disorder in which there are abrupt, jerky, purposeless, movements of the head, neck, or limbs. There are several variants, including Sydenham's chorea (which is often associated with children) and Huntington's chorea (more often associated with adulthood). There are many causes of chorea, including trauma, neoplasms, cerebrovascular disorders, infection, compromised immune system, metabolic disturbances, intoxications, and drugs (Padberg & Bruyn, 1986). Some forms are linked to hereditary causes.

Huntington's chorea is a disease of the basal ganglia, with an incidence of 4 to 7 per 100,000 people (Merritt, 1979). It has a genetic basis; the child of an affected person has a 50% chance of developing the disease. It usually appears in the 3rd through 5th decades of life (average age of 38 years) (Brin, Fahn, Blitzer, Ramig, & Stewart, 1992), although it has been reported to appear as early as age 5 and as late as age 70 (Merritt, 1979). The basic signs are choreiform movements and progressive mental deterioration. The abnormal movements appear to increase with heightened emotional levels, are dramatically reduced during sleep, and affect any voluntary movements. Mentally, a patient with Huntington's chorea experiences a progressive loss of memory

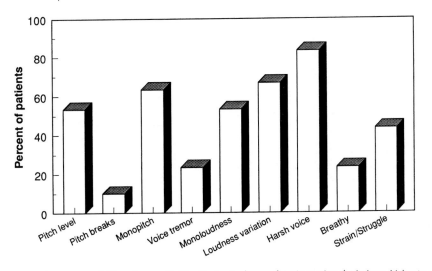

Figure 5.17. Percentage of 30 patients with Huntington's chorea showing voice deviations. Voice tremor was rated during contextual speech.

and intellectual capacity. Ramig (1986) reasoned that generalized instability of muscle contraction (involuntary contractions, variable tone or tremor) would be expected to affect the muscles of the larynx. Therefore, disorders of phonation associated with Huntington's chorea would be likely.

Perceptual Voice Signs and Symptoms

The most prominent perceptual voice sign is harshness, followed by monopitch and strain/struggle voice quality (Aronson, 1990; Aronson, Brown, Litin, & Pearson, 1968a). Figure 5.17 presents the percentage of patients exhibiting the various voice signs rated by Darley et al. (1969a).

Acoustic Signs

Jarema, Kennedy, and Shoulson (1985) studied some acoustic characteristics in 12 adults with Huntington's chorea. There were seven women, with a mean age of 44 years, and five men, with a mean age of 42 years. The authors also collected these data for a normal-speaking group. They measured habitual (mean) fundamental frequency and intensity during sustained vowel production and obtained estimates of phonational range and maximum phonation time. Their data on fundamental frequency and vocal intensity are summarized in Table 5.7. No statistically significant difference was found between the patient and normal-speaking groups on habitual fundamental frequency. Although there were some restrictions at both ends of the patients' phonational and dynamic ranges, the differences compared with the normal control group were not statistically significant. The male patients in the study were found to produce shorter maximum phonation times (15 seconds) than the normal male speakers (23 seconds), but this difference was not statistically significant. However, the female patient phonation times (14 seconds vs. 23 seconds) were significantly shorter than those for the normal group.

Ramig (1986) also measured some acoustic features in the speech of eight patients, four males and four females. She noted frequent abrupt low-frequency segments

Table 5.7. Fundamental Frequency and Intensity Characteristics of the Speech of
Patients With Huntington's Chorea

	Female		Male	
	Patient	*Normal*	*Patient*	*Normal*
Fund Frequency (Hz)				
Habitual	166	182	106	103
Low	155	143	92	83
High	592	716	390	422
Intensity (dB SPL)				
Habitual	71	71	74	72
Soft	68	66	71	66
Loud	100	108	104	106

during a sustained vowel (sudden drop of fundamental frequency, then a return to almost the same fundamental frequency), voice arrests, and reduced duration of the sustained vowels /ah/, /ee/, and /oo/. Voice arrests (370–510 msec in mean duration) occurred in six of the eight patients. Mean vowel durations for the patients ranged from 0.50 to 9.75 seconds, whereas mean normal vowel durations on the same task were 14.61 seconds.

A later report by Ramig et al. (1988) reported further acoustic data on these eight patients. The patient group did not show large cycle-to-cycle variation but rather abrupt drops of fundamental frequency. Low-frequency segments occurred 102 times in the 27 vowel segments produced by these patients. Furthermore, another group of patients at risk for Huntington's chorea showed 34 instances of low-frequency drops in 90 vowel segments. These abrupt low-frequency segments support the hypothesis of increased phonatory instability in these patients.

Another study (Zwirner, Murry, & Woodson, 1991) compared measurements of fundamental frequency, standard deviation of fundamental frequency, jitter, shimmer, and SNR of 13 patients with Huntington's chorea. There was no statistically significant difference between the patients and normal controls on fundamental frequency. Frequency variability was much greater for the patient group, as was jitter. Shimmer and SNR were different from the normal group, but the difference was not statistically significant. Another interesting finding was the lack of a significant correlation between perceptual ratings of voice severity and any measure of perturbation or variability (standard deviation of fundamental frequency, jitter, shimmer, SNR).

We have observed in a recording of a patient producing a sustained vowel /ah/ (Fig. 5.18) an abrupt change in phonation approximately in the middle of the vowel and a loss of the ability of the analysis program to track the pitch. Note the gap in the pitch trace (dark line just below the dotted line in the figure). There was a noticeable quality change during the brief segment.

Measurable Physiological Signs

Few measurable physiological data have been reported on voice in chorea. Jarema, Kennedy, and Shoulson (1985) measured airflow rates during sustained vowel production for their 12 adults with Huntington's chorea and found much higher flow rates (220 mL/sec for women, 320 mL/sec for men) than for their normal control subjects

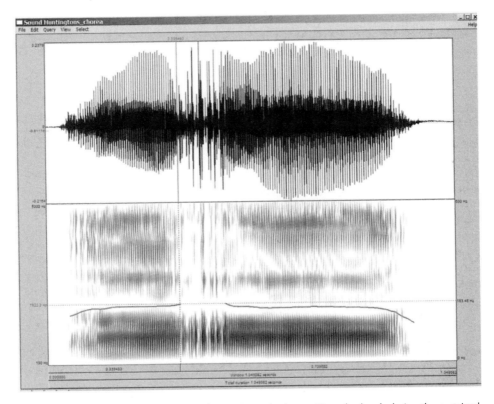

Figure 5.18. Spectrogram of a patient with Huntington's chorea. Note the break during the sustained vowel.

(178 mL/sec for women; 254 mL/sec for men). These data would suggest increased breathiness in patients with Huntington's chorea.

Ramig (1986) suggested that the previously noted voice arrests had to be associated with sudden adductory or abductory movements of the vocal folds, because they occurred much too fast to be produced by articulatory movements. This could be seen as indirect evidence of either hypertense or hypotense vocal folds.

Observable Physiological Signs

Usually, the larynges of patients with Huntington's chorea appear normal (Aronson, 1990). However, close observation may show short periods of adductory or abductory movement, especially in patients exhibiting voice arrests. Sudden shifts of fundamental frequency (usually downward) may be accompanied by jerky movements of the vocal folds. Further research is needed on the laryngoscopic signs of Huntington's chorea. No data have been reported on the stroboscopic signs in Huntington's chorea. Because the movements in Huntington's chorea are very jerky and irregular, visualization of the larynx with stroboscopy might be difficult in some patients.

Pathophysiology

The jerky, sudden, and abrupt movements of Huntington's chorea would seriously interfere with the production of smooth, controlled sound. Patients have decreased phonatory stability. Sudden adduction of the vocal folds may result in intensity bursts or voice arrests. Sudden abductory bursts would be accompanied by excessive airflow and breathiness or aphonic episodes. It is possible for a patient to exhibit both conditions, although one or the other characteristic will probably be the most prominent.

Supranuclear or Pseudobulbar Palsy

PRIMARY VOICE SYMPTOM: HOARSENESS OR HARSHNESS

Description and Etiology

Two major pathway systems converge on the lower motor neurons for control of muscles that affect voice and speech. These are the pyramidal and extrapyramidal tracts. Selected damage to the extrapyramidal or indirect pathway[3] usually results in spasticity and increased muscle reflexes. Selected damage to the direct or pyramidal pathway results in a loss of function, especially for skilled movements. The pyramidal system is said to be the newer system phylogenetically. Both pathways are located very close to each other anatomically, and lesions in these pathways would most likely affect both pathways and voluntary movement in four ways: spasticity, weakness, limitation of range, and a slowing of movement. The disease known as pseudobulbar palsy results when lesions affect these two systems.

Pseudobulbar palsy is actually a misnomer. The symptoms of the problem are in some instances very similar to those of bulbar disease (muscle weakness), and yet the evidence for bulbar lesions is equivocal. Langworthy and Hesser (1940) recommended the term *supranuclear bulbar paralysis*. Aring (1965) agreed, believing that the term had an anatomical basis, locating the lesions rostral to the appropriate cranial motor nerve nuclei. However, the term *pseudobulbar palsy* has remained in use.

Pseudobulbar palsy results from progressive lesions that occur bilaterally in the corticobulbar tracts. These lesions occur most frequently in the internal capsules (Aring, 1965; Langworthy & Hesser, 1940), although there may be pontine or midbrain lesions. These lesions are usually the result of a stroke, although other reported causes have been cerebral palsy, brain injuries, multiple sclerosis, and arteriosclerosis (Darley, Aronson, & Brown, 1975; Langworthy & Hesser, 1940). The chief symptoms are difficulties with speech and swallowing, plus emotional lability. The latter presents a unique feature of this problem. Patients may show bursts of laughter or crying in the presence of very mild stimuli or no stimuli at all. It is as if the patient's higher centers have released their control of these responses, and they appear uncontrolled. Kreindler and Pruskauer-Apostol (1971) documented these unusual behaviors, and Aronson (1990) emphasized that reduced thresholds for crying and laughter are critical cues in the diagnosis of this disorder.

Perceptual Voice Signs and Symptoms

A major sign of pseudobulbar palsy is dysarthria of speech, as documented by Darley and his colleagues (Darley, Aronson, & Brown, 1969a, 1969b, 1975). They grouped perceptual signs into clusters of the dysarthric symptoms that best characterize a particular type of neurological dysfunction. The important perceptual signs in pseudobulbar

---

[3] Indirect refers to the fact that information traveling along this pathway encounters many synapses or connection points along its way to the final destination. The direct pathway or pyramidal system has a single, continuous pathway from the motor cortex to the lower motor neurons in the spinal cord or nuclei in the brainstem.

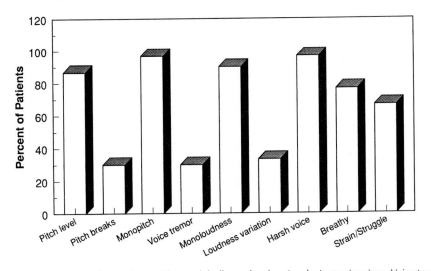

Figure 5.19. Percentage of 30 patients with pseudobulbar palsy showing deviant voice signs. Voice tremor was rated during contextual speech.

palsy are reported to be (using Darley, Aronson, and Brown's terminology) (a) prosodic excess (relates to rate and stress characteristics of speech); (b) prosodic insufficiency (monopitch, monoloudness, reduced stress, short phrases); (c) articulatory–resonatory incompetence (imprecise consonants, distorted vowels, hypernasality); and (d) phonatory stenosis (harsh voice, strain/struggle, pitch breaks).

Aronson et al. (1968a) rated the voice characteristics of 30 patients with pseudobulbar palsy (Darley, Aronson, & Brown, 1969a, 1969b) and found that 97% of the patients were considered to have monopitch and harsh voices, 87% had a too-low pitch level, 67% demonstrated considerable strain and struggle in phonation, and 30% exhibited pitch breaks and voice tremor. (These voice signs of pseudobulbar palsy are shown in Fig. 5.19.) Aring (1965) commented that the speech of a patient with pseudobulbar palsy is nasal and monotonic, with soft intensity and rapid rate, making it difficult to understand.

Acoustic Signs

Few data have been reported on the acoustic characteristics of patients with pseudobulbar palsy other than a study by Kammermeier (1969), who reported a mean fundamental frequency of 124.1 Hz in male subjects with a mean age of 61.7 years. When compared with the mean fundamental frequency (F_0) values reported for normal adult male speakers by Mysak (1959) (mean frequency, 124.3 Hz; mean age, 73.3 years) and Hollien and Shipp (1972) (mean frequency, 112 Hz; mean age, 64.6 years), the pseudobulbar subjects produced fundamental frequencies that were equal to or slightly higher than those of normal speakers. Kammermeier (1969) reported reduced variability of fundamental frequency in pseudobulbar patients, as well as reduced intensity variation. These findings may be related to the perception of monopitch and monoloudness. Patients with pseudobulbar palsy appear to exhibit normal or near-normal average fundamental frequency, reduced fundamental frequency variation, and reduced intensity variation.

Measurable Physiological Signs

We know of no data on the measurable physiological characteristics of the speech of patients with pseudobulbar palsy. Higher than normal subglottal pressures might be expected because of the hypertonicity and strain/struggle characteristics of the voice. If breathy, the patient would probably exhibit greater than normal airflows. If the range and force of movement of the vocal folds are affected, this might be reflected in slow opening and closing times of the vocal folds and perhaps a short closed phase because of the inability to maintain sufficient muscle forces.

Observable Physiological Signs

Laryngoscopy.   According to Darley et al. (1975), no laryngeal abnormalities have been reported. However, it is possible that vocal fold hyperadduction as well as hypofunction of other laryngeal structures might be observable, using the improved instruments available today for laryngoscopic examination. Further study of these characteristics is needed.

Stroboscopy.   Again, no reports exist on stroboscopic signs in patients with pseudobulbar palsy. When vocal fold hypertonicity is present, typical findings, according to Kitzing (1985), would include reduced vocal fold amplitudes, diminished mucosal waves, and excessive glottal closure. However, if the muscles have reduced force and movement, glottal closure may not be complete, and there may be asymmetry and aperiodicity of vocal fold movement.

Pathophysiology

Pseudobulbar palsy results in a loss of muscle coordination and a release of inhibition of the lower centers. The latter condition results in hyperactivity of the muscle reflexes and spasticity. In speech, pseudobulbar palsy patients show a reduction in the force and range of the muscle movement (Darley, Aronson, & Brown, 1969b). In addition, the release of the lower motor centers results in hypertonicity of the vocal folds. Pseudobulbar palsy seems to be a condition in which both muscle weakness and muscle hyperactivity coexist, with differential effects on the motor act being performed. Hypertonicity would be consistent with the perception of harshness in the voice, as well as the strain and struggle to speak. It is not necessarily consistent with the perception of a low pitch level or the findings that the fundamental frequency of these patients is within the normal range. These findings might be understood by hypothesizing that the cricothyroid is minimally affected in pseudobulbar palsy but that the other adductors or abductors of the larynx are affected differentially. Breathiness (noted in 14 of 30 patients with pseudobulbar palsy studied by Darley et al. [1969b]) would be produced by excessive opening of the vocal folds or perhaps by hypertonicity of the abductor muscle of the larynx (posterior cricothyroid). Hyperactivity in the adductors would have an effect similar to hypertonicity and would be consistent with strain/struggle quality, as well as excessive hoarseness or harshness. The specific voice signs (perceptual, acoustic, or physiological) noted in a patient with pseudobulbar palsy may reflect lesions at different locations along the long pathway from the brain to the ultimate motor neurons controlling the muscles of the larynx.

PHONATORY STABILITY

SHORT-TERM

Most patients with a neurological problem affecting the voice may show increased jitter and shimmer, especially if they exhibit hoarseness.

LONG-TERM

Amyotrophic Lateral Sclerosis (ALS)

PRIMARY VOICE SYMPTOM: HOARSENESS OR STRAIN/STRUGGLE

Description and Etiology

Amyotrophic lateral sclerosis (ALS or Lou Gehrig's disease) is a progressive, degen-erative disease of the CNS that involves both upper and lower motor neurons. As a result, the patient with ALS may have symptoms such as spasticity (upper motor neuron symptom) along with muscle weakness (a symptom of lower motor neuron lesions). The lower motor neuron lesions usually affect the ventral horn cells. The incidence of ALS is approximately 0.4 to 1.8 per 100,000 people (Janzen, Rae, & Hudson, 1988). The initial manifestation is muscle weakness, cramps, and fasciculation. The disease usually affects people later in life, although reports of early onset are known. The rate of progression of the disease may vary.

In the study by Carpenter, McDonald, and Howard (1988), 28% of 123 patients with ALS presented with symptoms in the head, neck, larynx, or voice. The mean age of these patients was 61 years, and the ratio between men and women was approximately equal. Of the patients presenting head/neck symptoms, 68% exhibited slurred speech, 14% had hoarseness, and 13% presented with dysphagia. On physical examination, the patients presented muscle weakness and fasciculation in various areas, as shown in Table 5.8. In many patients, excessive drooling may exist and presents unique problems for management. In the latter stages of the disease, it is likely that 100% of patients exhibit severe respiratory, speech, voice, and swallowing difficulties. Most require res-piratory assistance and augmentative speech systems.

Speech signs in ALS include flaccid dysarthria or spastic dysarthria or both. A more detailed list of speech signs is presented in Table 5.9. There are many possible causes for this condition. Aronson (1990) listed infection, malignancy, and genetic defects. Janzen et al. (1988) added toxins, autoimmunity problems, and metabolic deficiencies. There is no effective treatment, although certain drugs have been used to ease the symptoms.

Perceptual Voice Signs and Symptoms

The early primary symptom is hoarseness or harshness, with slurred speech as an additional symptom. In their classic study of the perceptual characteristics of dysarthria, Darley et al. (1969a) listed imprecise consonants, hypernasality, harsh voice, slow rate, and monopitch as the prominent speech characteristics in their group of 30 subjects

Table 5.8. Percent of ALS Patients Presenting With Physical Abnormalities in the Head and Neck Region

Area	Weakness	Fasciculations
Tongue	66	54
Extremities	66	30
Neck	412	10
Face	2	38
Palate and pharynx	2	32
Masseter muscle	8	2

Table 5.9. Frequency of Speech Deviations in Patients With ALS

Speech Deviation	Percent
Harsh voice	79.75
Hypernasality	74.68
Breathy voice	64.56
Voice tremor	63.29
Strain/struggle voice	59.49
Imprecise consonants	56.96
Reduced intelligibility	46.84
Slow rate	46.84
Phonemes prolonged	45.57
Audible inspiration	40.51
Continuous phonation	37.97
High pitch	37.97
Phrases short	36.71
Inappropriate silences	32.91
Nasal emission	30.28
Vowels distorted	24.05
Low pitch	7.59
Fast rate	2.53

with ALS. Figure 5.20 presents a summary of the voice signs and symptoms found in a group of patients with ALS, as reported by Aronson et al. (1968b). Similar speech and voice symptoms were reported by Carrow, Mauldin, and Shamblin (1974). One limitation of these early studies is the lack of information about the stage of the disease in the subject groups. Because this is a progressively deteriorating disease, all symptoms become increasingly severe and debilitating with time.

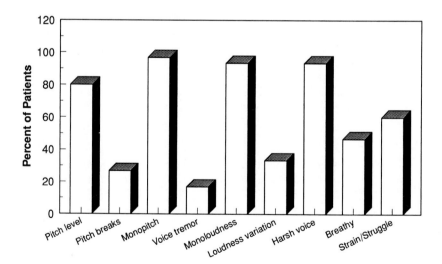

Figure 5.20. Percentage of 30 patients with amyotrophic lateral sclerosis showing voice deviations. Voice tremor was rated during contextual speech.

Table 5.10. Acoustic Measures in ALS

	Males		Females	
	ALS	Control	ALS	Control
Fundamental frequency	127.4	112.8	179	194.5
Jitter (msec)	0.11	0.12	0.24	0.07
Shimmer (%)	5.3	7	18.53	2.61
SNR (dB)	19.32	16.87	13.08	21.38

Acoustic Signs

Caruso and Burton (1987) reported that the stop gaps in stop consonant syllables and vowel duration were much longer in the speech of patients with ALS than in normal speakers. Voice onset time in the two groups was very similar. These authors suggest that laryngeal structures may move more slowly in ALS than in normal speakers. They point out that because the nucleus ambiguus is often affected, the neural control of adduction and abduction by the vocal folds may be impaired.

In a study primarily concerned with patients with other neurologic problems, Ramig et al. (1988) reported on the changes of F_0, jitter, shimmer, and harmonics-to-noise ratio (HNR) of a 69-year-old man recorded 4 times over a period of 6 months. Shimmer and HNR were most sensitive to the changes that occurred over the 6-month period. At the end of the recording sessions, the subject displayed greater acoustic instability. Additional data on this subject were reported by Ramig et al. (1990). The coefficient of amplitude and the coefficient of frequency, measures that reflect the long-term stability of phonation, were also greater for the patient than for his control. These data are consistent with the notion that ALS patients exhibit decreased phonatory control that is exacerbated by the progression of the disease.

Kent et al. (1991) reported abnormalities of fundamental frequency and perturbation in their group of 10 female patients with ALS. Kent et al. (1991) found that the fundamental frequency of their male patients with ALS (n = 32) was somewhat higher than the normal controls (127.4 Hz vs. 112.8 Hz) (Table 5.10).

Strand, Buder, Yorkston, and Ramig (1993) also reported on fundamental frequency, intensity, jitter, shimmer, and SNR of four adult females with ALS. Although the patient data were different from the normal controls, the patients did show considerable variation of fundamental frequency both in sustained phonation and in phrase samples. All four patients exhibited greater jitter and shimmer than the control subjects. One interesting facet of this study is the report of the perceptual voice characteristics of the four patients that should be considered when interpreting the acoustic data. One patient was characterized as having a strain/struggle voice quality, whereas another exhibited breathy phonation with low volume. The other two subjects exhibited harsh voice quality with fluctuations of intensity and frequency. The group was heterogeneous, and one should expect variation in the acoustic data. Such was the case in this report. ALS speech is characterized as a mixed dysarthria; some patients can exhibit symptoms characteristic of spasticity, whereas others can exhibit a flaccid dysarthria. The acoustic features of each type of dysarthria are very different.

Measurable Physiological Signs

No data have been reported on the physiological characteristics of the speech of ALS patients. However, EMG studies have been reported on nonlaryngeal muscles and reveal sporadic action potentials, a reduction in the number of potentials, and fibrillation. Similar findings might be expected in the laryngeal muscles.

Observable Physiological Signs

The larynx in ALS usually has a normal appearance (Aronson, 1990). However, it is possible to observe hyperadduction if the major component in the disease is spasticity. If the major component is flaccidity, one might expect incomplete closure, bowing, or slower speed of vocal fold movement.

No data have been reported on stroboscopic signs specifically in ALS patients. However, signs typical of flaccid paralysis (reduced mucosal wave, incomplete closure) or those associated with problems affecting the upper motor neurons (spastic characteristics such as hyperadduction) would be consistent with the nature of the effects of the disease.

Pathophysiology

Amyotrophic lateral sclerosis impairs CNS control of the muscles of the larynx (as well as most muscles in the body). Furthermore, if the lower motor neurons are affected, muscle tone and strength are affected. Patients may exhibit spastic phases or flaccid phases depending on the precise areas affected. Spastic effects might result in a strain/struggle type of voice, whereas flaccid effects might reduce the efficiency of glottal valving.

Essential Tremor

PRIMARY VOICE SYMPTOM: TREMOR

Classification of Tremor

Various types of tremor may have differing causes (central, peripheral, or both), characteristic timing features, and unique characteristics of presentation. Tremor may be present as an isolated symptom or it may be one characteristic of a more generalized neurological disorder.

Tremor is characterized by relatively regular, involuntary movements of the distal or proximal muscles. Everyone has some degree of normal tremor, which ranges in frequency from 6 to 12 Hz. Abnormal tremor has a lower frequency range, larger amplitudes, and may interfere with purposeful movements. Tremor may occur while a structure is at rest (resting tremor) or in action (action tremor). Action tremor may consist of postural tremor (when holding a structure in position), contraction tremor, or intention tremor (Brin, Fahn, Blitzer, Ramig, & Stewart, 1992). It may be focal or more generalized. Essential tremor is a disorder of the CNS that may result in tremor in the head, limbs, tongue, palate, and larynx. It tends to start in the hands and then progresses to the arms, head, neck, face, and so on (Brown & Simonson, 1963). "Essential tremor is typically absent at rest, maximal during maintenance of a posture, attenuated during movement, and often accentuated at the termination of movement" (Brin, Fahn, Blitzer, Ramig, & Stewart, 1992; Emanuel & Sansone, 1969). Typically, the frequency of tremor in patients with essential tremor is between 3 and 7 Hz (Brin, Fahn, Blitzer, Ramig, & Stewart, 1992).

Description and Etiology

In some patients, voice tremor may be the primary or sole characteristic. In the Brown and Simonson study (1963), only 6 of 31 essential tremor patients exhibited isolated voice tremor, whereas the remaining 25 had tremor in the head, tremor of the extremities, or both, in addition to voice tremor. Some have reported voice tremor in 10% to 20% of their patients (Brin, Fahn, Blitzer, Ramig, & Stewart, 1992). Lou and Jankovic (1991), reporting on 350 patients with essential tremor, found only one case of voice tremor as the sole symptom, gradual onset of tremor, and frequent occurrence of family members with some kind of tremor. Seventeen patients had associated neurological signs, including a positive sucking reflex, spasmodic torticollis, bilateral facial spasms, incoordination, and diadochokinesis.

Larsson and Sjogren (1960) reported that essential tremor occurred more frequently in men than in women, with a mean age of onset of 48 years. Aronson and Hartman (1981) reported the mean age of onset at 57 years. They also found extralaryngeal tremor in 93% of their patients. In their study of 678 patients with essential tremor, Koller, Busenbark, and Miner (1994) found that approximately 49% were female and 51% male. The average age of onset was 45.3 years. Approximately 90% of the patients had tremor affecting either hand; approximately 20% had head tremor, with smaller numbers of patients with tremors of the leg, chin, trunk, and tongue.

Thus, essential tremor seems to be associated with aging, although the reasons for this are unclear. The highest prevalence is in the 7th decade of life. Heredity may affect the development of the tremor. Approximately half of patients with essential tremor have a history of an affected family member (Young, 1986). In sudden-onset cases, Brown and Simonson (1963) suggested that some kind of arterial disease may have been responsible.

It is difficult to determine the locus of the CNS lesion that causes essential tremor. Critchley (1949) suggested that the extrapyramidal system is involved, but it is possible that other structures might be affected. Brin et al. (1992) suggest that tremor may be the result of oscillation in the olivocerebellar tracts. Young (1986) noted that a ventrolateral thalamotomy reduced or eliminated the tremor. There may be a possibility of dysfunction in the cerebellum as a cause of the tremor (Young, 1986).

Perceptual Voice Signs and Symptoms

The most prominent voice symptom and sign is tremor, a regular modulation of frequency or intensity that is most noticeable during prolonged production of a vowel but is also apparent during contextual speech. In 100% of their patients with essential tremor, Aronson et al. (1968b) reported tremor on a sustained /ah/ vowel (only tremor in contextual speech is shown in Fig. 5.21), as well as harshness and strain/struggle. Figure 5.21 presents a summary of the voice symptoms in essential tremor as reported in the Aronson et al. (1968b) study.

In general, the voice of essential tremor patients may be described as sounding quavery and tremulous. Some patients will have a relatively constant and noticeable tremor during speech. Some may have such severe tremor that stoppage of voice occurs, as reported by Ardran, Kinsbourne, and Rushworth (1966).

Acoustic Signs

Few data exist many of the acoustic signs in essential tremor. Most studies have concentrated on the variation of amplitude during sustained vowel production. Brown and Simonson (1963) measured the rate of tremor from oscillograms of 23 patients. Tremor frequencies of 5 to 6 Hz were measured in most patients. Ardran et al. (1966) reported spectrographic evidence of low-amplitude noise during the production of monosyllabic words by a single patient. This noise, they suggested, gave evidence of breathiness in the patients' speech. Aronson and Hartman (1981) analyzed the tremor in oscillograms

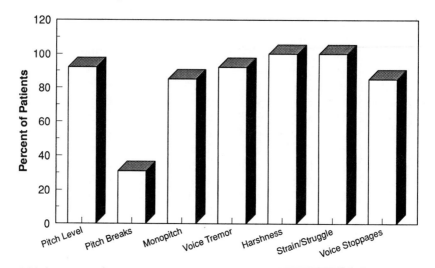

Figure 5.21. Percentage of 26 patients with essential tremor showing voice deviations. Voice tremor was rated during contextual speech.

of 14 patients with essential tremor and reported a mean tremor frequency of 5.7 Hz. Lebrun, Devreux, Rousseau, and Darimont (1982) reported a tremor frequency of 4 Hz in the voice of their 84-year-old patient. They also observed erratic voice breaks and arrests. Figure 5.22 shows a spectrogram of a male patient producing a sustained vowel /ah/. Note the rhythmic variations of intensity in the waveform along the top of

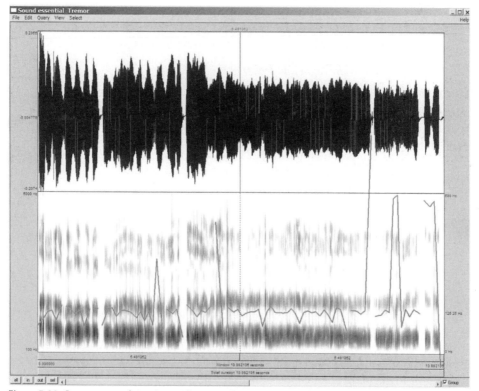

Figure 5.22. Spectrogram of a patient with essential tremor producing a sustained vowel.

the figure and the variations of fundamental frequency (shown by the gray line in the spectrogram).

Measurable Physiological Signs

Little data have been reported on the measurable physiological characteristics of patients with essential tremor. Ardran et al. (1966) performed electromyograms on the cricothyroid and hyoglossus muscles of a 72-year-old female patient. They showed that, at rest, both muscles had regular variation in activity at a rate of approximately 5 to 6 Hz. They comment that this was low-level activity that did not result in movement of the structures. This variation in muscle activity was not entirely regular and disappeared occasionally. Furthermore, the variation of activity between the hyoglossus and the cricothyroid muscle was not synchronized. There was also resting tremor in the EMG of the pectoralis major and external intercostal muscles in this patient. However, these disappeared when the patient contracted these muscles.

Observable Physiological Signs

By and large, the larynges of patients with essential tremor will show normal structure and movement. Rhythmic movement of one or more laryngeal structures sometimes may be observed during phonation or at rest. Brown and Simonson (1963) reported normal-appearing larynges in 13 of their essential tremor patients and vocal fold bowing in one patient. However, 17 of their patients were not examined laryngoscopically.

We know of no data on the stroboscopic signs in essential tremor. It has been our experience that obtaining stroboscopic imaging of sufficiently acceptable quality from which to make reliable interpretation of stroboscopic signs has not been possible. The tremor makes tracking of the fundamental frequency difficult. However, newer stroboscopic equipment appears to be able to track vibration in the presence of tremor.

Pathophysiology

The rhythmically changing activity in the muscles of the larynx create varying degrees of tension in the vocal folds and lead to a rhythmic change in fundamental frequency. Furthermore, the degree of adduction varies systematically in synchrony with the variation of muscle activity, creating a rhythmic change in the force of adduction. This results in variations of subglottal air pressure and thus of vocal intensity. If the tremor is severe, the adductory force could become large enough to completely stop voice production. Voice stoppages are also characteristic of SD. As discussed earlier (see "SD, Other Considerations"), Aronson and Hartman (1981) and others have suggested that some forms of SD may have essential tremor as their cause. Medication has been used to treat essential tremor with mixed results. Propranolol (sometimes in conjunction with diazepam), primidone, and clonazepam have been used. Brin, Fahn, Blitzer, Ramig, and Stewart (1992), however, report limited success in using these drugs to treat essential tremor. The voice tremor characteristics of patients with SD and those with essential tremor are different (Brin, Fahn, Blitzer, Ramig, & Stewart, 1992).

PHONATORY INCOORDINATION/ VOICED–VOICELESS DISTINCTION

Abductor SD

Abductor SD involves the muscle of abduction of the vocal folds and results in an intermittently breathy voice quality. Some authors (Hartman & Aronson, 1981; Shipp, Mueller, & Zwitman, 1980) have suggested that abductor SD is so dissimilar to the adductor type that it should be given a name more indicative of its pathophysiology. Hartman and Aronson (1981) have suggested the term *intermittent breathy dysphonia*, whereas Shipp et al. (1980) advocate the term *intermittent abductory dysphonia*. Ludlow (1995), believing the cause of the symptoms to be a failure in the execution of smooth transition from abductory to adductory posture during speech, has argued that this form of SD represents a problem of coordination.

Perceptual Voice Signs and Symptoms

Descriptions of the abductor type of SD vary. Some authors describe intermittent episodes of breathy dysphonia, drops in pitch, and vowel prolongations (Hartman & Aronson, 1981; Merson & Ginsberg, 1979; Zwitman, 1979). Aronson (1973, 1990) states that in many respects it is the mirror image of adductor SD. Ludlow (1995) describes the perceptual attribute characteristic of the abductor type of SD as a delay in voice onset after production of voiceless consonants. Pitch breaks may occur in some patients. Close attention to the episodes of voice interruption in these patients confirms the preponderance of difficulty associated with the transition from voiceless (i.e., /h/, /s/, /f/, /p/, /t/) to voiced phonemes.

Acoustic Signs

Fundamental Frequency.   Merson and Ginsberg (1979) reported mean fundamental frequencies of 161.3 Hz and 203.8 Hz for two female patients with abductor SD reading a sentence.

Vocal Intensity.   Hartman and Aronson (1981) reported the amplitude variations observed in the speech of 17 abductor SD patients. They found a steady but random variation of amplitude in some patients, rhythmic variation in other patients, and evidence of moments of breathiness in still other patients. We know of no data on vocal intensity in the abductor type of SD. It has been our experience, however, that some of these patients use much-reduced intensity levels in conversation, even to the point of aphonic whisper. This is perhaps a compensatory behavior adopted to avoid voice stoppages.

Few other data have appeared in the literature about the acoustic characteristics of abductor SD. Wolfe and Bacon (1976) reported some spectrographic findings for a patient with what appears to be abductor SD, in which there is evidence of interruptions of voicing, as well as irregularly spaced vertical striations indicating a variation of voicing associated with the strain and struggle to speak. Zwitman (1979) reported similar findings for two patients with abductor SD. He also reported that voiceless stops seem to be distinguished from voiced stops by a sustained frication during the voiceless stops. Some of the spectrographic features of abductor SD can be seen in Figure 5.16.

Ludlow and her colleagues reported the most extensive analysis of the acoustic features. An illustration of the delay in the onset of phonation often observed in patients with abductor SD is shown in Figure 5.23. The upper panel is the waveform of the sentence, *Do queens eat honey?* The lower panel shows the spectrogram of the same sentence along with the trace of fundamental frequency (the light gray line running in about the center of the spectrogram). The lightly colored rectangle at the end of the sentence brackets the word *honey*. Note the initial period of silence/breathiness corresponding to the /h/ in honey, followed by a very brief voiced segment, followed by breathiness for the remainder of the word.

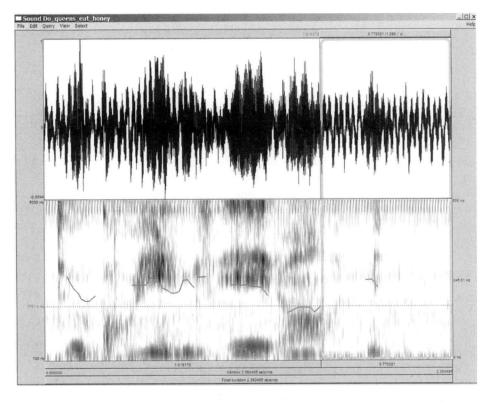

Figure 5.23. Spectrogram of a patient with abductor SD producing the sentence "Do queens eat honey?" The upper panel is the acoustic waveform, whereas the lower panel shows the spectrogram and the fundamental frequency trace (dark broken line). The light-colored rectangle at the end of the sentence shows the acoustic changes that occurred when the patient produced the word *honey*. Note the long noise duration followed by a very brief voiced segment.

Measurable Physiological Signs

One would expect large airflows to be associated with abductory SD. Indeed, Merson and Ginsberg (1979) reported such large flows in two patients (e.g., 321 mL/sec on a sustained /ah/ vowel, 400 mL/sec and 435 mL/sec) during sentence production.

Observable Physiological Signs

Laryngoscopy and Stroboscopy. There are few data on the laryngoscopic and stroboscopic characteristics unique to abductor SD.

Pathophysiology

In abductor SD, the spasm results in a sudden increase of airflow and relatively short closed times. The combination of rapid airflows and short closed time would be expected to produce much less energy in the higher frequencies of the spectrum. The voice will be perceived as intermittently breathy and weak. Again, there are periods of normal vocal fold vibration, but it is the sudden, unexpected stoppages that create havoc in the production of voice and speech.

MIXED DISORDERS

Cerebellar Ataxia

PRIMARY VOICE SYMPTOM: HOARSENESS

Description and Etiology

Cerebellar ataxia is a disorder of the cerebellum. Its accompanying speech disorder is called ataxic dysphonia or, more generally, ataxic dysarthria. A lesion in the cerebellum results in a loss of muscle coordination and movement. Fulton and Dow (1937) considered two kinds of speech defects in cerebellar lesions: (a) errors in the rate, range, direction, and force of movements; and (b) hypotonia. Kent, Netsell, and Abbs (1979) presented some acoustic evidence for "scanning speech" and suggested that it may be the result of the inability of the cerebellum to properly integrate movements, or it may be due to an alteration in the motor programming plan of the cerebellum. In their study of ataxic dysarthria, Brown, Darley, and Aronson (1970) concluded that excess and equal stress plus irregular articulatory breakdown were the speech scales most suggestive of this condition.

The cause of dysphonia in ataxic dysarthria is varied. In their study, Brown et al. (1970) reported that three patients had a neoplasm, one had experienced trauma, one had an infarct, one was thought to have multiple sclerosis, and 24 were diagnosed with cerebellar degeneration. They suggested that the important areas of the cerebellum serving speech were the vermis and the adjacent paravermis. Lechtenberg and Gilman (1978) implicate the left cerebellar hemisphere as important for the control of speech. Based on that implication, Kent, Netsell, and Abbs (1979) hypothesized that the right cerebral hemisphere must send its information to the left cerebellar hemisphere, making both hemispheres responsible for the control of speech prosody. If true, one might expect patients with ataxic dysarthria to have greater difficulty in the control of the suprasegmental features of speech (i.e., stress and intonation), both of which involve the vocal folds.

Perceptual Voice Signs and Symptoms

In their rating study of the speech of patients with various kinds of neuromuscular diseases, Aronson et al. (1968a) noted the voice features of harshness, monopitch, too-low pitch, strain/struggle, and pitch breaks as prevalent in ataxic dysarthria. The percentage of patients showing these perceptual signs of the voice is shown in Figure 5.24.

Aronson (1990) noted that some ataxics may exhibit normal voice quality but that many show harshness, monopitch, and monoloudness as characteristic perceptual features.

Acoustic Signs

Kent, Netsell, and Abbs (1979) reported a study on the acoustic characteristics of the speech of five ataxic patients. They found abnormally long vowel and segment durations and strongly suggested that there were aberrations in the control of fundamental frequency. In an earlier study, Kent and Netsell (1975) reported on the speech characteristics of a female ataxic patient. Among other variables, they examined fundamental frequency contours during the production of words and sentences. They noted that many fundamental frequency contours had a monotone appearance, whereas others

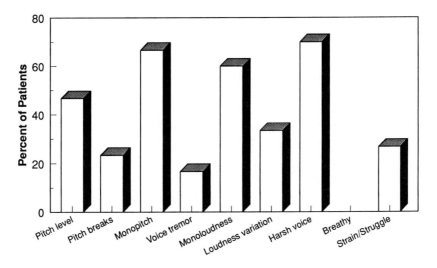

Figure 5.24. Percentage of 30 patients with ataxic dysarthria showing voice deviations. Voice tremor was rated during contextual speech.

had marked variability of fundamental frequency. They suggested that ataxics may have more difficulty controlling fundamental frequency during speech than they have in articulating the phonemes. They also noted spectrographic evidence of harshness or vocal fry.

The fundamental frequency of ataxic dysphonics is very similar to that of normal speakers (Zwirner, Murry, & Woodson, 1991); however, the standard deviation of fundamental frequency of these patients was over three times as large as that of normal speakers (1.3 vs. 6.1 Hz). Jitter was also much larger than normal. Patients also showed a difference of shimmer and SNR compared with the normal controls, but the differences were not statistically significant.

These data support the notion of Kent and Netsell (1975) that persons with cerebellar ataxia have difficulty controlling fundamental frequency. Both the standard deviation of fundamental frequency and jitter reflect frequency variability, and both are much larger than normal. Patients with cerebellar ataxia can produce the desired fundamental frequency, but they have difficulty controlling it.

Measurable Physiological Signs

No data appear to be available in the literature concerning the measurable physiological characteristics of the voice of ataxic patients. In their single-subject analysis, Kent and Netsell (1975) reported that cineradiographic analysis of the oral cavity during speech revealed abnormal but small anteroposterior lingual adjustments. Furthermore, they found that the patient's articulatory movements were longer in duration than normal movements. Thus, valving movements of the vocal folds might show abnormally long durations.

Brown et al. (1970) reported that electromyographic recordings were made on 6 of their 30 patients with ataxic dysarthria but failed to specify which muscles were studied. They reported normal EMG patterns in two patients, evidence of a motor lesion in one patient, and evidence of a peripheral neuropathy in three patients. Similar abnormalities might be found in the laryngeal muscles, although not in all patients.

Observable Physiological Signs

Aronson (1990) expects to find a normal-appearing larynx in patients with ataxic dysphonia. Evidence of reduced speed of adduction or abduction during valving and movements of the vocal folds might be observed on careful study. There are no reported data on the stroboscopic signs in patients with ataxic dysphonia.

Pathophysiology

Ataxic dysphonia or dysarthria seems to be characterized by hypotonia and an incoordination of muscles. Hypotonia manifests itself as a delay in the generation of a force, a reduced rate of muscular contraction, and a reduced range of movement (Brown, Darley, & Aronson, 1970; Kent & Netsell, 1975; Kent, Netsell, & Abbs, 1979). Reduced muscle activity may account for the reduced fundamental frequency range during conversational speech, because, to increase vocal pitch, cricothyroid muscle activity must be increased. Reduced muscle tone also may account for hoarseness in ataxic voices because of tension differences between the two vocal folds. Hypotonicity will have a similar effect on the control of intensity, although few data have been reported on this acoustic variable. Incoordination of phonation may be manifested by difficulty in controlling the magnitude and extent of laryngeal movements as well as the control of the magnitude and extent of articulatory movements.

Multiple Sclerosis

PRIMARY VOICE SYMPTOMS: IMPAIRED LOUDNESS CONTROL AND HOARSENESS

Description and Etiology

Multiple sclerosis (MS) was first described by Charcot (1881), who referred to it as disseminated sclerosis. It is a disease characterized by multiple scarring (sclerosis) of the white matter in the brain, brainstem, and spinal cord. The initial symptoms of the disease may be very mild. As it progresses, the severity of the symptoms may increase, yet intermittently there may be long periods of remission or latency during which the person may seem well. It is very likely an autoimmune disorder, but the evidence is not clear on this (Corboy, Goodin, & Frohman, 2003). In the United States, the incidence of multiple sclerosis is approximately 50 per 100,000. It is much more common in the temperate regions of the northern and southern hemispheres, with the incidence dropping markedly close to the equator. The male–female ratio is about 1.7–2.1 in the United States. The disease frequently develops in young adulthood, although it has been suggested that the onset of the very slowly progressing symptoms occurs in childhood but only becomes apparent in the adult (Millar, 1971).

Approximately 50% of patients with multiple sclerosis initially seek medical attention because of ENT symptoms, including vertigo (25%), nystagmus (40%–70%), dysarthria (20%), or dysphagia (10%–15%) (Garfinkle & Kimmelman, 1982; Ward, Cannon, & Lindsay, 1965). Bilateral abductor paralysis of the vocal folds also may occur. Noffsinger, Olsen, Carhart, Hart, and Sahgal (1972) documented many of the

Table 5.11. Neurological Signs in Multiple Sclerosis

Neurological Sign	Percent
Finger to finger/toe to finger tests	82
Dysdiadochokinesis	71
Impairment of posterior column sense	60
Pyramidal signs (sucking reflex, Hoffman's sign, Babinski's sign, increased muscle stretch reflexes)	92
Muscular weakness	9

auditory and vestibular system dysfunctions in patients with multiple sclerosis. Of course, a patient may present with multiple symptoms.

Most patients present a relapsing–remitting form of multiple sclerosis (RRMS) that most often develops into a progressive deterioration of various brain functions. Approximately 10% present a progressive disease from the start with little or no evidence of remission (Corboy, Goodin & Frohman, 2003).

The reported loci of CNS involvement are not consistent. In a study of 234 multiple sclerosis patients, 85% were reported to have pyramidal involvement, followed by cerebellar (77%) and brainstem (73%) involvement (Kurtzke, Beebe, Nagler, Auth, & Kurland, 1972). Multiple system involvement was also noted by Garfinkle and Kimmelman (1982). Patients with multiple sclerosis present a variety of neurological signs. Some of these are summarized in Table 5.11, based on the data presented by Darley, Brown, and Goldstein (1972).

It has been stated that the cardinal signs of multiple sclerosis are scanning speech, nystagmus, and intention tremor (Ivers & Goldstein, 1963). However, available data suggest that speech/voice problems, although sometimes present, are not pervasive. Darley et al. (1972) found that 59% of their 168 patients presented normal speech patterns, and another 29% had minimal speech impairment. Table 5.12 presents a summary of the speech and voice symptoms in their patients. These authors also noted that the severity of speech difficulty increased with an increase in the severity of the neurological deficit. They concluded that dysarthria was not characteristic of MS speech, nor

Table 5.12. Speech Deviations in Multiple Sclerosis

Speech Deviation	Percent
Normal speech performance	59
Defective speech performance	41
Impaired loudness control	77
Harshness	72
Defective articulation	46
Impaired emphasis	39
Impaired pitch control	37
Hypernasality	24
Inappropriate pitch level	24
Breathiness	22

was scanning speech. Kurtzke et al. (1972) reported that scanning speech was present in only 18.9% of their 525 male patients with MS.

Treatment of MS may involve a variety of drugs that have shown promise for the relief of some of the symptoms of MS, including interferon-beta-1a and interferon-beta-1b as well as other drugs (Corboy, Goodin, & Frohman, 2003). Some have suggested the use of alternative medicines for the relief of some symptoms, although the use of such drugs has shown only slight improvement of some symptoms (Bowling & Stewart, 2003). Others (Bever, 1999; Bielekova & Martin, 1999) have discussed additional treatment options for patients with MS, including traditional therapy for the relief of pain, fatigue, and mood changes.

Perceptual Voice Signs and Symptoms

The primary voice symptoms associated with multiple sclerosis are impaired loudness control and harshness (Darley, Brown, & Goldstein, 1972; Farmakides & Boone, 1960; Hartelius, Buder & Strand, 1997). Hypernasality is also prominent (Farmakides & Boone, 1960), whereas impaired pitch control, inappropriate pitch level, and breathiness can occur less frequently. Speech characteristics include a slowing of speech rate, defective articulation (Darley, Brown, & Goldstein, 1972; Jensen, 1960), impaired emphasis (scanning speech), and occasionally poor respiratory control (Table 5.12).

Acoustic Signs

The range of fundamental frequencies produced by patients with MS appears to be very similar to that of normal speakers, with the possible exception of a slightly greater fundamental frequency range and larger variability of fundamental frequency (Zemlin, 1962). In their study of five MS speakers, Hartelius, Nord & Buder (1995) found little difference of fundamental as compared with their normal controls and published data. These authors also noted that their MS speakers exhibited considerable variability in the various measurements they made.

Hartelius, Buder, and Strand (1997) analyzed the sustained vowel productions of 20 individuals with MS and compared the results with 20 age- and gender-matched controls. Their method of analysis focused on the stability (i.e., variation) of both fundamental frequency and intensity. One unique acoustic analysis involved analyzing the sustained phonations for fundamental frequency and intensity contours and then analyzing the results of those analyses for low-frequency spectral components. One measure they derived involved looking at the magnitude of the frequencies present in three low-frequency bands, 0 to 4 Hz, 4 to 6 Hz, and 16 to 19 Hz. They demonstrated distinct differences between the MS patients and their controls for the low- and high-frequency bands. These authors concluded that this type of fine analysis of variability and stability could be useful in helping to differentiate MS patients from normal controls before any evidence of dysarthria was discernible.

Measurable Physiological Signs

We know of no data on the measurable phonatory physiological characteristics of patients with MS. If harshness is present, suggestive of vocal fold hypertonicity, low flows and high subglottal pressures might be expected. The vibratory cycle of the vocal folds is probably highly variable because of the harshness and impaired muscle control.

Observable Physiological Signs

In most patients, the larynx would be expected to appear normal. In patients with abductor paralysis, vocal fold opening should be impaired, and the patient may present problems related to air intake. There may be reduced range of motion of the vocal folds and momentary stoppages of vocal fold motion.

We know of no data on the stroboscopic signs in MS. We might expect to find good closure of the vocal folds (unless the patient is very breathy), but there may be a reduction of the amplitude of vibration and perhaps poor phase symmetry.

Pathophysiology

Multiple sclerosis is characterized by increasing incoordination, spasticity, and weakness of the muscles in the body. When the laryngeal musculature is affected, these same characteristics might be evidenced by impaired phonatory coordination and control and by reduced range and force of movement. Spasticity and muscle weakness will affect the ability of the vocal folds to adduct smoothly and to maintain the proper adductory forces needed for phonation. Weakness of vocal fold adduction may mean an inability to produce the proper subglottal pressures needed for speech. This will manifest itself in reduced vocal loudness. The spastic characteristic of multiple sclerosis may impair the ability to maintain control over vocal fold adduction and therefore may result in uneven vocal loudness. Poor coordination of the vocal folds may produce aperiodicity of vibration and lead to greater perceived hoarseness/harshness. The rate of movement of the vocal folds also may be impaired similarly to the impaired rate of speaking (Jensen, 1960).

Treatment may involve various drugs to produce relief of symptoms such as spasticity, fatigue, neurobehavioral disorders, paroxysmal disorders, pain, bladder dysfunction, and cerebellar dysfunction (Mitchell, 1993). Immunotherapies also may provide benefits (Rolak, 2001).

MISCELLANEOUS DISORDERS

Arnold-Chiari Malformation (Chiari II Malformation)

The Arnold-Chiari malformation is a congenital anomaly of the hindbrain in which the brainstem and cerebellum are squeezed into the cervical portion of the spinal column, causing injury to the cerebellum, medulla, and lower cranial nerves (Bralley, Bull, Gore, & Edgerton, 1978; Merritt, 1979). It was first described by Arnold (1894) and more extensively by Chiari (1896). There are actually four types of malformations originally discussed by Chiari. Types I and II are often referred to as the Arnold-Chiari type (Bamberger-Bozo, 1987; Salam & Adams, 1978). Type I is one in which only the cerebellar tonsils are displaced. Types III and IV are much more severe and in some cases incompatible with life. In type II, malformation of the medulla, cerebellum, and mesencephalon are encountered, usually with a lumbar meningomyelocele. Interestingly, many of the clinical manifestations of type II occur after birth (Bamberger-Bozo, 1987). Infants usually have difficulty swallowing, apneic episodes, laryngeal paralysis, stridor, and occasionally arm weakness. Most laryngeal paralysis is the abductor type.

In some cases, this malformation can result in vocal fold paralysis (Rullan, 1991), in which voice symptoms will appear that are similar to cerebellar ataxia (discussed earlier) or to lesions affecting the medulla or the peripheral nerves as they leave the cranium, causing flaccid paralysis. In the latter case, perceptual, acoustic, and physiological signs as seen in recurrent nerve paralysis would be expected (see "Peripheral Nerve Lesions" for a more complete discussion.)

Gilles de la Tourette Syndrome

Gilles de la Tourette syndrome develops in early childhood, usually between ages 2 and 13. It is characterized by twitching and grimacing, with tics of the face and eyes being the most common symptom (Golden, 1977; Merritt, 1975). The tics may later spread to the limbs. The speech of these individuals is characterized by unusual noises, explosive outbursts, and may include unexpected utterance of profanities. Contrary to most beliefs, coprolalia (foul explicatives), and echolalia are not frequently heard in childhood. The disease increases in severity during childhood, but the symptoms may diminish in adulthood. The disease can usually be controlled by the use of the drug haloperidol, although there have been reports of unwanted side effects in some patients. Lang and Marsden (1983) reported a case in which SD developed during the use of haloperidol and persisted after removal of the drug.

Gilles de la Tourette syndrome, although interesting and unusual, does not present any unique challenges for the speech pathologist insofar as the voice is concerned. The symptoms are not under voluntary control and cannot be altered or controlled through a behavioral approach. Pharmacological treatment can be effective in reducing or eliminating the symptoms.

SUMMARY

Vocal fold vibration depends on an intact neurological system to maintain the proper tension in the vocal folds, produce the proper airflow and air pressures needed for voicing, and adduct or abduct the vocal folds in accord with the requirements of the speaking act. Disruption of this control will affect the normal vibration of the vocal folds. This disruption may occur either in the central or the peripheral nervous system. When lesions occur in the peripheral nervous system, the phonatory system will show signs of denervation and flaccidity. The muscles controlled by the nerves will fail to receive the proper innervation and will not contract.

When lesions occur within the CNS, the phonatory system may show signs of flaccidity or hyperfunction depending on the site of the lesion(s). Lesions high in the CNS but not in the cortex affecting the pyramidal or extrapyramidal systems will produce hypertonia and exaggerated reflexes. Lesions in the cerebellum will produce deficits in the control of muscles, especially groups of muscles needed for the complex motor act of speech. The signs and symptoms of phonatory difficulty that develop will depend on the site of lesion. A good working knowledge of the appropriate physical signs and symptoms as well as the voice signs and symptoms is needed before the clinician can properly diagnose or understand the nature of the difficulty presented by a patient. In this chapter, we have presented an overview of many different neurological problems in which voice may be affected, including Parkinson's disease, myasthenia gravis, ALS, Shy-Drager syndrome, multiple sclerosis, cerebellar ataxia, SD, essential tremor, and many of the problems that may affect the recurrent and superior laryngeal nerves when they exit the CNS or as they travel in the neck and thorax to their ultimate destinations.

Chapter 6

Voice Problems Associated With Organic Disease and Trauma

The conditions discussed in this chapter represent organic disease states that have an effect on phonation. The cause of these conditions is unrelated to ways in which the voice has been used, and their treatment is primarily medical or surgical. It is important for clinicians to be familiar with these conditions and their effect on phonatory physiology, and to be prepared to offer the appropriate level of service as the need for it becomes timely. Often the speech–language pathologist provides presurgical treatment counseling, and secondarily is called on to provide voice therapy along with or subsequent to medical or surgical intervention. The conditions include keratosis, granulomas, pachydermia laryngis, ankylosis of the cricoarytenoid joint, papillomas, carcinoma and other malignancies, blunt or penetrating trauma, and chemical or heat trauma.

BENIGN LESIONS

Keratosis

PRIMARY VOICE SYMPTOM: HOARSENESS

Description and Etiology

Keratosis refers to epithelial lesions in which there is abnormal tissue growth on the vocal folds (Fig. 6.1). This usually originates in epithelium but may enter the superficial layer of the lamina propria. Other terms may be used to describe this condition, including leukoplakia, hyperkeratosis, keratosis with cellular atypia, and dyskeratosis. According to Frangez, Gale, and Luzar (1997), leukoplakia is a clinical term that describes a whitish patch on the laryngeal mucosa, whereas keratosis is a histological term indicating a pathological condition and the accumulation of keratin on the epithelial surface. Two kinds of lesions may be seen: flat, white, plaque-like lesions (leukoplakia) or irregular growth of epithelium that results in a warty lesion (papillary keratosis). A full spectrum of premalignant laryngeal tissue changes are observed in smokers that are not seen in nonsmokers (U.S. Dept. of Health and Human Services, 1985). These lesions must be carefully monitored.

Smoking, environmental pollutants, and other factors have been implicated in the development of keratotic epithelium on the vocal folds. These lesions tend to occur more often in men than in women. Gastroesophageal reflux disease (GERD) has also

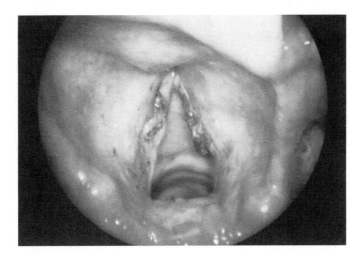

Figure 6.1. Hyperkeratosis of the vocal folds. See color plate.

been implicated as a cause of these tissue changes (Koufman, 1991; Cohen, Bach, Postma, & Koufman, 2002). The lesions may be unilateral or bilateral but are usually asymmetric in appearance. The glottal edge is often rough.

Perceptual Signs and Symptoms

The primary symptom is hoarseness or roughness in the voice.

Acoustic Signs

Few data are available on the acoustic characteristics of patients with keratosis of the vocal folds. Because of the growths on the vocal folds, greater than normal frequency and amplitude perturbation as well as greater than normal spectral noise would be expected.

Measurable Physiological Signs

Minimal measurable physiological data exist on patients with keratosis of the vocal folds. Iwata, von Leden, and Williams (1972) reported a mean airflow rate of 227 mL/sec for patients with leukoplakia of the vocal folds. Lesions that might have a similar effect (papilloma, epithelial hyperplasia) also show greater than normal airflows (see Table 3.6 in Hirano, 1981b).

Observable Physiological Signs

In patients with leukoplakia, there will be whitish plaque-like lesions on the mucosal surface of the vocal folds. These may be limited in extent or may cover almost the entire vocal fold. Ballenger (1985) reports that another form of this lesion, papillary keratosis, may show a piling up of small, reddish epithelium or an irregular mucosa covered by keratin.

Because these lesions can be so variable in extent and in location on the folds, their stroboscopic appearance will vary. Vocal fold edges may be rough and result in an irregularly shaped glottic chink on vocal fold closure. There will be asymmetric behavior and aperiodicity. In extensive lesions, diminished amplitude of lateral vocal fold excursion and limited mucosal wave, especially over the sites occupied by the lesion, are seen. Colden et al. (2001) studied the amplitude of vocal vibration and the mucosal wave in 62 patients with a diagnosis of keratotic lesion. The lesions of 45 of these patients were subsequently identified as intraepithelial keratosis and 17 as cancer. Four judges blind to the diagnoses rated the amplitude of vibration and lateral extent of the mucosal wave. Only two of the intraepithelial lesions were rated as normal with respect to both amplitude of vibration and lateral extent of the mucosal wave. According to the authors, neither reduced amplitude of vibration nor reduced mucosal wave were predictive of the presence of cancer. They conclude that the presence of a mucosal wave probably indicates that the vocal ligament is not extensively involved.

Pathophysiology

Keratotic-type lesions, for the most part, affect the cover, increasing its mass and stiffness.

Laryngeal Granulomas

PRIMARY VOICE SYMPTOM: HOARSENESS

Description and Etiology

Laryngeal granulomas most commonly are a complication of intubation (Fig. 6.2). Their development may be an early complication occurring at some point between intubation and extubation, or a late complication, the morbid sequelae of extubation (Balestrieri & Watson, 1982). The passing of an intubation tube between the vocal processes may be necessary to provide access to the airway for purposes of delivering anesthesia and maintaining appropriate oxygenation during a surgical procedure. Intubation also may be necessary in nonsurgical situations to maintain adequate oxygen supply for persons in need of respiratory assistance. Contact between the tube and the vocal processes may occur at the time of intubation or with the tube in situ. During such contact the mucosal perichondrium of the vocal processes may be traumatized, causing a small ulcer to appear on the vocal process. The bare process will eventually be covered by granulation tissue, which will become epithelialized and present as a granuloma. The condition is surprisingly uncommon in light of the frequency with which intubation is required, and spontaneous resolution occurs within a few weeks in most cases. The incidence of granuloma is dependent on factors such as duration of intubation, the method of intubation, the patient's age and general condition, nursing techniques, and other factors. All reported cases have occurred in patients 15 years of age or older, and women are more prone to develop an intubation granuloma because of small laryngeal size and a thinner mucosal layer covering the vocal processes (Snow, Marano, & Balogh, 1966).

Endotracheal intubation is being accepted for longer and longer periods. Although it is not a benign procedure, mortality and morbidity rates, when compared with the option of tracheotomy, are much lower. Weymuller (1988) presents a thorough review of the pertinent factors relating to endotracheal injury, its nature, the biomechanical factors of the tube itself, and the efforts made to prevent injury from the procedure.

Perceptual Signs and Symptoms

The symptoms of granuloma are breathiness and hoarseness. Some may not affect phonation because of their location.

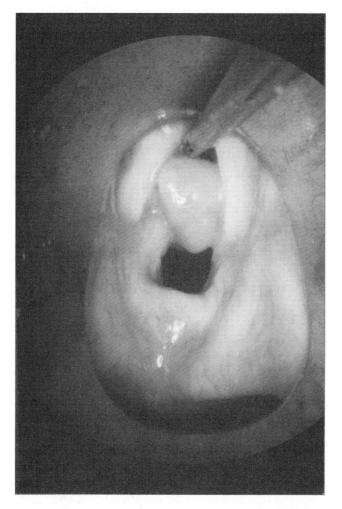

Figure 6.2. Contact granuloma involving the posterior part of the glottis. See color plate.

Acoustic Signs

No data are available on the acoustic characteristics of patients with granulomas. Greater than normal frequency and amplitude perturbation would be expected, and, depending on the severity of the hoarseness, greater than normal spectral noise could be present.

Measurable Physiological Signs

Normal airflow rates have been reported in patients with contact granulomas (see Table 3.7 in Hirano, 1981b). Few other physiological data are available on the physiological characteristics associated with granulomas of the vocal folds.

Observable Physiological Signs

Granulomas manifest themselves laryngoscopically as irregularly shaped masses of tissue either at the site of the vocal processes of the arytenoids (if an intubation granuloma) or elsewhere on the vocal folds or larynx.

The vocal folds will show normal stroboscopic signs unless the granuloma appears on the vocal fold margins. In that case, glottic closure may be incomplete, and we would expect to see reduced amplitude of lateral excursion of the affected vocal fold(s) and some degree of disturbance of the mucosal wave.

Pathophysiology

Intubation granulomas primarily affect the mucosa of the vocal processes of the arytenoids.

Vocal Process Granuloma (Contact Ulcer)

PRIMARY VOICE SYMPTOM: HOARSENESS

Description and Etiology

Vocal process granuloma is a benign lesion affecting the vocal process of the arytenoid cartilage. These lesions have been given a variety of names in the literature, including contact ulcer, contact granuloma, arytenoid granuloma, and vocal process granuloma. We prefer the term *vocal process granuloma* to refer to all of these type lesions, as suggested by Hoffman et al (2001). Usually, a small ulceration develops on the medial surface of the vocal processes of the arytenoid cartilages. The ulceration may be unilateral or bilateral and may present a "cup and saucer" appearance, with a protuberance on one side and a crater or concavity on the other. Continued irritation results in an ulceration on one side and the production of granulation tissue on the other.

The thinking about the etiology of vocal process granulomas has undergone major change within the recent past. The traditional view had been that they occurred predominantly in men with an average age of 50 years (Peacher, 1947), who engaged in a great deal of forceful, aggressive speaking, the so-called type A personality.

In support of that view, von Leden and Moore (1960) described some of the anatomical and physiological variations of phonation that could contribute to the formation of a vocal process granuloma. They pointed out that at low pitches the arytenoids oscillate vigorously, in a rocking-type motion. Thus, at low pitches it is more likely that the arytenoids would be subjected to greater trauma. They also observed that at low pitches there is greater vocal fold approximation, the approximation is prolonged, and it tends to persist beyond the vibratory phase of the vocal folds. Greater loudness also will increase the degree of approximation as well as its duration. Harsh, guttural sounds will increase the force of approximation of the vocal folds, as will other non-phonatory acts (throat clearing, etc.). Voice therapy was a treatment course often followed but with little documentation of its efficacy. Vocal process granulomas often were surgically excised, but they showed a propensity to recur.

In a study relating gastric reflux to vocal process granulomas, Cherry and Margulies (1968) studied three patients who showed evidence of peptic ulcer. All were treated with antacids, reduced food intake at night, and elevation of the head during sleep, and all experienced resolution of the ulcer. Delahunty and Cherry (1968) demonstrated that continued exposure of the arytenoid vocal processes to stomach acids would create ulcers and granulation tissue in dogs in about 1 month's time. Histologically, these lesions exhibited epithelial necrosis with an organized fibrous exudate beneath. Submucosal edema and nonspecific inflammation were also described. In a control condition, saliva was applied to the arytenoids over the same period, with no development of granulation tissue. Ward, Zwitman, Hanson, and Berci (1980) reported that vocal process granulomas result from constant throat clearing that is secondary to irritation of the mucosa caused by gastroesophageal reflux (regurgitation of peptic acids, especially at night), and with less frequency to irritation from nasal secretions (postnasal drip). They further reported that of 28 cases, only two failed to respond to medical treatment. Feder and Michell (1984) divided ulcers into two groups, hyperfunctional and hyperacidic. Watterson, Hensen-Magorian, and McFarlane (1988) reported that 51% of their patients with a vocal process granuloma also exhibited a hiatal hernia. Hiatal hernia and GERD were thought to be two parts of the same problem. According to Bozymski (1993), most hiatal hernias are now thought to be normal variants of the anatomy. Thus, it would appear that the cause of vocal process granulomas may be primarily related to reflux, with hyperfunctional vocal abuse being a contributory factor.

Benjamin and Croxson (1985) reported clinical and histological similarities between vocal process granulomas and other laryngeal granulomas. They studied 16 patients, of whom seven had postintubation granulomas and the remainder contact ulcers. The most common symptom of all patients was hoarseness. They concluded that vocal process granuloma was not a precursor to granulomas because the history of the problems was different and the patient with a granuloma did not present the profile of a patient with a vocal process granuloma. Recent literature has even more strongly implicated GERD as the primary cause of vocal process granuloma, and, furthermore, postnasal drip is also thought to be related to the same process of mucosal irritation resulting from the reflux of gastric juices (Bozymski, 1993; Deveney, Benner, & Cohen, 1993; Gaynor, 1991; Koufman, 1991; Wilson, Pryde, Cecilia, & MacIntyre, 1989).

Perceptual Signs and Symptoms

The primary perceptual symptoms of a vocal process granuloma are low pitch, throat clearing, and vocal fatigue. There may be a breathy voice with some hoarseness, accompanied by discomfort or even severe, stabbing pain. The pain is usually unilateral and located in the area of the greater horn of the thyroid. The pain may radiate to the ear. There is usually the constant feeling of something in the throat, which accounts for the continual throat clearing.

Acoustic Signs

Depending on the severity of the voice symptoms, some increased frequency perturbation and spectral noise may be present in the voice. Several investigators have reported lower than normal fundamental frequency of vibration (Hillman et al., 1989; Ylitalo & Hammarberg, 2000). If the voice is hoarse, greater than normal frequency and amplitude perturbation would be expected, but Ylitalo and Hammarberg (2000) reported no significant changes of frequency perturbation in a group of 19 male patients. Little or no abnormal acoustic characteristics also may be present. Verdolini, Hoffman, and McCoy (1994) reported on one patient whose only abnormal finding was higher than normal phonatory effort during singing.

Measurable Physiological Signs

Isshiki and von Leden (1964) reported a mean flow of 144 mL/sec for their group of patients with contact ulcers. This value is not much higher than would be expected in normal speakers. However, Hillman et al. (1989) found significantly higher airflows in their two patients with a contact ulcer. Both patients also had higher than normal open quotients when phonating at normal loudness. Hillman et al. (1989) also reported that subglottal air pressures were within normal limits for their two patients. Muscle activity levels should be within normal limits.

Observable Physiological Signs

Laryngoscopically, a vocal process granuloma will be visible as a buildup of pink or pinkish-white tissue on one of the vocal processes of the arytenoids. This usually occurs at the tip of the process, but it is possible to find such an outgrowth elsewhere on the vocal process or on the lower base of the arytenoid. On the contralateral process, there may be injection of the mucosa or a depression. This has been described as the "cup and saucer" appearance, because the two processes fit together in that way. Inflammation of the arytenoids and the posterior pharyngeal wall may be seen. In the early stages of vocal process granuloma development, even before tissue outgrowth, a strand of mucus may be seen between the two processes. This is referred to as a vocal process granuloma diathesis.

Unless there are abnormal voice symptoms, normal stroboscopic features would be anticipated.

Pathophysiology

Because the vocal process granuloma does not involve the membranous vocal fold, there will be little change in the mass or stiffness of the cover, transition layers, or body.

Pachydermia Laryngis

PRIMARY VOCAL SYMPTOM: HOARSENESS

Description and Etiology

This is a relatively rare problem whose cause is unknown. Some suspect smoking to be the major cause, and others suspect irritation caused by GERD. Pachydermia laryngis is characterized by a thickening of the epithelium with acanthosis and keratosis (Ballenger, 1985). Clinically it appears as a whitish mass of tissue in the interarytenoid space. The membranous vocal folds may also be injected and thickened. Conservative treatment usually consists of cessation of smoking and alcohol use as well as treatment (behavioral and pharmacological) of the GERD. Surgical removal may be necessary.

Perceptual Signs and Symptoms

Hoarseness will be a primary perceptual sign of this disease.

Acoustic Signs

Few data are available on the acoustic signs for this vocal problem. A lower fundamental frequency may be expected if the vocal folds are thickened sufficiently.

Measurable Physiological Signs

We have no knowledge of physiological data on this vocal problem. One might expect that if the lesion interfered with glottal closure, excessive airflows would result.

Observable Physiological Signs

On direct or indirect laryngoscopy, the vocal folds may look thickened and rough, and there is an excess of rough, uneven tissue present in the interarytenoid space.

We know of no data concerning the stroboscopic signs associated with pachydermia laryngis. However, we would expect that glottal closure might be compromised, and mucosal wave and amplitude may be reduced because of the thickened mucosa.

Papilloma

PRIMARY VOICE SYMPTOM: HOARSENESS

Description and Etiology

Papilloma is a rather common benign tumor that starts in the epithelium and is thought to be caused by a virus, usually the human papilloma virus types 6 and 11. It occurs in both children and adults. In children, it is referred to as juvenile papilloma. There are an estimated 4.3 cases per 100,000 population, and it is very resistant to eradication. Surgical excision is required, because papillomas tend to proliferate and can obstruct the airway. Children with this problem may require multiple surgical excisions before the condition runs its course. If juvenile papilloma persists or begins in adulthood, it continues to be a condition that is highly resistant to treatment. Adult papilloma occurs in approximately 1.8 cases per 100,000 population.

The papilloma may occur in various parts of the larynx: subglottally, at the level of the vocal folds, and supraglottally. It is sometimes necessary for children with aggressive papilloma growth to undergo tracheotomy. When the papillomas have ceased recurring, or perhaps between episodes of recurrence, voice therapy may be appropriate to maintain or restore the best possible voice production. The prognosis will depend largely on the state of the vocal fold mucosa.

Perceptual Signs and Symptoms

Hoarseness is the primary symptom and sign of the voice disorder caused by this condition. Other symptoms include low pitch, breathiness, and a strained voice in the adult patient. In the child, there may be a weak cry, chronic cough, swallowing difficulties, and stridor.

Measurable Physiological Signs

We know of no measurable physiological data reported for individuals with papillomas of the vocal folds. However, because of the increased stiffness of the cords, we might expect greater expiratory air pressures.

Observable Physiological Signs

Laryngoscopy. A papilloma typically presents as a whitish cluster of tissue, somewhat comparable in texture to a raspberry. An example of the laryngoscopic appearance of a papilloma is shown in Figure 6.3. In Figure 6.4, multiple papillomas are evident, illustrating the potentially extensive nature of the disease.

Stroboscopy. Papillomas often interfere with glottal closure. To what extent this is true will depend on the extent of the lesion. The increased stiffness created by the lesion will impede horizontal excursion of the folds, and mucosal wave will be absent in the area of the lesions. When multiple surgical excisions have been required for vocal fold papilloma, the membranous cover of the vocal folds may have been sufficiently damaged to interfere with amplitude and vibratory behavior.

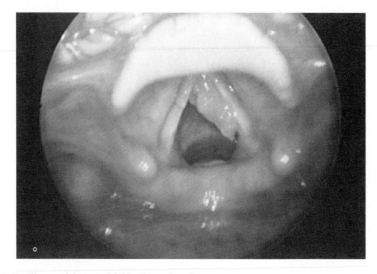

Figure 6.3. Papilloma of the vocal folds. See color plate.

Pathophysiology

Papillomas affect vocal fold vibration by increasing the mass and the stiffness of the vocal folds and altering the biomechanical characteristics of the mucosa. Although they can be removed surgically, the lesions tend to recur, especially in children (Bastian, 1986). Surgery is usually the treatment of choice and includes traditional knife surgery as well as CO_2 laser (Simpson & Strong, 1983). Various other treatments have

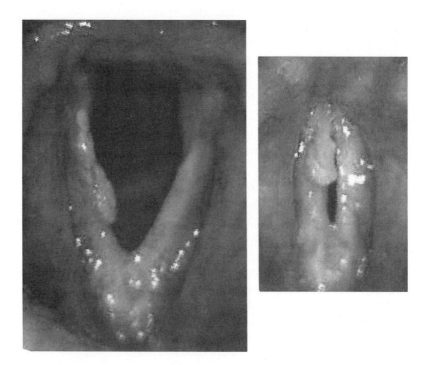

Figure 6.4. Multiple papillomas of the vocal folds. See color plate.

been tried, including interferon (Benjamin, Gatenby, Kitchen, Harrison, Cameron, & Basten, 1988; Leventhal, Kashima, & Mounts, 1991; Sessions, Dichtel, & Goepfert, 1984; Sessions, Goepfert, & Donovan, 1983), photodynamic therapy (Abramson, Shikowitz, & Mullooly, 1994), and various drugs (indole-3-carbinol, ribavirin, acyclovir, and others; Avidano & Singleton, 1995).

Ankylosis of the Cricoarytenoid Joint

PRIMARY VOICE SYMPTOM: HOARSENESS

Description and Etiology

Fixation of the cricoarytenoid joint may be attributable to several causes, including arthritis, trauma, or joint disease. Ankylosis of the cricoarytenoid joint is sometimes difficult to distinguish from paralysis of the vocal folds. Clinically they appear very similar (Cummings, 1986). However, pain may be a symptom of ankylosis caused by arthritis and would usually not be a symptom of paralysis. An attempt to manipulate the joint under direct laryngoscopy may be necessary to distinguish between the two conditions. Treatment of ankylosis requires surgical arytenoidectomy or arytenoidopexy (Ballenger, 1985). Voice therapy is usually not helpful.

Perceptual Signs and Symptoms

The primary perceptual symptoms of unilateral arytenoid fixation are hoarseness and breathiness secondary to the anticipated inadequacy of posterior vocal fold closure. In the event that the condition is bilateral, stridor may be present, and the patient may display symptoms of dyspnea.

Acoustic Signs

We know of no experimental data concerning the acoustic characteristics of voice in the presence of cricoarytenoid ankylosis. In unilateral ankylosis, these might include increased frequency and amplitude perturbation (jitter and shimmer), reduced phonational and dynamic ranges, increased spectral noise, and reduced phonation time. Acoustic signs in bilateral ankylosis may be minimal.

Measurable Physiological Signs

Physiological signs of ankylosis are not documented. As with unilateral vocal fold paralysis, if the glottis is not fully adducted during phonation, we would expect increased airflows and a glottogram that would show the incomplete closure and reduced closed time. Conversely, in the bilateral condition, airflows might be expected to be reduced, and the glottogram should reveal minimal vocal fold opening phase.

One also would expect normal electrical activity of the muscles of the larynx.

Observable Physiological Signs

As noted previously, the laryngeal appearance of ankylosis might be difficult to distinguish from vocal fold paralysis. If unilateral, we would expect to observe lack of movement of the arytenoid and incomplete glottal closure. In bilateral ankylosis, the position of both arytenoids would be fixed and unmoving, resulting also in lack of either adduction or abduction of the folds. We have observed that, in paralysis, movement in the opening of the pyriform sinuses may be absent, whereas in ankylosis such movement continues to be present. If the cause of ankylosis is an arthritic condition (usually rheumatoid arthritis), mucosal edema, inflammation, or both may be seen in the area of the cricoarytenoid joint.

We know of no data on the stroboscopic signs of a fixed arytenoid. One might expect to see incomplete glottal closure but minimal aberrations in the vibratory motion of the vocal folds.

Pathophysiology

The movement of the ankylosed arytenoid cartilage(s) is reduced or absent. The glottis may be incompletely adducted, or, in the case of bilateral ankylosis, it may be neither fully adducted nor abducted.

VASCULAR DISORDERS

Hemorrhage

PRIMARY VOICE SYMPTOM: HOARSENESS, OCCASIONAL OR INTERMITTENT APHONIA, AND LOSS OF PITCH RANGE

Description and Etiology

Hemorrhage into the vocal fold is usually unilateral, although it may be bilateral. It can involve the full length of the vocal fold or portions of the fold. The hemorrhagic area appears reddish, with significant swelling. Hemorrhage is most frequently the result of a single episode of traumatic voice use or laryngeal trauma. It also can result from the combination of heavy voice use and use of anticoagulants and salicylates (such as aspirin) or extended use of inhaled steroids. Neely and Rosen (2000) reported on the case of an opera singer taking Coumadin who developed a hemorrhage that seriously restricted her ability to sing.

Perceptual Signs and Symptoms

Patients may complain of pain, particularly at the time of the precipitating event. Dryness, vocal fatigue, and loss of upper range are among the perceptual symptoms that accompany the primary symptom and sign of hoarseness. Depending on the severity of the bleed, the voice may be intermittently aphonic, and it may require added effort for voicing to be produced. Vocal fold hemorrhage occurs more frequently in women than in men and usually in adults (Lin, Stern, & Gould, 1991).

Acoustic Signs

Although no data have been reported for this population, we would anticipate increased shimmer and jitter related to the hoarseness that is perceptible. We would also expect decreased signal-to-noise ratio, and restricted pitch and dynamic ranges.

Measurable Physiological Signs

We would expect subglottic air pressures to be increased because the patient must exert greater effort to produce phonation. Increased air flows also may be noted as a result of the limitations in laryngeal valving caused by stiffness of the hemorrhagic cord.

Observable Physiological Signs

As noted in the description, hemorrhage is visible when the vocal folds are visualized by the apparent redness of the area of the fold involved, the significant swelling present, and the stiffness of the cord. A prominent blood vessel may be seen.

Under stroboscopic observation, stiffness of the hemorrhagic vocal fold or part thereof is apparent with reduced amplitude of the involved fold and absence of mucosal wave in the area of the hemorrhage. Glottal closure may vary in degree, depending on the amount of stiffness and swelling. The vocal fold edge usually remains straight as long as the hemorrhage has not organized into a specific lesion such as a hemorrhagic polyp. Because the lesion is usually unilateral, asymmetry of movement between the vocal folds would be apparent, as would aperiodicity.

Pathophysiology

Rupture of blood vessels results in bleeding into the submucosal layer. This produces extreme swelling of that area, decreasing the efficiency of the vibratory behavior of the vocal folds. The mass and stiffness of the cover are increased.

Varix and Ectasia

PRIMARY VOICE SYMPTOM: HOARSENESS

Description and Etiology

A varix is seen as a prominent, distended, lengthened, and tortuous blood vessel on the surface of the vocal fold. The location of a varix may be either on the superior surface of the fold or on the free edge of the fold. A varix is often visualized after resorption of a hemorrhage or in conjunction with a hemorrhagic polyp. We have also observed varices in the absence of a known previous hemorrhage. The cause seems to be related to vocal abuse or trauma and usually results from a single or focused short-term episode of abuse.

Ectasia is defined as a dilation of a small vessel. Occasionally, vascular microectasias are seen on the surface of the vocal folds, which may affect vibration in that location.

Acoustic Signs

These signs vary depending on the size and location of the varix or ectasia. When hoarseness is present, we would anticipate increased shimmer and jitter magnitudes.

Measurable Physiological Signs

Airflow should not necessarily show any change from normal unless the varix is large or ectasias are extensive enough to create vocal fold stiffness and interfere with glottal closure.

Observable Physiological Signs

Laryngoscopy. Varices and ectasias may be seen on the surface of the vocal folds as increased vascularity not normally present. When a hemorrhagic polyp is present, it is often possible to visualize a prominent blood vessel leading directly to the polyp, suggesting that the vessel is "feeding" the polyp and is a factor in its presence.

Stroboscopy. The area of the varix or the ectasia may appear stiffened, with reduced mucosal wave. The effect on vibratory behavior of the fold will be in direct relation to the location and the extent of the varix or the ectasia. A small varix on the superior surface of the fold may have minimal effect on the vibratory characteristics of that fold, whereas a large vessel along the edge or even on the superior surface of the fold will limit mucosal wave and perhaps amplitude of lateral excursion of the fold. Glottal closure pattern will also vary depending on the size and location of the lesion.

Pathophysiology

The varix is usually in the submucosal layer, and the amount of distortion of that layer will depend on its size. A large varix or large cluster of small vessels will increase stiffness and mass of the cover. If a varix is the residual effect of a hemorrhage, full resorption of the hemorrhage may not have occurred, and the behavior of the fold will be affected by that as well.

Laryngeal Web

PRIMARY VOICE SYMPTOM: HOARSENESS

Description and Etiology

Laryngeal webs often are congenital, the result of incomplete maturation of the developing larynx. Webs are often manifested as a sheet of tissue between the vocal folds, usually at the anterior end. Typical symptoms in the child include a weak cry, difficulty breathing, and stridor. In the adult, the complaint is hoarseness, high pitch, and perhaps shortness of breath. Small webs at the anterior commissure may present few problems, whereas extensive webs could necessitate a tracheotomy. Treatment typically consists of surgery to split the web, but unless the surgery is carefully performed, the possibility of a refusion of the web is very possible.

Perceptual Signs and Symptoms

Typically, the major signs are hoarseness and a high pitch. In a child, there may be a weak cry. The high pitch may be attributable to the shortening of the effective vibrating length of the vocal fold because of the attachment of the web between the two vocal folds. The web also will interfere with the normal vibratory movements, resulting in the hoarseness.

Acoustic Signs

Few data exist on the acoustic signs of a laryngeal web. One would expect acoustic features consistent with increased frequency and amplitude perturbation. If the patient has a higher-than-normal pitch level, a higher-than-normal fundamental frequency of phonation would be expected.

Measurable Physiological Signs

We know of no data concerning the airflow or air pressure characteristics of children or adults with a laryngeal web. Because the web would restrict the vibratory amplitude of the vocal folds, a decreased airflow might be expected. Air pressure could be elevated if the patient is trying to force vibration.

Observable Physiological Signs

Stroboscopically, the patient with a web would show decreased amplitude of vibration and no mucosal wave in the area of the web. If the voice is hoarse, the periodicity of vocal fold vibration would be affected.

Pathophysiology

The attachment of tissue to the margins of the vocal folds would limit their vibratory motions and produce instability. Moreover, the attachment of the web would limit the effective vibrating length of the vocal folds, producing a higher than normal pitch. Often, voice symptoms take a back seat to establishing an airway or making it easier for the patient to breathe.

Blunt or Penetrating Trauma

A variety of traumatic injuries may affect the larynx. These may include attempted strangulation, a penetrating neck wound, blunt trauma resulting from a blow to the neck or from the body's being hurled with force, and the neck's striking an object. In severe trauma, the structures of the larynx may be fractured or severely damaged, compromising the airway and resulting in vocal difficulty. An example of the effects of trauma to the vocal folds is shown in Figure 6.5.

Most cases of blunt or penetrating trauma require medical/surgical treatment. The most urgent concern is management of the airway. Subsequently there will be an attempt to repair or reconstruct the damaged structures. Voice restoration, following the completion of the repair, may be very difficult. A speech–language pathologist may be asked to help the patient achieve the best possible voice. In these cases, the speech–language pathologist should ask for and expect to receive detailed information about the altered laryngeal anatomy, to understand the constraints on the system and to be able to plan the treatment approach accordingly.

Inhalation and Thermal Trauma

There is a paucity of information in the literature about the long-term laryngeal and phonatory sequelae of the inhalation of gases, smoke, or steam. Inhalation injuries are usually referred to as chemical tracheobronchitis, a term that seems to exclude laryngeal and supraglottal effects of such injury even though they occur as frequently and almost always with greater severity (Hunt, Agee, & Pruitt, 1975; Miller, Gray, Cotton, & Myer, 1988). Hot fumes cause reflex closure of the glottis, which, in combination with the cooling capacity of the upper respiratory tract, protects the trachea and lower tract (Miller et al., 1988). Acute airway obstruction can result from either supraglottal or laryngeal edema, or both. Hunt et al. (1975) point out that laryngeal and supraglottal structures tend to show massive amounts of edema in a short period because of the loose attachment of the surface mucosa to the underlying basal layers.

During the acute stage, those who suffer inhalation injury are frequently at risk for survival, making their medical condition and treatment of the utmost urgency. The severe edema of the respiratory tract may appear immediately or may develop within a matter of hours and can quickly lead to airway obstruction and to death (Crapo, 1981; Cudmore & Vivori, 1981). Intubation or tracheotomy may be required. A risk of intubation is the possibility of damage to the already compromised mucosal tissue. Symptoms of inhalation trauma include swelling, inflammation, burns, or soot around

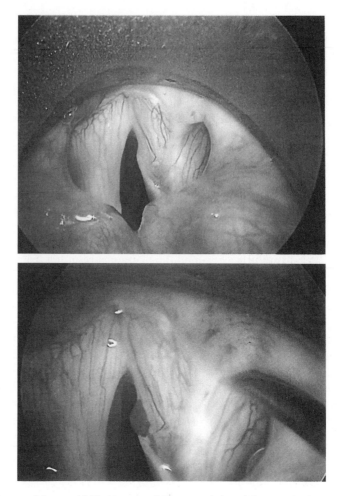

Figure 6.5. Trauma of the vocal folds. Note the obliteration of clear definition of either vocal fold caused by the formation of a web that has grown after trauma. There is also excessive vascularization of the folds. See color plate.

the nose and mouth and in the oropharynx (even with minimal body surface injury), respiratory distress, stridor, wheezing, and hoarseness (Crapo, 1981). The symptoms depend on the severity of the trauma, the type of fumes or gases inhaled, and the stage of the body's response to the trauma. The trauma may result not only from heat but also from the particles and toxic chemicals released as the burning material breaks down, and from the reduction in oxygen. The heat capacity of steam is 4,000 times greater than that of air; thus, steam inhalation can quickly produce thermal burns of the respiratory tract. Steam inhalation burns may occur with a scald injury in young children. According to Cudmore and Vivori (1981), inhalation of hot, dry gases causes damage primarily to the upper airway (including the larynx), because there is a rapid decrease in temperature of the gases as soon as they enter the airway. Chemical damage to the entire airway results from inhalation of smoke. Smoke from the combustion of polyurethane foams is reported to be especially damaging (Dyer & Esch, 1976). This fact is all the more disturbing in view of the increased numbers of house fires resulting in more inhalation burns in children (Chisnall, 1977) and the increased use of plastics and polyurethane foam in homes.

Voice can only become a concern after the patient has survived the acute stage of trauma and has completed the major portion of treatment for the injuries sustained. If there has been extensive body surface burn in addition to the inhalation injuries, treatment may be quite lengthy. Only when the patient is sufficiently recovered is it appropriate to focus on aspects of vocal recovery. However, during the recovery period, consultation by the speech–language pathologist may be helpful in establishing the most efficacious means of communication for patients whose ability to communicate has been significantly compromised.

As noted previously, there is little documentation of the long-term effects of laryngeal trauma. Close, Catlin, and Cohn (1980), reporting on the chronic effects of ammonia inhalation burns, cite one case in which breathy phonation was present and showed some improvement with voice therapy. In another instance, severe and progressive hoarseness noted in the early post-trauma stage apparently resolved spontaneously. Recently, 22 patients who had been treated in the regional burn unit at University Hospital of the Upstate Medical University over a 10-year period were examined for voice problems (Casper, Clark, Kelly, & Colton, 2002). Of these, 11 (50%) were judged by an experienced voice clinician to show some degree of voice abnormality that, according to patient reports, was not present before the trauma. Although most of the patients so identified had been either intubated or tracheotomized or both, some patients had not experienced either of these procedures. Thus, injury resulting from intubation or tracheotomy cannot fully account for the resulting voice abnormality.

In view of these findings, we suspect that more residual voice problems occur in inhalation burn survivors than have previously been recognized. The pathophysiology is not well understood and may differ from patient to patient. There are many unanswered questions relative to phonatory function in this population, such as whether problems result from changes in laryngeal mucosa, peripheral nerve damage from the burn or from subsequent surgery, or central nervous system damage caused by hypoxia.

Our experience in voice therapy with this population is very limited. Nevertheless, the case study of C.H. is instructive.

Case Study

C.H. was a 17-year-old young man who had suffered extensive burns of the head, neck, face, hands, and upper body after the crash of an ultralight plane that he had been flying alone. He also suffered inhalation injury. His treatment course included two periods of intubation, the first for a week and the second for 4 days, with a 2-day intervening period. He survived a long and painful course of treatment and surgeries. Although now he was being followed up as an outpatient, he faced further surgery in the future. He was in constant physical pain and discomfort, and his emotional pain because of his grotesquely deformed appearance was perhaps even greater. He was essentially aphonic, as he had been throughout the entire post-trauma course. Ear, nose, and throat examination was reported to be negative, with no observable reason for the aphonia. The vocal folds were reported to show good movement, although they did not adduct completely during speaking.

C.H. responded minimally to questions, offered no information spontaneously, and did not make eye contact with the clinician. He generally kept his eyes downcast or looked out of the window. Several sessions were required to work through this resistance and to establish a relationship. As he began to open up, C.H. talked more about the crash, and also about his parents, who were divorced. He was living with his mother; he would have preferred to have been with his father, but the accident had occurred during a time spent with the father, who was apparently finding the guilt related to the event overwhelming. C.H. was supposed to be returning to school but had thus far been resisting that because he saw himself as a "monster" whom others saw as disgusting. As therapy progressed, C.H. was increasingly willing to attempt voicing. Indeed, he was able to produce voice, but with a hoarse and somewhat breathy quality. The sound of this voice was just one more abnormality that he could not deal with, and his response had been to be aphonic. Work with C.H. continued for a time, during which he began to use voice routinely and with some improvement in quality. He was clearly in need of psychological counseling but had previously refused to consider such referral. Leading him to an acceptance of such counseling had been one of the goals of therapy, and, indeed, after his experience with us he was able to accept the support that had been offered and to recognize his need for continuation of such support. Although his voice quality was not "normal," C.H. was using voice routinely and finding that communication was easier.

The reason for C.H.'s hoarse voice quality was never fully understood. However, more testing, given his initial level of resistance and the subsequent determination of his very vulnerable psychological state, was not entirely necessary and might result in his withdrawal from further therapy. He made sufficient progress so that his voice was entirely usable, and although still hoarse, was not severely so. The reason for his aphonic presentation appeared to be primarily psychological. This case highlights the need to be alert to more than a single problem being present at one time, especially when there may be an obvious cause that might explain the problem.

CARCINOMA AND OTHER TUMORS

Carcinoma

PRIMARY VOICE SYMPTOM: HOARSENESS

The primary voice symptom of laryngeal cancer is hoarseness. Indeed, this is recognized as one of the seven warning signs of cancer.

Description and Etiology

Cancer is one of the diseases that may affect the structures of the oral cavity, pharynx, and larynx. If allowed to proceed unchecked, it is life threatening. The incidence of laryngeal cancer is reported to be between 2% and 5% of all malignancies. Persistent hoarseness is well known as one of the primary symptoms of cancer. If a malignant lesion affects one or both vocal folds directly, hoarseness will result. Figure 6.6 shows a cancer involving both vocal folds. Laryngeal lesions that do not affect the vibratory characteristics of the vocal folds will not necessarily result in a change in the voice.

Many possible causes exist for cancer, including smoking, environmental irritants, chemicals and other contaminants, metabolic disturbances, and unknown causes. According to the Surgeon General's report (U.S. Department of Health and Human Services, 1985), "Cigarette smoking is a major cause of cancers of the lung, larynx, oral cavity and esophagus" (p. vi). Furthermore, 50% to 70% of oral and laryngeal cancer deaths are associated with smoking. The report also states that a synergistic effect is

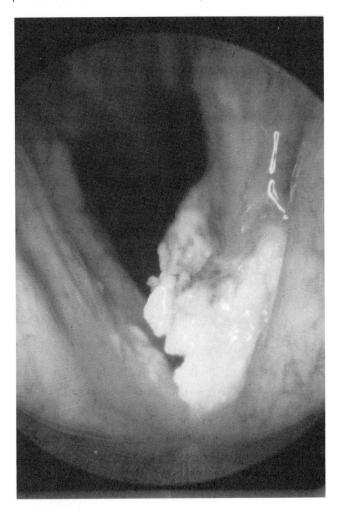

Figure 6.6. Carcinoma of the vocal folds. See color plate.

created by the use of alcohol in conjunction with smoking that greatly increases the risk of oral and laryngeal cancers. The ratio of men to women who develop these cancers was reported to be 5 to 1 in 1985 (Ballenger, 1985), but that ratio has been narrowing steadily for the past 20 years. The carcinogenic effects of cigar and pipe smoke are similar to those of cigarette smoke.

The severity of the malignancy is evaluated using the "TNM" system or its variants (American Joint Committee for Cancer Staging and End Results Reporting, 1983). The T refers to the site of the primary tumor, the N indicates the involvement of lymph nodes, and the M signifies spread of the lesion to other parts of the body (metastasis). Low numbers associated with each code indicate a lesser involvement; the numbers increase as severity or extent increase (Table 6.1). Thus, a patient described to have a T1N0M0 lesion has a locally confined tumor with neither node involvement nor any distant metastasis. Where the values of N and M are zero, the description is often truncated (e.g., T1 or T2 carcinoma) (Fig. 6.7).

Table 6.1. Classification of Glottal Cancers

T: Location of Primary Tumor

Tx	Cannot be staged
T0	No evidence of tumor
Tis	Carcinoma in situ
T1	Confined to vocal folds
T2	Supraglottal or subglottal extension, normal or impaired mobility
T3	Confined to larynx but with fixed cord
T4	Massive tumor

N: Involvement of Regional Lymph Nodes

Nx	Cannot be assessed
N0	No involvement
N1	A single small node on one side
N2	A single large or multiple small nodes on one side
N3	Massive nodes on one or both sides

M: Distant Metastasis

Mx	Cannot be assessed
M0	No known metastasis
M1	Metastasis present

Perceptual Signs and Symptoms

Hoarseness is the primary sign and symptom (Stoicheff, Ciampi, Passi, & Frederickson, 1983). Other signs of cancer of the larynx may include (a) a lump in the neck, (b) a broadening of the larynx, detected on palpation; and (c) tenderness in the neck. Other symptoms may include dysphagia, odynophagia (pain on swallowing), and dyspnea.

Acoustic Signs

Cancer will affect the vibration of the vocal folds and therefore will affect the acoustic characteristics of the voice. The magnitude of the effect will depend on the extent of the carcinoma. Frequency and amplitude perturbation will be increased. For their sample of five cancer patients, Hecker and Kruel (1971) reported pitch perturbation quotients similar to normal (patients, 13.6 vs. normal, 13.0) but much greater directional perturbation quotients (patients, 48.9; normal, 33.3). Lieberman (1963) had reported large perturbation values in an earlier study. Murry, Bone, and von Essen (1974) reported lower than normal phonational ranges for their one male subject with T1 carcinoma of the vocal folds. Colton, Reed, Sagerman, and Chung (1982) reported slightly higher fundamental frequencies for the vowels /ah/ and /ee/ for males with T1 or T2 carcinoma and much larger fundamental frequencies for both vowels produced by female patients with T1 cancer of the vocal folds (Fig. 6.8). Pitch perturbation quotients were increased in both vowels for both male T1 and T2 cancer classification groups. However, female patients tended to show lower pitch perturbation quotient (PPQ) for the vowel /ah/ and similar PPQs for the vowel /ee/ when compared with the normal control group (Fig. 6.9). Spectral noise levels are also increased. Colton, Sagerman, Chung, Young, and Reed (1978) reported elevated spectrum levels, especially in the higher frequencies, for their sample of five cancer patients. Similar findings were reported for

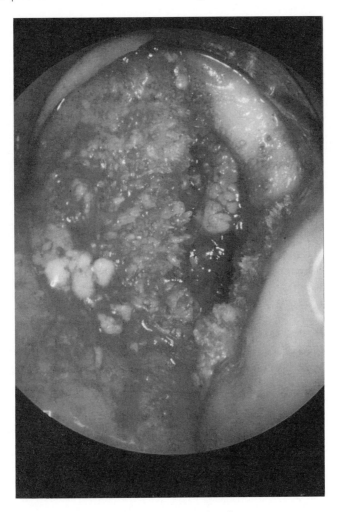

Figure 6.7. Extensive carcinoma involving both folds. See color plate.

a much larger group of patients with cancer (Colton et al., 1982). In the same study, both phonational and dynamic ranges were found to be lower in patients with laryngeal cancer than in normal control subjects (Fig. 6.10).

Measurement of the noise energy in the voices of patients with laryngeal cancer may be predictive of the severity of the cancer (Kasuya, Ogawa, Mashima, & Ebihara, 1986). Noise levels were measured in sustained vowels, and a measure called normalized noise energy (NNE) was calculated for 64 samples of normal voice and 57 samples of patients with carcinoma of the vocal folds. NNE was effective in detecting 91% of the normal voices. In voices with carcinoma, NNE was effective in detecting T1 cancer approximately 77% of the time and always detected T2, T3, or T4 cancer. Thus, measurement of noise levels may be a very useful clinical technique for documenting the magnitude of the voice change of cancer patients and for following effects of treatment.

Leeper et al. (2002) also studied some acoustic characteristics of patients receiving irradiation for their T1 cancer. They recorded their voices over five sessions during

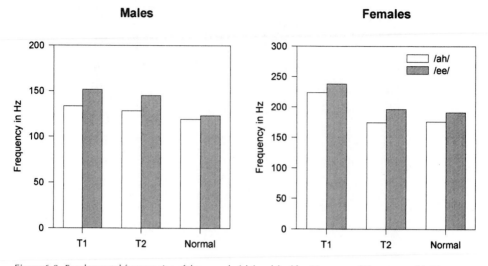

Figure 6.8. Fundamental frequencies of the vowels /ah/ and /ee/ for 38 men and 5 women with T1 cancer classification and 13 men and 7 women with T2 cancer classification compared with a normal control group of 35 men and 27 women.

and after the treatment and found greater harmonics-to-noise ratios (HNR), and lower NNE levels, across the five recording sessions. Perceptual judgments of hoarseness systemically decreased over the same period. Dworkin et al. (1999) found many of their patients receiving irradiation showed values of jitter, shimmer, and HNR within normal limits.

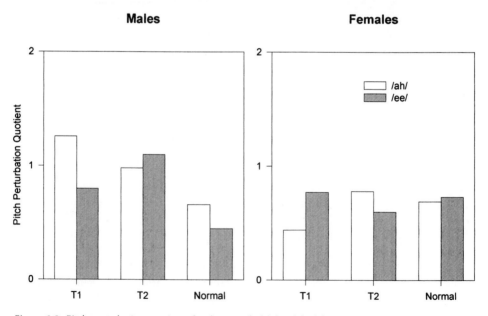

Figure 6.9. Pitch perturbation quotients for the vowels /ah/ and /ee/ for 38 men and 5 women with T1 cancer classification and 13 men and 7 women with T2 cancer classification compared with a normal control group of 35 men and 27 women.

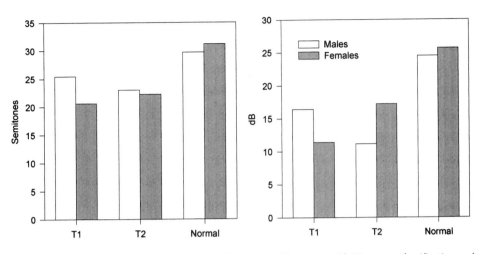

Figure 6.10. Phonational and dynamic ranges of 38 men and 5 women with T1 cancer classification and 13 men and 7 women with T2 cancer classification compared with a normal control group of 35 men and 27 women.

Measurable Physiological Signs

Very few data exist on the measurable physiological characteristics of patients with cancer. Airflows are generally increased, with large leakage flows associated with large tumors that prevent complete vocal fold closure. Mean airflow rates are increased (Murry, Bone, & von Essen, 1974). Electroglottogram (EGG) recordings will reflect reduced time of closure. Subglottal air pressures may be increased because of the increased stiffness of the vocal folds.

Observable Physiological Signs

Laryngoscopy. Laryngoscopic examination may reveal anything from a small, well-defined tumor to a large and diffuse one involving any part of the larynx or vocal folds. Precise diagnosis of carcinoma usually requires biopsy and histological analysis. Most carcinomas of the larynx arise from the epithelium and are of the squamous cell variety. As the severity of the lesion increases, it becomes more invasive in nature as well as more extensive in size.

Stroboscopy. Early carcinoma in situ can be more readily diagnosed using stroboscopy than other methods of examination. The distinguishing feature is the presence of a small lesion that has a markedly negative effect on vibratory vocal fold behavior (Sessions et al., 1989). It has been suggested that stroboscopy can be used to detect cancer by its effect on the mucosal wave or amplitude of vibration. Colden et al. (2001) tested that hypothesis by rating extent of mucosal wave and amplitude of vibration in 52 subjects with pre-malignant appearing lesions and then related the strobe results to the actual extent of the lesion found after surgery. They concluded that stroboscopy was not a reliable method for determining the presence of cancer nor the depth of the lesion. A variety of benign as well as precancerous lesions would affect the vibratory characteristics in a similar manner. Stiffness of any kind would affect the mucosal wave and the amplitude of vibration. Thus, stroboscopy may not be a viable technique to help differentiate a cancer from a noncancerous lesions. However, stroboscopy may be used to detect the return of a mucosal wave after the suspected lesion has been treated with radiation therapy (Tsunoda et al., 1997).

Pathophysiology

Cancerous lesions invade the tissue and destroy the normally behaving cells. Depending on its location and size, the tumor may affect vocal fold closure. Invasion of the tumor into the various levels of the lamina propria and muscle results in greater stiffness of the tissue, resulting in reduced horizontal excursion of the affected fold and often of the contralateral fold and restricted or absent mucosal wave.

Treatment

There are several approaches to cancer treatment. These include surgery, radiation therapy, and chemotherapy. Their use depends on many factors and is determined on a case-by-case basis. Spector and Ogura (1985) have discussed some of the considerations in the diagnosis and treatment of carcinoma. Patients who undergo radiation therapy as the primary treatment mode may experience some alterations in voice during the course of the treatment (Colton, Sagerman, Chung, Young, & Reed, 1978; Finizia et al., 1999; Fung et al., 2001; Leeper et al., 2002). Depending on the extent of the lesion, a patient may still have a normal-sounding voice after radiation therapy. Voice therapy is usually not necessary or indicated.

There are a variety of surgical approaches in the treatment of laryngeal cancer, which may involve excision of the lesion, of up to half of the larynx, of supraglottal structures only, or of the entire larynx (Cassisi, Sapienza, & Vinson, 1996; Franco & Zeitels, 2002). The effect on voice production capability will depend on the extent and the nature of the surgery performed. In addition to concerns about voice, patients who have had extensive surgery also may have difficulty with swallowing. A full discussion of the problems of dysphagia and those associated with the total absence of the larynx is beyond the scope of this book. These topics are well covered in the literature.

The voice problems associated with partial laryngeal excisions vary a great deal. Both voice problems and dysphagia will require the assistance of a speech–language pathologist. The role of the speech–language pathologist is to assist the patient in producing the best possible voice. To do so, the speech–language pathologist must be completely informed about the specifics of the surgical procedure. It is important to know what structures remain intact, how the anatomy is altered, and what functional skills remain relative to phonation. Some patients with laryngeal cancer have extremely extensive disease that requires excision of not only the larynx but also of other structures essential to the production of speech, such as the tongue. The speech–language pathologist also should be involved with these patients in an effort to provide a means of communication.

Other Tumors

A variety of benign and malignant tumors may be found in the laryngeal or neck area in both children and adults. Such tumors may obstruct the airway directly, or they may occupy space and place pressure on the trachea or larynx, thereby creating airway problems indirectly. The effect on the voice will depend on the position of the tumor. These lesions require medical or surgical treatment. In many cases of small or benign tumors, surgery is a viable treatment option. In cases of extensive malignant tumors, radiation therapy or chemotherapy or a combined protocol may be possible treatment choices. Rarely is there need for speech therapy services unless the tumor (or surgery) has compromised vocal or speech function. Tumors that are frequent in children include cysts, hemangiomas, and lymphangiomas; malignant neuroblastomas and lymphomas also occur. Many of these same tumors also may be found in adults.

SUMMARY

In this chapter, some organic problems that may affect the voice have been reviewed. The cause of these problems is not related to voice use. However, their effects can drastically alter voice production. A variety of medical and surgical approaches are the primary treatment modalities. Vocal rehabilitation may be helpful in establishing the best voice the patient is capable of producing. A section on geriatric voice discusses physical changes attributable to aging that may affect phonation and stresses the need to distinguish between age-related changes and those attributable to associated disease states.

Chapter 7

Voice Problems Associated With the Pediatric and the Geriatric Voice

THE PEDIATRIC VOICE

Dysphonia in children deserves careful consideration by the speech–language pathologist. Many congenital conditions that affect the larynx are diagnosed at birth because of difficulty breathing, stridor, or abnormal cry. However, conditions that have more subtle effects may go unrecognized until later. In our own practice, for example, identification of school-age children with webs and even laryngeal paralyses that appear congenital or related to a birth injury occasionally occurs. Parents may become aware of an unusual voice as the child experiences greater vocal and speech development. Interestingly, however, it also may be a teacher or speech–language pathologist who initially questions the child's voice quality. Parents of these children sometimes report that the child's voice has "always sounded this way" and consequently has not been a source of concern. Children can experience many of the same laryngeal pathological conditions more frequently diagnosed in adults, including nodules, papilloma, cysts, polyps, and ulcerative lesions likely related to laryngopharyngeal reflux (Benjamin, 1990; Dejonckere & Lebacq, 1984; Michaels, 1984; Morrison & Rammage, 1994; Tucker, 1987). A pathological condition that produces dysphonia requires accurate diagnosis, as well as assessment in terms of its impact on the child's speech–language and social development. Thus, hoarseness in children warrants appropriate attention by the speech–language pathologist and other care providers. Pertinent to this objective is an understanding of the unique characteristics of the pediatric larynx and voice. The intent of this section is to review laryngeal and vocal development in children, as well as both congenital and acquired conditions that may produce voice disorders in the pediatric population.

LARYNGEAL AND VOCAL DEVELOPMENT IN CHILDREN

Normative data for various measures of phonatory function in children are few. Their collection is beset by a number of problems, including a need for data that account for respiratory and phonatory structures and processes that are continually changing. Not only is the pediatric larynx different from the adult larynx, but it also is in a continual state of change throughout childhood. These changes are particularly rapid in the first 2 to 3 years, then decelerate until puberty.

Larynx Position

In a newborn, for example, the larynx is high in the neck, with the lower border of the cricoid cartilage approximately at the level of the 3rd or 4th cervical vertebrae (C3–4) (Hirano, Kurita, & Nakashima, 1983; Magriples & Laitman, 1987; Roche & Barkla, 1965; Symington, 1881). It will descend to approximately C5 by age 2 years, and to C6–7 by 15 years. This descent is associated with increasing separation between the hyoid bone and the thyroid cartilage, which are contiguous at birth. The higher position of the larynx in the child's neck before age 2 years suggests that vertical adjustments of the larynx are limited. In addition, cartilages are more elastic in children, becoming more osseus with aging. If either or both of these factors are associated with less stability in the laryngeal framework, they may have implications for adjustments of structures that lie within it, such as the intrinsic laryngeal muscles. From a clinical perspective, the higher, more anterior position of the pediatric larynx makes it more difficult to intubate when required for any surgical procedure.

Vocal Fold Histology

The pediatric larynx is also less complex structurally than the adult larynx. Tissues of the vocal fold cover are loose and elastic and not composed of the multiple layers characteristic of the adult. The cover is also thicker, relative to the length of the membranous vocal fold, than in adults. Hirano, Kurita, and Nakashima (1983) have suggested that the three connective tissue layers of the lamina propria are apparent at puberty but continue to become more differentiated until at least 16 years. According to Hirano et al., the vocal ligament, comprising the intermediate and deep layers of the cover, may appear by age 4 years, but again, continues to develop through puberty. Other authors (Ishii, Yamashita, Akita, & Hirose, 2000) have described a lamina propria distinguished by superficial and deep layers in children older than 10 years, with differentiation of superficial, intermediate, and deep layers complete by age 17 years. This evidence is supported by Hammond, Gray, Butler, Zhou, & Hammond (1998). These authors investigated the presence of elastin, which is characteristic of the intermediate layer of the lamina propria, in larynges representing the age span from infant to geriatric. Elastin content between the epithelium and vocalis muscle was significantly less in infant specimens, consistent with the lack of a well-defined intermediate layer.

The differentiated layers of the lamina propria are a hallmark of the adult larynx, and the relatively undifferentiated cover of the pediatric larynx may impact the child's ability to make fine adjustments necessary for certain vocal behaviors—for example, to produce voice in different registers or phonatory modes. The implications of a less well-differentiated and relatively thicker cover also may extend to the child's ability to regulate vocal intensity or to generate a mucosal wave. Clinically, the denser and more vascular character of the pediatric cover make it more susceptible to inflammatory or post-traumatic edema.

Neuromuscular Development

Neuromuscular differences between the pediatric and adult larynx also have been described. Young children have a higher proportion of type II muscle fibers in the vocal fold, which are fast acting, consistent with airway protection, and not as capable of prolonged contraction, which is likely critical to the development of phonation. By puberty, a preponderance of type I fibers, capable of slow, prolonged contraction, is noted (Kersing, 1986). There are also fewer muscle fibers in the child's vocal folds, and some muscles share attachments. Konig and Von Leden (1961) have reported that the development of the vocalis muscle continues to at least the third year of life.

Changes in neural structures and neural control with growth also have an impact on laryngeal and vocal behavior. Both the superior and recurrent laryngeal nerves demonstrate an adult pattern of distribution even at the end of the embryonic period (Muller, O'Rahilly, & Tucker, 1985). However, nerve fibers continue to increase in size, in myelination, and in the number and extent of both dendritic and axonal endings until approximately age 3 years. One study has described motor end plates in the intrinsic laryngeal muscles of infants innervated by either single or multiple axons. In adults, only single axon innervation was identified (Perie, St. Guily, & Sebille, 1999). These authors further noted that both the size and axonal complexity of motor end plates were increased in the adult specimens they investigated, as compared with fetal and infant larynges.

Central laryngeal mechanisms also demonstrate developmental effects. For example, in the fetus and newborn infant, chemical stimuli that pose a threat to the airway induce laryngeal constriction, apnea (cessation of breathing), and swallowing among other responses. The laryngeal chemoreflex (LCR) that mediates these behaviors develops in an environment of amniotic fluid, which poses an aspiration risk to the airway. Swallowing is thus a primary means of airway protection at this stage of development. With maturation, infants appear to transition from apnea and swallowing responses to cough, reflecting the change in environment (Thach, 2001). Laryngeal control, reflected in the speed, range, and accuracy of various laryngeal adjustments required for vocal behavior, may be directly related to neural maturity, and this is not complete in the child.

Anatomical Changes

Exactly how such changes influence the child's emerging vocal skill is not clear, but we might expect that mass/length/tension adjustments, and particularly the fine co-ordination among them, undergo similar development. The voice source at birth is shorter and thicker, and more circular, and with growth becomes longer, thinner, and more ovoid. The overall length of the vocal folds, including both cartilaginous and membranous portions measured from the anterior commissure to the posterior laryn-geal ventricle, may change from approximately 3 mm at birth, to 13 to 16 mm at age 10 years, to perhaps 20 to 30 mm for adult women and men, respectively. Hirano, Kurita, and Nakashima (1983) have postulated that, in general, vocal control improves as the ratio of membranous vocal fold to cartilaginous vocal fold increases (from 1–1.8 in newborns to 3–6 in adults) and as the proportion of cover thickness to membra-nous vocal fold length decreases (from approximately 0.4–0.5 in newborns, to 0.1 or less in adults). As the membranous portion of the vocal fold increases in length, the vibratory source becomes a better, more stable oscillator. It has been further suggested (Dejonckere, Wieneke, Bloemenkamp, & Lebacq, 1996) that these changes may ac-count for decreased perturbation in the voice associated with development. In short, the larynx at birth serves respiratory and airway protection purposes particularly well, whereas more complex vocal behaviors associated with speech and singing may not be fully mature until adulthood.

Voice Physiology

Given the complexity of the issue, it is not surprising that the relation between laryngeal development and vocal development has not been thoroughly elaborated. Longitudinal studies involving large numbers of subjects, dependent variables that adequately reflect the maturing larynx, and the use of measures beyond central tendencies are few. Most available data are cross-sectional, describing children in particular age groups, and often involve a limited number of subjects. In studies that have been performed, large intrasubject and intersubject variability is typical. A major problem with these types of studies, in fact, is that intersubject variability is often larger than the age-related changes being investigated (Bennett, 1983). These cautionary statements notwithstanding, some evidence is available that may be useful for documenting phonatory function in children.

FUNDAMENTAL FREQUENCY CHARACTERISTICS

Change in fundamental frequency associated with growth and development is the variable most often investigated in developmental studies (Kent, 1976; Baken & Orlikoff, 2000). In general, the data available suggest a rapid lowering of frequency in the first 2 to 3 years of life, and then a more gradual drop until puberty. At birth, the fundamental frequency (F_0) of cry is approximately 500 Hz. Between 5 and 8 years, we would expect F_0s to be in the mid to high 200s. From 8 years to puberty, F_0 is likely to drop to the lower 200s. At puberty, gender differences begin and are much more pronounced in boys than in girls. In particular, the angle of the thyroid cartilage becomes more acute (from approximately $120°$ to $90°$) in males, and this is accompanied by a marked increase in vocal fold length and pharynx size. Adult F_0s will be approximately 200 to 220 Hz for women and approximately an octave lower for men. Other studies have described fundamental frequency ranges in children of ages 9 and 10 years to be on the order of 21 to 25 semitones (Flatau & Gutzman, 1908; McAllister, Sederholm, Sundberg, & Gramming, 1994). Further evidence suggests that children's voices may demonstrate slightly greater frequency perturbation than adult voices (Cheyne, Nuss, & Hillman, 1999; Dejonckere et al., 1996).

It is well known that F_0 in adult speakers (nonsingers) tends to increase with increases in intensity. Titze (1996) has postulated that these changes may be greater in children, because of the shorter length of the vocal folds. In excised larynges, the author found that folds with a membranous portion of 5 mm in length produced a 40-Hz increase in fundamental frequency with a doubling of subglottal pressure. In larynges of 10 mm in length, a doubling of subglottal pressure produced only a 5-Hz increase in F_0. To our knowledge, the model has not been tested in children.

AERODYNAMIC CHARACTERISTICS

Other studies have reported age-related differences in aeromechanical properties of voicing. For example, mean airflow rates for maximally sustained vowel sounds (Beckett, Thoelke, & Cowan, 1971) and oral flow rates for consonant productions (Stathopoulos & Weismer, 1985) have been reported to be less in children than in adults. Interestingly, differences in phonation threshold pressure, defined as the minimal subglottal pressure required to produce the softest possible phonation at a particular fundamental frequency, also have been reported (Stathopoulos & Sapienza, 1997). At both conversational and loudest levels of phonation in the lowest part of their F_0 ranges, children's threshold pressures were found by these authors to be 2 to 4 times greater and 4 to

8 times greater, respectively, than values predicted for a mean speaking F_0 of 250 Hz. At higher F_0s, children's threshold pressures were similar to those predicted for adult female voices. The authors suggested that the structure of the vocal folds in children 8 to 11 years of age may demand relatively higher subglottal pressures to vibrate. Other data indicate that mean subglottal pressures at normal conversational loudness levels also may be somewhat higher in children than in adults (Stathopoulos et al., 1985).

Changes in subglottal pressure also may affect vocal intensity somewhat differently in children as compared with adults. Stathopoulos and Sapienza (1997) reported that doubling subglottal pressure yielded a 16-dB SPL (sound pressure level) increase in intensity in a group of 8-year-old children, but only an 11-dB gain in adults. In a second study, these authors found that doubling subglottal pressure produced a 10-dB SPL gain in 10-year-old children, results that are quite similar to data reported for 8- to 11-year-old children by McAllister & Sundberg (1998). These differences are reasonable if the smaller vocal folds of children, in particular those younger than 10 years of age, undergo greater vibratory displacement, and hence greater closing speeds, than the longer vocal folds of adults.

MAXIMUM PHONATION TIMES/DURATIONS (MPT, MPD)

The appropriateness of tests of maximum performance in clinical evaluations has been questioned (Kent, Kent, & Rosenbek, 1987). Nevertheless, some of these measures continue to be widely used, in particular, to assess treatment effects in individual patients. Maximum phonation duration (or time), for example, is frequently included in tests of vocal function for this purpose. Harden and Looney (1984) examined maximum duration of sustained vowels /i/, /a/, and /u/ in 160 children with an average age of 6.2 years. No differences according to gender were identified, and children with voice disorders achieved significantly shorter durations than control subjects. The authors also identified a significant vowel effect, with /i/ sustained for longer times than either /a/ or /u/. Finnegan (1985) reported maximum phonation times in children ranging in age from 3 to 17 years. Each subject performed 14 trials of sustained /a/ and was provided with visual feedback and encouragement in an attempt to maximize performance. Data were based on the 3 longest times obtained for each subject. In contrast to Harden and Looney (1984), Finnegan identified gender differences at several age levels. The range of maximum times from the youngest to oldest subjects was 7.92 seconds to 28.7 seconds in males and from 6.28 seconds to 21.99 seconds in females. Our own experience suggests that the use of repeated trials and careful attention to producing the same vowel at the same fundamental frequency and intensity levels contributes to the utility of MPT in assessing treatment effects in both children and adults.

Another duration measure that is frequently used is called the s/z ratio. To determine the ratio, the subject first sustains /s/ for as long as possible and then repeats the task sustaining /z/. The assumption, which to our knowledge has not been validated, is that the amount of air expelled during phonation should be equal for each phoneme in normal subjects, so that the resulting ratio is "1." In the event of a mass on one or both vocal folds, however, excessive airflow on the /z/ might be expected to reduce its duration with a resulting ratio larger than "1." One study has investigated the maximum duration of /s/ and /z/ in children of ages 5 years, 7 years, and 9 years of age (Tait, Michel, & Carpenter, 1980). The authors reported no significant differences in the s/z ratio by age or gender. However, they did find a significant increase in the maximum duration of both /s/ and /z/ with increased age. Carefully obtained, the s/z ratio may be useful in assessing treatment effects in an individual patient. However, the measure does not differentiate laryngeal from respiratory components of voicing.

VOICE RANGE PROFILE (VRP) CHARACTERISTICS

Also referred to as phonetograms, VRPs have been investigated for some age groups of children. Having the subject produce a sustained vowel sound at the softest and loudest intensities possible at selected intervals within his or her F_0 range generates these profiles. In a study of 10-year-old children, McAllister, Sederholm, Sundberg, and Gramming (1994) found that both pitch range, in semitones, and maximum dynamic range, defined as the difference between SPL at a given fundamental frequency, were generally compressed in children. According to the authors, differences in the higher contour of the profile, which was reduced in children, may reflect a restricted ability of the vocalis muscle to resist the high subglottal pressures required to produce loud voice at a high pitch. Differences in the lower contour, which was elevated in the children investigated, were attributed to a need for greater subglottal pressure to initiate vibration in children's vocal folds. The authors recommend the VRP as a useful means not only of differentiating adult and pediatric voices, but also of differentiating normal and dysphonic voices in the pediatric population.

Heylen, Wuyts, Mertens, DeBodt, Pathyn, Croux, and Van de Heyning (1998) have described voice range profiles obtained for a large number of children with and without vocal fold pathological conditions. Subjects were between 6 and 11 years of age. Based on a discriminant analysis that identified VRP characteristics most sensitive to vocal pathological conditions, the authors constructed a Voice Range Profile Index for Children (VRPIc). Calculation of the Index uses a combination of the child's age, the highest vocal fundamental frequency produced, the softest intensity produced, and the slope of the upper VRP contour. According to the authors, the VRPIc may be used as a screening tool for voice disorders, or to assess the effects of time or treatment on a child's vocal performance.

EGG CHARACTERISTICS

Another measure with potential for documenting vocal function in children has been described by Cheyne, Nuss, and Hillman (1999). These authors investigated 164 children between the ages of 3 and 16 years, using electroglottography (EGG). The authors reported no significant differences for age or sex for the variables of open quotient, closing quotient, opening quotient, and jitter. Jitter values, or relative average perturbation for frequency, were somewhat larger than those reported for adults, and open quotient values were more similar to those reported for adult men than for adult women. Fundamental frequency data, which also can be obtained from EGG, were reportedly similar to other literature reports. The apparent lack of sex or age effects suggest that some elements of vibratory timing are maintained across growth of the larynx, and the authors speculate that this may be critical to the perception of normal vocal quality in children.

CONDITIONS AFFECTING THE LARYNX AND VOICE IN CHILDREN

Congenital Anomalies

Some congenital conditions affecting the larynx may be resolved with time or intervention, whereas others may have long-term effects on voice. Furthermore, some conditions can be either congenital or acquired. The treatment may differ depending on the age of emergence.

Laryngomalacia, which is the most common congenital laryngeal disorder (Tucker, 1987; Morrison et al., 1994), involves immature development of cartilaginous structures that allows soft tissues to collapse and obstruct the airway, particularly during inspiration. Because a primary clinical sign is stridor, this condition is typically identified at birth or shortly thereafter. Although surgery to protect the airway may be required, the condition often resolves with growth and development and does not generally come to the attention of the speech pathologist.

Subglottic stenosis identified at birth is usually associated with respiratory difficulty (Tucker, 1987; Benjamin, 1990; Dejonckere, 1984). The condition may represent a failure in the development of vestibulotracheal tract that becomes the airway, and can involve soft tissues only or cartilage. Other stenoses may be the consequence of an inflammatory process (Benjamin, 1990). If respiration is significantly affected, surgical reconstruction is likely to be required, and there can be long-term consequences for voice (Macarthur, Kearns, & Healy, 1994; Smith, Marsh, Cotton, & Myer III, 1993). Stenosis involving soft tissues may resolve spontaneously during childhood (Schultz-Coulon, 1984).

Laryngeal paralyses present at birth can occur as a consequence of birth trauma, abnormalities in cardiac, pulmonary, or other structures that impact laryngeal innervation, or in association with central nervous system damage. Bilateral paralyses are typically related to central nervous system conditions and thus more likely to be permanent (Michaels, 1984). Effects on respiration and voice will, of course, be dependent on the specific type of paralysis. If the paralysis is bilateral and the folds are fixed in an adducted position, respiratory difficulty and stridor would be expected. If one or both folds are fixed in an abducted position, weak and breathy or aphonic cry, and aspiration, may result. Bilateral vocal fold paralysis frequently accompanies Arnold-Chiari malformation, which involves displacement of the cerebellum and brainstem into the cervical spinal canal through the foramen magnum with subsequent injury to the medullary respiratory center and cranial nerves IX and X.

Congenital webs involving the true vocal folds may produce respiratory difficulty or stridor that leads to their subsequent identification. Webs are a consequence of anomalous embryological development and recently have been related to specific chromosomal abnormalities (Milczuk, Smith, & Everts, 2000). In the embryological development of the larynx, the vestibule and laryngeal lumen are at one time composed of an epithelial lamina that fuses the primordial epiglottis and arytenoid cartilages. Reestablishment of the supraglottic and infra-glottic airways involves the eventual regression of this epithelial tissue. A failure of this process can lead to webs at various sites. When the true vocal folds and glottis are significantly involved, early identification is more likely. If the web is thin and membranous, surgical correction may result in good voice quality (Benjamin, 1983). However, surgical excision of thicker, more fibrous webs is likely to have serious implications for voice quality. As noted previously, webs and paralyses may not be recognized until much later, particularly if their functional consequences are subtle.

Congenital cysts of the vocal folds are apparently rare. In a series of 657 congenital anomalies of the larynx, Holinger and Brown (1967) reported only three cases of cysts. However, some congenital cysts may not be identified at birth but rather become apparent later. In other series of benign laryngeal pathological conditions, cysts have been reported in young children, though again, infrequently (Kawasaki, Kuratomi, & Mitsumasu, 1983). In a description of an intracordal cyst identified in an infant, Smith, Callanan, Harcourt, and Albert (2000) described episodic stridor, respiratory distress, and feeding difficulties. The symptoms were resolved by excision of the cyst. Congenital cysts are most often epidermoid (Milutinovic & Vasiljevic, 1992) and may represent remnants of the fourth and sixth branchial arches that become trapped in the vocal fold cover (Bouchayer et al., 1985). Tucker (1987) notes that simple cysts are likely a consequence of obstruction of ducts associated with mucous, serous, or minor salivary glands. Entrapment of air or secretions in the anterior portion of the laryngeal ventricles, or saccule, can produce laryngoceles that may become enlarged during pneumatizing activities, such as crying or straining at stool. Cysts that interfere with respiration or voicing are more likely to be identified at birth or shortly thereafter.

Papilloma in the larynx is of viral origin, often recurring and requiring surgical or medical management strategies or a combination thereof. When papilloma directly affects the vocal folds and requires surgical excision, dysphonia may be marked, and therapy directed at optimizing functional oral communication may be of value.

This is also true for children who have sustained laryngeal injuries from frequent or prolonged intubations.

INTUBATION INJURY

The child who requires a long-term tracheotomy from birth to maintain the airway presents unique challenges to the speech–language pathologist. With a tracheostomy tube in place, air enters and exits the airway below the level of the vocal folds. In perforated tubes, occlusion of the tube with a finger during exhalation will divert air across the vocal folds to produce voice, assuming the true vocal folds are capable of this function. Passy-Muir valves respond to increases in pressure (consistent with voicing) to close the tracheostomy tube and divert air with no external manipulation, and have been used in pediatric patients with good pulmonary function (Morrison et al., 1994). In children with a long-term compromised ability to vocalize, for whatever reason, a key role of the speech–language pathologist is to maximize both the child's functional communication skills and his or her development of speech and language.

Signs and Symptoms of Congenital Laryngeal Disorders in Children

In general, the primary signs of a congenital laryngeal abnormality include dysphonia, difficulty breathing, and stridor during respiration. Feeding difficulty also may be noted, indicated by coughing, choking, and cyanosis (bluish discoloration of skin and mucous membranes due to reduced hemoglobin in the blood). Observation of the larynx endoscopically, and perhaps with radiographic studies, is likely to produce at least a preliminary diagnosis of the specific pathological condition. To our knowledge, there is little experimental evidence that specifically addresses the differentiation of dysphonias associated with congenital laryngeal anomalies according to acoustic or perceptual characteristics of voice or cry. Nor are we aware of measurable physiologic variables that are used to differentiate congenital anomalies of the larynx. Tucker (1987) noted that careful attention to voice, however, may be helpful in directing diagnostic efforts. For example, the presence of inspiratory and expiratory stridor, as well as weak or muffled cry, suggests a web, whereas the presence of stridor with a normal voice points to stenosis.

Acquired Pathological Conditions

VOCAL NODULES

The most common laryngeal pathological condition associated with voice disorders in children is vocal nodules, possibly accounting for 50% of voice disorders in this population (Fig. 7.1) (Herrington-Hall, 1988; Morrison et al., 1994). Most often, these lesions are attributed to excessive voice use or habitual vocal hyperfunction. However, reports exist in the literature of nodules even in infants, and it has been suggested that these may be related to laryngopharyngeal reflux, that is, acidic material that is refluxed from the esophagus onto the structures of the larynx (Halstead, 1999). Typically, nodules are bilateral and occur at the mid-membranous point of the true vocal folds, which is the site that experiences the greatest contact forces during voicing. In newborns and infants, the composition and position of the larynx differs markedly from those of adults and older children. At birth, the cartilaginous portion of the vocal folds constitute approximately half of their length from the anterior to posterior commissure, with the membranous portion responsible for the remainder (Hirano et al., 1983). This is in contrast to adults, in whom the posterior cartilaginous processes constitute approximately 40% of the anteroposterior length of the true vocal folds. Nodules therefore may be more anteriorly located in children than in adults. Histologically, they appear as fibrotic thickenings or swellings of the mucosa. They may be soft or

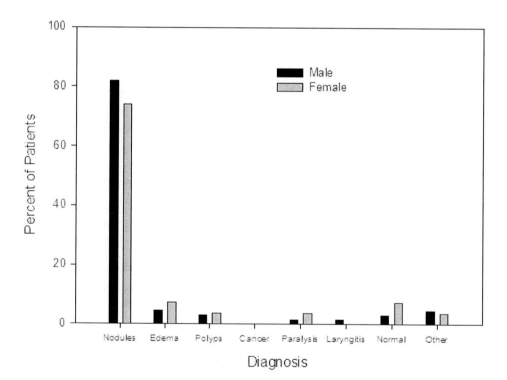

Figure 7.1. Prevalence of Voice Problems in children 0–14 years. Data are from Herrington-Hall, B. L., Lee, L., Stemple, J. C., Niemi, K. R., & McHone, M. M. (1988). Description of laryngeal pathologies by age, sex, and occupation in a treatment-seeking sample. *Journal of Speech and Hearing Disorders, 53,* 57–64.

firm, depending, in part, on how long they have been present. With greater chronicity, thickened epithelium contributes to the fibrotic character of the nodule.

Vocal nodules rarely require surgical excision. Most contemporary otolaryngologists writing about nodules in children (Tucker, 1987; Morrison et al., 1994; von Leden, 1985) suggest that only in rare cases, for example, when oral communication or social development is significantly affected and when conservative measures, including voice therapy, have failed, would surgery be considered. One reason for this is that, at puberty, growth of the larynx typically changes the point of maximum compressive forces of the vocal folds. With a reduction in the collision forces acting on them, the nodules may resolve spontaneously. In addition, vocal behaviors that produced the nodules are likely to attenuate with increasing maturity of the individual.

Conservative management is the recommended treatment for vocal nodules in children. In our experience, focus is directed to the identification and modification of those behaviors considered most excessive or hyperfunctional, such as screaming and yelling or imitating machine or animal noises. In all cases, a team approach directed to achieving stable voice quality (no vocal fatigue) and reinforcing appropriate voice use by parents, teachers, and other care providers appears to have the best chance of being effective. The intent is not to criticize communicative behavior, but to minimize excessive or inappropriate vocal behaviors. The older the child, the more possible it is to discuss directly the need for modification of vocal behaviors, and strategies for achieving this objective.

In our clinical experience, adults who present with vocal nodules or other voice use–related pathological conditions sometimes report frequent episodes of dysphonia when they were children or teenagers. On reflection, they may acknowledge to us that they have consistently engaged in excessive or hyperfunctional vocal behaviors throughout their lives. These patients often note that they were not treated for dysphonia at an earlier age, possibly because of the intermittent nature of the hoarseness. Based on these experiences, we believe it may always be worthwhile to engage in at least some counseling of parents and of older children regarding the nature and cause of the child's vocal nodules. Our hope, of course, is that these early educational efforts may prevent the individual from having difficulty as an adult.

VOCAL FOLD PARALYSIS

Non-congenital unilateral vocal fold paralysis may be seen in children, perhaps most often as a consequence of trauma (Daya, Hosni, Bejar-Solar, Evans, & Bailey, 2000). In some cases, trauma may be related to surgery, for example, as in the repair of a congenital heart anomaly that damages a recurrent laryngeal nerve. Depending on the likelihood that a unilateral vocal fold paralysis may be permanent, and on the severity of symptoms produced, surgical intervention may be required. If so, careful consideration must be given to treatment choices, and the same options available to adults may not be applicable to children. For example, augmentation procedures used to medialize a fixed vocal fold may reduce the size of the airway, particularly if the augmentation material is over-injected to compensate for anticipated resorption. Though the added mass usually does not present a problem for adults, it could produce respiratory difficulty in the smaller pediatric airway. Treatment alternatives that could interfere with the continuing growth and development of the larynx are also avoided. Voice therapy in such cases may be of value in maximizing optimal vocal fold function, and in preventing hyperfunctional compensatory behaviors that could develop in response to the paralysis. Acquired bilateral vocal fold paralyses resulting from trauma would be expected to produce immediate consequences for respiration or airway protection, and to require immediate intervention.

LARYNGOPHARYNGEAL REFLUX

Reflux of material from the esophagus into the pharynx and larynx has become increasingly recognized as a source of laryngeal tissue change and subsequent chronic dysphonia in children (Halstead, 1999; Kalach, Gumpert, Contencin, & Dupont, 2000). In a study of 17 chronically hoarse children between 2 and 12 years of age, laryngeal findings included interarytenoid erythema or edema with vocal fold granuloma or nodules in 13 cases, and isolated granuloma or nodules in 3 cases (Kalach et al., 2000). Only one subject had a normal-appearing larynx. Twenty-four-hour dual-probe pH monitoring was performed in all children and showed abnormal findings in 15 of the 17 subjects. The possible role of gastroesophageal reflux in the development of a wide range of pediatric upper airway disorders also has been investigated (Halstead, 1999). Results of pH probe testing, laryngeal examination, and bronchoalveolar lavage suggested reflux as a causative factor in subglottic stenosis, recurrent croup, apnea, and chronic cough, and as an inflammatory co-factor in chronic sinusitis/otitis/bronchitis, laryngomalacia, and possibly true vocal fold nodules (Halstead, 1999). Otolaryngologists and voice clinicians routinely consider reflux as a causative or exacerbating influence on laryngeal pathological conditions in adults; it would appear that similar attention should extend to dysphonic children as well.

PHARMACEUTICAL CAUSES

Children as well as adults may take medications that affect the vocal folds in ways that may contribute to voice change. In our own clinic, for example, the number of children who are using corticosteroid inhalants for asthma appears to be on the rise. The effects of these drugs in adults have been frequently described and include mucosal changes of the vocal folds, fungal infections, and adductor myasthenia (Lavy, Wood, Rubin, & Harries, 2000). We would therefore urge clinicians to be as thorough in reviewing pharmacological regimens in their pediatric patients as they are in evaluating adults.

Signs and Symptoms of Acquired Laryngeal Disorders in Children

The acquired laryngeal disorder that has been most investigated in children is vocal nodules, and consequently, most of the available experimental evidence regarding signs and symptoms, as related to voice, pertains to this population. This information is reviewed here.

PERCEPTUAL SIGNS AND SYMPTOMS

McAllister, Sederholm, Sundberg, and Gramming (2000) described perceptual characteristics in a group of 60 normal children who underwent laryngeal examinations. Although 10% of the group were found to have vocal nodules, 14% were perceived as demonstrating hoarseness on two separate occasions. At least one subject with vocal nodules was perceived as having a normal voice. The authors note that, in particular, the perception of breathiness, which is often associated with laryngeal pathological conditions in adults, may not be perceived as unusual in children.

In a much earlier study, Silverman (1975) found that listeners perceived 23% of 162 school-age children screened for speech and voice abnormalities as hoarse. Again, of the hoarse children who underwent laryngeal examinations, not all were identified with laryngeal pathological conditions. It would seem, thus, that not all children with vocal nodules experience significant voice change; similarly, some children perceived to have normal voice quality also may have vocal nodules. Of course, those children with perceived hoarseness, or abnormal voice quality, come to the attention of the voice clinician. In our opinion, children who demonstrate chronic hoarseness are candidates for laryngeal examination. Though factors other than laryngeal pathology may contribute to perceived hoarseness in children, for example, tissue changes related to asthma medications or to allergies, the only means of ruling out pathological conditions is by laryngeal examination.

ACOUSTIC SIGNS

Hufnagle (1982) reported an increase in the habitual fundamental frequency of boys with vocal nodules, as compared with a group of boys without laryngeal pathological conditions. The groups were matched for age and size, and fundamental frequency measurements were obtained from narrow band spectrograms magnified to expand the spectrum from 0 to 1,300 Hz. The group with vocal nodules had significantly higher fundamental frequencies (mean of 301 Hz) than the normal group (246 Hz). Using the Voice Range Profile described previously, McAllister, Sederholm, Sundberg, and Gramming (1994) reported a decrease in fundamental frequency range in 10-year-old children with vocal nodules (19 semitones), as compared with a control group (25 semitones). These authors did not find a difference in the two groups for maximum dynamic range (lowest to highest intensity at a given fundamental frequency), however.

Heylen, Wuyts, Mertens, DeBodt, Pathyn, Croux, and Van de Heyning (1998) investigated 94 normal children and 130 children with laryngeal pathological conditions, primarily vocal nodules (118/130), using a number of variables derived from the Voice Range Profile. The authors found that the two groups, matched for age, differed significantly on all measures considered with the exception of the lowest fundamental frequency produced. Both fundamental frequency range and maximum dynamic range were significantly reduced in children with pathological conditions. Interestingly, in contrast to the Hufnagle study, modal fundamental frequency was found to be lower in the pathology group. The authors suggest that the presence of mass-adding lesions is likely to interfere with more rapid vibratory rates of the vocal folds, thus limiting the high end of the fundamental frequency range. In addition, nodules or other mass-adding lesions affecting the vocal folds are likely to require greater driving pressures to initiate and maintain phonation, affecting, in particular, the generation of intensities at the lower end of the maximum dynamic range. As noted previously, from their preliminary testing, the authors constructed for each subject a Voice Range Profile (VRPIc) using a combination of age, highest fundamental frequency produced, lowest intensity produced, and the slope of the upper VRP contour. The measure was found to demonstrate good sensitivity (90%) and specificity (83%) in differentiating the normal group from the group with laryngeal pathological conditions.[1]

---

[1] Sensitivity refers to the proportion of dysphonic children correctly identified by the test; specificity, to the proportion of normal children correctly identified.

Campisi, Tewfik, Pelland-Blais, Hussein, and Sadeghi (2000) examined a number of measures from the MultiDimensional Voice Program (MDVP) (Kay Elemetrics, Lincoln Park, NJ) in boys with and without vocal nodules. The two groups were matched in age and ranged from 7 to 12 years. Boys with vocal nodules were found to have statistically significant elevations in absolute jitter, jitter percent, relative average perturbation, pitch period perturbation quotient, smoothed amplitude perturbation quotient, and fundamental frequency variation. These findings suggest, not surprisingly, that cycle-by-cycle variability in vocal fold vibration is increased by the presence of nodules.

One other acoustic measure that has been considered in children with vocal nodules is the noise-to-harmonics ratio (NHR). Pereira, Cervantes, Abrahao, Parente Settanni, and Carrara de Angelis (2002) described higher NHR values in a group of boys with laryngeal pathological conditions, including vocal nodules, as compared with a group of boys without laryngeal pathological conditions. The NHR does not differentiate sources of noise in the voice, which may be related to turbulence, increased cycle-to-cycle amplitude or frequency variability, voice breaks, or possibly to other factors. However, in the case of vocal nodules (or other mass-adding lesions), we might reasonably expect that any one or all of these factors may account for the finding of greater noise in the acoustic signal produced.

MEASURABLE PHYSIOLOGICAL SIGNS

Sapienza and Stathopoulos (1994) examined respiratory and laryngeal measures in children and women with vocal nodules and in control subjects without pathological conditions. Higher peak and minimum airflows were found in the nodule subjects, as well as larger lung volume excursions. We have found, clinically, that airflows may be particularly elevated in children with vocal nodules during syllable repetition tasks and may be accompanied by elevations in subglottal pressure estimates, as well. Interestingly, this has not always been our experience in adults with laryngeal pathological conditions. Although some adults with lesions demonstrate similar elevations in airflow and subglottal pressure, others appear able to manipulate respiratory behavior, that is, to significantly reduce expiratory airflow, possibly in an attempt to preserve durational characteristics of speech (as number of syllables per exhalation).

Characteristics of different types of vocal initiation in children with vocal nodules were investigated by Leeper (1976), using both acoustic and aerodynamic measures. Results showed consistently longer voice initiation times and greater air volume expenditure during the initial few hundred milliseconds of phonation in the children with vocal nodules, as compared with the control group. This was true for three types of vocal initiation, including hard, soft, and breathy.

OBSERVABLE PHYSIOLOGICAL SIGNS

Laryngoscopy

As noted previously, nodules are more anteriorly located in young children than in adults. However, as in adults, they are typically bilateral. Closure of the vocal folds on phonation may be incomplete, particularly on either side of the pathological condition. If the nodules are of recent origin, there may be accompanying edema and erythema. In our experience, nodules are often broad-based in children, appearing as a fibrous thickening or swelling of the mucosa. They may be soft or firm, depending, in part, on how long they have been present. With greater chronicity, thickened epithelium contributes to the fibrotic character of the nodule.

Stroboscopy

In our experience, stroboscopic examination of the larynx in children can be somewhat compromised. Even when the child's true vocal folds can be visualized easily, it may be difficult to elicit sustained sounds of the several seconds' duration required for good stroboscopic imaging. This appears to be true in children, in general, whether they do or do not have a laryngeal pathological condition. Extent or duration of the closed phase and symmetry from right to left may be difficult to judge. Our impression, however, is that stroboscopic findings in children with nodules would generally be comparable to those in adults. That is, the mucosal wave is likely to be affected by the size and character of the pathological condition, being unaffected or minimally affected with soft lesions and reduced significantly with firmer lesions. Similarly, degree of closure will vary depending on size and compressibility characteristics of the pathological condition.

Case Study: Dysphonia of Unclear Origin in 7-Year-Old Child

A 7-year-old girl (N.S.) was referred to the Voice Clinic by an outside otolaryngologist. He indicated that the child's parents had consulted him on the advice of the speech–language pathologist (SLP) at N.S.'s school. The SLP had noted hoarseness on a screening examination and was concerned that it may be related to an underlying laryngeal pathological condition. The otolaryngologist had performed an indirect laryngeal examination on the child and found the true vocal folds to be normal in appearance and function. However, he noted that N.S. was using her false vocal folds on phonation and thought that her marked dysphonia was functional in origin. The remainder of the HEENT (head, eyes, ears, nose, throat) examination was normal. The otolaryngologist referred N.S. to the Voice Clinic for voice therapy.

N.S. presented to the Voice Clinic as a happy child who enjoyed friends, family, and many activities. She appeared small for her age. Voice quality was soft, low in pitch, and judged as severely hoarse. Her history was significant for a 3-month premature birth requiring respiratory assistance for 1 month. The parents did not recall whether this involved intubation. N.S. required frequent hospitalizations during her infancy for pneumonia, and at age 3 years underwent an adenotonsillectomy. At 5 years, a tympanoplasty was performed. She had been diagnosed with attention deficit disorder, for which she was currently taking medication. She was enrolled in a special education classroom at her school and was making good progress. Her parents reported that N.S. had sounded the same since she began talking, and they were not particularly concerned about her voice quality until recently. They also described their daughter as active, but generally quiet. They felt she in no way fit the profile of a child whose voice use is excessive or hyperfunctional. Her teachers described N.S. in a similar manner.

Phonatory function testing showed an average speaking fundamental frequency of 233 Hz, and a range of 11 semitones (215–405 Hz). Maximum phonation time on a sustained vowel was 12 seconds. Perturbation measures for both frequency and amplitude were mildly elevated, and the noise-to-harmonics ratio was 0.32. Laryngeal function testing showed reduced airflow for a sustained sound (<25 cc/sec). On a syllable repetition task, however, airflow was extremely high (>400 cc/sec), with a subglottal pressure estimate of 4.52 dyne/cm^2. The estimate of glottal resistance was so high as to be invalid. Though maximum dynamic range was not tested, N.S. appeared unable to produce voice at loud intensities. A pulmonary screening examination suggested a moderate restriction, although neither the parents nor N.S. reported respiratory difficulties.

On laryngeal examination with rigid endoscopy, our initial impression was that the larynx was within normal limits. However, on phonation, the impression was that the false folds medialized, almost completely obscuring the underlying true folds. In exploring this behavior further, we continued to observe the larynx over a wide range of vocal and vegetative tasks—an evaluation strategy we refer to as a phonoscopic examination. N.S. was compliant with the laryngeal examination, and the prolonged observation was productive. During this testing, it became clear that N.S. had a laryngeal web. The web was above the level of the true folds, and it appeared to originate from the anterior commissure and extend into the laryngeal ventricles between the false and true vocal folds (see Fig. 7.2). When her true vocal folds were abducted (Fig. 7.2A), the web retracted and was not apparent; however, as the vocal folds moved to an adducted state (Fig. 7.2B), the web moved posteriorly until it formed a cover over the true vocal folds (Fig. 7.2C and 7.2D). By observing the vocal folds carefully, and on slow motion replay of the videotaped examination, we were eventually able to make this determination.

Whether the visualized web was congenital or came about as a consequence of intubation or other trauma was not clear. However, it did explain N.S.'s marked dysphonia, and probably most of the unusual findings on phonatory and pulmonary function testing. For example, during the production of a sustained sound, the web covered the true vocal folds to the extent of markedly reducing any airflow. On a syllable repetition task, requiring rapid abduction and adduction gestures of the true vocal folds, airflows were greatly elevated, possibly reflecting a tethering effect of the web.

The case of N.S. reminds us that not all laryngeal pathological conditions in children are related to vocal nodules, and that long-standing hoarseness in children needs to be explained. In this instance, a number of clues in her case history suggested the possibility of a congenital pathological condition or early trauma to the larynx. Similarly, N.S. did not appear to fit the profile of a child we might suspect of developing vocal nodules related to excessive or hyperfunctional voice use. Both the phonatory function and pulmonary screening results were unusual, and the careful, phonoscopic examination of the larynx over a broad range of tasks was critical to the eventual diagnosis. Excision of the web required surgery, and both N.S.'s parents and the voice team thought that, if performed, it should be carefully timed to optimize results. Factors such as N.S.'s small size for her age, her apparent lack of respiratory signs and symptoms related to the web, and her own awareness of the unusual quality of her voice were given careful consideration in the decision-making process.

THE GERIATRIC VOICE

In this section, the biological and voice characteristics of the geriatric voice are discussed. Here *geriatric* refers to individuals 65 years of age or older. Aging is a process that results in a progressive decline of the multiple control mechanisms needed for daily life (Barry & Eathorne, 1994). All organs are affected, although the change may be prevented or minimized by physical activity, diet, and lifestyle. There may be a large difference between the chronological age of an individual and his or her biological age. We do not all age at the same biological rate. Individuals with identical chronological ages can be very different in their biological abilities. In his preface to the book *Geriatric Otolaryngology*, Dr. Jerome Goldstein (1989) reported on several geriatric individuals

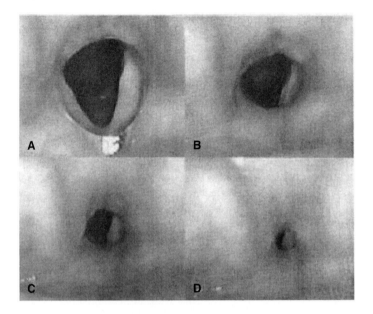

Figure 7.2. Seven-year-old girl with supraglottic web. In **A**, true vocal folds appear within normal limits when fully abducted. In **B**, as folds begin to adduct, the web can be seen to move posteriorly. Coverage of true vocal folds becomes more extensive in **C**, and is nearly complete in **D**.

to demonstrate that even at 72, 76, or 81 years of age, an individual can be very active and biologically fit. One of his examples was an 81-year-old female power lifter who dead-lifts 245 pounds, squat-lifts 148 pounds, and works out daily with running, swimming, and lifting (Goldstein & Salmon, 1978). Clearly, we do not all age at the same rate; we merely count the number of years from birth in the same way. A very good review of the effects of aging on communication may be found in Linville (2001). A brief review of the current understanding and treatment of the voice of the elderly can be found in *Current Opinions in Otolaryngology* (Casper & Colton, 2000).

Theories of Aging

The following is a brief discussion of some of the major theories of aging. Some of these theories share similar concepts and information, suggesting that we are still awaiting the development of a theory that will account for all of the processes involved in aging and will help us understand what aging is and how we might control it.

PLANNED OBSOLESCENCE THEORIES

The focus of these theories is DNA and the effect genetics has on the aging process. We all have our own unique DNA code, a code that determines all of our physical characteristics and may even determine how long we will live as well as what kinds of diseases we may experience. DNA can be easily damaged by outside influences such as diet, lifestyle, environmental pollutants, and many other factors. Gene damage appears to occur when the gene repairs itself after being damaged. The gene duplicates itself incorrectly, eventually leading to dysfunction of the cell. Other factors that may damage the DNA molecules include the lack of important enzymes used in DNA repair and the presence of free radicals produced as a byproduct of the process used to extract oxygen from the air we breathe.

A variant of this type of theory is the Telomerase Theory of Aging (Ahmed & Tollefsbol, 2001; Boukamp, 2001; Djojosubroto, Choi, Lee, & Rudolph, 2003; Kipling & Faragher, 1999). Telomeres are repeating sequences of nucleic acids extending from the end of a chromosome. When a cell divides, the length of the telomere is shortened. When the length reaches a critical value, the cell can no longer replicate and ultimately dies. In a way, the telomere is a biological clock that eventually winds down to cause death. However, there is some skepticism about this theory, because some animals have rather long telomeres but have relatively short life spans.

FREE RADICAL THEORY

This theory was developed by Denham Harman (Harman, 1992; Harman, 1998; Harman, 2001) and later popularized by others. Normal cell metabolism produces a byproduct, generally known as free radicals. Free radicals are molecules with an extra electron. These free radicals cause damage to the cell's DNA structure, other proteins, and mitochondria. The extra electron causes the molecule to try to bind with other balanced molecules. Thus, a free radical attacks other cells in the attempt to become balanced. This attack in turn creates waste products that interfere with normal cell function. Antioxidants are scavengers that bind to free radicals and reduce their effects. They help to remove these free radicals and have been part of the popular herbal medicine culture. Some researchers have suggested that antioxidants actually work to suppress appetite. Reduced caloric intake has been shown to increase the life span of animals.

NEUROENDOCRINE THEORY

This theory focuses on the endocrine system and the role hormones may play in the aging process. As we grow older, the hypothalamus loses its ability to precisely regulate the hormones circulating through our bodies. This results in the receptors for the hormones becoming less sensitive, which in turn results in less of the hormones being manufactured. The theory was first introduced by Vladimir Dilman (Dilman & Dean, 1992; Dean, 1999; Dean, 2003) and has been advanced by Ward Dean (Dean, 1999; Dean, 2003). Dean claims that over 85% of deaths of the middle-aged and elderly may be attributed to this faulty neuroendocrine regulation. He believes that replacement of essential hormones and other substances involved in the regulatory process could extend life. Dean recommends drugs that can reestablish some degree of regulatory ability to the various structures involved in this regulatory control.

MEMBRANE THEORY

This theory was introduced by Imre Zs-Nagy, who postulated that age-related changes in cell membranes interfered with the ability of the cell to interchange chemicals, heat, and oxygen with the external environment (Zs-Nagy, 1997). Cell membranes become less watery, thereby impeding the efficiency of membrane transfer. Waste products and toxins may accumulate within the cell that could result in cell death. Substances exist that improve the ability of the membrane to transfer waste products, needed chemicals, and other substances.

MITOCHONDRIAL DECLINE THEORY

Mitochondria are the energy-producing structures of the cells (Beckman & Ames, 1998; Cadenas & Davies, 2000; Kowald, 2001). They are responsible for the production of adenosine triphosphate (ATP) needed for everyday function. ATP cannot be stored in the body; the mitochondria must constantly replenish the supply. Mitochondria are susceptible to free radicals, which are also produced by them and against which they have few defenses. As the production of ATP declines because of mitochondrial damage, there is less energy for organ function. Each organ has its own set of mitochondria, and when they are damaged, the organ itself may become damaged and fail. Antioxidants can be used to minimize the free radical damage of the mitochondria.

There are other theories of aging, many of which are variants on the basic themes presented above. A single unified theory will no doubt emerge in time as more is learned about the process of aging. That single theory will need to account for all of the effects described above and generate methods to control the aging process and extend life.

Anatomical and Physiological Changes in the Larynx

Aging in the larynx affects cartilages, connective tissue, blood supply, glandular secretions, and muscle. Changes in the lamina propria include loss of collagenous and elastic fibers, atrophy of submucous glands, disorganization of collagen fibers, increased fibrosis, and atrophy of the muscles (Gracco & Kahane, 1989; Kahane, 1987; Kahane, 1981a; Kahane, 1981b). Structural changes include ossification of the thyroid cartilage and changes in the articular cartilages. Blood supply decreases, the types of cells present and their proportional quantities are altered, and generalized increased stiffness and decreased flexibility occur. Presumably, these anatomical changes affect the vibratory characteristics of the vocal folds and thereby alter the perceptual, acoustic, and physiological voice signs. Table 7.1 presents a summary of the age-related changes in various parts of the body for men and women.

Anatomical changes that may occur in the brain and spinal cord may have an impact on the neurological control of the vocal muscles. Luschei et al. (1999) studied the electrical activity of cricothyroid, thyroarytenoid, and lateral cricoarytenoid muscles in aged men and women (>65 years). They reported lower firing frequencies of the thyroarytenoid in aged men and suggested that a change in the morphology of motor units may account for these differences. Similar findings were reported for a non-laryngeal muscle (first dorsal interosseous) by Erim et al. (Erim, Beg, Burke, & De Luca, 1999), who reported a decrease in firing rates, decreases in fluctuations of firing rates, increased delays between motor unit firing rates, and lower starting firing rates for their geriatric subjects.

PERCEPTUAL SIGNS

Extensive reviews of acoustic and perceptual features of the geriatric voice have appeared in the literature (Casper et al., 2000; Colton, 1989; Linville & Fisher, 1985a; Linville, 1987a; Linville, 2001; Linville & Rens, 2001; Linville, 2002; Shindo & Hanson, 1990), and only a brief review is presented here. Perceptually, listeners can identify a geriatric voice and can do so from a recorded sample with surprising accuracy. Some of the major features of the geriatric voice include hoarseness, low pitch, imprecise articulation, breathiness, and long pauses (Hartman & Danhauer, 1976). In another study (Ryan & Capadano, 1978), the important perceptual features of the

Table 7.1. Summary of Significant Changes Due to Aging

Morphologic Changes in Connective Tissue	Male	Female
• Edema within superficial layer of lamina	X	X
• Fiber density decreases, leading to thinning of muscle and vocal ligament	X	X
• Loose connective tissue replaces myofibrils	X	X
• Decrease in number of fibroblasts that control synthesis of elastin and collagen, leading to decreased synthesis of fibrous components in lamina propria	X	X
• Elastic fibers in lamina propria no longer smooth or uniform in size; become rough and variable in size	X	X
• Elastic fibers no longer aligned parallel to free edge; run in various directions as a branched network	X	X
• Elastic fibers in superficial layer degenerate and atrophy, affecting stiffness of vocal fold	X	X
• Increase in density of collagen fibers	More	Less
• Slow turnover and repair rates of elastic fibers	More	Less
Mucosal Changes		
• Mucous membrane becomes thinner and atrophic	X	
• Mucous membrane thickens in postmenopausal women (edema, polypoid)		X
• Underlying tissue becomes infiltrated with fatty tissue	X	X
• Fatty tissue and keratosis lead to graying and yellow discoloration	X	X
Cartilaginous Changes		
• Ossification of cartilages	More	Less
• Arthritic changes of cricoarytenoid joint	X	X
• Thinning of articular joint surfaces; irregularities, breakdown in collagen fiber organization	X	X
Muscle Changes		
• Atrophy	More	Less
• Stiffening	More	Less
• Apoptosis, programmed cell death occurs in TA muscle	X	X
• Proportion of regenerating fibers increases with age, but the properties of those fibers is not known	X	X
• Decrease in surface density of certain muscle fibers	X	X
• Increase in atrophy factor of certain muscle fibers	X	X
• Decrease in ratio of satellite cells to myonuclei	X	X
Vascular Changes (Animal Studies)		
• Mucosal blood flow probably decreased as result of atrophy and increasing fibrous characteristic of aging vocal folds	X	X
• Decreased flow in PCA, TA, and CT	X	X
Sensory Changes		
• Decrease in number of small myelinated fibers in the superior laryngeal nerve (animal)		
• Peripheral neuropathy (human)		

Continued.

Table 7.1. (continued)

Respiratory Changes		
• Decreased elasticity of respiratory tissues	X	X
• Decreased vital capacity of lungs	X	X
• Changes in chest wall structure	X	X
• Irregular respirations	X	X
• Phonation initiated at higher lung and ribcage volumes	X	X
• Higher lung and ribcage excursions	X	X
• Trachea softens and widens; prebronchial muscle atrophy	X	X
Neuromuscular Control Changes		
• Vocal instability	X	X
• General slowing of CNS functions	X	X
• Increase in muscle fiber type grouping	X	X
Glandular Changes		
• Decreased number of mucous glands due to atrophy	X	X
• Decreased number of lymphatic channels	X	X
Hormonal Changes		
• Decrease in thyroid hormone	X	
• Decrease in sex hormones		X
Systemic Changes		
• Increased incidence of gastroesophageal reflux	X	X
• Decreased auditory acuity	X	X

From Casper and Colton, 2001.

geriatric voice included pitch, volume, speed, clarity, and authority. According to this study, geriatric voices sounded less clear and less flexible. Table 7.2 presents some of the perceptual changes that occur as a result of aging for both men and women.

ACOUSTIC SIGNS

Acoustically, several features of the voice change as a result of aging (see Table 7.2). Fundamental frequency tends to rise as a function of age in men (Benjamin, 1981; Hollien & Shipp, 1972) and decrease in women (Brown, Jr., Morris, & Michel, 1989; Linville et al., 1985a). Hollien (1987) postulated the male–female coalescence model of voice change, in which, as they age, men and women become more alike, at least vocally. The model predicts that the fundamental frequency of a male voice will increase substantially as it ages, whereas the female voice will show a slight downward change of fundamental frequency or no change at all. These predicted changes are thought to be the consequence of the pronounced changes within the larynx of a male voice but the fewer or less pronounced changes in the female larynx.

Fundamental frequency variability is also affected by aging. Mysak (1959) reported larger values for men, and Stoicheff (1981), Linville and Fisher (1985b), and Morris and Brown (1994) for women. Fundamental frequency range is also reduced both in men (McGlone & Hollien, 1963; Ptacek, Sander, Maloney, & Jackson, 1966) and women (Linville, 1987b).

Fundamental frequency perturbation may be affected in aging. Orlikoff (1990) reported much higher jitter values for his group of old subjects (0.728) versus the young group (0.461). Conversely, others (Brown, Jr. et al., 1989; Casper, 1983; Linville, 1987a;

Table 7.2. Summary of Physiological Changes Attributable to Aging

Perceptual	Male	Female
Determine age from voice sample	X	X
Classify into age groups	X	X
Pitch changes	X	X
Hoarseness	X	X
Breathy	X	X
Slow rate	X	X
Acoustic		
Average fundamental frequency changes	Higher	Lower
Variability of fundamental frequency	Greater	Greater
Frequency perturbation	Greater	Greater
Fundamental frequency range	Smaller	Smaller
Average intensity level	Greater	?
Variability of intensity	Smaller	Smaller
Intensity range	Smaller	Smaller
Speaking rate	Slower	Slower
Spectral changes	Yes	?
Physiological		
Vital capacities	Smaller	Smaller
Lung pressure	Lower	Lower
Peak airflow rates	Greater	
Leakage airflow rates	Greater	
Open quotient	Greater	
MFDR	Less	
Muscle Electrical Activity		
Thyroarytenoid-firing frequency or /s/	Reduced	Reduced
Cricothyroid-firing frequency or /s/	Same	Same
Lateral cricoarytenoid-firing frequency or /s/	?	?

From Casper and Colton, 2001.

Linville, 1987b; Ramig & Ringel, 1983) reported no difference of jitter between young and geriatric subjects.

It has been reported by some that the intensity of a geriatric voice may be slightly greater than that of a young voice (Brown, Jr. et al., 1989; Ryan, 1972), although the differences are small. Conversely, Hodge, Colton, and Kelley (2001) found that their elderly speakers produced slightly lower SPLs at selected percentage points of their total intensity range. Morris and Brown (1994) reported smaller variability of intensity for their old group (mean age, 79.4 years) versus their young group (mean age, 27.5 years). These results suggest that the geriatric population has stiffer, less flexible vocal folds. Amplitude perturbation or shimmer is generally higher in the geriatric speaker (Biever & Bless, 1989; Ramig et al., 1983; Ringel & Chodzko-Zajko, 1987).

OBSERVABLE PHYSIOLOGICAL SIGNS

Laryngoscopic changes also have been reported, including bowed vocal folds, atrophy or apparent thinning of the vocal folds, edema, and a posterior glottal gap (1980). Segre (1971) noted a yellowish discoloration of the vocal folds, atrophy of the ventricular folds, loss of normal tension, and a fissure in the middle or anterior third of the glottis. A vocal fold sulcus has been noted in some elderly subjects (Honjo & Isshiki, 1980; Mueller, Sweeney, & Baribeau, 1984).

Stroboscopic signs studied in the geriatric voice mostly have been concerned with glottal closure configuration (Biever & Bless, 1988; Biever et al., 1989; Linville, 1992; Södersten & Lindestad, 1990). Most young men show complete closure of the vocal folds during the closed phase of the vocal fold vibratory cycle (1992). Geriatric men appear to show a greater incidence of incomplete vocal fold closure (Honjo et al., 1980), but the data are based on a small number of subjects. In the female voice, Biever and Bless (1989) reported that 90% of their 20 geriatric subjects exhibited some kind of glottal gap. However, 80% of their group of 20 young men also exhibited some form of a glottal gap. Most of the young women with glottal gaps had a posterior chink, whereas the older subjects had mid-membranous or anterior gaps in addition to a posterior chink. Linville (1992) also reported a high incidence of glottal gaps in her sample of 10 patients (79%). Most common was an anterior chink (27%), but she also noted configurations such as posterior chink (13%), spindle (11%), and incomplete closure (5%). Linville also reported that 86% of her group of 10 young subjects had some form of a glottal gap. The presence of a glottal gap, at least in women, appears not to be a significant feature of aging. However, the precise form of the gap may help to differentiate the elderly from the young, at least in women.

Other stroboscopic features studied in older individuals include mucosal wave, amplitude of vibration, asymmetry, and stiffness. In their study of 20 geriatric females, Biever and Bless (1989) reported that 85% showed aperiodicity of vocal fold vibration, 45% to 55% had some mucosal wave changes on either vocal fold, 50% to 55% showed decreased amplitude of vibration for either vocal fold, and between 5% and 10% of the patients showed some apparent increase of stiffness of either vocal fold. Their young female subjects showed much smaller percentages of these signs. Thus, aging may result in physical changes that produce changes in the vibratory characteristics of the vocal folds.

PATHOPHYSIOLOGY OF THE GERIATRIC VOICE

Aging affects the structures of the larynx in varied ways and at varied times during the aging process (Tables 7.2 and 7.3). Although there is a general trend toward age-related decline of function in many body systems, the decline may be ameliorated or exacerbated by other factors such as lifestyle, diet, and amount of physical activity. Similar comments may be said about the voice itself. Singers who continue singing as they age can produce wonderful tones well into their 70s and, in rarer cases, even into their 80s. Concomitant with increased age is the likelihood that an individual will contract some kind of disease or suffer some kind of accident. Herrington-Hall

Table 7.3. Summary of Social and Interpersonal Communication Changes Due to Aging

Psychosocial Change	Male	Female
Hearing loss	X	X
Social Isolation	X	X
Reduced Communication	X	X
Depression	X	X

From Casper and Colton, 2001.

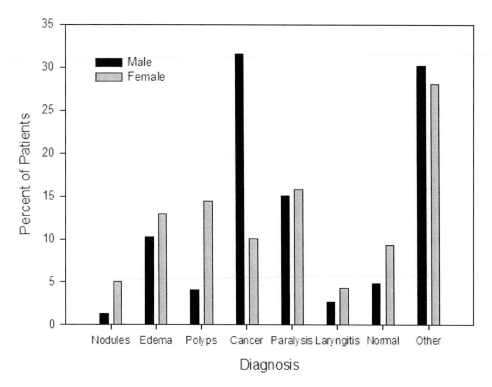

Figure 7.3. Prevalence of voice problems in geriatric patients. Data are from Herrington-Hall, B. L., Lee, L., Stemple, J. C., Niemi, K. R., & McHone, M. M. (1988). Description of laryngeal pathologies by age, sex, and occupation in a treatment-seeking sample. *Journal of Speech and Hearing Disorders, 53,* 57–64.

et al. (1988) reported the prevalence of voice problems in their sample of 285 subjects aged 65 years and older (Fig. 7.3). Of the men in their sample, some type of cancer affecting the voice constituted the largest group, followed by those with paralysis and then edema. The female patients tended to present with paralysis followed by polyps and then nodules. Cancer was present much more often in men (approximately 32%) than in women (approximately 10%).

In our clinic, most geriatric patients with a voice disorder have had a physical or neurological problem associated with their voice disorder (1992). The most common diagnosis among our group of 151 geriatric patients was vocal fold paralysis followed by cancer (see Fig. 7.3). Voice disorders thought to be caused by the aging process itself accounted for only approximately 4% of the patients. Many progressively deteriorating neurological conditions typically affect people in the 6th to 7th decades of life. Many of these have serious implications for voice production and communication problems.

Thus, aging per se may not result in voice problems. However, geriatric individuals in poor physical condition may experience more communication problems than those of the same age who are in good physical condition. We believe that voice problems that might be attributable to aging can be minimized and improved by proper attention to lifestyle, diet, and physical condition. Exercise is known to maintain or improve heart rate, blood pressure, muscle strength, and bone mass as well as many other bodily functions (Lowenthal, Kirschner, Scarpace, Pollock, & Graves, 1994). Prevention of communication problems in the geriatric population may be the best course of action. Vocal rehabilitation techniques for this population are discussed in Chapter 10.

SUMMARY

The chapter began with a review of the anatomical changes that exist during a child's development and how these characteristics compare with those of adults. Some of the anatomical changes may help to explain some of the physiological characteristics of children's voices. Congenital and acquired conditions that affect the larynx and the voice are presented. Vocal nodules are the most frequently seen vocal pathological conditions in children, but fortunately they tend to resolve with maturation and, if needed, voice therapy designed to reduce the abusive behaviors that may have caused them. The pediatric section concludes with the presentation of a 7-year-old child with a laryngeal web.

The section on the geriatric voice in this chapter begins with a brief discussion of a number of theories on the aging process. No single theory has yet been found to be adequate. Organic problems that may affect the voice of the geriatric population have been reviewed. The cause of these problems is not typically related to voice misuse but rather to illness. The effects of these problems can drastically alter voice production. A variety of medical and surgical approaches are available to address these problems (see Chapter 9), and vocal rehabilitation also can be effective.

Universal age-related physical changes in laryngeal structures also affect phonation. The need to distinguish between age-related changes and those attributable to associated disease states is stressed.

Chapter 8

The Voice History, Examination, and Testing

VOICE HISTORY

The clinical skills of the practitioner are critical when working with a patient with a voice problem. The interview with the patient, the search for information, and the elicitation of the history require a combination of art and science. The art is the skill of the clinician with the interview process and in fitting together the various pieces of information. The science is the knowledge base that guides the selection of questions and informs the interpretation of responses. The two are inseparable, and there is a constant interplay between them throughout the interview and the treatment. It is not enough to know what questions to ask, if there is no skill in the asking. It is not enough to know what questions to ask, if there is no understanding of their implications or of why it is important to ask. It is not enough to know what questions to ask, and to have skill in the asking, without adequate knowledge and understanding for interpretation of the responses.

Another way to distinguish between what we have referred to as art and science is to think of them as process and content (Reiser & Schroder, 1980). All communication between people involves a process level. It is at this level of communication that many associations, silent questions, and feelings are expressed by both the patient and the professional through both verbal and nonverbal means. The content level of the interview refers to information specific to the problem.

The Interview Process

Teaching the skill of interviewing and the art of communication with patients is woefully neglected in the training of most speech–language pathologists and physicians. Aronson (1985) states:

> Any in-depth study of voice disorders forces us to conclude that so long as clinicians obtain privileged information from patients; so long as people have voice problems because of life stress and interpersonal conflict; so long as voice disorders produce anxiety, depression, embarrassment and self-consciousness; so long as patients need a sympathetic person with whom they can discuss their distress, will speech pathologists and physicians [author's addition] need to consider their training incomplete until they have learned the basic skills of psychological interviewing and counseling. (p. 271)

Aronson presents further rationale for the need for good interviewing and counseling skills and also discusses the personal characteristics clinicians must bring to the process. Although Aronson targets his discussion on the interaction of the clinician with patients whose voice problems are largely of psychological origin, we believe the concepts are pertinent to interactions with all voice patients.

During the past decade, the field of medicine has shown an increasing awareness of the emotional components of disease processes. Furthermore, it has been recognized that effective treatment of these components occurs when there is a positive relationship between the patient and the health professional (Bernstein & Bernstein, 1985). The initial interview, usually the history-taking session, establishes the patient–clinician relationship. It is the foundation on which the success of treatment may depend (Bernstein & Bernstein, 1985; Hersen & Turner, 1985).

An interpersonal relationship by definition involves the dynamic interaction of at least two people, each of whom brings emotions, expectations, experience, and knowledge to the process. How these two sets of "baggage" match up, or fail to do so, will determine how well the process unfolds. Indeed, some studies have indicated that the breakdown in this relationship may be a major cause of malpractice suits (Blum, 1960; Rosenthal, 1978).

The clinical interview is an interaction of a particular type. Its specific purpose is to explore the nature and history of the patient's presenting symptoms. Unfortunately, it occurs within set time limits and a busy office environment. Despite these limitations, the interaction need not and must not be allowed to become rigid with preset boundaries.

Before we become clinicians, we are people who have been socialized into avoiding certain topics of conversation, not asking overly personal questions of relative strangers, and not probing when a topic appears to make our conversational partner uncomfortable. As clinicians, we must recognize that clinical interviews are different from social conversations. The professional has not only the right but indeed the obligation to ask personal questions and to probe gently when areas require further exploration. A patient's indication of discomfort or avoidance may be a very important sign to the skilled clinician who knows how to probe without shutting off the flow of information. A clinician can only do this successfully by reaching a level of self-comfort in discussing sensitive areas.

WHAT THE PATIENT BRINGS TO THE PROCESS

The patient comes to an evaluation or examination with a heightened sense of anxiety. The patient brings a personal history not only of the current problem but also of previous problems, previous contacts with members of the health professions, relationships, education, social ease, personal needs, and culture. The patient's ethnic background may shape attitudes toward illness and affect interaction with professionals (Bernstein & Bernstein, 1985). The patient also may have need for support and guidance in understanding the current problem. All of these factors will fashion the patient's behavior and responses.

WHAT THE PROFESSIONAL BRINGS TO THE PROCESS

The most obvious contribution of the professional is expertise with a body of knowledge concerned with voice production. The professional also brings a history of encounters with many patients, relationships with peers as well as with family and friends, personal needs, and the pressures of time. In the current climate of frequent litigation, the practitioner also may bring a sense of anxiety or wariness to the process, perhaps generating a defensive posture toward the patient.

Bernstein and Bernstein (1985) identify the following as the responsibilities of the professional in the interview process:

1. Assume responsibility for the conduct of the interview.
2. Avoid control and rigidity that inhibits or intimidates the patient.
3. Keep the interview in focus.
4. Maintain flexibility.
5. Remain sensitive to the patient's feelings expressed both verbally and nonverbally.
6. Do not permit expression of subjective, personal feelings.
7. Remain open and accepting of the patient even when the patient is hostile or uncooperative.

To that list we would add that the professional must be able to speak in language tailored to the individual patient-language that the patient can understand and that is neither insulting to the patient's intelligence nor patronizing in manner.

LISTENING

Although we cannot fully explore all of the crucial aspects of interview skills in a single chapter, the art and skill of listening demands more discussion. A frequent request of beginning clinicians, or of those who have not developed a level of understanding of a particular area sufficient to allow them to be comfortable with it, is for a checklist of questions to ask. Indeed, forms providing such questions are readily available (Boone, 1983; Darley & Spriesterbach, 1978; Wilson, 1987; Wilson & Rice, 1977). They will, however, prove to be of little help to the inadequately trained clinician. For the trained and skilled practitioner, a form is a convenient way to organize the interview, but it is not cast in stone. The value of a form is directly dependent on the skill of the clinician in conducting the interview and extracting the relevant information.

Attentive and sensitive listening on the part of the professional, rather than extensive talking, is the key. Some argue that engaging in note taking during an interview is disruptive to the process of attentive listening. Furthermore, patients may be influenced to focus on specific areas if the clinician's note taking appears to indicate those as areas of importance. Others, however, believe that patients are made to feel confident about the importance of their reporting when they observe the practitioner taking notes. Whichever system a given clinician uses, it is important that the taking of notes be done in such a way as to minimize interference with active and attentive listening.

Listening is more than hearing the spoken words. It involves observation of facial expressions, both as one's questions are heard and during the response. It involves observation of body language. It involves attention to the sound of the voice, the suprasegmentals of stress and inflection and prosody. And it involves hearing messages sometimes hidden behind the words, the well-known "listening with the third ear" (Reik, 1948), and using the sixth sense of feelings or intuitions (Browne & Freeling, 1976). If the clinician is focused on self or the next question to be asked, all of this will be missed. Indeed, much information will never be elicited.

As a component of developing good listening skills, it is necessary to develop a tolerance for moments of silence. The beginning or insecure clinician tends to abhor silence, and the very busy and rushed clinician has no time for it. Moments of reflection, of allowing the patient to provide additional information or sometimes to raise a new point, can be exceedingly valuable. The silence must be a comfortable one, however, in which the clinician must nonverbally project a sense of ease and of understanding.

Listening well need not be a lengthy process. Good listening skills enable the clinician to shape and control the interview. A balance must be maintained between the patient's need to talk and the clinician's need to elicit pertinent information. The clinician learns to pick up the important cues, to follow them while always targeting the problem, to ask directed questions when indicated, and to refocus responses when necessary. Patients will usually provide all the information needed by the professional, if they can be helped to express it in their own way in an environment of understanding and acceptance.

It is difficult to learn the skill of interviewing by reading about it. Our intent here is not to exhaust the topic but rather to raise it and recognize its importance. It is so extremely important when dealing with voice patients because of the very close linkage between voice and personality and emotional states. Readily available resources provide skills training in listening and in interview skills. We would strongly urge that all academic courses in voice disorders incorporate such skills training as part of the curriculum. Suggested readings on interviewing may be found at the end of this chapter.

Before leaving this topic, we must not ignore the use of history questionnaires that can be completed by patients before their appointments. There is some value in the use of such questionnaires because they make it possible for patients to review personal medical records, to validate their impressions against those of other family members or friends, and to think about the issues raised by their answers. However, if questionnaires are taken at face value, they clearly eliminate the immensely important interview process and abort the establishment of a relationship between the patient and the clinician. If such forms are to be used, their contents must be reviewed verbally, allowing the patient to elaborate and clarify, and opening the door for further probing by the clinician.

Content of the Interview: The Case History

THE PROBLEM

After initial introductions and review of identifying and demographic data, it is usually appropriate to begin the interview by asking the nature of the problem that has brought the patient for the examination. Not only is this a natural place to begin the interview, but the patient's response may hold a vast amount of information. The clinician will begin to get an impression of how aware the patient is of the problem, how articulate the person is in providing descriptive information, and what the patient's level of concern or motivation is relative to the problem. These early impressions should be recognized as just that—impressions that need to be verified or altered as the interview progresses. Indeed, what eventually results from the interview and subsequent examination may be quite different from the concerns voiced initially. Nevertheless, having this starting point is important.

Some patients will provide an almost nonstop narrative in response to the very first question, whereas others will have to be prodded and asked many questions. Either type of patient will require that the clinician manage the questioning skillfully so as to obtain all of the important information without being either drowned by trivia or blinded by an absence of response. Asking many open-ended questions, in an attempt to elicit information without putting words into the patient's mouth, is important. For example, the open-ended request, "Tell me about the problem that brought you to see me today," may bring a more complete response than, "I understand you are here because you have a polyp on your vocal folds."

In response to the question concerning the nature of the problem, it is helpful to obtain the patient's description of the sound of his voice and how it differs from other voices or from his own premorbid voice. We have found that patients often are accurate in describing the problem and that their statement of the primary symptom is an important one.

It is instructive to ask what patients believe may have caused the problem or what they have been told about the problem by others they have consulted. Patients frequently indicate a lack of understanding, or perhaps a misunderstanding, of information received from the physician. It is not unusual for a patient to say, "My doctor said I have polyps or something growing in my throat, but I don't know what that means or what it has to do with my being sent to you." Other patients, of course, can quote the dates of office visits, procedures that were done, and their outcome. Despite what they have been told, or in the absence of having been given any information, patients often have their own ideas about the cause of the problem. Frequently heard comments include, "It's this postnasal drip," "It's probably my sinus condition," and "I think I'm allergic." It is important for the clinician to recognize that patients frequently have difficulty giving up such ideas, even when they are unsubstantiated, and that the inability to do so may compromise the treatment program. Therefore, it will be important for these issues to be raised at the appropriate time in the process, and for the patient to be provided with information that is understandable and acceptable. The nature of the clinician–patient relationship established during the initial contact will have an important impact on this subsequent interaction and the patient's acceptance of new ideas.

EFFECT OF THE VOICE PROBLEM

If the patient has not spontaneously commented on the effect of the voice problem on his life, it is important to ask about this as a follow-up question. Once again, this information will help the clinician understand the degree of importance the patient attaches to the problem. Voice problems may exert profound effects on people, including depression, anxiety, withdrawal, embarrassment, and self-consciousness. Indeed, a voice problem may have a profound effect on the individual's total being. On the other hand, for some the voice problem may be a minor embarrassment or have little effect on lifestyle. The severity of this reaction is not always directly proportional to the severity of the voice problem. Equally as important is information as to what effect the problem has had on family members, on work-related activities, and on coworkers or superiors; that is, on all aspects of the person's life. Some patients may express denial of a problem and a lack of personal concern. Such statements must be fully explored before they are accepted as valid. Feelings expressed by the patient in this discussion must be listened to carefully. The clinician must use skill in helping the patient to discuss feelings openly without fear of being judged or humiliated.

DEVELOPMENTAL HISTORY OF THE PROBLEM

Very valuable information may be obtained from this section of the case history. It is important to learn as much as possible not only about the onset of the current episode but also about how it has developed. Information relative to previous episodes of voice difficulty and any prior treatment and outcome must be known. When patients suggest dissatisfaction with the outcome of previous treatment, it is well to inquire whether there is any litigation in progress or in planning. This information may sometimes be obtained in an oblique or indirect manner rather than by a direct, confrontational question. In some instances, patients may have been referred by a lawyer specifically for a second opinion. This knowledge may have little impact on your assessment of the patient, but it is helpful to know it in advance, and it may have some impact on the degree to which the entire interaction is documented.

Onset

The onset of a voice problem may be gradual or precipitous. Why is this a critical piece of information? In understanding the natural history of the development of laryngeal pathological conditions, we know that certain problems will most likely develop over time, whereas others may have a very sudden onset. Although some patients can provide only rather vague information about the onset of the problem, others will provide the date, time, and exactly what they were doing at the very moment that the problem began. Clues to the diagnosis may be contained in each of these types of responses, as well as in the host of responses that lie between these two extremes. Patients frequently date the onset of the symptoms of a problem to another stressful occurrence in their lives. This is a natural tendency that can sometimes be misleading if accepted without full and careful exploration. Another common report is the association of an episode of laryngitis or upper respiratory infection with the onset of the current problem. This event may indeed have some bearing on the problem, but it requires verification.

Most laryngeal lesions develop over time. An exception to that would be the apparently rapid development of a polyp or vocal fold hemorrhage coinciding with a specific episode of excessively strenuous voice use. Patients have reported the sensation of a sudden, sharp pain during shouting or loud, stressful singing, with the subsequent finding of a hemorrhage or hemorrhagic polyp. We know that professional singers may show evidence of beginning nodules immediately after a performance; these usually resolve spontaneously if the voice is allowed to rest in a state of less strenuous use.

Most patients with laryngeal growths that affect the vibratory behavior of the vocal folds (and thus the sound of the voice) report a gradual onset of voice symptoms over a period of weeks, months, or even years. Often they describe early episodes of voice change lasting only brief periods, with return to what they describe as normal voice. The episodes increase in frequency and in duration over time, and the normal voice does not return. By the time they seek medical attention, the problem may have become chronic and may be worsening.

Voice changes that result from vocal misuse, including increased musculoskeletal tension, also tend to run a gradual course even though observable laryngeal pathological conditions may not be present. Indeed, patients may be totally unaware of when or how a problem developed. Small, gradual changes tend not to be noticed, and persons unaware of these minor changes show little or no concern until a more obvious change is noticed by either themselves, a friend, or a family member.

Neurologically based voice problems may have either a sudden or a gradual onset. Progressive deteriorating neurological diseases that affect the voice tend to do so in a gradual manner, whereas the precipitous nature of a stroke or a head injury may have an equally precipitous effect on voice production. Recurrent laryngeal nerve paralysis is not an uncommon result of severing the nerve during thyroid surgery (Johns & Rood, 1987). Obviously, the resulting voice problem will be immediately noted postoperatively. However, the history provided by patients with idiopathic recurrent laryngeal nerve paralysis is not so clear. Some patients report a slight voice change at first, with worsening of the voice symptoms over a relatively short period. Others report a very sudden change that neither worsens nor improves.

The voice of the adolescent male that fails to lower in pitch despite normal laryngeal growth no longer sounds exactly like it did before laryngeal growth, but it usually takes months, or more likely years, for it to be recognized as unusual.

Sudden, marked vocal change that can be pinpointed as to date and time, in the absence of other symptoms suggestive of an organic origin, is often the first clue of a psychogenic dysphonia. Once again, the process of differential diagnosis involves the exploration of all facets of a problem and does not allow for premature conclusions. Clues such as this must be viewed as only one piece of a puzzle, and the clinician must be careful to maintain an open mind so as not to overlook important information that might not fit a preconceived notion.

Duration

When a voice problem has occurred in a sudden manner, its effect on the person is usually more disturbing than a gradual change, and, as a result, consultation may be sought more quickly. Nevertheless, it has been our experience that a period of months has usually elapsed from the onset of the problem to the time the person is referred for a voice evaluation. The pattern usually involves a period of consultation and treatment with the family physician, pediatrician, or other practitioner, followed by referral to an otolaryngologist. Another period of treatment may ensue, and if the problem persists, referral is made to a voice management team, to an otolaryngologist who specializes in laryngeal problems, or to a speech–language pathologist.

As noted previously, many problems have a gradual onset or may have been tolerated at a low level of dysfunction for lengthy periods. Often determining how long a condition has been present is not possible. The germane question, then, is, does it matter? The answer is yes—and maybe. Obviously, if the patient's problem involves a malignant lesion, time is of the essence. The earlier a malignancy is identified, the more positive the prognosis and the less traumatic the treatment. Early identification of any organic condition is, of course, a desired goal. Obtaining resolution of a small, soft, new nodule is easier than for one that has become increasingly fibrotic. It is also easier to change damaging habits that have not had a lengthy period to develop. Early identification of certain neurological disease processes may allow early treatment of symptoms, if possible, although such treatment may not change the course of the disease. Early diagnosis and treatment of psychogenic dysphonias may shorten the period during which the patient must be dysfunctional.

The clinician needs to obtain the best estimate possible of the duration of the problem. This information, put into context, will help the clinician plan a treatment protocol.

Variability Versus Consistency

The reporting of the variability or the consistency of a voice problem is very important. It is unlikely, for example, for a person with paralysis of the recurrent laryngeal nerve to report much variability in voice production from hour to hour or day to day. Some minor worsening of symptoms might occur with extensive or strenuous voice usage. (Recognize, however, that return of nerve function and thus return of normal voice may occur in cases of idiopathic paralysis. This would not constitute variability of symptoms so much as a change or improvement of voice.) We would not expect a person with a mass lesion to experience periods of normal voice. Such a patient may report improved voice for periods, but if questioned carefully it will become apparent that improved does not mean a return to normal voice. However, that same patient may experience worsening of symptoms associated with voice use. Another caution here is that patients who have experienced months or years of disordered or changed voice may no longer have a very clear auditory memory of how they used to sound, nor be sensitive to minor variability.

Variability in voice production can be understood in the light of certain neurological disorders. For example, patients with myasthenia gravis may experience periods of entirely normal voice production but will report a gradual worsening of voice with prolonged speaking and increased fatigue. Patients with voice disorders of psychological origin frequently report much variability in voice production. This variability, usually unpredictable, may occur throughout the day, from day to day, or for other intervals.

Some patients report that their voices are at their worst in the morning, for the first hour or two after arising. Such report should raise the suspicion of gastroesophageal reflux disease. Such reflux frequently occurs while the person is sleeping in the prone position, allowing acidic stomach contents to actually wash up over the posterior laryngeal areas, including the arytenoids.

Variability of voice production may be situation related, use related, or related to general physical well-being. Voice-disordered patients frequently report a worsening of vocal function when under stress and when physically fatigued. Both of those states have a tendency to exacerbate any existing condition, but the clinician must not assume psychological causation based on such reports. When patients report variability in symptoms, they should routinely be asked to describe those things that seem to make the problem better and those that make it worse.

Once again, to understand the implications of information received, the clinician's knowledge base must include awareness of the ways in which phonation can be affected by pathological conditions and use factors.

Associated Symptoms and Sensations

Always ask patients about any other symptoms they may have experienced that they associate with the voice problem. These may include difficulty in swallowing, slurring of speech, loss of fluids through the nose, weight loss, excessive coughing, increased fatigue, heartburn, and the like. In addition, inquiring about sensations in the neck, throat, and larynx, either accompanying phonation or at other times, is important. Patients with patterns of increased musculoskeletal tension frequently report the sensation of pain localized lateral to the larynx and a feeling of fatigue. A patient may say, "I just feel my throat is too tired to talk." Some patients with mass lesions or laryngeal irritation report the sensation of a constant lump in the throat and a need to strain to produce voice loud enough to be heard. A feeling of dryness in the mouth and throat is often reported. Reporting of many other sensations may be provided by the patient. Such reports may be helpful not only in the diagnostic process but also as useful indicators of change in response to treatment.

Patient History

VOICE USE

Exploration of how much a person talks and of where and how the voice is used constitutes a crucial part of the total history. An individual's job and lifestyle may not give indication of excessive or damaging voice use until it is discovered that she is or was a cheerleader, or he is the soloist in a church choir, or she performs with an amateur theater group.

There are specific concerns relative to voice use and, indeed, the entire voice history, if the patient is a professional voice user, a person whose profession is dependent on use of a "good" voice (e.g., a singer, actor, teacher, lawyer, minister, or public speaker). Of major importance is whether the person has had professional voice training. It has been our experience that among the most difficult patients to treat are singers who have had no vocal training but who have had a few years of success in singing with a small group or choir, or in amateur theatrical productions. They have not recognized their traumatic vocal behavior, which now has "caught up with them," often resulting in laryngeal tissue changes. It is difficult for these patients to understand or accept that what they have been doing constitutes the problem.

Vocal performers work in a variety of settings and environments and engage in many styles of performance. Some must sing above the sound of amplified music, and others perform in large areas without adequate amplification; some use a belting style, some sing rock, some perform in smoke-filled rooms, and some may be performing at night after rehearsing all day. The vocal demands of actors' scripts vary from job to job. All of these factors must be explored. Not to be forgotten, however, are the nonperformance vocal demands and voice habits of professional voice users. Well-trained performers who have learned their art may use their voices well when singing or on stage but show little transfer of those habits to everyday speaking behavior. In addition, professional voice users are not immune to phonotrauma when engaging in noisy post-performance parties, loud talking backstage, teaching, and during other strenuous uses of the speaking voice. Sataloff (1981, 1986, 1987a, 1987b) presents a thorough discussion of the voice history to be used with professional singers, as well as samples of case history forms.

As noted earlier, any individual whose livelihood depends on the use of voice can be considered a professional voice user. Lawyers who must effectively argue cases before juries present with their own particular sets of phonatory demands and issues. These must be explored along with the individual's total patterns of voice use in and outside of a court room. Clergy often present unique problems because of the constant demands on voice use—preaching, teaching, community meetings, person-to-person interactions—and all to be done without the benefit of voice training. The individual's preaching style must be explored thoroughly by reviewing recordings of actual preaching or obtaining a truly representative sample. The vocal demands placed on teachers are often heavy and compounded by lunchroom and recess duty, extracurricular activities, parent–teacher meetings, dusty environment (from chalk) with poor ventilation, difficult room acoustics, and the added demands on voice outside of school. All of these factors must be thoroughly explored during the initial information-gathering session.

Children constitute another group for whom the voice use history must be carefully investigated. Some children may use their voices at appropriate levels and in acceptable ways much of the time, but the voice of the playground may be excessively loud, or making "weird sounds" may be a hobby. There are, of course, children who use their voices loudly and aggressively much of the time.

The voice and the manner of voice usage demonstrated in the office situation during the initial visit may not be an accurate reflection of potentially damaging voice use on the job, at the playground, or in the home. Explore all of these areas thoroughly during the interview and perhaps pursue them further during the voice evaluation.

HEALTH

Because the voice is such an integral part of the whole person, it serves to reflect not only emotional states and personality but also physical states. We recognize the weak voice of the very ill, the lifeless voice of the pharmacologically subdued, or the tired voice of the physically exhausted. It has been said that the whole person "is considered to be greater than the sum of its parts; each part can only be understood in the context of the whole; a change in any one part will affect every other part" (Papp, 1983). For these reasons the voice history must explore a patient's health history. The vital importance of the proper functioning of all body systems for the professional singer has been described by Sataloff (1981, 1986, 1987a, 1987b), who provides as one example the effect a broken leg may have in altering the singer's posture, thereby affecting abdominal support for singing.

Inquiring first about the patient's present health status is most appropriate. We are most interested in whether the patient has any neurological problems, respiratory problems, problems affecting the gastrointestinal tract, allergy-related problems, or psychiatric problems; suffers from any chronic conditions such as arthritis; has any congenital anomalies or hearing loss; or has any other current health problem. The past health history, which may be relevant to the present vocal difficulty, is also important, as is the patient's history of surgeries and hospitalizations. It is important to know the nature of surgical procedures that the patient has undergone, particularly those that may have some connection to the present difficulty, such as laryngeal, head and neck, thoracic, or cardiac surgery. For example, a history of appendectomy at 4 years of age may not be pertinent in the case of a 35-year-old patient. However, the history of cardiac surgery in that same patient should be explored to determine whether any sequelae of that surgery were directly related in time to the onset of the voice problem. What kind of sequelae may accompany such surgery? The most obvious might be hoarseness after intubation. However, recalling the course of the left recurrent laryngeal nerve, injury to that nerve also might be a possible sequela of cardiac surgery.

When exploring the surgical and hospitalization histories of a patient, learning either from the patient or from medical records whether the patient was intubated and, if so, whether it was a difficult or traumatic intubation, the duration of the intubation, and whether there is a time relationship between the procedure and the present voice problem, is important.

Another related area to be explored is whether the patient has experienced any trauma, the effects of which might have an impact on the structure of the larynx or the mucosa. Some possible categories of such trauma would be blows to the neck, knife or gun wounds, automobile or other vehicular accidents, chemical ingestion or inhalation, and body burns or smoke inhalation.

A thorough history of substance use is important and takes some skill to elicit truthfully and completely. Substance abuse, that is, excessive use of alcohol or illegal drugs, is often not readily admitted. Questions about these areas must be asked in the same manner as inquiries into all other areas. The clinician must, however, be prepared to pursue vague responses or to probe further if there is reason to believe that the patient may be withholding information. It is often necessary for patients to be reassured about the confidential nature of the interaction. But patients do not seem to be reticent in divulging a history of tobacco use even when it is quite excessive.

There is widespread use of over-the-counter and prescription drugs in the treatment of illness or various physical discomforts. Because drugs work systemically, they often have an effect on all mucosa or tissues, not just that being targeted. For example, diuretics are used in many conditions in which release of fluids from body tissues is desired. However, recognize that the laryngeal mucosa is not exempt from the diuretic action. Whereas release of excess body fluid may be very helpful to a person with certain medical conditions, the associated drying of laryngeal mucosa may have a negative effect on phonation.

Because the effect of various drugs on the laryngeal mucosa and laryngeal motor control is such an important yet relatively unreported area, additional information on it was presented in Chapter 4.

VOCATIONAL

It is not sufficient to simply obtain a person's occupation. It is necessary to discuss the nature of the work done, the environment in which it is done, the need for an adequate voice to carry out the job requirements, interactions with coworkers and superiors, and the level of job satisfaction. In this area, as well as throughout the history taking, open-ended questions such as "Tell me about your job and the people with whom you work" may elicit more complete information than closed questions such as "Do you need to talk as part of your work?"

SOCIAL

The focus of questioning in this area is designed to obtain information about the patient's lifestyle, family constellation, and even living arrangements. Environmental factors such as lack of adequate humidification or the use of a wood stove may have adverse effects on laryngeal tissues. People often do not recognize vocally abusive behavior that may occur in the home when yelling to the children or pets who are out in a large backyard or upstairs in another part of a house. Perhaps a hard-of-hearing person is a member of the family, requiring louder than usual voice usage. Home life is replete with examples of the need to raise the intensity level of the voice: talking above the television or music, talking above the level of others' speech to gain their attention, arguments. If the lifestyle includes much entertaining of large groups or frequenting of bars where extremely loud music is a constant background noise, phonotrauma may well be involved in the voice problem. Relationships with family members or "significant others" may be a source of stress or anxiety, which may be reflected in a problem with the voice.

RECREATIONAL

Certain recreational activities may have implications for the voice. For example, the weightlifter who strains mightily while lifting, simultaneously producing harsh, grunting phonation, is placing considerable stress on the laryngeal tissues; so, too, the golfer or tennis player who phonates with each swing of the club or racket. Forceful phonation accompanying strenuous exercise of any type may constitute abusive behavior.

PSYCHOLOGICAL

Placing this information at the end of this section should not suggest that it has the least importance. Indeed, psychological factors may be of utmost etiological importance. Furthermore, as stated previously, all disease processes carry components of emotional stress.

Throughout this chapter, and elsewhere in this book, frequent reference is made to the close link between voice and personality, voice and self-identity, voice and emotions.

After our physical appearance, it is the voice that sets us apart from others and serves to identify us to others. It reports about our physical condition as well as our emotional state and well-being. How often during a phone conversation have you commented to a friend that she sounds tired or depressed or, perhaps, really happy? Because of this close linkage, the voice also may be the primary reflector of inner turmoil. The importance of recognizing stress-related voice usage and the need to explore the patient's social interactions and interpersonal relationships cannot be overstated. The skilled clinician will be alert to indications, both verbal and nonverbal, of psychological stress factors. A patient's history of previous or current involvement in counseling or psychotherapy is valuable information.

EXAMINATION OF THE VOICE

Examination of the larynx and testing of its performance can be carried out through a variety of techniques. It is our bias that no one or two procedures are enough to provide the best and most complete information about a person's vocal functioning. Furthermore, each procedure adds to our understanding of normal voice production and of the deviations that alter the normal state. We are well aware that many assessment techniques are not immediately available to many speech–language pathologists or voice coaches, nor to all practicing otolaryngologists (Feder, 1986). However, within the past decade an explosion of interest in the voice and a concomitant development of voice laboratories has occurred. These laboratories often can provide testing, examination, and diagnosis by an interdisciplinary team of voice specialists. Full information is therefore highly likely to be obtainable from sources within the community or in close geographic proximity, if it is sought. Making diagnoses of voice disorders without adequate data is no longer acceptable. Claiming lack of immediate availability of equipment is akin to a physician failing to obtain an x-ray because he does not own radiology equipment.

Examination Procedures

Many procedures can be used to examine the larynx and vocal folds. Some involve direct visualization of the vocal folds, whereas others record some of the aerodynamic, vibratory, or acoustic events in the larynx. Direct examination of the larynx usually requires the insertion of a device to transmit light to the folds and receive the image back. This involves invasion of the airway of the patient with potential risks to both the patient and the examiner. Anyone who examines patients must be aware of the potential risk of infection or injury and follow universal precautions during the examination. Gloves should be worn by the examiner when manipulating any part of the patient's anatomy, particularly those areas where the examiner could come into contact with body fluids such as saliva, blood or blood products, or other fluids. Any instrument that is inserted into the patient's oral cavity or nasal cavity should be properly cleaned and disinfected after use. If the instrument touches any blood product, it must be sterilized.

Oral or nasal endoscopes used for continuous or stroboscopic light examinations need to be disinfected (Rutala, Clontz, Weber, & Hoffmann, 1991). A solution of glutaraldehyde such as found in Cidex is often used to disinfect endoscopes. This solution will not harm the components of the endoscope (unless allowed to soak for very long periods) and can be effective in eliminating most bacteria and viruses. Read and follow the directions on the product to determine the effective concentration and length of time the endoscope should be immersed. Being knowledgeable about guidelines for infection control that may be in use within your employment setting is essential. Private practitioners should also have such guidelines in place and insure adherence to them by all employees.

Face masks are often used to collect information about the airflows during speech. Although these do not usually come into contact with blood or even mucus, they should be disinfected. Although glutaraldehyde solutions could be used, we are not certain about their effects on the individual components of face masks, especially the rubber seals that surround the circumference of the mask. We routinely use a diluted solution of common household bleach to disinfect all parts of our face masks. A 25:1 dilution is recommended (Rutala, 1990) and should be effective for about 30 days. However, because bleach is so inexpensive, we mix fresh solutions every week or so. Thoroughly clean all parts of the mask with a water/soap solution (Hibiclens, Stuart Pharmaceuticals, Wilmington, DE) to remove any foreign matter on the mask. Immerse the mask and its parts for at least 20 minutes in the bleach solution. Rinse off and allow to dry before use. (For more information on disinfecting face masks, see Colton, 1994.) If spirometry is routinely used in your clinic, you should be aware of the potential risks of transmission of airborne pathogens via the instruments used (Rutala, Rutala, Weber, & Thomann, 1991).

INDIRECT LARYNGOSCOPY

Indirect laryngoscopy is the traditional means of examining the larynx by using a laryngeal mirror. This technique requires that the tongue be pulled forward as the mirror is introduced into the oropharynx and positioned in such a way as to reflect the image of the vocal folds. Pulling the tongue forward has the effect of moving the epiglottis forward, thereby allowing visualization of the laryngeal structures. The patient is then asked to produce a high-pitched /ee/ sound. The choice of the /ee/ vowel enhances visualization of the larynx during phonation because its production is usually characterized by superior and anterior movement of the dorsum of the tongue and the epiglottis. The reasons for the use of a high pitch are (a) the vocal folds are expected to lengthen in the phonation of a high pitch, and this lengthening maneuver tends to "open" the larynx to view, and (b) there is usually some degree of upward vertical movement of the larynx in the production of a high pitch, which brings the structures closer for viewing.

Indirect laryngoscopy is thought of as a fairly noninvasive procedure because it does not require anesthesia or surgery, nor does it cause any pain or other trauma to the patient. It does, however, have some limitations. Some patients have very active gag reflexes and are unable to tolerate the presence of the mirror deep in the oropharynx. Anatomical variations not infrequently make it difficult to visualize the larynx adequately with the mirror examination. Visualizing the larynx of a young child through indirect laryngoscopy is especially difficult because of the anatomical relationships of the structures, which are different from and smaller than those of the mature adult. Another limitation is the inability of the patient to speak in a normal manner in the position required for this examination, thus limiting the information available relative to laryngeal physiology. Indeed, the unnatural positioning required and the tension created in the patient may actually alter the typical laryngeal behavior of an individual, thereby rendering a less than accurate impression of phonatory behavior.

Despite these limitations, indirect laryngoscopy continues to be a useful means of examining the larynx, especially in conjunction with other visualization techniques.

DIRECT LARYNGOSCOPY

Direct laryngoscopy is perhaps the most invasive of the laryngeal examination proce-dures. It is usually a hospital-based procedure requiring that the person be anesthetized. Direct laryngoscopy permits more detailed examination of laryngeal structures, in-cluding their actual manipulation. It is required when it becomes necessary to obtain a biopsy of a lesion and in attempts to determine the extent of a lesion. Manipulation of the arytenoid cartilages may be helpful in making the distinction between a diagnosis of arytenoid ankylosis versus vocal fold paralysis.

The disadvantages of direct laryngoscopy are its invasive nature, its cost, and the inability to observe laryngeal function. Before the relatively recent explosion of other imaging techniques, direct laryngoscopy was sometimes necessary as the only means to examine the larynx in persons for whom indirect laryngoscopy was unsuccessful.

FLEXIBLE FIBEROPTIC LARYNGOSCOPY

The advent of fiberoptic technology has opened much of the human body to view in ways never before possible. Fiberscopes are used in many branches of medicine as diagnostic tools. A fiberscope, in simple terms, is a bundle of flexible fibers, some carrying light to the object to be examined and others carrying the image back to the viewer. The flexible laryngeal fiberscope was introduced in the late 1960s (Sawashima & Hirose, 1981). To examine the larynx, the fiberscope is passed through the nasal cavity, over the soft palate, and into the oropharynx and the hypopharynx, as shown diagram-matically in Figure 8.1. Its moveable lens tip can be angled (the degree depending on the particular instrument), and the fiber bundle can be rotated to view the full larynx. The tip of the scope is usually positioned vertically, slightly above the epiglottis, but it can be moved closer to the vocal folds for more detailed visualization. One of the

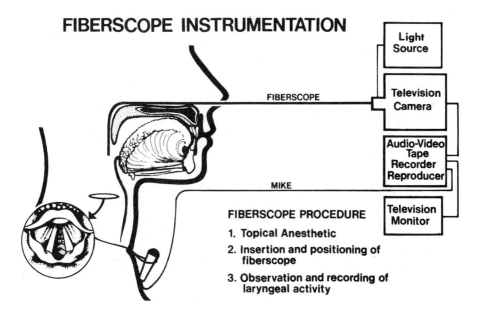

Figure 8.1. Schematic of instrumentation used in a fiberoptic examination of the larynx. The procedure used during the examination is listed.

benefits of this instrument is the flexibility possible in the positioning of the scope in the vertical dimension so as to allow visualization not only of the larynx but also of supraglottal structures and even of the velopharyngeal mechanism. Within the larynx, it is usually possible to view the anterior commissure, which is difficult to do with a mirror examination. The use of wide angle and zoom lenses also adds to visualization capabilities. The zoom lens allows for a closer look at specific laryngeal structures without discomfort to the patient, and the wide angle lens permits visualization of the entire larynx and supraglottal structures as well (depending on the vertical placement of the scope within the vocal tract). An example of a fiberoptic view of the vocal folds during respiration is seen in Figure 8.2, and Figure 8.3 shows the same larynx during phonation.

This examination method has many advantages. Although it may be characterized as invasive because the scope is introduced into the body, it causes only minimal discomfort as the scope is passed through the narrowest part of the nose. As the diameter of the scope has decreased in size (and will perhaps continue to do so), discomfort to the patient has decreased. The fiberscope can be used to successfully visualize laryngeal structure and function in all but a relatively few patients. It is used with all age groups, including infants, and it allows visualization of the larynx in persons with hyperactive gag reflexes and those in whom the anatomical relationships are only minimally distorted. It is possible to have the instrument coupled to a video camera, thereby allowing for visualization of an enlarged image on a television monitor during the examination and for videotaping the examination for careful subsequent review. The image can be observed simultaneously by a number of people and has been used by some as a feedback tool during therapeutic intervention (Bastian, 1987). Videotaping provides the addition of visual documentation to the traditional verbal description and can make comparison of laryngeal conditions over time, or over a course of treatment, much more reliable. A method for computer-assisted measurement of fiberoptic images has been described by Conture, Cudahy, Caruso, Schwartz, Brewer, and Casper (1981)

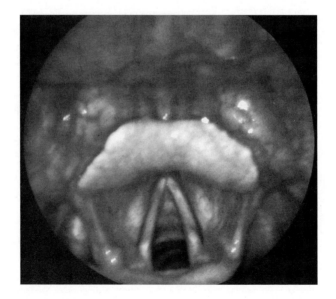

Figure 8.2. A normal larynx during respiration. See color plate.

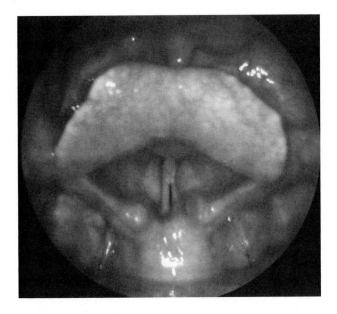

Figure 8.3. A normal larynx during phonation. See color plate.

and was demonstrated to be useful in measuring and documenting actual intrasubject change in laryngeal physiology accompanying the use of therapeutic techniques (Casper, Brewer, & Conture, 1981). Digital acquisition of flexible fiberoptic images now permits the use of digital manipulation and analysis techniques on these images (Colton, Casper, Brewer, & Conture, 1989). Kay Elemetrics (Lincoln Park, NJ) offers a stroboscope that features software to perform measurements of vocal fold amplitude, glottal area, and lesion size. A major advantage of fiberoptic laryngeal examination is that the patient is able to speak, sing, whistle, play a wind instrument, or simply to sit at rest, with minimal interference created by the presence of the fiberscope. This makes observing the patient's phonatory and nonphonatory laryngeal and supraglottal behavior possible. Speech tasks tend to move the scope because of the movements of the soft palate, and occasionally structures in the larynx may displace the instrument. Rarely does the presence of the endoscope result in excessive nasality.

The quality of the fiberoptic examination will be influenced by the quality of the equipment used. Casper, Brewer, and Colton (1987b) cautioned that imaging of laryngeal structures also will be affected by factors inherent in the equipment, such as the wide angle lens distortion effect, particularly at the periphery of the image, and distortions created by the angling of the scope tip. Although these effects are not of sufficient degree to deny the overall effectiveness of the instrument, they must be taken into account when interpreting observed structural or behavioral deviations. Hibi, Bless, Hirano, and Yoshida (1988) have described the distortions as systematic and have suggested a mathematical procedure that corrects for the distortions. In addition to knowledge of the capabilities of the equipment and the skill of the examiner in handling the fiberscope, consider the sample of laryngeal and supralaryngeal behavior elicited from the patient. One of the primary advantages of this technique is that it allows such a diversity of behaviors to be explored. In examining singers who are having difficulty in a particular portion of their range or in some aspect of their singing technique relative to phonatory behavior, watching the larynx and vocal tract as they "perform" is possible. For examination of the voice-disordered patient, a complete protocol of speech and nonspeech activities designed to elicit habitual speech behavior, flexibility of pitch adjustments, adductory nonspeech behavior, resting state, and any other behaviors of interest, must be well thought out. To obtain the best visualization of the larynx during speech, stimulus sentences should be heavily loaded with the /ee/ and /oo/ vowel sounds. Whistling, a nonphonatory activity, frequently provides the opportunity to observe abductory–adductory vocal fold behavior at a slower rate than occurs in speech. A suggested examination protocol can be found in the Appendix. This protocol may serve only as a starting point, after which activities designed to elicit a particular behavior of interest or to attempt to change a laryngeal gesture may be added. The person who performs this aspect of the fiberoptic examination must be skilled in "reading" the image, in understanding the physiology, and in knowing the types of vocal maneuvers that might elicit the desired changes in behavior. That person is frequently the speech–language pathologist skilled in diagnosis of phonatory function, referred to by some as a phonoscopic examination (Leonard, 2001).

One of the limitations of the fiberoptic technique with a continuous light source is that vibratory behavior of the vocal folds cannot be seen. The technique does not alter the speed of movement of the structures beyond what is visible with the human eye. Thus, in a certain sense, fiberoptic examination provides a relatively gross look at phonatory behavior at the vocal fold level. It can be used to assess the valving function of the vocal folds and, of course, to visualize any pathological conditions. It also can be used to assess vibration if it is used in conjunction with a stroboscopic light source (as described below).

Who should perform fiberoptic endoscopy? Naturally, any ENT physician should have the necessary training and experience to perform this procedure and to be able to handle any potential problems that might arise. Speech–language pathologists in increasing numbers are receiving the training necessary to perform these procedures. ASHA has issued guidelines to be followed by speech–language pathologists who are engaged in the use of this and other imaging techniques (American Speech-Language-Hearing Association, 1992). It is incumbent on the practitioner to receive adequate training and gain supervised experience before performing this or any other procedure for the examination of the larynx.

STROBOSCOPY

Stroboscopy is a procedure that has been used to examine the larynx since the late 1800s. It is now the primary technique used to view the behavior of the vocal folds in most clinics, hospitals, and doctors' offices in many European countries, Japan, and the United States. During the past 10 years or so, sophisticated and easy-to-use equipment has become available. Hirano (1981b) states that "stroboscopic examination, as a routine clinical test, is the most practical technique for examination of the vibratory pattern of the vocal folds." Stroboscopy, indeed, permits visualization of vibratory behavior in a way otherwise not possible with the human eye, and in so doing enhances understanding of the physiological basis of voice disorders. Kitzing (1985) further points up the benefits of the stroboscopic technique for early detection of neoplasms and for differential diagnosis of laryngeal paresis and its outcome. Stroboscopy has been helpful in differentiating between functional voice problems and those caused by subtle structural abnormalities of the larynx (Bless & Brandenburg, 1983; Woo, Colton, Casper, & Brewer, 1991).

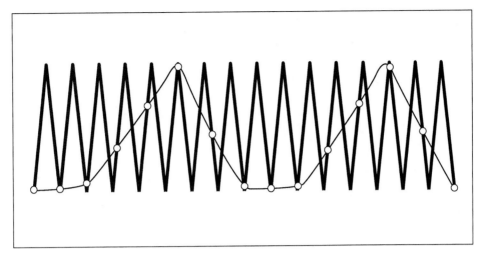

Figure 8.4. Basic principle of stroboscopy. When a rapidly moving object (represented by the high-frequency waveform) is strobed by flashes at a lower frequency (curve with open circles), the rapidly moving object appears to move more slowly.

The stroboscopic light emits rapid pulses at a rate that can be set by the examiner or controlled by the fundamental frequency of the vocalization. If the frequency of the light pulse is the same as the vocal frequency, the resulting image will appear to be static, and the vocal folds will seem to be at a standstill. At a frequency slightly less or greater than the frequency of vocal fold vibration (often between 1 and 2 Hz), the image is, in effect, sampled at different points in the vibratory cycle and over several successive cycles takes on the appearance of slow motion movement of the vocal folds. Each pulse of light illuminates a different point of the vibratory cycle, as schematized in Figure 8.4. These fragmented sections become fused because of the phenomenon of Talbot's law, that is, the persistence of an image on the human retina for 0.2 seconds after exposure.

Thus, stroboscopy differs from ultra-high speed photography in that it creates an optical illusion of slow motion and does not show details of each vibratory cycle, whereas high speed photography captures parts of each vibratory cycle at a very rapid rate, which appears as slow motion when the film is projected at a normal rate of 24 frames per second.

The clearest images are obtained by using a rigid endoscope, a straight tube in which the light-carrying and image-carrying fibers are encased. At the end of the scope is a prism that directs light and receives the image at various angles depending on the specific endoscope in use. Common angles are 90° and 70°. The flexible endoscope also can be used with the stroboscopic unit. Recent developments by some equipment manufacturers have dramatically improved the clarity and brightness of the images obtained with flexible fiberoptic endoscopy.

Another development made by manufacturers is the introduction of digital technology to record and store the stroboscopic images. Digital storage of these recordings allows greater ease of retrieval and side-by-side viewing of two different recordings. Digital recording techniques also allow for greater ease of editing recordings for teaching purposes and the analysis of the recordings using digital image processing techniques.

At the start of the examination with the rigid endoscope, the patient is asked to protrude his or her tongue, which is held by the examiner outside the oral cavity with a gauze pad. The endoscope is then inserted into the mouth until its end is in the pharynx (but not touching the velum or posterior pharyngeal wall, which may cause gagging). The exact position of the endoscope needs to be altered slightly as the examination progresses to bring the vocal folds into view. The technique is not difficult and can be learned rather quickly. Possible dangers are gagging, bruising (if the endoscope is pushed hard against the delicate mucosa) or chipping of the teeth. Practice can increase the skill of the examiner in obtaining good examinations even with wide variations of anatomy and patient cooperation.

It is possible to carry out a stroboscopic examination using a rigid endoscope, a flexible fiberoptic laryngoscope, or both. Kitzing (1985) also describes the use of stroboscopic light in the operating microscope, combining good magnification and "superb optic resolution" while providing stereoscopic evaluation of the mucosal wave.

The method for obtaining stroboscopic images is not difficult. A microphone is placed or held on the patient's neck along the lateral aspect of the thyroid lamina to record the voice signal from which the fundamental frequency is extracted and to control the rate of firing of the stroboscopic light. The rigid or flexible scope is introduced, the stroboscopic light is switched on (usually by a foot pedal), and the patient is asked to sustain phonation of the vowel /ee/. The patient needs to produce a sufficiently long sample to permit the stroboscopic unit to track the phonation and produce reliable stroboscopic light pulses. Because vocal fold vibratory behavior will vary with frequency and loudness, it is important to obtain samples of phonation produced in various ways. The following conditions should be a part of the examination: (a) a minimum of 2 seconds (4 seconds is better) of sustained vowel phonation at the patient's habitual pitch and loudness level; (b) another phonation at a higher pitch; (c) another phonation produced at a pitch lower than the habitual pitch level; (d) production of sound at habitual pitch but at much louder than habitual loudness level; and (e) phonation on inhalation. Often patients will initially produce a vowel higher than their habitual pitch or loudness level. With coaching and practice, they will be able to produce a phonation more typical of their habitual pitch and loudness. Sometimes, additional samples of phonation may be requested such as a string of the vowel /ee/ with intervening silences, or a pitch glide. Samples of speech are not appropriate for stroboscopic examination.

Interpretation of the Stroboscopic Image

The stroboscopic image provides information about the following areas: symmetry of movement of the vocal folds, regularity or periodicity of successive vibrations, glottal closure, amplitude (horizontal excursion) of the vocal folds, presence and adequacy of the mucosal wave, phase closure (open/closed phase), presence of any non-vibrating portions of the vocal folds, and additional observations relative to the presence of lesions and their apparent effect on the vibratory behavior. Although all of these parameters can be systematically rated, most clinicians place considerable importance on glottal closure, the mucosal wave, and the presence of any non-vibrating segments. Observations of the stroboscopic image must be based on a thorough understanding of laryngeal anatomy and physiology, as well as of the changes in the mechanical characteristics of the vocal folds that result from variations in frequency and intensity. Interpretation of the observations requires understanding and knowledge of laryngeal pathological conditions.

Symmetry of Vocal Fold Vibration

The judgment of symmetry refers to the timing of the opening and closing of the folds relative to each other, as well as to the extent of lateral excursion of the folds. If the folds are functioning equally, they are said to be symmetric and are mirror images of each other. When there is phase asymmetry, one fold may appear to move out of phase or the vocal folds may appear to be following one another. It is important to remember that if one fold is abducting, the other fold should be abducting also. Furthermore, to be symmetrical in movement, they should be abducting at about the same speed.

Aperiodicity

As noted previously, when the stroboscopic light flashes are synchronous with the fundamental frequency, the image appears to be static. Under this synchronous condition, any visible movement is evidence of irregularity of successive vocal fold vibratory cycles, or aperiodicity. Aperiodicity may be present always or the vibration of the folds may be intermittently irregular, in which case the image appears static part of the time, moving at other times. It is not necessary to stop the stroboscopic light at a specific part of the cycle to judge aperiodicity. The judgment can be made from the typical stroboscopic image by using the slow motion feature of the playback and observing the clarity of the image. If the image is clear, the vocal folds are reasonably periodic; if the image is fuzzy or unclear, even momentarily, the frequency of phonation is more variable. Hoarseness is usually associated with periodicity of vibratory behavior. When aperiodicity is constantly present, it may not be possible to obtain a stroboscopic image or, if obtained, it would be difficult to interpret the images obtained.

Glottal Closure Configuration

Judgments about glottal closure (the extent to which the vocal folds approximate each other) and glottal configuration during the closed phase are made during observation of phonations of normal pitch and intensity level, that is, at the patient's normal or comfortable pitch level. Bless, Hirano, and Feder (1987) have described seven categories of glottal closure that seem to encompass the possible variations (complete, anterior chink, irregular, bowed, posterior chink, hourglass, incomplete). Complete closure occurs when the vocal folds close completely during each vibratory cycle. Anterior chink or gap is a noticeable opening in the anterior portion of the vocal folds. Irregular refers to the appearance of several points of contact with openings in between along the length of the vocal folds. Bowing refers to a pattern in which the folds close anteriorly and posteriorly but not in the midsection. It is possible for one cord to be bowed and the other straight. Posterior chink or gap, as described by Bless et al. (1987), is an opening at the posterior area of the folds. We have observed variations in the size and configuration of this chink. In some it appears as a Y formation with a relatively small gap at the vocal processes. In others, it has the appearance of a V with the opening or chink tapering down as far anteriorly as two thirds of the length of the vocal folds. Hourglass closure pattern looks just like an hourglass, a noticeable narrowing of opening at about the midpoint of the vocal folds. Incomplete closure is when no portion of the vocal folds touches another. Although the primary judgment of closure is made during the speaking pitch and comfortable loudness condition, it is also advisable to note any changes that occur during the other conditions of voicing, particularly loud voice.

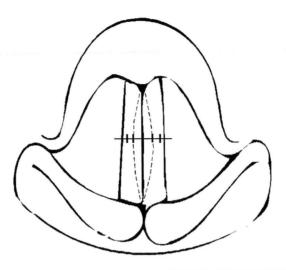

Figure 8.5. Schematic of the larynx to illustrate rating horizontal excursion of the vocal folds. The solid line between the folds illustrates no horizontal movement; the first mark along the dotted line illustrates normal horizontal excursion, and the second mark outside of the dotted line illustrates greater movement.

Horizontal Excursion of the Vocal Folds

Amplitude is defined as the extent of horizontal (lateromedial) excursion of the vocal folds during vibration. Each vocal fold is rated independently for this parameter. The absolute amplitude is contingent on the size of the vocal folds; thus, it tends to be larger for adults. The amplitude of the horizontal excursion is approximately one-third the width of the visible part of the vocal fold in normal subjects (Fig. 8.5). During abnormal vibration, the amplitude of movement may be less than normal or greater than normal. We rate amplitude as normal; slightly, moderately, or severely decreased or increased; or absent. It is important to remember that with increased loudness there will be greater lateral excursion, and with high pitch lateral excursion will be reduced. Therefore, when interpreting stroboscopic examinations, judgments of amplitude should be made during the habitual pitch, habitual loudness condition.

Horizontal Excursion of the Mucosal Wave

The mucosal wave, a ripple-like wave of mucosa, originates in the subglottal area and follows the contour of the vocal fold. In stroboscopy, we see, and thus rate, only the horizontal excursion across the superior surface of the fold. It often appears as a ripple along the surface much like the ripple on the surface of a body of water. Sometimes it can be visually tracked as a light reflection traveling along the upper surface.

Normal refers to the range and size of the mucosal wave for phonation produced at habitual pitch and loudness levels. The extent of the wave varies, but it normally traverses at least a third of the width of the visible part of the vocal fold. If a wave is visible on only part of the fold, the rating should be based on the overall impression of the wave travel.

Vocal Fold Edge

This judgment pertains to the straightness and smoothness of the edge of each vocal fold individually. This is rated on a 4-point scale, where 1 is smooth and 4 is extremely rough. This rating can be affected by the particular point in the cycle chosen for making the judgment. If the tape is advanced frame by frame through a cycle, it is possible to see an edge that appears smooth on full abduction, whereas on partial adduction a lesion may clearly be present. With this understanding, it may be important to routinely make the judgment at a given point in the cycle. This parameter refers to the smoothness of the medial edge and should not be confused with the appearance of a bowed vocal fold, which, despite the convexity of shape, nevertheless has a smooth edge.

Phase Closure

Phase closure refers to the approximate proportion of time the vocal folds are open. On a 5-point scale, 3 refers to normal phase closure with an open phase of approximately 40% to 60% of the total cycle. A rating of 1 refers to a wide open phase, as one might find during a whisper, whereas 5 indicates hyperadduction or a condition in which the closed phase predominates. Phase closure will depend on the loudness, effort, and pitch as well as mode of phonation. It is important that this rating be made on a phonation that is appropriate. Phase closure can be estimated by counting the number of video frames during the open phase and the number for the entire cycle and computing an approximate open quotient. Because there can be much cycle-to-cycle variability, it is well to sample more than a single cycle. Ten to twelve open frames out of a 20-frame cycle is considered normal. Ratings made using this slow motion or stop frame counting procedure may differ from those based on an overall gestalt using regular tape playback speed.

Vibratory Behavior

This is a judgment of whether the entire vocal fold is seen to vibrate. We rate vibratory behavior independently for each fold. It is sometimes difficult to distinguish between mucosal wave and vibratory behavior. Indeed, we probably judge vibratory behavior by the presence of mucosal wave. For a complete rating of all phonatory conditions, a 5-point rating scale can be used; 1 is always fully present, 2 is partial absence sometimes, 3 is partial absence always, 4 is complete absence sometimes, and 5 is complete absence always (totally immobile fold).

Based on our experience with judging stroboscopic images, we are aware of a number of unresolved questions with respect to this process. Among them are the following:

1. What criteria should be used in selecting the sample for judging?
2. Should judgments be made on the overall gestalt without attention to a specific sample?
3. Is it better to use slow motion to rate mucosal wave, amplitude, and phase symmetry, or is viewing at regular speed adequate?
4. How much of the length of the vocal fold must be visible to judge glottal closure, mucosal wave, vibratory behavior, and amplitude?
5. Which of the parameters that we are rating actually make a difference clinically? There is redundancy in the information obtained. What information is most valuable?

Diagnostic Probing During Stroboscopic Examination

The rigid scope limits but does not totally eliminate the use of diagnostic probes. Indeed, such probing may yield the most important information of the examination. Patients can be instructed to vary or manipulate pitch or loudness of the vowel being produced. Producing the vowel /ee/ on inhalation provides interesting information that can be helpful in differentiating among nodules, cysts, polyps, and other benign lesions (Behlau et al., 1999).

ULTRA-HIGH-SPEED PHOTOGRAPHY

This technique was developed by scientists at the Bell Telephone Laboratories in 1937, and since that time many scientists have modified and used the technique to observe vocal fold vibratory events in both normal and pathological larynges (Baer, Löfqvist, & McGarr, 1983a, 1983b; Childers, Naik, Larar, Krishnamurthy, & Moore, 1983; Hirano, Kakita, Kawasaki, Gould, & Lambiase, 1981; Hirano, Yoshida, & Matsushita, 1974; Hirose, Kiritani, & Imagawa, 1991; Metz, Whitehead, & Peterson, 1980; Moore, 1975; Moore, White, & von Leden, 1962; Rubin & LeCover, 1960; Timcke, von Leden, & Moore, 1958, 1959; von Leden, LeCover, Ringel, & Isshiki, 1966; von Leden & Moore, 1961, von Leden, Moore, & Timcke, 1960). Although this technique is capable of providing excellent information about the vibratory behavior of the vocal folds, it has not found widespread acceptance clinically for a number of reasons. It requires an expensive array of equipment, the technical expertise to operate it, and the expenditure of much time both in the examination procedure and in subsequent analysis of the films; it also involves a procedure that is difficult, if not impossible, for many patients.

The primary piece of equipment is a camera capable of taking pictures at a rate of 3,000 frames per second or more. When films taken at these high speeds are viewed at a regular speed of 24 frames per second, the recorded events are seen in ultra-slow motion. The technique for obtaining high-speed films (Hirano, 1981b) requires that the patient be able to position herself onto a fixed laryngeal mirror. The mirror must be positioned in such a way as to permit visualization of the vocal folds. The laryngeal mirror is used in a manner similar to indirect laryngoscopy, with the difference being that the patient must be capable of moving forward onto a fixed mirror rather than the mirror being moved into a stationary patient. An example of a high-speed motion film sequence is shown in Figure 8.6.

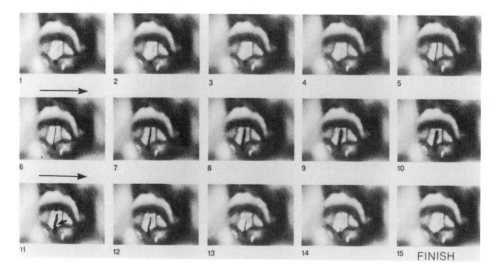

Figure 8.6. Example of a high-speed motion picture sequence. This plate is a single cycle of vibration produced by a female speaker sustaining the vowel /ee/ at about 275 Hz. The film was exposed at a rate of 4,000 frames per second.

Hirose and his colleagues (Hirose, 1988; Hirose, Kiritani, & Imagawa, 1987, 1988, 1991a, 1991b) have described a variant of high-speed photography technique. Instead of recording the high-speed image on film, it is captured using a digital image array that is sampled and stored in the computer. They are able to obtain images at a rate of 1,000 per second and can display the image sequence immediately after capture. Furthermore, because they are dealing with a digital image to start with, they can use digital techniques to track desired aspects of vibration almost in real time. The technological problems discussed previously remain the same for this technique.

The information obtained from high-speed films is glottal area over time. That is, we can determine the amount of opening of the vocal folds during the vibratory cycle. It is also possible to determine the vibratory movement of each vocal fold, as well as the pattern of their opening.

As valuable as the information obtained from high-speed films is to our understanding of the vibratory characteristics of the vocal folds, it does not seem to be a tool appropriate for routine use in the diagnosis and treatment of voice problems.

VIDEOKYMOGRAPHY

Videokymography is a technique for tracking a line from a video image and plotting the intensity gradient of that line as a function of time. In the United States, video is created by sequentially scanning an image very rapidly so that the eye fuses the 525 scanned lines into moving pictures. This scanning process is repeated so that an entire frame is replaced at approximately 1/30th of a second. By selecting only one of these scanned lines and plotting its intensity level as a function of time, one can obtain a trace that shows the variation of intensity as a function of time.

In the case of the vocal folds, the intensity variation may represent the variation of glottal area as a function of time. The technique was first described and developed by Svec and Schutte (Svec & Schutte, 1996; Schutte, Svec, & Sram, 1998). To produce a videokymogram, a video line is selected from a displayed image of the larynx. As the video is played (or phonation occurs live), that line is displayed on the video monitor. A typical picture of the spatial image and the videokymographic image is shown in Figure 8.7.

The videokymograph is a valuable addition to the tools used for image acquisition and analysis. It permits the acquisition of small details as a function of time and furthermore permits the clinician to vary where on the image the desired detailed analysis takes place. With further work and experience, it should become a valuable tool for use in the voice clinic.

ULTRASOUND

Ultrasound is an imaging technique in which a high-frequency current is passed through a portion of the body and partially reflected back when it strikes a change in body composition. Analysis of these reflections can be used to create an image of the part of the body of interest. It is a relatively safe procedure because the currents and frequencies used are low.

Ultrasound has been little used in the analysis of voice function. A few reports concerned with the analysis of normal voice function are available (Hamlet, 1981). Few voice clinics or laboratories possess the costly equipment and have personnel with the expertise to use it properly.

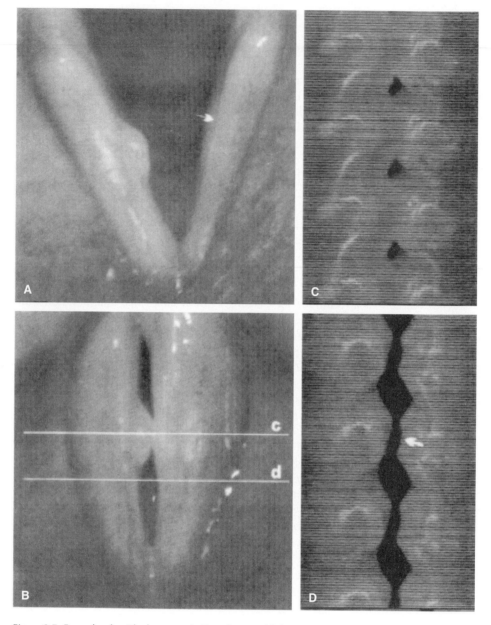

Figure 8.7. Example of a videokymograph. From Svec and Schutte, 1996.

LABORATORY TESTING

Acoustic Studies

FUNDAMENTAL FREQUENCY

Fundamental frequency is an acoustic measure that directly reflects the vibrating rate of the vocal folds. The term "fundamental frequency" refers to the component in the vocal fold tone with the lowest frequency or to the frequency spacing between the component frequencies. The unit of measurement is Hertz (Hz).

Fundamental frequency may be measured in a variety of ways and using any of several types of speech samples. The phonatory tasks may include sustained vowel phonation, reading, and conversational speech. The simplest of these is the sustained vowel phonation, in which the patient is instructed to produce and sustain a vowel (most commonly /ah/ or /ee/) at a comfortable, natural pitch and loudness level. The advantages of using a sustained vowel are that it can usually be sustained in a steady manner and for an adequate period. The uncomplicated nature of the task makes it possible to obtain accurate measures with relatively simple and inexpensive equipment. The use of a reading passage or conversational speech as the phonatory task will usually introduce greater variability of fundamental frequency, thereby making extraction of fundamental frequency a slightly more complex procedure or one that requires more expensive instrumentation. There is not full agreement as to whether the speech sample used has a significant influence on the actual measured fundamental frequency (Hirano, 1981b).

A variety of methods are available for the measurement of fundamental frequency, ranging from the very simple to the complex and elaborate. Subjective judgments can be made through a matching procedure, but such judgments often are incorrect. Indeed, subjective perception of fundamental frequency, particularly in persons with disordered voice, may be misleading (Murry, 1978). Objective measurement of fundamental frequency from sustained vowel production can be carried out very simply with the aid of a frequency counter and a low-pass filter (available for less than $500). Without the filter, the frequency counter would attempt to count the many frequencies that a vowel contains. A low-pass filter, when appropriately set, will remove the higher components of the laryngeal tone, leaving only the fundamental frequency. The output of this equipment provides objective documentation that can be used to demonstrate and chart change.

A commercially available and easy-to-use pitch meter or analyzer is available (Visi-Pitch, Kay Elemetrics Corp., Lincoln Park, NJ). A sustained vowel or a speaking or reading sample using the patient's live voice or a recorded segment is fed into the instrument, and the fundamental frequency as a function of time is displayed on the screen. It is possible to control the total time to be displayed and thus to obtain a detailed fundamental frequency trace for short periods, or a less detailed trace of fundamental frequency over longer periods. This instrument can provide measures of other voice and speech parameters as well.

Computer programs, such as Computerized Speech Lab (CSL, Kay Elemetrics Corp.), CSpeech (a Windows version of this program called TF32 is also available), EZ Voice, and Dr. Speech (Tiger Electronics), that run on IBM or IBM-compatible computers extract fundamental frequency from sustained vowels or longer speech samples. A very good freeware program that can extract fundamental frequency, Praat, is also available. For the Macintosh computer, SoundScope can be used. These programs can perform many more measurements than simple frequency measurements and are relatively simple to use. An example of a fundamental frequency analysis using the Praat program is presented in Figure 8.8.

Three summary statistics of frequency data that are useful for comparing patients with normal speakers or with themselves over a course of treatment are mean fundamental frequency, the standard deviation of fundamental frequency (pitch sigma),

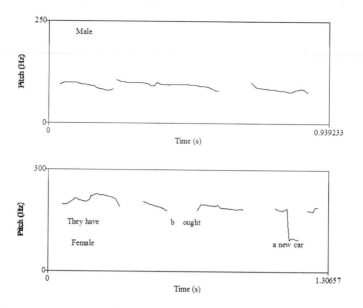

Figure 8.8. Fundamental frequency during the production of a sentence produced by a normal male speaker. The sentence was "They have bought a new car." The average fundamental frequency of the sentence was 120.45 Hz, with a standard deviation of 12.28 Hz. The minimum fundamental frequency was 81.79 Hz; the maximum, 153.32 Hz. Total time of the sentence was 1.3 seconds. Analysis was made using Praat.

and frequency range. Clinically, these measures are helpful diagnostically and as documentation of pre- and post-treatment status. Mean fundamental frequency is useful to estimate the appropriateness of frequency level for the patient's age and sex. The other two statistics help to assess and document variation of fundamental frequency during speech or lack thereof. Speakers who are judged to be monotonic would be expected to have small standard deviations and small ranges of speaking fundamental frequency.

PHONATIONAL RANGE

Another useful measure of the frequency characteristics of a patient's voice is phonational range, that range of frequencies from the highest to the lowest that a patient can produce. The highest and lowest frequencies are defined as the absolute limits of frequency that a patient can produce, usually of short duration (approximately 1 second), without regard to intensity level or voice quality. Phonational range is said to reflect the physiological limits of the patient's voice. It is expressed in either Hertz or semitones and can be measured by using any of the instrumentation discussed in the preceding section and also by using the phonetogram.

The absolute limits of frequency may be obtained by asking subjects to produce the highest and then the lowest sounds they can, or by using a singing scale progressing upward and downward in a stepwise fashion. Whichever technique is used, it is usually necessary to practice this task, encouraging the person to keep extending the range in both directions. The lowest and highest frequencies produced can be plotted, as shown in Figure 8.9. Kent, Kent, and Rosenbek (1987) have noted that intra- and intersubject variability on maximum performance tasks is large and may be affected by practice, motivation, or instructions. These caveats hold true for measurement of phonational range.

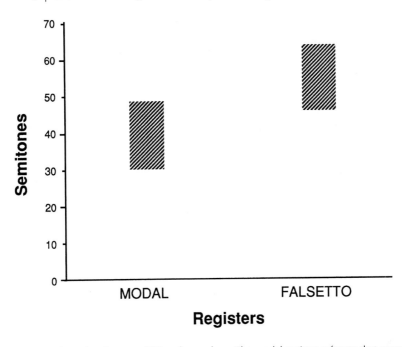

Figure 8.9. Mean phonational range of 35 male speakers. The modal register refers to that range of frequencies used most often during speech. Falsetto is a voice quality usually produced at high fundamental frequencies.

Voice Range Profile (Phonetogram)

The voice range profile is an extension of the idea behind phonational and dynamic range. A patient phonates at frequencies from the lowest to the highest frequency he or she can produce. At each frequency, the patient produces his or her loudest and softest phonation. These extremes are plotted on a graph that is often referred to as a phonetogram. The task is very laborious and time consuming, although software programs exist to reduce the time and labor needed (see the Kay Voice Range Profile program or the Dr. Speech Phonetogram program). An example of a phonetogram is shown in Figure 8.10.

The voice range profile has been investigated in a number of different populations and has been shown to yield useful information (Coleman,1993; Damste, 1970; Giger, 1984; Gramming, 1988; Gramming & Akerland, 1988; Heylen, Wuyts, Mertens, & Pattyn, 1996; Pabon, 1991). However, we believe that the time and effort involved in its generation may be too great for routine clinical use.

VOCAL INTENSITY

Measurement of vocal intensity is useful in documenting the dynamics of the voice. Mean intensity correlates with the perception of vocal loudness, and the variability of intensity would presumably correlate with a patient's loudness variations.

Clinically, the mean intensity level of a patient's voice is usually a more meaningful measure than the absolute limits of intensity. However, the intensity range, frequently referred to as dynamic range, may be diagnostically important and helpful in documenting change. Patients whose mean intensity level is lower than expected for age

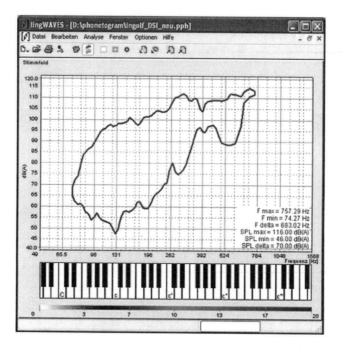

Figure 8.10. An example of a phonetogram.

(see Chapter 14 for some normative data on vocal intensity) and whose vocal intensity range is markedly reduced need very careful and complete examination, including, of course, audiological assessment. The procedure for establishing intensity or dynamic range requires that the person produce the very softest /ah/ possible and, at the other extreme, the very loudest /ah/. Patients should be asked to produce both of these sounds at a natural and comfortable frequency because frequency level will have an influence on intensity level (Coleman, Mabis, & Hinson, 1977; Colton, 1973). An example of plotting the highest and lowest sustainable intensity is shown in Figure 8.11.

Intensity can be measured from sustained vowels or connected speech. A simple intensity measurement device can be found on most tape recorders (e.g., the VU volume unit meter). However, this provides a very rough measure because these meters usually lack calibration in traditional intensity units (dB sound pressure level). A sound level meter that is so calibrated can be purchased at reasonable cost (Radio Shack). A digital version is also available at slightly higher cost. The patient is asked to sustain a vowel at a normal loudness level with the microphone of the sound level meter held at a given distance from the mouth, and the intensity of the phonation in decibels is read from the meter. This device is of little use, however, for measurement of vocal intensity during connected speech.

The Visi-Pitch can be used to measure and to visually display vocal intensity during connected speech. CSL, CSpeech, EZ Voice, Dr. Speech, and Praat will display the intensity of speech production over time. It is also possible to obtain summary statistics such as average intensity level and standard deviation from these instruments and programs. The microphone used must be capable of responding to all of the frequencies present in the tone whose intensity is to be measured. All sound level meters have microphones that can respond to those frequencies expected in the speech signal, as does the Visi-Pitch. In computer programs, the sampling rate of the speech signal

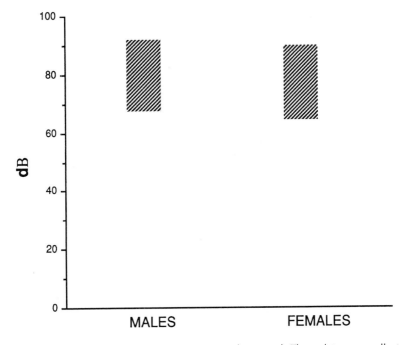

Figure 8.11. Example of intensity range measurement and portrayal. These data were collected on a sample of 35 older males (mean age, 56.17 years) and 27 females (mean age, 57.48 years) while they were phonating the vowel /ah/ at 40% of their modal register frequency range.

determines the frequencies present in the waveform and should be high enough to accurately reproduce frequencies of at least 5000 Hz (i.e., a sampling rate of 10,000 samples per second).

Another consideration when measuring vocal intensity is the distance between the speaker's lips and the microphone. The actual distance is not as important as that it be documented and consistent. Remember, sound intensity will be reduced by the square of the distance. That means a doubling of the distance will produce an intensity difference of 6 dB. The noise level of the room in which phonation is measured also must be taken into account. It is not necessary to have a sound-isolated room, although that would be ideal. It is important to have a reasonably quiet room and to know its noise characteristics. Most rooms will have a considerable amount of ambient noise below 60 Hz. Because most speech exhibits frequencies above 100 Hz, the use of a simple high-pass filter will attenuate the energy below 100 Hz and permit valid measurements to be made. Many sound level meters possess a weighting function that, in effect, carries out this filtering process. The presence of heavy drapes and floor carpeting helps to reduce noise and yield usable recordings.

Once again, it must be noted that the variability of maximum performance measures may be large. Thus, caution must be used in the interpretation of measures obtained.

PERTURBATION

Perturbation refers to the small, rapid, cycle-to-cycle changes of period and amplitude that occur during phonation. These changes reflect the slight differences of mass, tension, and biomechanical characteristics of the vocal folds, as well as the slight variations in their neural control (Baer, 1979). Perturbation correlates with perceived roughness or hoarseness in the voice (Wendahl, 1963, 1966), so that patients with voice problems

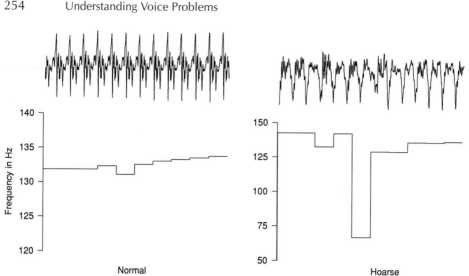

Figure 8.12. Example of frequency and amplitude perturbation in a sustained vowel produced by a normal (left panel) and a hoarse voice (right panel). These waveforms were produced using CSpeech.

manifesting roughness or hoarseness would be expected to show a large amount of both frequency and amplitude perturbation.

Perturbation must be measured from sustained vowel phonations in which the subject is instructed to produce a steady pitch level. Connected speech confounds the measure because linguistically produced frequency variations cannot be separated from frequency variations produced by the biomechanical characteristics of the vocal folds.

An example of frequency perturbation within a sustained vowel /ah/ is shown in Figure 8.12. In the left panel an example of normal, sustained phonation is shown. The acoustic waveform is shown in the upper portion of this panel, and the results of a CSpeech analysis of fundamental frequency is shown in the lower portion of the panel. The average fundamental frequency is 133.02 Hz, with a standard deviation of 1.0 Hz. The frequency did not vary more than 4 Hz. The percent jitter value was 0.30, and percent shimmer was 2.11. In contrast, an example of hoarse voice is shown in the panel on the right. Note the greater irregularity both in the period of the raw acoustic waveform shown at the top of the panel and in the amplitude of the phonation. The lower-frequency track shows large swings of fundamental frequency in what is supposed to be a steady-state sustained vowel. The mean fundamental frequency is 132.67 Hz with a standard deviation of 17.67 Hz. The largest frequency variation was approximately 76 Hz. The percent jitter value was 3.335, and percent shimmer was 11.82. The differences of perturbation between the normal and hoarse voice is very striking, suggesting that frequency and amplitude perturbation should be an important acoustic measurement to make on pathological voices.

Frequency perturbation, also called jitter, is obtained by measuring the period of each cycle of vibration, subtracting it from the previous or succeeding period, averaging the differences, and dividing by the average period. If the result is multiplied by 100, jitter can be expressed as a percent change of period relative to the average period. That measure is referred to as the jitter factor. There are several other formulations for computing frequency perturbation, which make comparison of data somewhat difficult (Casper, 1983). Titze (1995) recommends the use of some form of ratio measurement of jitter.

Frequency perturbation can be measured by the Visi-Pitch, which reports it as a ratio measurement. These measures are helpful for comparison of intra- or intersubject data when the same measure is being used for that comparison. The computer programs CSL and CSpeech calculate frequency perturbation and report their results in a variety of ways. For example, CSpeech reports jitter results both as the average absolute change of period in milliseconds and as percent change of frequency. It is possible to make the measurement of frequency perturbation from oscillographic recordings, but this requires much hand measurement and is a tedious and impractical task.

Amplitude perturbation, or shimmer, refers to the small cycle-to-cycle changes of the amplitude of the vocal fold signal. As was the case for the measurement of frequency perturbation, the amplitude of each glottal cycle is measured, subtracted from the previous or following period, and averaged over all differences. Shimmer is most often expressed in average change in decibels although percentage and ratio measurements may be reported and may be preferred (Titze, 1995).

Amplitude perturbation can be obtained directly from the CSpeech program, CSL, as well as from a number of other software programs. The measure of amplitude perturbation from the speech signal emitted at the lips is determined not only by the vocal folds but also by the resonance characteristics of the vocal tract. Thus, a measure of amplitude perturbation probably reflects the effect of the vocal tract on the speech signal, as well as the effect of the vocal folds.

SPECTROGRAMS

Spectrograms reflect the properties of the source of sound (the vibratory characteristics of the vocal folds) and the resonator (the vocal tract). To compare spectral characteristics of a given phonation, it is important to use the same vowel. It is also necessary to have a good working knowledge of the acoustic characteristics of normal speech to properly interpret spectrograms obtained from voice patients.

Spectrograms are useful for analyzing and showing changes in the spectral characteristics of the vocal fold sound. Noise and weak sounds will exhibit characteristics that can easily be studied from a spectrogram. As shown in Figure 8.13, the spectrum of a hoarse voice (right panel) has considerable noise energy in the higher frequencies, whereas the normal voice on the left has little high-frequency noise energy but strong

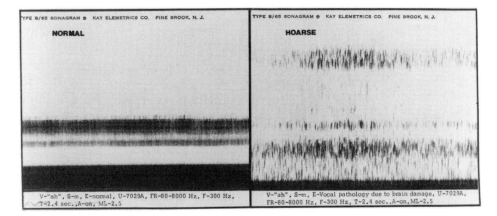

Figure 8.13. Spectrogram of a normal voice (left panel) and a hoarse voice (right panel).

low-frequency periodic energy. Amplitude sections can be taken at selected points and a detailed analysis made of the spectral characteristics of the sound. Spectrograms can be stored in the patient's record for analysis and comparison with later phonatory samples.

One useful measure that can be obtained from spectrograms is harmonics-to-noise ratio (also called signal-to-noise ratio). This is a measure of the energy in the harmonics of the voice signal (i.e., the frequencies produced by the vibrating vocal folds) and the noise energy in the signal. Abnormal voices will exhibit greater noise either directly (i.e., produced at the vocal folds) or indirectly as greater perturbation (Klingholz & Martin, 1985). On a spectrogram of an abnormal voice, there would be greater noise and less energy in the harmonics of the sound. The harmonics-to-noise ratio is a convenient measure to express this relationship. For example, the normal sustained vowel shown in Figure 8.12 had a signal-to-noise ratio of 22.4 dB, whereas the signal-to-noise ratio for the hoarse voice was 11.61 dB. After treatment, the spectrogram of a voice patient would exhibit greater harmonics-to-noise ratio because greater energy in the harmonic components of the sound would be expected, along with less noise energy.

Several computer software programs produce acceptable spectrograms (CSL, Kay Elemetrics; Cspeech [Windows version is called TF32], Paul Milenkovic; Dr. Speech, Tiger Electronics; Praat, Paul Bosma; SoundScope [Mac], GW Instruments). The use of these programs makes it possible to obtain spectrograms routinely on voice patients and greatly speeds the process of measurement. It is also possible to compute a harmonics-to-noise ratio via computer analysis (Kitajima, 1981; Kojima, Gould, & Lambiase, 1979; Kojima, Gould, Lambiase, & Isshiki, 1980).

ACOUSTIC SPECTRUM

Acoustic spectrum is a plot of the energy in each of the frequencies present in a complex tone. The amplitude section from a spectrograph is an example of acoustic spectrum. Acoustic spectrum may be determined directly from the speech signal, using special purpose spectrum analyzers or appropriate computer programs. Special purpose spectrum analyzers are very expensive, but several computer programs are available that are not only less expensive but also more practical for clinical application. An example of a spectrum analysis produced by the CSpeech software program is shown in Figure 8.14. Such spectral profiles can be printed out for inclusion in a patient's file. Of course, it is important that the patient produce the same vowel or sound under similar conditions for each profile to properly interpret any spectral changes that might be obtained.

Another variant of spectrum analysis is computation of the one-third octave spectrum of the speech sample. One advantage of a one-third octave spectral analysis is that it produces a small, manageable number of distinct frequency bands. In normal speech, one expects to find energy in frequencies from 100 to 5,000 Hz. In a one-third octave display, the spectrum is analyzed into 10 to 20 different frequency bands, depending on the frequency range desired. Furthermore, there is a well-documented and internationally accepted body of data concerning standardization of one-third octave spectra and the characteristics of the filters. Another advantage of one-third octave analysis is that it is similar, although not identical to, the way in which the ear analyzes sound. In view of this, the results of a one-third octave analysis may correlate best with perceptual measurements of voice. Unfortunately, few data are available on this relationship. In our judgment, the one-third octave or some variant seems to be the best choice at this time for analyzing the spectral characteristics of normal and abnormal voices.

Several expensive one-third octave spectrum analyzers are available for performing these measurements. It is also possible to extract one-third octave information from a computer-generated spectrum.

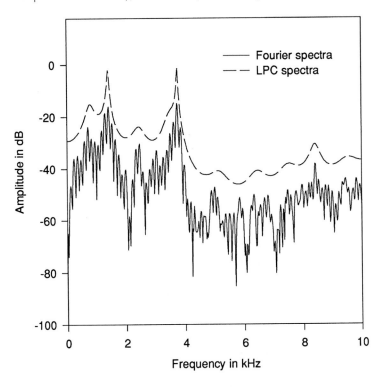

Figure 8.14. Spectral plot of a vowel produced by a normal speaker. These data were produced using CSpeech. A Fourier analysis produces a plot of all of the frequencies present in the phonation. An LPC analysis is used to compute the formant frequencies of the utterance.

Physiological Studies

ELECTROGLOTTOGRAPHY

Electroglottography (EGG) is a technique for the measurement of vocal fold contact area based on the principle that tissue conducts current. A high-frequency, low-current signal is passed between the vocal folds via electrodes located on the external neck over the thyroid lamina. When the vocal folds touch, a greater current flows than when they are open. There is a proportional variation of current when the vocal folds are less than maximally open or closed. Electroglottographic recordings can be used to determine when the vocal folds are closed and how fast they are closing. If carefully interpreted, determining characteristics of the opening of the vocal folds from an electroglottographic recording is possible. An example of an EGG waveform is shown in the bottom trace of Figure 8.15.

Devices to record the electroglottographic signal are readily available. Currently these include the Voiscope and Laryngograph (Laryngograph, Ltd., London, UK), the single channel SC1 or the dual channel MC2-1 (Glottal Enterprises, Syracuse, NY), and the unit from FJ Electronics (Surrey, UK). For a full discussion of the measurement technique, see Baken (1987). The electrical output of the electroglottograph can easily be converted to hard copy by using an oscillograph or similar graphic recording device, or from a computer-generated display.

The literature on EGG is primarily qualitative in nature, based on interpretation of the waveform.

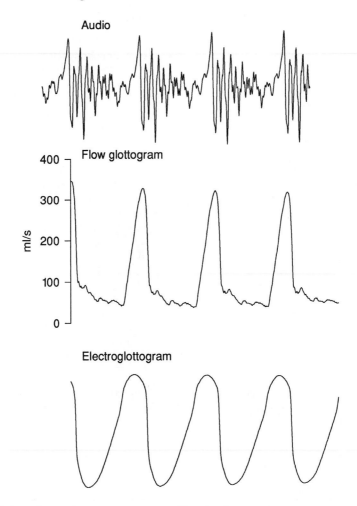

Figure 8.15. Acoustic waveform (top trace), inverse filtered airflow (middle trace), and electroglottograph waveform (bottom trace) of a normal speaker. In this plot, vocal fold contact is indicated by a downward deflection in the electroglottogram waveform.

Several studies have related the shape of the EGG waveform to the underlying physiology of vocal fold vibration (Childers, Moore, Naik, Larar, Krishnamurthy, & Moore, 1983; Dromey, Stathopoulos, & Sapienza, 1992; Hicks, Larar, Moore, & Childers, 1985; Houben, Buekers, & Kingma, 1992; Kiritani, Imagawa, & Hirose, 1986; Painter, 1988; Rothenberg, 1981; Titze, 1984, 1990; Titze & Talkin, 1981). Information also has been reported on characteristic waveforms in patients with vocal pathological conditions (Berry, Epstein, Fourcin, Freeman, & MacCurtain, 1982; Berry, Epstein, Freeman, MacCurtain, & Noscoe, 1982; Borden, Baer, & Kenney, 1985; Chevrie-Muller, Arabia-Guidet, & Pfauwadel, 1987; Childers, Alsaka, Hicks, & Moore, 1986; Colton, Brewer, & Rothenberg, 1983; Dejonckere & Lebacq, 1985; Gerratt & Hanson, 1987; Haji, Horiguchi, Baer, & Gould, 1986; Hanson, Gerratt, Karin, & Berke, 1988; Jentzsch, Unger, & Sasama, 1981; Karnell, Li, & Panje, 1991; Kaszniak, Garron, Fox, Bergen, & Huckman, 1979; Kitzing & Löfqvist, 1978; Sataloff, Spiegel, Carroll, Darby, & Rulnik, 1987; Scherer & Titze, 1987; Sorin, McClean, Ezerzer,

& Meissner-Fishbein, 1987; Swenson, Zwirner, Murry, & Woodson, 1992; Trapp & Berke, 1988; Ward, 1990; Wechsler, 1976; Wirz & Anthony, 1979). Many attempts have been made to quantify the electroglottograph signal (Brodie, Colton, & Swisher, 1988; Higgins & Saxman, 1993; Karnell, Li, & Panje, 1991; MacCurtain & Fourcin, 1982; Moore & Childers, 1984; Scherer & Titze, 1987; Singh & Ainsworth, 1992; Titze & Talkin, 1981; Rothenberg & Mahshie, 1988; Rasinger, Neuwirth-Riedi, & Kment, 1986; Wendler, Köppen, & Fischer, 1986; Wendler & Köppen, 1988).

EGG reflects the state of the vocal folds in a way that can be easily demonstrated and interpreted to patients. However, a limitation of the technique is that it cannot be used with all patients. Because the technique depends on vocal fold contact, the signal is considerably diminished or even absent in patients with lack of good contact, such as those with unilateral paralysis or aphonia. It also may be difficult to obtain a clear waveform in the presence of severe hoarseness. The thick or large necks of some patients hinder transduction of the current and result in a poor EGG tracing. Manufacturers of EGGs have greatly enhanced its clinical value. For example, the MC2-1 EGG made by Glottal Enterprises uses two identical circuits and two sets of electrodes. The output of each electrode pair is compared and displayed on a meter. When the meter reading is 0, the output of the two channels is identical and the vocal folds are centered between the two electrode pairs. This simple monitoring device helps to insure the proper placement of the electrodes and an optimal EGG signal.

PHOTOGLOTTOGRAPHY

Photoglottography is a technique designed to obtain estimates of variations of glottal area during phonation. Light is directed from above, usually from a fiberoptic light source passed through the nose. The light passes through the glottis and is detected by a light-sensitive device usually positioned over the skin of the trachea immediately beneath the vocal folds. As the vocal folds vibrate, their area of opening will vary and so will the amount of light passing through the glottis. It is a simple, relatively noninvasive device that yields a good, but not exact, approximation of glottal area. The photoglottographic technique is complementary to the EGG signal (Baer, Löfqvist, & McGarr, 1983a, 1983b).

Several measurements can be made from photoglottographic recordings. The first, speed quotient (SQ), is the speed of the opening phase of the vocal folds divided by the speed of their closing phase. The second, open quotient (OQ), is the time of the open phase of the vocal folds divided by the total period of vibration. This term is somewhat analogous to the term "duty cycle" used in engineering. Open quotient and speed quotient reflect efficient vocalizations, although which values are produced with maximally efficient phonations is unclear. Titze concluded that an OQ of approximately 0.50 resulted in efficient vocalization (1994).

A few studies relate photoglottographic results to different kinds of speech and voice production (Gerratt, Hanson, & Berke, 1988; Gerratt, Hanson, Berke, & Precoda, 1991; Gerratt, Hanson, Hunt, & Karin, 1985; Hanson, Gerratt, & Ward, 1983; Hanson, Ward, Gerratt, Berci, & Berke, 1989; Sonnesson, 1959; Vallancien, Gautheron, Pasternak, Guisez, & Paley, 1971). The waveform obtained from this technique may not be an entirely accurate representation of the actual glottal area waveform (Wendahl & Coleman, 1967). However, it may be useful for extracting measures such as SQ or OQ, which are known to be affected by disorders of the vocal folds (von Leden, Moore, & Timcke, 1960).

INVERSE FILTERING

In the inverse filtering procedure, the voice signal emitted at the lips is analyzed to remove the resonant effects of the vocal tract, producing an estimate of the waveform produced at the vocal folds. According to the acoustic theory of speech production (Fant, 1970; Stevens & House, 1961), speech is the product of a sound source and a filter. That is, the sound output of the vocal folds is modified by the resonant characteristics of the vocal tract. If the resonant characteristics of the vocal tract are known, it should be possible to retrieve the characteristics of the output of the vocal folds from the orally emitted speech signal.

Inverse filtering has been performed on the acoustic sound pressure waveform (Hillman & Weinberg, 1981; Miller & Mathews, 1963; Sondi, 1975), and on the airflow waveform (Rothenberg, 1973, 1977, 1981). We have used the airflow waveform for inverse filtering of normal and voice-disordered subjects (Brodie, Colton, & Swisher, 1988; Casper, Colton, & Brewer, 1985; Colton & Brewer, 1985; Colton, Brewer, & Rothenberg, 1983). We routinely record the EGG signal simultaneously with the inverse filtered airflow signal to extract information about the vibratory characteristics of the vocal folds during the complete cycle. The techniques complement each other in that airflow often will not be present during the closed phase of the vocal folds, but the EGG provides information about vibratory characteristics of the vocal folds during that phase. Thus, with both techniques, we are able to obtain a more complete picture of vocal fold vibratory characteristics during speech.

The result of inverse filtering of the oral airflow waveform is called a flow glottogram, and an example is shown in Figure 8.15. Four channels are collected directly into the computer using CSpeech. These are the (a) acoustic waveform, (b) raw oral airflow waveform, (c) EGG waveform, and (d) intraoral air pressure pulses associated with the stop plosives in the utterance (not shown in Figure 8.15, but see Figure 8.16). The oral airflow waveform is inverse filtered using CGlott, a computer program separate from but complementary to CSpeech. The result is the inverse-filtered or flow glottogram shown in Figure 8.15. An explanation of the analysis of the intraoral air pressure traces may be found in the next section.

Collection of electroglottographic and inverse filtered airflow waveforms is routine in our clinic. The following measures are obtained from computer-assisted analysis of the waveform: (a) each cycle's minimum (or leakage) and ac (or fluctuating flow) airflows; (b) the ratio of the time of the airflow pulse relative to the total period (airflow duty cycle); (c) the ratio of the closing and opening slopes of the airflow pulse (airflow speed quotient); (d) the ratio of the open time to the total period of the electroglottographic waveform (abduction quotient); (e) the closing time of the electroglottogram waveform; and (f) lung pressure (described later). Each cycle's measurements are added to the other cycles in the data and averaged. Patient data are thus available for comparison with data collected on a small group of normal speakers.

SUBGLOTTAL (LUNG) AIR PRESSURE

Proper interpretation of the airflow rates through the vocal folds requires knowledge about the driving pressure beneath the vocal folds, often called subglottal pressure (and sometimes by a variety of other names such as lung pressure, tracheal pressure, etc.) Various techniques are available for the measurement of the air pressure beneath the vocal folds, including the esophageal balloon technique and intratracheal puncture.

In the esophageal balloon technique, a small, latex balloon attached to a catheter is swallowed and positioned in the esophagus immediately behind the trachea and

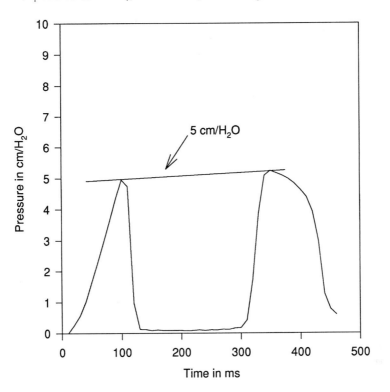

Figure 8.16. Air pressure traces during the production of the syllable /bœp/. The line drawn between each peak represents an estimate of the subglottal air pressure during the production of the vowel.

inferior to the cricoid cartilage. The posterior wall of the trachea is composed of smooth muscle, and any pressures in the trachea are reflected through this muscle wall into the esophagus. The balloon reflects these pressure changes, which are converted to a recordable voltage by a pressure transducer at the other end of the catheter. Several potential problems and pitfalls are present in the use of this technique (Kunze, 1964) but, with care, reliable and accurate measurements can be made (Schutte, 1980).

The second technique used to measure subglottal pressure is a tracheal puncture. A small needle attached to a catheter is inserted through the skin/tissue between a tracheal ring, usually the second or third ring. The pressure in the trachea is recorded using a pressure transducer. With both techniques, appropriate calibration maneuvers are performed to be able to relate pressure magnitude to the level of the electrical signal.

A third way of measuring subglottal pressure is by recording the intraoral air pressure variations as a speaker produces stop plosives (e.g., /b/, /p/). The theory is that the pressures produced behind the oral constrictions are the same as the pressures in the rest of the respiratory tract because the tract is a closed system. Thus, the intraoral pressure magnitudes will be similar to the subglottal air pressure magnitudes, at least during the production of the consonant. During the actual production of the vowel after the consonant, intraoral pressure drops markedly; however, there still is subglottal pressure because now the constriction is at the vocal folds. However, the intraoral pressures are good estimates of the subglottal pressure during the vowel (Hixon & Smitheran, 1982; Rothenberg, 1982; Smitheran & Hixon, 1981). An illustration of the technique for obtaining subglottal air pressure estimates from intraoral air pressure traces is shown in Figure 8.16. In our system, the peak pressures before and after the vowel are measured, averaged, and used to estimate the subglottal or lung pressures.

ELECTROMYOGRAPHY

Electromyography (EMG), a technique in which electrodes are inserted into specific muscles to measure their electrical activity, is used routinely by neurologists for the study of peripheral muscle function in various neuromuscular and neurological diseases. EMG is invasive and requires expertise; precautions must be taken to safeguard the patient's well-being. For these reasons, EMG has enjoyed limited use in the diagnosis and management of voice disorders. EMG of the vocal muscles requires detailed knowledge of head and neck anatomy, along with considerable experience in manipulating needles or needle carriers within the pharynx and larynx. The muscles involved in phonation are not readily accessible. Electromyographic recording equipment is available from a variety of manufacturers and has been engineered to be medically safe. The output of the equipment, an electromyogram, is a detailed tracing of muscle activity. An example of an electromyogram is shown in Figure 8.17.

Interpretation of electromyographic recordings requires experience and practice. Onset or offset of muscle activity, the pattern of muscle activity, and the overall amplitude of muscle activity are the parameters that provide the most valuable information. Electromyographic patterns of neurologically disordered patients show greater or lesser than normal amplitudes of muscle activity, extraneous bursts of muscle activity, and slower or faster than normal muscle activation. Laryngeal electromyograms may be helpful in those patients with voice problems of suspected neurological or neuromuscular origin. Another use for EMG is to verify excessive muscle activity before injection of Botox for symptom relief of spasmodic dysphonia. The needle used to

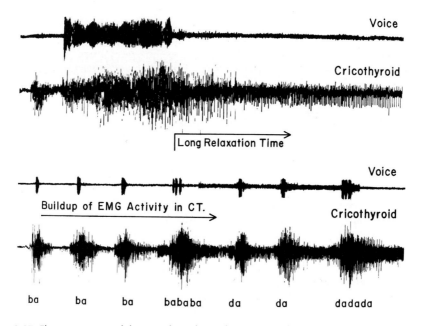

Figure 8.17. Electromyogram of the cricothyroid muscle in an elderly speaker during sustained vowel production (upper trace) and consonant–vowel syllable production (lower trace).

inject the Botox is used as an electrode whose electrical activity is monitored aurally to assist in the placement of the toxin in muscle. An EMG study can be helpful in differentiating vocal fold paralysis from arytenoid ankylosis.

Respiratory Studies

AIR VOLUMES AND CAPACITIES

Many clinicians advocate the analysis of a patient's respiratory function, including studies of lung volumes, vital capacity, residual capacity, and phonation volume. Others doubt the necessity for obtaining these data and question their value provided the patient is able to maintain adequate air volumes and airflows needed for speech. There is no controversy concerning the helpfulness of this information when dealing with professional voice users, particularly singers and actors. There are, of course, research issues for which such information is important.

The wet spirometer is the most common instrument used for the analysis of respiratory volumes. This device consists of an upper and a lower canister, each with an open end. The lower canister is filled with water. The open end of the upper canister fits into the mouth of the lower so that an airtight seal is produced. The two canisters are now effectively sealed, partially filled with known volumes of air and of water. A pipe, into which the patient breathes, connects to the air within the sealed canisters. When the patient exhales, air is forced into the sealed lower canister, the upper portion of which is allowed to move to accommodate the increased air volume. A pen or other marker attached to the vertically moving drum records the movement of the drum in response to the patient's breathing. Since the relationship between the air volume change and the movement of the pen is known, it is possible to obtain the volume of air used by the patient. Common measurements obtained from voice patients include tidal volume (the volume of air in an average breath), vital capacity (the volume of air that can be maximally exhaled after maximum inhalation), and total lung capacity (the total volume of air in the lungs). Other volumes that may be measured are inspiratory reserve volume (the amount of air that can be inspired from the end-expiratory level of a tidal breath) and expiratory reserve volume (the amount of air that can be expired from the end-expiratory level of a tidal breath). Respiratory physiologists are also concerned with reserve volume and gas exchange, but such measurements are not performed routinely for voice patients.

A certain amount of air volume, flow, and pressure is required for speech. The respiratory system, however, can provide considerably more volume, flow, or pressure than is required for speech or even for singing. Only a small portion of the total available volume is normally used in speaking. Thus, it would seem unnecessary, and perhaps unproductive, to spend inordinate amounts of time gathering information about lung volumes for most voice patients. Information that may be more valuable is that concerning the control of the respiratory system during speech. It is necessary and vitally important that informed decisions be made concerning the relative contributions of respiratory versus laryngeal function to the presenting voice problem.

RESPIRATORY MOVEMENTS

Assessing control of respiratory movements may be important in some voice patients. Assessment of the movement of the thorax and abdomen during speech may provide important information about the control exerted by a voice patient. Analysis of these movements is possible using a variety of tools, including mercury-filled strain gauges (Baken, 1987), the respiratory inductive plethysmograph (Bless, Hunker, & Weismer, 1981; Sackner, 1980; Watson, 1979), and magnetometers (Hixon, 1987). Bless et al. (1981) provide a comparison of these techniques. Although their methods vary, all of these tools are able to monitor the movements of the chest and abdominal walls using noninvasive external devices. All are available from commercial manufacturers; there is some variation in the expertise required for their operation.

A typical recording of the movements of the chest wall and abdomen is shown in Figure 8.18. Note that the rib cage (upper trace) shows a steady decrease of

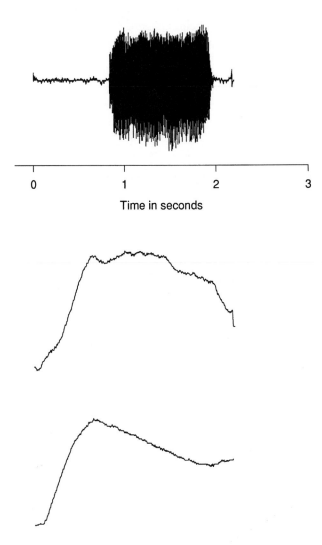

Figure 8.18. Examples of traces obtained with an inductive plethysmograph. The top trace is the acoustic signal, the middle trace reflects the circumferential changes occurring in the chest wall, and the bottom trace shows changes occurring in the abdomen. The speaker was a male who inhaled normally and produced a sustained vowel /œ/. Because we were only interested in time events, the rib cage and abdomen traces reflect voltage changes and not volume changes.

circumference as exhalation progresses, with irregular but decreasing changes noted in the abdominal channel. These curves can be calibrated to produce estimates of lung volume.

NONINSTRUMENTAL TESTING

Critical Listening and Description

Although we have presented the voice history as a separate section, in practice there can be no separation between history taking and the voice evaluation. The initial interview, during which the history is elicited, is the point at which the evaluation begins. It affords the clinician the opportunity to listen critically not only to the content of the message but also to the vocal output. Because patients are referred for voice therapy from various sources after laryngological examination, the speech–language pathologist should always have this question in mind: Are the vocal symptoms consistent with the referral diagnosis? The voice clinician's ears must always be turned on and tuned in. Picking up very significant clues about the presenting problem before the patient is aware that the examination is in progress is not unusual.

Case Study

A 35-year-old woman who complained of having lost her voice several weeks previously was answering all questions put to her in an aphonic whisper. During her aphonic explanation of the effect of this problem on her work, she cleared her throat. The clinician noted the entirely normal sound of the throat clearing. What information did this present?

While listening critically, the clinician should make observations about the consistency or variability in the sound of the voice and about its stability. When the voice exhibits variability or instability, it is important to be aware of the nature or pattern of that variability. For example, is the voice clear and strong initially, with gradual worsening over time? Does this happen with each sentence or two or over a more extended period? What is changing: quality, pitch, or loudness?

Making a perceptual judgment of vocal pitch is appropriate, but such judgments must be made with caution and later verified with objective data. Perhaps the most important perceptual judgment to be made relative to pitch is whether its level is appropriate for the age and sex of the speaker. Perceptual impressions of fundamental frequency in the presence of laryngeal pathology tend to suggest lower than expected levels; however, it has been shown (Murry, 1978) that the fundamental frequency of some voice problems does not differ systematically from the norm, with the exception of reduction in phonational range in laryngeal paralysis. Another aspect of pitch to which the clinician must attend is its variability. Variations in pitch are used linguistically to mark the meaning of utterances. In the English language, pitch is expected to fall at the end of a declarative sentence and to rise to mark a question. Voices that show pitch variability are generally thought to be more "interesting" and less apt to lull the listener.

Case Study

While taking the history from a 65-year-old man, the clinician was struck by an absence of inflection and a monotonic, flat, and unvarying delivery. Questions and statements were undifferentiated by the usual pitch changes. This observation, combined with noticeable slurring of speech, alerted the clinician to look for additional signs of neurological involvement. What would this absence of pitch variability suggest to you, and what other signs might you expect to find?

The loudness level of the patient's voice during assessment in presumably quiet surroundings should be another focus of the clinician's critical listening. The salient judgments to be made are whether the voice is too loud, too soft, or out of control. The consistency or variability of the loudness level are also important to note.

Case Study

Another observation made about our 65-year-old patient mentioned previously was the tendency for the loudness level of his voice to remain constant, with some decay at the end of an utterance. When asked to count and to alternate loud and soft voice for each successive number, the patient was able to comply with only the first three numbers, after which the loudness level became constant. Is this consistent with our previous observation, and why?

Descriptions of voice quality are most difficult to make. Many adjectives are used to describe voice quality, but they are difficult to quantify, and no widespread agreement exists on the meanings of voice quality terms. Some perceptions of quality can be checked against objective measures. For example, in the presence of hoarseness, there is the expectation of increased frequency perturbation (Coleman & Wendahl, 1967). Scaling of perceptions is perhaps the most valid approach to assigning a degree of objectivity to subjective judgments. Various types of scales are discussed later in this chapter.

Those aspects of speech referred to as suprasegmentals may hold information about voice production or may add to other findings in the search for the diagnosis. The rate of speech is one such aspect. Excessively fast or laboriously slow rates may be suggestive of neurological involvement or may simply be a reflection of personality. Persons who tend to talk very rapidly often tend also to stretch vocalization to the last bit of air they can squeeze out. This style of speech is often characterized by increased tension in the respiratory and laryngeal systems. Prosody of speech may be disturbed by vocal behavior, as is the case with spasmodic dysphonia. If the clinician is aware of a disturbance of prosody, determining the nature of that disturbance and describing it as accurately as possible are important.

Attention must be paid to any unusual vocal characteristics, such as stridor, grunts, and vocal tics. Of particular importance is the observation of stridor, inspiratory or expiratory noise. The presence of stridor suggests obstruction somewhere in the airway, subglottally, glottally, or supraglottally. It may be a sign of a laryngeal web, an obstructing lesion, severe inflammation, or abductor vocal fold paralysis. In infants, inspiratory stridor is usually symptomatic of laryngomalacia. Yet another cause of stridor may be fixation or ankylosis of the cricoarytenoid joints as a consequence of rheumatoid arthritis.

Case Study

J.W., a 41-year-old nurse, presented for a voice evaluation with a 10-year history of vocal difficulty and shortness of breath. She denied concern about her voice quality, which she claimed was unchanged. She believed that her vocal pitch was perhaps slightly higher than it had been but not enough to be of concern. Perceptually, we were in agreement with these judgments. Her main vocal complaint was the inability to complete a whole sentence on one breath. J.W. has continued to work during this 10-year period but admitted to shortness of breath in climbing stairs or during other physical exertion. Throughout this history taking, the examiner was aware not only of her obvious shortness of breath and the disruption in the prosody of speech caused by frequent interruptions to renew breath supply but also of her characteristic thrusting forward of the mandible during inspiration and of audible inspiratory stridor. J.W. was immediately referred for laryngological examination, which revealed abductor vocal fold paralysis, probably as a consequence of a viral infection.

Vocal tics are characterized by sudden, unexpected, and involuntary vocalizations. They are usually thought to be a symptom of a neurological disorder. Other unusual vocal manifestations that may suggest a neurological origin include grunts, barking sounds, and echolalia.

Critical Observations and Descriptions

The clinician must maintain eye contact with the patient and be in visual contact so as to be able to make observations of behavior that may not be audible. This requires that note taking be kept to a minimum, freeing the clinician to take full advantage of all diagnostic clues. After completion of the examination, the clinician should describe all observations made.

Watch facial expression and body language. Do they match the words being spoken? How do they change in response to questions? Is the person comfortable, anxious, tense, or fidgety? Is eye contact made and maintained? Are there extraneous facial or body movements? Is there tremor of the head, the hands, the jaw? Can you observe signs of neck, face, or laryngeal tension or strain? What is the emotional affect being projected? Does the person make adequate use of mouth opening and lip movement?

We suggest that observations of respiratory behavior be made during the period of eliciting the history and before asking the patient to engage in any specific vocal or respiratory tasks. Observing respiratory behavior both during speech and at rest is important. Does the person have sufficient air supply to complete sentences? Does the person habitually speak until the air supply is exhausted? Does the person release exhalation before voice onset, or do you observe a holding of the breath in anticipation of speaking with an abrupt, sharp voice onset? Where do you observe the greatest amount of respiratory activity when the person is speaking, and when at rest? Is it clavicular, midthoracic, or abdominal/diaphragmatic?

Diagnostic Testing Probes

The procedures used in this part of the evaluation cannot be rigidly specified because they often depend on the symptoms presented by the patient and the observations made by the clinician up to this point. The objectives of this part of the evaluation are to explore the patient's response to different ways of producing voice, to attempt to elicit an improved voice, to test the patient's ability to manipulate parameters such as pitch, loudness, and resonance, and to test the limits of the voice. Sometimes this involves making sounds and noises that create some self-consciousness. Patients with psychogenic voice disorders often appear frightened and threatened when asked to produce "different" sounds, perhaps because they are uncertain of their ability to maintain control over such phonations. Each step of this process must be carried out with sensitivity and encouragement. The clinician also must demonstrate the task being required of the patient. If the patient is being asked to produce a grunt, it will ease self-consciousness if the clinician models the grunt as the patient is to do it.

The following are some diagnostic testing tasks that might be useful.

PRODUCTION OF REFLEXIVE SOUNDS

These include coughing, laughing, clearing the throat, and the vocalized pause "uh-huh." The clinician's ears should have been tuned in to hear these sounds if they occurred spontaneously during the interview. It is interesting then to compare the quality of the sound produced spontaneously with that elicited during this task. The rationale for using this task is to determine the quality of the phonation produced in a nonspeech task. Judging whether this elicited quality differs from the voice heard in speech in quality, pitch, or loudness is most important. Often you must work with the patient on these tasks until you are satisfied that the best sound that person is capable of, or is willing to produce, has been heard.

ALTERING PITCH

Before attempting to obtain a phonational range, it is helpful to work with patients on the concept and on their ability to change pitch upward and downward. Some patients are unable to succeed on this task for reasons having to do with the nature of their problem. Others seem unable to carry it out because of difficulty in discriminating pitch changes and difficulty in matching pitches. It is important to try, during this diagnostic therapy period, to determine which of these is operative. It is helpful to engage in this activity as a practice for the actual testing of phonational range that may be carried out later. When patients exhibit difficulty in either matching a pitch or spontaneously altering pitch, we have found it useful to have them imitate animal sounds, such as the high-pitched meow of a kitten, the squeal of a mouse, or the howl of a wolf. Once again it is important to emphasize that such activities often create feelings of self-consciousness, which must be allayed by the clinician. One of the most effective methods of accomplishing this is through humor as the clinician models the desired sounds. The rationale for this activity is to test one of the limits of the voice, to explore whether the patient is capable of copying a model presented by the clinician, and to determine whether there is an overall improvement in the clarity of the sound at any point in the range. (Caution: This is not a search for an optimal pitch, which we do not believe is a viable concept, but rather an attempt to understand the physiology responsible for the vocal behavior.)

SUSTAINING STEADY, PROLONGED PHONATION

As in the previous activity, it is helpful to allow the patient some practice on this task before the taking of measurements. An increased level of tension is often generated in patients when they know an activity is being timed, and it is not unusual to find that they perform better in a more relaxed activity. The vowel of choice is usually /ah/. It is important for the clinician to observe carefully how the patient prepares to carry out this task and how natural or strained the phonation is, as well as noting the steadiness and length of the phonation. The rationale for this activity is to observe the patient's ability to control phonation and respiration. Vocal tremor, if present, will become more obvious on this task than during connected speech. The patient may be asked to produce such a phonation at various pitch levels as a means of continuing to explore vocal capacity.

ALTERING VOCAL LOUDNESS

Eliciting a very quiet sound is usually not difficult, but people are often quite reticent to produce the loudest phonation of which they are capable while seated in a quiet office. Therefore, it may be necessary to pursue increments of loudness in steps, with the clinician providing the model. Clearly, if the patient has been referred with the diagnosis of a vocal fold lesion, inflammation, or edema, this activity should not be carried out. Some persons who have habituated very loud voice use find it difficult to lower the loudness level and ask with incredulity whether they can be heard. The rationale for this activity is to further test the limits of voice production and explore the patient's ability to manipulate isolated vocal parameters and match a model.

PHONATION WITH EFFORTFUL GLOTTAL CLOSURE

This activity must be used wisely and only with those patients for whom the activity itself will not be harmful. A variety of techniques elicit effortful closure of the glottis: grunting, isometric pushing together of the palms of the hands held chest height, isometric pulling apart of linked hands held chest height, lifting a very heavy object, and attempting to raise a chair while seated on it. The person is required to phonate while tension is maintained during the activity. The rationale for the use of such a stressful phonatory act is to attempt to force vocal fold adduction and elicit a nonspeech sound that is difficult to control voluntarily. This is an activity that we have found helpful in eliciting a lowered pitch level in young boys who present with puberphonia and an improved voice in some patients with psychogenic dysphonias. Use of this procedure in therapy is discussed in Chapter 10. The intent here is to use the technique as an exploratory measure as part of the total assessment.

"PLACING THE VOICE"

This is often referred to as placing the voice in the mask, or voice focus. As a diagnostic task, it constitutes one of the methods used in the search for the best voice a patient can produce. This technique is discussed more completely in Chapter 10.

Noninstrumental Objective Measurements

MAXIMUM PHONATION TIME

An individual's ability to sustain phonation provides some information about the control of respiratory function, glottal efficiency, and laryngeal control. When respiratory function is compromised, there will be either reduction in the amount of air available to support phonation or a problem in the control of the airflow. If the problem is at the laryngeal level, glottal resistance to airflow may be reduced because of inadequate glottal closure, or increased because of obstruction or hyperadduction. Certain problems affecting motor control of phonation may not inhibit or restrict maximum phonation time but may affect the quality of the phonation. The task is designed to test the limits of function and as such may uncover weaknesses that are not apparent at lower levels of function. Thus, for example, in the case of an individual with essential tremor, a vocal tremor may become increasingly obvious as phonation is sustained, although it may have escaped notice during speech.

The patient should be instructed to take a deep breath and sustain the vowel /ah/ for as long as possible. This should be done at pitch and loudness levels that are comfortable for the patient. A stopwatch should be used to obtain the measure, and patients should be asked to repeat the task at least three times (Hirano, 1981b), with the greatest duration being adopted as the maximum phonation time. Kent et al. (1987) caution, however, that the database for this, as well as many other maximum performance measures of speech production, may not be adequate for confident clinical use. Although Stone (1983) and others (Finnegan, 1984, 1985; Lewis, Casteel, & McMahon, 1982; Neiman & Edeson, 1981) have reported instability of the maximum phonation time measure over as many as 15 trials, Bless and Hirano (1982) found that three trials were adequate if subjects were given adequate instruction and practice in the task. Corroboration of this can be found in the report that coaching and instruction led to a mean increase in maximum phonation time of 5.2 seconds for a group of 3rd-grade girls (Reich, Mason, & Polen, 1986). The available normative values for sustained phonation may be found in Chapter 14.

The ability to sustain phonation is developmental and increases from childhood to adulthood. It is logical that this should be the case in view of the physical growth of the body and increased lung capacity. Significant differences in maximum phonation time exist between the sexes, but that difference does not begin to appear until puberty, when growth spurts between the sexes differ in degree (Hirano, 1981b). An overall reduction of pulmonary function with aging, as well as a lessening of laryngeal efficiency, occurs (Kent, Kent, & Rosenbek, 1987), resulting in a decrement in maximum phonation time in the geriatric population.

S/Z RATIO

As noted previously, both respiratory and laryngeal factors play some role in determining maximum phonation time. However, the measure of maximum phonation time does not provide sufficient information to differentiate between deficits in respiratory support versus laryngeal inefficiency. Boone (1977) introduced the s/z ratio as an expansion on the measurement of maximum phonation time. The underlying theoretical construct suggests that individuals with normal larynges should be able to sustain vocalization (i.e., /z/) for a period of time equal to that of sustained expiratory airflow without vocalization (i.e., /s/), resulting in a ratio that approximates 1. If the respiratory system is compromised and the laryngeal system is intact, there should be an equal reduction in expiratory airflow for the voiceless /s/ and the voiced /z/ components of the task, which again would yield a ratio approximating 1. However, reduced vibratory efficiency of the abnormal larynx should result in air wastage, with reduction in the ability to sustain phonation but without a reduction in duration of expiratory airflow in the absence of phonation. Thus, the s/z ratio would be greater than 1 in the presence of laryngeal abnormality. Eckel and Boone (1981), in a study of dysphonic adults with and without laryngeal pathological conditions, obtained results that support this notion. Ninety-five percent of patients with vocal fold margin pathological conditions studied by Eckel and Boone had s/z ratios above 1.4, whereas the ratios for both the normal control group and those patients with dysphonia without pathological conditions approximated 1.

Two studies have been reported investigating the use of the s/z ratio with children, and the results have not supported the previous research. In a study of 16 children with vocal nodules, Rastatter and Hyman (1982) report s/z ratios of 1, similar to expectations in the normal population. Similar findings are reported by Hufnagle and Hufnagle (1988) in a larger study of 123 dysphonic children, of whom 69 had vocal fold nodules. Based on the results of these studies, the s/z ratio appears not to be sensitive to the presence of vocal fold pathological conditions in children, nor does it separate dysphonic children (with or without pathological conditions) from normals. Although the reason for the difference between adults and children on this measure is not entirely clear, it is theorized that the size and stiffness of the pathological condition may have been greater in the adult subjects than in children, all of whom in the Hufnagle and Hufnagle study were reported to have had small to moderate-sized nodules that were soft in consistency. Measures of maximum duration of production of both /s/ and /z/ have been reported by Tait, Michel, and Carpenter (1980) for 53 children aged 5, 7, and 9 years with normal voices. Their results are shown in Figure 8.19. As one might expect, the older children had longer maximum phonations than the younger children, reflecting perhaps greater lung capacity or greater phonatory control. The maximum duration times for both /s/ and /z/ reported by Rastatter and Hyman (1982) and by Hufnagle and Hufnagle for their subjects who had vocal fold nodules or were dysphonic were lower than those reported by Tait et al. for their normal subjects.

The procedure for measuring the s/z ratio is very straightforward. The patient is instructed to take a deep breath and then sustain an /s/ for as long as possible. The examiner should model the task, although it is not necessary to sustain the model maximally. The task should be repeated at least twice by the patient, with the longest duration taken as the score. The same procedure is carried out for sustaining the /z/. It is best to use a stopwatch in obtaining these measures. The ratio is obtained by dividing the maximal /s/ value by the maximal /z/ value. Available normative s/z ratio data are presented in Chapter 14.

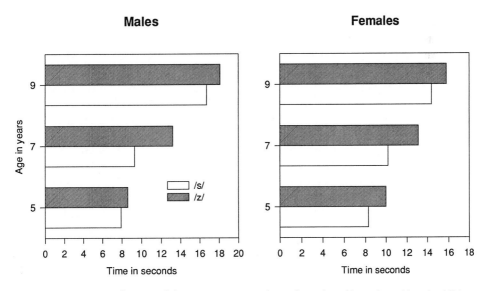

Figure 8.19. Maximum duration of phonation in sustained vowels produced by male and female children ages 5, 7, and 9 years.

Although this measure has been demonstrated to have some validity for adults, the cautions discussed relative to maximum phonation time measures also apply here. The s/z ratio should be used primarily as a screening measure or as one test among many others. A diagnosis of a pathological condition should never be made based on the result of this procedure alone. However, it may alert a clinician to the need for medical examination, if that has not been done, or, conversely, it may raise questions about a diagnosis of a pathological condition if the results are not consistent. The validity of this measure for children is still open to question, and thus it should be used in that population with even greater caution.

The apparent simplicity of this measure may be somewhat deceiving. Clinically we have found that it is necessary to teach this task to patients and to allow them adequate practice before taking formal measures (Chapter 14).

SCALING

Perceptual judgments of various aspects of voice, quality in particular, are usually described as being subjective and with the implication that such judgments are not valid. However, perceptions can be quantified using well-established techniques of psychophysics and the procedure of scaling. The simplest type of quantification of qualitative or categorical variables is at the level of the nominal scale. The fundamental principle of nominal scales is equivalence; that is, all observations placed within the same category are considered to be equal. For example, voice qualities can be assigned names such as harsh, breathy, hoarse, or strident, which constitute categories. The perceptual judgment task may be to place voice samples within categories along that scale. No judgments are made or implied as to quantity or severity of the quality perceived. This is simply, as the name of the scale implies, a naming task.

However, we are usually interested in more than naming. Perhaps we want to make judgments about the degree of a quality that is present. Using our group of subjects who were nominally scaled as having hoarse voice quality, we can now rank order them according to severity using an ordinal scale. In this scale, numbers are used to express order of magnitude of the perception. The rank order means that higher numbers have a greater amount of a feature than lower numbers. Thus, the voice quality given a rank order of 1 has been judged to have less hoarseness than that with a rank order of 15. Ranks do not tell us how much of a feature is present or how much difference there is between ranks or even if the difference between ranks are equal. The only information we have is that at a given rank there is less or more of a feature than at the ranks above or below.

Interval scales are very common in voice quality scaling because we can use them to determine how much of a feature is present in one quality compared with another. The refinement over an ordinal scale is that the distance between adjacent points on the scale has meaning, and a given interval between measures has the same meaning anywhere along the scale. Common examples of this type of scale are degrees of temperature and calendar years. In the latter, we know that as much time elapsed between 1790 and 1800 as between 1970 and 1980. The interval scale thus has a defined unit of measure. However, it does not necessarily have a defined beginning or a meaningful zero point.

The ratio scale has all the properties of the interval scale, with the added benefit of an absolute zero. Such a scale makes it possible to talk meaningfully about ratios. Examples of this type of scale are measures of length.

A visual analog scale simply presents a continuum between two anchor points, such as an undifferentiated 5-inch line-scale along which a mark is made representing the quantity of a feature judged to be present. Such a scale does not use any verbal descriptors along it and is reported by some to produce more reliable and valid judgments because it permits finer discriminations to be made (Kempster, 1984). For scoring purposes, the 5-inch line in the example above could be converted into a 100-point rating scale.

The most complex scaling method is referred to as multidimensional scaling, a method for identifying the perceptual attributes of complex stimuli such as voice quality (Kempster, 1984; Schiffman, Reynolds, & Young, 1981). Algorithms of multidimensional scales represent stimuli as points on a spatial map. The difference between points is then a reflection of the judged similarity or dissimilarity of the stimuli. The closer the points, the greater the similarity of the feature being judged.

CAPE-V PERCEPTUAL RATING FORM

The Consensus Auditory-Perceptual Evaluation of Voice (CAPE-V) system was developed at a consensus meeting in 2002 sponsored by Division 3, Voice and Voice Disorders, of ASHA and the University of Pittsburgh. Speech–language pathologists, voice scientists, and other scientists interested in sound perception met to discuss the current state of the art for the perceptual rating of voice and to create a system that could be used for the routine perceptual rating of disordered voices. The intent was to develop a standardized procedure for rating, to define the basic qualities of the voice that should be rated, and to recommend the development of a standardized training system. The CAPE-V was the outcome of that meeting and is currently in its testing and evaluation stage (see form in the Appendix).

The scale identifies six core perceptual attributes of the voice: overall severity, roughness, breathiness, strain, pitch, and loudness. The degree of each attribute is indicated on a 100-mm line, where the left end indicates normal or a very mild severity and the extreme right end indicates severe amount of the attribute. The rater also may indicate whether the attribute is consistent or intermittent in the voice sample rated. For pitch and loudness, the rater is to indicate the nature of the abnormality as well as the rating. There is also space for two additional but unnamed attributes to be added by the clinician and rated. There is also space for comments about resonance as well as any other perceptual features observed in the sample.

The ratings are to be made after the completion of several tasks, including sustained vowels, sentences, and spontaneous speech. The clinician marks the amount of the deviancy on the 100-mm line and, after completion of the ratings, measures the distance from the left end of the line to the mark and writes the value in the column labeled __/100. For example, if the distance of the line for Overall Severity is 57, then the notation 57/100 would appear. The clinician also may use descriptive words such as mildly deviant, moderately deviant, or severely deviant.

The consensus group expects that there will be modifications to the basic reporting form as more clinicians begin using the form and further experience is gained.

Scaling of Pitch

Perceptual judgments of voice quality are often confounded by other perceptual attributes of the voice sample and may not always be related to a simple acoustic correlate. For example, let us examine the perception of pitch. Wolfe and Ratusnik (1988) have shown that listeners will rate the pitch of rough vowels much lower than the pitch of normally produced vowels. Consequently, vowels produced by a patient with a hoarse voice may be expected to be perceived as lower in pitch than their measured fundamental frequencies would predict. Furthermore, Wolfe and Ratusnik reported that the pitch matches they obtained were related to the acoustic measures of noise energy level and jitter ratio rather than to fundamental frequency. Thus, with respect to pitch, other abnormal perceptual (e.g., roughness, hoarseness) or acoustic (e.g., jitter, noise level, spectrum) attributes may result in inaccurate judgment. This may account for some of the discrepancies that have been noted between perceptual pitch judgments of abnormal voices and the measured acoustic correlate of fundamental frequency. Wilson, Wellen, and Kimbarow (1983) suspect that there is a skill in discriminating pitch differences in the speaking voice that is not easily developed. Their judges, described as trained and untrained, performed at chance level on a pitch discrimination task until there was at least a 20- to 29-Hz difference present between paired voice samples.

Another factor affecting the reliability and validity of perceptual judgments is the experience of the listener. Many studies in which perceptual judgments were reported used experienced listeners or listeners with extensive exposure to normal and abnormal voice qualities. How much experience is needed to produce reliable judgments is somewhat unclear. Bassich and Ludlow (1986) conducted a study using four judges who required 16 half-hour training sessions before reaching 80% agreement with one another. Perhaps the lack of training or experience may account for the lack of difference between groups of trained and untrained listeners in distinguishing pitch differences between pairs of children's voices in the Wilson et al. (1983) study. The trained group consisted of 10 graduate students in speech–language pathology, of which only 4 had had previous experience in working with patients with voice disorders.

Graduate students with only a brief exposure to voice disorders (usually a single academic course and perhaps an actual patient in clinic) would be unlikely to be able to reliably and accurately rate attributes of the voice such as pitch, loudness, and tremor. In a study reported by Colton and Estill (1981) concerned with the identification of four distinct voice qualities, the group of six speech–language pathologists performed slightly worse than the group of 15 "naive" listeners (66% vs. 68%). Singers and individuals who played a musical instrument performed somewhat better than these two groups (73% for singers, 75% for instrumentalists). Although the differences between the groups were not large, these results suggest that experience in music may help a listener to make judgments concerned with voice quality attributes. At the very least, musicians may attend better to the nonlinguistic aspects of the speaker's utterance.

Perceptual judgments of vocal pitch are sufficiently unreliable to cast doubt on their use in planning treatment strategies. Determinations of the appropriateness of pitch level should be made on the measurement of its acoustic correlate, fundamental frequency, for which normative values appropriate for age and sex are available for comparison. Whenever measurable acoustic correlates of vocal attributes are available, their use is encouraged in preference to reliance on the perceptual feature.

Scaling Vocal Effort

The effort a patient uses to vocalize may be important to assess in the exploration of a voice problem. Many patients report that at the end of a day of prolonged talking, they feel vocally fatigued. They also may report that they need to expend more energy in talking than they did before the onset of their vocal problem. It is difficult for the clinician to know how to assess such reports and what value to give them. However, such "feelings" can be measured, and such measures can be helpful therapeutically and in assessing the efficacy of treatment and of specific treatment techniques.

How does the clinician quantify the vocal effort a patient uses during phonation? Simply ask the patient to produce a vocalization and afterward ask that patient to assign it a number that represents the amount of effort used. Subjects can scale their own effort levels with this simple procedure (Colton & Brown, 1973; Irwin & Mills,

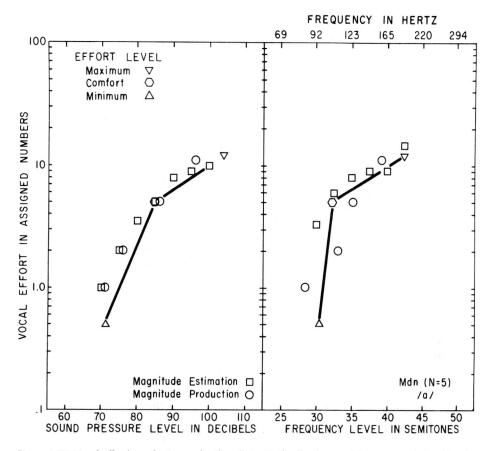

Figure 8.20. Vocal effort/sound pressure level and vocal effort/fundamental frequency relationships for five normal speakers.

1965; Lane, Catania, & Stevens, 1961; Wright & Colton, 1972a, 1972b). Wright and Colton (1972a, 1972b) asked speakers to produce the vowel /ah/ at their minimum, most comfortable, and maximum effort levels. The fundamental frequency and the sound pressure level of each phonation was measured during each vocalization. The subjects were then asked to assign a number that represented the amount of effort used. They could use any number they wished, with the understanding that greater effort levels would be associated with higher numbers. This procedure is often referred to in the psychophysical literature as the method of magnitude estimation. Median results for the group are shown in Figure 8.20. The left panel shows vocal effort in assigned numbers versus SPL in decibels. In the right panel, vocal effort is compared to fundamental frequency. The solid lines connect minimum, most comfortable, and maximum effort levels. The data points between these three effort levels (squares) were generated by asking the subject to produce a phonation whose effort was halfway between minimum and most comfortable or most comfortable and maximum. Each of these intervals then was bisected again to produce the estimates of vocal effort shown in this figure. Note how consistent the subjects were in producing and rating their effort levels, especially for effort versus SPL. The data points for magnitude production (shown by circles) were obtained by providing a number to the subject and asking him to produce a phonation with an effort level representative of the number supplied. These data are very similar to the data obtained in the magnitude estimate phase of the experiment. The vocal effort/fundamental frequency data show somewhat more variability between magnitude production and estimation than the vocal effort/SPL data. It is abundantly clear, however, that individuals can rate the effort they use to produce voice and that variations of vocal effort are manifested acoustically by variation of SPL and fundamental frequency.

The data of Figure 8.20 clearly show that an increase of vocal effort is accompanied by an increase of both intensity and frequency. Colton and Brown (1973) have shown that speakers also exhibit systematic increases of intraoral air pressure with an increase of vocal effort. In simple consonant–vowel syllables, intraoral air pressure can be a good estimate of the pressures driving the vocal folds (Hixon & Smitheran, 1982; Rothenberg, 1982; Smitheran & Hixon, 1981). Thus, suspecting that the magnitude of subglottal air pressure, accompanied by the consequent tension of the vocal folds, contributes to the judgments of vocal effort is not unreasonable.

Verdolini-Marston and her colleagues (Verdolini-Marston, Burke, Lessac, Glaze, & Caldwell, 1995) reported using vocal effort scaling in their study of the effectiveness of two kinds of therapy for vocal nodules. Before therapy, five subjects who received the confidential voice therapy protocol had a mean rated effort level of 115 (a judgment of comfortable level of effort while talking was assigned the number 100), whereas the three subjects who received the resonant voice therapy protocol have a mean rated effort level of 142. After a 2-week, concentrated period of voice therapy, the confidential therapy group reported a mean effort level of 90; the resonant therapy group, an effort level of 105. These measures were obtained 2 weeks after therapy had ended, and both therapy groups had a mean effort level of 97. These results suggest that monitoring vocal effort may reflect the physiological changes that occur as a result of therapy and may monitor the vocal usage by patients with voice disorders.

Listeners also can rate vocal effort from recorded samples of speech (Brandt, Ruder, & Shipp, 1969; Lane, Catania, & Stevens, 1961; Moll & Peterson, 1969; Warren, 1962), but the ratings are not simply ratings of the vocal loudness (Brandt, Ruder, & Shipp, 1969). Listeners apparently use the increase of energy in the higher frequencies as cues for their judgments of vocal effort as well as the greater sound pressure levels that accompany increased effort levels. They also may internalize what they hear and relate their judgments to their own perceived efforts. Increased tension in the adducted vocal folds results in greater subglottal air pressure and also results in the production of increased energy in the higher frequencies. Thus, listeners and speakers appear to use similar cues; only the speaker has access to the significant physiological variable, air pressure, whereas the listener must depend solely on its acoustic manifestation, increased high-frequency energy.

The concept of vocal effort, as well as its measurement, have implications for the management of voice problems, for monitoring progress, and for assessing treatment efficacy (see Chapter 10).

Voice Sample Recording

One of the easiest and simplest ways of testing a subject is to obtain a voice recording. Even if no further analysis of the recording is performed, the recording itself can be invaluable. Recording makes repeated listening possible, allowing the voice clinician further opportunities to learn about the person's voice characteristics. A voice recording during the initial assessment provides a baseline record of the voice before intervention. This documentation can be helpful for demonstrating progress or change as a result of treatment and for judging the efficacy of treatment. A baseline recording is highly important when medical–legal issues arise. Surprisingly, however, very little attention is generally given to the techniques and equipment needed for producing good-quality recordings. The material presented in the following sections is based both on personal experience and on discussions by Izdebski (1981, 1983).

TAPE RECORDERS

Several kinds of voice recorders can be used to make audio recordings of patient vocalizations: (a) reel-to-reel, (b) cassette, (c) videotape recorders, (d) DAT recorders, (e) minidisc recorders, and (f) direct-to-CD recorders. The reel-to-reel models have an excellent frequency response and a wide dynamic range but are not often found in most voice clinics. Manufacturers of reel-to-reel units include Nigra, Ampex, and Revox. Cassette recorders are much more popular and offer the conveniences of portability and use of cassette tapes. Although inexpensive cassette recorders are available, they rarely have good frequency response or adequate dynamic range, do not produce good recordings, have high tape instability (wow and flutter), and are prone to breakdown. These inexpensive recorders are not recommended for clinical use. There are many cassette recorders costing $200 to $600 that have good to excellent characteristics and are easy to use. We include videotape recorders in this category, because many of the medium-priced models, as well as the higher-priced ones, have excellent frequency and dynamic ranges in the audio range, very low tape instability, and can store considerable data. Furthermore, many can record and reproduce in stereo.

Two additional recording devices have become available in recent years whose price and performance warrant consideration for routine and even critical clinical use. The DAT recorder is very similar to a cassette recorder except that the analog voice signal is digitized and recorded on tape. The cassette is approximately the size of a microcassette (the kind used in dictating equipment); however, depending on the tape quantity and the recording speed, up to 4 hours of high-quality signal can be recorded. At the fastest speed currently available, the quality rivals that heard on compact discs (CDs). DAT recorders are made by Sony, JVC, and Aiwa, among others. However, the popularity of a DAT recorder has waned in recent years and their availability is becoming limited. We use two models of Sony DATs. The first, the model TCD-D3, is approximately the size of a Walkman, operates from batteries or an AC line source, and is capable of recording with a sampling rate of 44.1 kHz (CD quality). At this rate, we can record up to 2 hours. Our second unit is a larger unit, the Sony DTC-700. Both units feature the ability to label each recording with a number permitting more rapid retrieval of desired recordings. Prices vary a great deal and may be less for new units or units produced by other manufacturers.

Minidisc recorders use a small disc approximately the size of the $3\frac{1}{2}''$ disc used in many computer systems. The recorder can record approximately 60 to 70 minutes of vocalization with CD quality. Sony makes a minidisc recorder that is approximately the size of a Walkman. Although perceptually, the recordings sound excellent, the frequency response may be limited because of circuitry used to pack the samples on the small disc. Thus, a minidisc recorder may not be suitable for critical clinical applications but is suitable if the intent is only to collect audio recordings for listening purposes. Beware of minidisc players that can play prerecorded minidiscs but have no record capability. However, Sony has introduced the MD Walkman MZ NHF800 minidisc recorder that features an option to record audio using the PCM Linear recording mode. Recording with this mode does not discard any parts of the frequency spectrum and would be comparable to DAT, cassette, or CD recordings. Since a recording will require a larger amount of disk space when recorded in this mode, only about 28 minutes can be recorded on a standard 80-minute minidisk. Sony has introduced a higher capacity minidisk, the 1 GB Hi-MD that permits recording up to 94 minutes even in the PCM mode.

One manufacturer, Marantz, has introduced a direct-to-CD recorder, the model CDR 300 portable CD recorder. With this unit, it is possible to record audio samples direct to a CD with very high quality. New recordings can be added at any time, and when the CD is full and finalized, it can be played in any computer system. Individual recordings can be identified on the CD and quickly retrieved for listening or analysis. Marantz has also introduced a solid-state digital recorder (PMD 670) that can record audio direct to Compact Flash storage cards typically used with digital cameras. High-capacity storage cards permit recordings of considerable length and, like the CD, allow for random retrieval of the audio material.

In addition to good recording equipment, using high-quality recording tape is important. High-quality tape has a number of advantages: (a) It is strong enough to withstand the starting and stopping required when many speech samples are recorded and played back, and (b) less of the oxide particles in the tape will rub off to affect the recording and playback heads and interfere with the motor and wheels that transport the tape. Cassette tapes are available in 30- to 120-minute lengths. The 120-minute tapes should be avoided because the tape is very thin and can break easily. Cassette tapes made by TDK, Maxell, Sony, Nakamichi, 3M, or similar manufacturers are of good quality. Tapes also may differ in type, for example, standard tape, chromium dioxide tape (a high-bias tape), or metal tape (also a high-bias tape). Most higher-priced tape recorders are able to play back all of these types of tape. Metal tape tends to have the best response characteristics, but at considerably greater cost. Many of the good to excellent cassette recorders have metal tape recording/reproducing capability.

Videotapes also come in various time lengths, usually ranging between 2 and 6 hours (VHS format). When using the tape to obtain good audio recordings, it is best to use the highest speed settings (2 hours).

DAT tapes are made by several manufacturers, including Sony, JVC, and Maxell. They are available in 30-, 60-, and 120-minute lengths. These tapes are considerably more expensive than standard cassette tapes but are of superior quality. Mini discs usually can record up to 70 minutes of information and are generally inexpensive.

Audio CDs typically can store approximately 80 minutes of recording with high quality. Avoid cheap blank CDs; even high-quality CDs are available at very reasonable prices.

MICROPHONES

Microphones should be selected on the basis of low distortion, low sensitivity, wide frequency response (50-16,000 Hz), directionality, stability, and cost. Good-quality microphones can be purchased for relatively low cost ($50–$100). A good source for microphones is Radio Shack. Many new microphones are of the electret type, which contain a small battery and pickup element that has very good frequency and dynamic response characteristics. Condenser and dynamic microphones have excellent characteristics at moderate cost. A pressure zone microphone, a relatively new type of microphone that permits recording large groups with good fidelity, is also worthy of consideration.

For voice work, a microphone attached to an earphone band works very well. It maintains a constant mike-to-mouth distance, and because it is very close to the source, can produce good recording levels even with a very quiet voice. However, the mic should be placed at an angle and to the side of the lips to avoid transient noises caused by the air flows produced during speech. One good head-mounted microphone is the AKG C420.

ENVIRONMENT

Recordings should be made in a quiet room, away from noisy corridors and windows that face onto busy streets. The room need not be completely soundproofed, however. Carpeted floors and walls and windows hung with fabric coverings serve to reduce noise level significantly. Of course, special acoustic absorbing panels can be installed, which will produce a very quiet room. The clinician should measure the noise levels within the room to make sure they are acceptable (less than 50 dB at the low frequencies) and periodically check these levels to ensure that the noise present is predominantly low frequency.

TASKS

Choose a variety of tasks for the patient to carry out that will sample the full range of the patient's vocal capabilities. Sustained vowels are useful for subsequent measurement of fundamental frequency, perturbation, and spectra. Syllables and sentences should be used to sample the patient's voice under more speech-like conditions and yet yield data that can be compared at different times. Testing of vocal limits, that is, phonational (frequency) range and dynamic (intensity) range, also can be recorded. We usually include a standard reading passage, the Rainbow Passage (Fairbanks, 1960), and a sample of conversational speech as part of our recording protocol. Also record any special or unusual characteristics of a patient's vocal behavior. The speech tasks from the protocol for fiberoptic examination in the Appendix may be used for any audio recording. One also could use the speech tasks recommended by the CAPE-V consensus group (see Appendix).

Quality of Life Evaluation

Voice evaluation has traditionally involved the use of perceptual, acoustic, aerodynamic, and other physiological measures. The intent of these tools is to allow the clinician to describe the voice, compare it with normal, document changes with time or treatment, and estimate the severity of the dysphonia present. Despite the extensive use of these instruments, however, many questions regarding their reliability and validity, as well as how they are obtained and interpreted, are unresolved (Kent, Kent, & Rosenbek, 1987; Karnell, Scherer, & Fischer, 1991; Karnell, 1991; Karnell, Hall, & Landahl, 1995; Kreiman & Gerratt, 2000; Gerratt & Kreiman, 2001). In recent years, increasing attention has been given to the patient's own assessment of the dysphonia and its impact on his or her life. The development of patient-view instruments for many disorders has been motivated by a number of factors.

With rising health care costs and increasing competition for limited available funds, it has become more critical to assess outcomes of treatment(s). Although health care providers have always been interested in the effects of their interventions, the ability to document these in meaningful and objective ways has become imperative. Institutions that manage health care services, insurers, and other funding sources scrutinize the relative effectiveness of treatments in an effort to determine the best use of resources and to establish standard of care guidelines. With the intense focus on outcomes research, there has been a growing realization that subjective information regarding the effects of disability on the individual patient represents an important addition to assessment batteries. Insights into the effects of a disorder on a patient's emotional and social well-being, and on his or her ability to function in real-world situations, such as in a work setting, are revealed in a manner not possible with clinician-view measures.

The impact of disability on "quality of life" (QOL) issues is reflected in a number of tools designed specifically for patients with voice disorders. Typically, these instruments take the form of a set of questions, or statements, that require a response from the patient. Though simplistic in form, good QOL instruments reflect the same rigorous development that is key to establishing the validity and reliability required of any assessment tool. (See Hogikyan & Rosen, 2002, for a review of subjective assessment.)

The Voice Handicap Index (VHI) (Jacobson et al., 1997), is one of the first, and perhaps most frequently used, QOL instruments specific to voice disorders. In its original form, the VHI included 85 items taken from patients' reports of the impact of their voice disorder on various aspects of their lives. These were then administered to 65 patients with voice disorders and the results subjected to tests for internal consistency and reliability. This testing identifies items that best represent the scale's content and contribute to its overall reliability. Through this process the original 85 items were reduced to 30. These 30 items were found to reflect three domains in equal proportions: a 10-item functional subscale, a 10-item emotional subscale, and a 10-item physical subscale. The items are expressed in first person, for example, "I use the phone less often than I would like." Patients respond to each item using a 5-point scale from "0," indicating that the particular item was "never felt," to "5," indicating that the item was "always felt." Scores are determined for each domain and for the total VHI. The higher the score, the more severe the dysphonia and its impact are perceived to be by the patient.

Differences in VHI scores before and after treatment reflects the "amount" of improvement, or lack thereof, the patient has experienced as a result of treatment. The VHI has proved useful not only in comparing patients' perceptions of disability before and after treatment, but also in comparisons of patients with different pathological conditions. Benninger, Ahuga, Gardner, and Grywalski (1998) recently reported results of VHI testing on patients with different vocal pathological conditions, as well as on patients with chronic, non–voice-related, diseases. The authors found that patients with vocal fold paralysis had the highest level of pre-treatment disability, as compared with patients with masses or edema. Interestingly, the authors also used another tool for assessing general (not specific to a particular disorder) QOL and found that dysphonia represented a significant disability even when compared with sinusitis, sciatica, mental health, and angina pectoris. Rosen and Murry (2000) compared performances on the VHI across patients representing three types of disorders, including muscular tension dysphonias, benign vocal fold lesions, and unilateral vocal fold paralysis. Consistent with the Benninger et al. study, these authors found that, both before and after treatment (surgery, voice therapy, or both), patients with paralysis demonstrated the highest self-perception of handicap, whereas patients with benign lesions demonstrated the lowest perceptions of handicap severity.

Murry and Rosen (2000) described the possible utility of voice-specific outcome measures in treatment planning. For example, a patient with a low score on the VHI and a benign laryngeal pathological condition may be best served by voice therapy or conservative treatment, whereas a patient with a similar pathological condition but a higher self-perception of handicap may be more quickly directed to surgical intervention. These authors (1999) investigated relative self-perceptions of severity of handicap in a group of patients who shared a diagnosis of vocal fold paralysis. One group included working professionals; the second group comprised individuals who were retired. Results indicated that the working professionals demonstrated greater self-perceptions of handicap than did the individuals who were retired. Although this result might be anticipated when looking at group evidence, it should not be taken to suggest that voice is not important to retired persons. Rather, the findings lend support to the value of individual assessment and QOL testing in treatment planning.

In another study, Rosen and Murry (2000) compared scores on the VHI in singers and nonsingers who demonstrated various types of laryngeal pathological conditions. Interestingly, the professional singers appeared to view their dysphonia as a less severe handicap than did the recreational singers. The authors suggested several reasons for the findings, including the possibility that the VHI may not reflect the unique features of dysphonia in a singer, such as a diminished pitch range, or inability to control voice while singing softly at high pitches. Singers also might have sought treatment very early in their dysphonia, whereas nonsingers may have waited until the dysphonia had reached a handicap level. The authors caution that results of the VHI must be considered in the context of the particular population with which it is used.

The Voice-Related Quality of Life (V-RQOL) is another instrument designed specifically to assess QOL in patients with vocal handicaps (Hogikyan & Sethuraman, 1999). The instrument tests three domains, including social–emotional, physical, and general. Patients are required to consider 10 statements, such as, "I have trouble speaking loudly or being heard in noisy environments"; "I avoid going out socially because of my voice." Items were reportedly based on interviews with patients and with the authors' clinical experience. Responses are on a 5-point scale where "1" indicates no problem and "5" indicates that the problem is as "bad as it can be." Both domain and overall scores are easily manipulated to form 0–100 scales, with "0" indicative of poor V-RQOL and "100" an excellent V-RQOL. As a part of the development of this instrument, the scale was administered to patients reflecting a wide variety of voice disorders, and reliability, construct validity (ability of the instrument to identify significant differences in populations with regard to predetermined a priori hypotheses), responsiveness to change, and burden (related to how "burdensome" the instrument is to potential responders) were investigated. The authors concluded that the V-RQOL met appropriate standards of validity and reliability, was sensitive to change, and did not, in its administration, represent an undue burden to patients.

The V-RQOL instrument has been used to assess patients with vocal fold paralysis and patients with spasmodic dysphonia. In one investigation, patients with untreated vocal fold paralysis were compared with patients with paralysis who had undergone thyroplasty (Hogikyan, Wodchis, Terrell, Bradford, & Esclamado, 2000). Differences between the two groups were significant, with the treated patients generating scores significantly higher than those of untreated patients. In the second study, (Hogikyan, Wodchis, Spak, & Kileny, 2001), 27 new patients diagnosed with adductor spasmodic dysphonia completed the V-RQOL before, and 6 to 8 weeks after, administration of botulinum toxin injections. Mean scores improved from 30 to over 80 between assessments. The authors concluded that the instrument is capable of documenting and differentiating the effects of voice disorders and their treatments, and continue to investigate its utility.

One other instrument that should be mentioned is the Voice Outcome Survey (VOS) (Gliklich, Glovsky, & Montgomery, 1999). The VOS includes five items, one of which is related to a general appraisal of the speaking voice, and four others that address specific effects of the voice disorder, such as, "To what extent does your voice now limit your ability to be understood in a noisy area?" In developing the VOS, the authors investigated 56 patients with uncompensated vocal fold paralysis. Patients underwent testing before, and 6 months after, treatment for their paralyses. They also underwent tests of objective voice measures, including maximum phonation time and average intensity. The authors reported that the VOS was more sensitive to changes associated with treatment than other measures administered, and recommend the VOS because of its sensitivity, but also because, in their opinion, it meets appropriate standards of validity and reliability, is quickly and easily administered, and is highly sensitive to change. This scale may be limited in applicability to patients with unilateral vocal fold paralysis. However, it does set a model for development of disorder-specific scales by using fewer items, but ones that may be unique to or typical of a particular disorder.

Hartnick (2002) used a modified version of the VOS to assess the impact of voice disorder in children who either had a tracheotomy or had achieved surgical decannulation. In this study, parents and caregivers of children responded to items on the assessment instrument. After analyses of the construct validity and reliability of the instrument, one item on the scale related to swallowing, "How often do you have trouble with food or liquids going 'down the wrong pipe' when you eat, or find yourself coughing after eating or drinking?" was removed. On the resulting 4-item scale, the instrument demonstrated good ability to assess voice-related QOL in children, at least as perceived by a parent or caregiver. It was able to discriminate between two subpopulations; that is, children who had undergone decannulation were perceived by their parents (or caregivers) as less vocally handicapped than children who had tracheotomies, and the authors suggested that the parent-proxy tool may play a valuable role in assessing the effect of pediatric voice disturbances on the child's overall QOL. We might question whether a 4-item scale would be sufficient to differentiate a wide range of pediatric dysphonias from each other; for the specific problem and populations investigated by these authors, however, the small number of items was apparently appropriate.

Yet another voice-specific rating tool recently described is the Voice Symptom Scale (VoiSS) (Deary, Wilson, Carding, & MacKenzie, 2003). In the first phase of this instrument's development, 133 consecutive patients reflecting a variety of disorders were asked to list all of their voice-related problems. A total of 467 responses was subsequently classified by WHO (World Health Organization) criteria into 24 impairments, 15 disabilities, and 15 handicaps. One item (reported by only one patient) was removed, and the remaining 53 items constituted the pilot scale. Each item had two 5-point response scales, the first dealing with frequency of the complaint—all the time, occasionally—and the second dealing with the severity of the complaint—unbearable, slight.

The pilot scale was then administered to a large number of patients reflecting, again, a variety of voice disorders, excluding those related to malignancy or surgical causes for dysphonia. A principal components analysis performed on the results indicated that not all of the items were independent, and the scale was revised to eliminate redundant items. Based on the large number of incomplete responses to the questionnaire, in particular, to the severity scale, the authors also thought the scale needed to be shortened. Modified with these findings and concerns in mind, the final questionnaire comprised 43 items that appeared best able to capture information pertinent to patients' voice-related perceptions of handicap. The five components of the scale consider the impact of dysphonia according to "communication problems," "throat infections," "psychosocial distress," "voice sound and variability," and "phlegm, " respectively. These components are of particular interest because, as noted, they were derived from complaints expressed by a large number of patients with voice disorders. The authors of VoiSS note that further empirical exploration may produce further changes in the scale. Though longer than the other scales described, the development of the instrument to date is impressive in its attention to the reality of patient complaints and in its exposure to a large number of subjects.

Other patient-view scales have been developed, or are in various stages of development, that are at least in part directed to the impact of voice disorders on an individual's workplace performance. Smith et al. (1998), for example, investigated work-related effects of spasmodic dysphonia and vocal fold paralysis. Their results provide interesting insights into both the perceived and real liabilities associated with vocal disability and success in the workplace. Difficulty performing required work and keeping a job, or having to change jobs, were reported significantly more often in individuals with spasmodic dysphonia and vocal fold paralysis than in individuals who had no vocal impairment. In addition, these individuals viewed their vocal disability as having a significant potential to adversely affect future career options. In another study, Smith et al. (Smith, Gray, Dove, Kirchner, & Heras, 1997) found that teachers had experienced more missed days of work than other occupation groups for problems related to voice. Perceptions that voice problems had affected or would in the future adversely affect their career options were also more common to teachers than to individuals in other occupations. Our understanding of the impact of a voice disorder on an individual's ability to work is rudimentary, and, in fact, little information is available regarding the prevalence of vocal disability among various occupational groups. Obviously, such data, and instruments that can elaborate on these issues, are needed.

Assessing the impact of a voice disorder on an individual patient is important not only for determining treatment outcomes, or for determining the degree of disability associated with various types of pathological conditions, but also for establishing the relative worth of vocal disability. In this country, annual claims for workmen's compensation and occupational disability involve huge amounts of money. As one example, in 1998, the California Workmans' Compensation System spent a total of $6.4 billion on disability claims. By 2003, the overall cost of the worker's compensation system in California was estimated to approximate $29 billion. The consequences of such costs spiraling out of control have broad-reaching implications, including increasing costs of insurance that are generally absorbed by employers.

The need for instruments that can provide realistic insights into the determination of vocal disability is particularly acute. Although work-related claims involving voice or speech are less common than other types of claims—such as those for back or hand injuries or noise-induced hearing loss—vocal function disability appears to be on the increase as well. Cellular telephones, voice-activated computer systems, open-office designs that add to ambient noise levels, and buildings that create hostile breathing environments may be contributing factors. Major differences exist between many other injuries and voice injuries. Voice injuries are less well known and are poorly understood; they are invisible and often do not involve physical pain. In some instances, they may vary in severity because they are affected by amount and type of voice use. Not surprisingly, another major difference between vocal injuries and many other injuries is the lack of well-established guidelines for determining vocal disability. Little information is available to help a physician or voice clinician determine or elaborate on a worker's level of impairment or to formulate appropriate restrictions and limitations on voice use.

Many states use guidelines that have been developed by the American Medical Association (AMA) for this purpose. For speech impairment, this organization recommends three criterion measures for determining disability—audibility, intelligibility, and functional efficiency. Each has five levels of disability, depending on severity. In terms of audibility, for example, a class 1 impairment implies that the patient can produce speech of sufficient intensity for most everyday needs, although this occasionally may require effort and occasionally may be beyond the patient's capacity. A class 5 impairment in audibility implies that the patient can produce speech of intensity sufficient for none of the needs of everyday speech communication. The determination is made on the basis of observing the patient, reports from others, and on the results of selected tasks. Interestingly, a patient classified as demonstrating maximum disability on all three criteria, according to the AMA, would have only a 35% impairment of the "whole person."

State guidelines may be even less delineated and may vary from state to state. Again using California as an example, the California Labor Code (California Labor Code, State of California) defines permanent disability as a "medical or mental condition that results in an inability or reduced ability to compete in the open labor market." Both subjective and objective measures are considered in determining disability. Objective factors are defined as "those findings on physical examination that can be directly measured, observed or demonstrated, and are not in the control of the patient." Unfortunately, no objective criteria exist for determining voice or speech disability, and only two levels of disability can be assessed: "difficulty speaking," which is rated as a 10% disability, and "complete loss of speech," rated as a 50% disability. Beyond this, the determination can be made by an otolaryngologist, or a general practitioner, neither of whom is required to have any background in voice or speech.

In short, commonly used guidelines for determining occupational disability related to voice (and speech) are inadequate, in particular, for those individuals whose occupations rely heavily on voice use. Objective measures of voice, including perceptual and acoustic, have not been particularly helpful in resolving this situation. There is not wide agreement on a particular set of measures that should be used for this purpose, and the selection of almost any particular measure available could be argued in terms of its relevance to voice use in a work setting. Quality of life measures that address this issue from the patient's perspective have the potential to play a valuable role in determining the impact of vocal disability on this very specific matter, that is, how handicapped is an individual, and to what extent does this impact the ability to maintain or resume his or her usual occupation?

As noted, years of attention to objective acoustic, perceptual, and physiological measures, although beneficial to other purposes, have not yet yielded robust measures that are universally used to provide objective indices of vocal disability, differentiate vocal impairment across types of voice disorders, or to document treatment effects in individual patients. Such data are necessary to demonstrate the benefit of voice therapy to third-party payers and others, to help establish meaningful guidelines for determining vocal disability, and for many other purposes. QOL measures seem uniquely able to demonstrate significant differences, are easily and quickly administered, and are easy for both patients and professionals to understand. They are a relevant and excellent inclusion in the voice clinician's evaluation battery and should be administered to each patient before and at the termination of treatment. At this time, the VHI and V-RQOL scales are probably the most commonly used.

SPECIAL TESTING

Psychiatric

The link between personality and voice cannot be overemphasized. It is expressed in a multitude of ways by all speakers. Second only to our appearance, the voice serves as our identity, as a means of identification even in the absence of the visual presence. It serves as our emotional escape valve as we laugh, cry, scream in fear, or shout in rage. It speaks of our well-being, of our energy level, of our emotional state. We use it to cajole, to seduce, to energize, to subdue, to question, to arouse, to soothe, to scorn, to demand, to plead; in short, to give special meaning to our words. We are called on to use our voices to impart information; to express opinions; to defend our property, our rights, ourselves; to intercede for others; to influence others; and simply to interact with others. Our voices are a road between people, the road on which the words we speak travel. Is it any wonder, then, that the road is sometimes subject to bumps and irregularities, that it becomes altered because of excessive tensions and stresses? In some cases these changes are minor, requiring only that someone understand the situation and arrive at a way to resolve it. However, other problems require extensive repairs and require specific types of expertise if they are to be attended to properly.

The analogies are obvious. For some people, excess tensions are felt most keenly in the laryngeal area. The effect of these tensions may take time to gradually become apparent and bothersome, or they may reach a significant level rather quickly. There is a continuum of effect, from the very mild hoarseness that tends to come on at the end of the day to the constant and all-pervasive lack of voice. However, that continuum should not be equated with the depth of the problem. The degree of the dysphonic symptoms is not necessarily correlated with the "severity" of the problem.

Clinically, patients with voice disorders of psychological origin constitute a fascinating group of people, for many of whom an almost magical return of voice is not infrequent. Skill, understanding, and patience are required, but the reward for the speech–language pathologist is an immediate gratification that comes rarely in the practice of the profession. Specific procedures for the treatment of these kinds of problems are discussed in Chapter 9.

For a significant number of patients, however, the basic problems are much deeper. The patient is unable to give up the symptom, or unable to do so permanently. Such cases present a clear need for referral for psychiatric or psychological consult or counseling. Indeed, such a referral is also often necessary and helpful for those persons who, with our help, may be able to abandon their symptoms, but for whom there continue to be problems that need attention.

Case Study

R.W., an overweight and not very attractive 16-year-old boy, was referred for voice therapy with a diagnosis of dysphonia in the presence of a normal-appearing larynx. It was very difficult to engage R.W. in conversation. He responded to all questions in as few words as possible. He made only fleeting eye contact. The dysphonia was in its third month, and he had been out of school for that entire period on doctor's orders. Before this referral, he had already been on a regimen of voice rest and through several courses of pharmacological treatment with no change in symptoms. R.W.'s voice sounded very strained and tense. Hoarseness was present. Working very slowly, with constant encouragement and praise, we were able to elicit a normal voice quality. R.W. refused to recognize this change at first, but slowly became willing to use the good voice more frequently. Within a few therapy sessions, R.W. had full return of normal voice and was ready to return to school.

During the therapy sessions, the need for R.W. to see a psychiatrist or psychologist was raised with both him and his mother. With return of normal voice, a direct referral for such additional treatment was made. A month later, R.W. returned. His voice had worsened, with a full recurrence of earlier symptoms. Our referral for psychiatric follow-up had not been carried out. R.W. was seen again for several sessions of voice therapy, during which he continued to be very closed in all respects. Once again voice was restored, and once again referral for psychiatric consultation was made, even more strongly. Two months later, R.W.'s mother wished to schedule another appointment because once again the symptoms had recurred. She was advised that it was not appropriate to continue voice treatment, because it was clear that numerous other problems were present and particularly in view of the lack of follow-up on our referral for psychiatric consultation.

Moving slowly is often necessary when referral for counseling or psychiatric examination is being considered. A sense of trust must be built between the clinician and the patient. The clinician must be sufficiently attuned to the patient's needs to be able to approach the referral in the manner that will be most likely to be accepted. Referrals made too abruptly may be totally rejected by the patient, who also may reject the person making the referral. When that occurs, the patient may be lost to follow-up or treatment of any kind for some time. This is what we were hoping to avoid in R.W.'s case. Unfortunately, even our best efforts sometimes do not bring about the desired result.

Consider all possible causes of a presenting problem before adopting the diagnosis of psychogenic voice disorder. A number of neurological disease processes have early symptoms that may be very similar to those presented by patients with emotionally based problems. Furthermore, the presenting symptoms and signs of psychogenic dysphonia sometimes may be similar to those of spasmodic dysphonia or musculoskeletal tension/hyperfunctional dysphonia. These patients present with minimal visible laryngeal changes, if any, and with symptoms that may be mystifying and histories that may be confounding.

Neurological

Case Study

J.R., a 37-year-old woman with intermittent dysphonia, had been examined and treated by several otolaryngologists over a period of months with no change in her vocal status. She was then referred for a trial of voice therapy. J.R. reported a rather troubled social history involving a very difficult recent divorce preceded by a number of years in an abusive marriage during which she had suffered attempted strangulation and blows to the neck. She and her 7-year-old son were now living with a friend as she was trying to put her life in order. Her voice symptoms began during the course of the divorce process. She described a "gravelly" quality that came on gradually with any extended period of talking but that cleared when she was able to rest and be silent for a while. She denied any other physical symptoms.

The history thus far seemed to suggest a classic voice disorder of psychological origin. During the initial evaluation, however, the clinician was impressed with this patient's attitude, forthrightness, and overall affect. Furthermore, we noted the gradual worsening of voice as the evaluation progressed, which J.R. attributed in part to having engaged in much conversation during a lengthy car trip from her home to our office. Trials of diagnostic therapy procedures were totally ineffective in eliciting improved voice quality. J.R. was subsequently referred for neurological examination, and a diagnosis of myasthenia gravis was made.

Referral for neurological examination is usually well accepted by patients. It should be considered when laryngeal findings are either negative or suggestive of disordered coordination of laryngeal function, when the voice symptoms are neither consistent with nor explained by the history, when changes in vocal output cannot be altered by behavioral approaches, and whenever there is a family history of neurological problems. Similarly, patients usually respond well when referred for further medical examinations, as might be indicated when gastroesophageal reflux is suspected as a key factor in the voice problem.

Imaging

The past decade has seen major growth and development of increasingly sophisticated imaging technology: computed axial tomography (CT scan), ultrasound, magnetic resonance imaging (MRI), and positive emission tomography (PET), to name a few. Although these techniques are being widely used to determine the location and extent of disease, data relevant to phonatory behavior are only beginning to appear. Baer and others (Baer, Gore, Boyce, & Nye, 1987; Baer, Gore, Gracco, & Nye, 1991; Lufkin & Hanafee, 1985; Stark, Moss, Gamsu, Clark, & Gooding, 1984) have applied the technique of MRI to the study of normal neck anatomy and the physiology of the vocal tract during speech acts. Leboldus and his colleagues (Leboldus, Savoury, Carr, & Nicholson, 1986) showed how MRI imaging could be applied to the diagnosis and treatment of ENT problems. Others (Shaefer, Freeman, Finitzo, Close, & Cannito, 1985; Swenson, Zwirner, Murry, & Woodson, 1992) have used MRI to study brain dysfunction in patients with spasmodic dysphonia. MRI and CAT images show considerable promise in the study of normal and disordered speech and voice. At this time the primary use of these techniques for the study of laryngeal function is in the realm of research. Clinical use is more limited, in part because of limitations of the equipment, limited equipment availability, and the cost of the procedures.

SUMMARY

The voice history is a critical part of the diagnostic process not only for the information obtained but also because of the relationship that is established between the clinician and the patient during the information gathering. The first section of this chapter was devoted to a discussion of the skill involved in the interview process. The content of the interview was presented in some detail and included the following sections: the problem and its effects, the developmental history of the problem, its onset and duration, the variable or consistent nature of the problem and associated symptoms, the patient's health history, and vocational, social, and recreational histories.

The array of techniques used in the examination and testing of the voice have been described in the second and third sections of this chapter. Examination of the larynx can be carried out through both direct and indirect methods. Technological advances have substantially increased our ability to visualize not only the structure of the larynx and supraglottal vocal tract but also the dynamic physiology of both phonatory and nonphonatory behavior. The examination procedures described include indirect laryngoscopy, direct laryngoscopy, flexible fiberoptic laryngoscopy, stroboscopy, ultra-high-speed photography, and ultrasound. Advantages and disadvantages of each are discussed.

Laboratory testing procedures provide documentable and measurable evidence of vocal function. These techniques sometimes provide indirect evidence about the functional status of the larynx. They include acoustic measures of fundamental frequency and its variability, functional limits of the voice relative to frequency and intensity, periodicity and stability of the voice as evidenced by measures of perturbation, and visual evidence of the acoustic components of the voice as displayed in a spectrogram or an acoustic spectrum. Physiological studies provide further evidence and information about the larynx and the voice. These include electroglottography, photoglottography, inverse filtering of airflow, and electromyography. Testing of respiratory function is another aspect of physiological function that can add to the total data pool in selected cases.

We have also included various forms of noninstrumental evaluation of the voice, usually carried out by the speech–language pathologist but useful to all who examine and work with the voice-disordered patient. These noninstrumental methods include critical listening, observation, and description. Formalization of the kinds of observations that should be made, both auditory and visual, will help to focus the examiner's careful attention to the variety of clues that can be obtained about vocal function through this approach. The clinical trial involved in a diagnostic therapy approach allows the examiner to test hypotheses and extend the observations.

Objective measurements that can be made without the benefit of any equipment more sophisticated than a stopwatch are also discussed. Although fairly simple to obtain, these measurements can be extremely useful in establishing baseline measures of vocal function and subsequently to chart progress or assess the results of treatment. Within this section we also have discussed the need for suitable audio recordings and the types of equipment that are appropriate to address this need.

The final section of this chapter dealt briefly with the need for referral for additional testing. Such testing may include psychiatric or psychological consultation, neurological examination, medical assessment for associated problems, and special imaging techniques.

SUGGESTED READINGS

Bernstein, L., Bernstein, R. S. (1985). *Interviewing, a guide for health professionals* (4th ed.). Norwalk, CT: Appleton-Century-Crofts.

Hersen, M., & Turner, S. M. (1985). *Diagnostic interviewing*. New York: Plenum Press.

Levinson, D. (1987). *A guide to the clinical interview*. Philadelphia: WB Saunders.

Maple, F. F. (1985). *Dynamic interviewing, an introduction to counseling*. Beverly Hills, CA: Sage Publications.

Chapter 9

Surgical and Medical Management of Voice Disorders

Three general approaches are used for the management of voice problems, no one of which necessarily excludes the others. These approaches are (a) surgical, (b) medical, and (c) behavioral.

The first two are discussed in this chapter; the behavioral approach is discussed in Chapter 10. Although these approaches are being presented separately, often ideal treatment requires the use of combined treatment modalities. For example, the patient who has sustained traumatic laryngeal damage in an automobile accident may first be a surgical candidate. However, after surgery and healing, this patient may well benefit from vocal rehabilitation to reestablish the best possible voice production. Many patients who present with vocal fold lesions also have reflux disease and poor vocal hygiene. All three modalities of treatment are required: surgically remove the lesion, medically control the reflux, and behaviorally correct vocal misuse.

Surgery is considered the more radical treatment approach because of the need to cut into tissues to remove abnormal growths, or to physically alter or augment the shape or position of structures. A review of surgical techniques that are being used in the management of laryngeal problems with a phonatory component is presented in the first section of the chapter. The medical approach to the treatment of voice disorders refers to techniques that are not as invasive or do not involve surgical ablation, reconstruction, or alteration; these are discussed in the second section.

SURGICAL MANAGEMENT

Introduction

Surgical management of the larynx is a broad topic by virtue of the multitude of pathological conditions that can affect the larynx. The main premise for whatever procedure is performed is that the function of the larynx be preserved or improved. For example, in a patient who has a poor voice because of a unilateral polyp, surgical removal should yield an improvement in the voice and possibly the respiratory airway. A patient with a unilateral immobile vocal fold who undergoes a medialization procedure should have improved voice and be able to swallow without aspiration.

Over the past 30 years, tremendous changes and advances have taken place in all aspects of vocal fold surgery. Indeed, 30 to 40 years ago, it was not unlikely for vocal fold lesions to be "plucked" or "stripped" using cupped forceps by either direct or indirect non-magnified laryngoscopy. Scarring of the vocal fold with subsequent dysphonia was not an uncommon result. Hirano (1981) helped usher in the modern age of vocal fold surgery by detailing the structure of the vocal folds in his "cover-body" theory. The concept that a delicate mucosa moves on a cushion of ground substance over a rigid ligament and muscle hundreds of times per second leads to the appreciation of the needed precision required in preserving this vibrating tissue.

Advances have been made in binocular microscopes, laryngoscopes, microinstrumentation, surgical techniques, and lasers. Complementing these surgical improvements have been advances in complementary medical and behavioral care of the larynx. Surgical treatment is often combined with medical and behavioral treatments to yield the best possible functional outcome for a patient. Certainly any laryngologist will attest to the importance of perioperative voice care to surgical outcome. Such care should include training in proper vocal hygiene, and medical control of reflux disease, asthma, or other causes of inflammation.

The goals of surgical management are to conserve, reconstruct, or improve laryngeal functions—phonation, swallowing, and respiration.

Surgical procedures may be divided into four major groups:

1. Endoscopic removal of pathological tissue (microphonosurgery)
2. Surgical correction of the position, shape, or tension of the vocal fold(s) by endoscopic approach or by external approach
3. Surgery directed at neuromuscular function of the vocal folds
4. Surgical repair or reconstruction for partial loss or deformity of the larynx. These abnormalities can arise from blunt or penetrating trauma, congenital abnormalities, acute or chronic diseases, or exposures.

History

The earliest laryngeal examinations and procedures done in the mid-1800s were performed indirectly by way of mirror visualization. The first direct laryngeal examinations were carried out in 1852 and in 1895. Kirstein laid out the advantages to this approach (discussed in Zeitels, 1995). The next half-century saw the introduction of suspension laryngoscopy; the Jackson laryngoscope with a sliding, removable blade; and the use of the microscope although still with monocular vision. Surgical procedures consisted of removal of lesions and vocal fold injections for paralyzed vocal folds. In the 1960s, binocular visualization was possible because of wider laryngoscopes commercially produced by Pilling and Storz. Von Leden first published the term *phonosurgery*, indicating the desire to have vocal fold surgery address a major function of the larynx: phonation (von Leden, 1991).

Over the next two decades, better understanding of laryngeal anatomy and physiology led to a greater appreciation of vocal fold function and need for newer techniques to address this expanded knowledge base. At the same time, technological advances in illumination led to better visualization and increased precision of surgery. The operative microscope was combined with the CO_2 laser (Jako, 1972), resulting in a potent new tool. Consistent improvement in voice results was continually sought.

In the 1990s, laryngology blossomed as a field, with advances in all aspects from the basic science of histology, wound healing, and pathophysiology to evaluation using stroboscopy to surgical refinements. Endoscopic visualization, development of fine micro-instrument sets, precision laser micro-manipulators, and newer materials for implantation all occurred. These advances have clearly resulted in improved surgical techniques and thereby also improved surgical outcomes. Quality of life scales and outcome studies have validated that voice disorders have a negative impact on an individual's functional, emotional, physical, and vocational life, all of which are significantly improved by intervention (Murry & Rosen, 2000).

MICROPHONOSURGERY

Instrumentation

To perform precise microlaryngeal surgery, proper state-of-the-art instrumentation is needed. Because of its anatomic location and differences in individual anatomic features, direct imaging of the larynx has historically presented a challenge. Several generations of laryngoscopes have been designed, each with the goal of giving the best view of the larynx. Anatomic factors that influence which particular scope may fit best include neck thickness, neck mobility, tongue size, mandibular arch dimensions, dentition, and mandibular mobility. Benefits of the later generation of laryngoscopes are the ability to adjust the dimensions of the scope in situ, the incorporation of suction channels and fiberoptic light carriers, and placement of these channels in such a manner as to reduce interference with passage of instruments through the scope. An example of a newer laryngoscope is shown in Figure 9.1. It features a triangular end to conform to the shape of the glottic introitus. The Zeitels glottiscope features a lateral recessed area near the mouth for easier instrument entry. It further provides the ability to slide out the floor of the scope, if intubation through the scope is needed, and permits interchangeable blades. It also can be used with a suspension gallows attached to the operative table, giving true suspension (Fig. 9.2). Most laryngoscopes are retained on a Mayo stand or the patient's chest by a torsion–fulcrum method (Fig. 9.3).

Instrument sets have also been refined over the past decade. The Ossoff-Pilling microlaryngeal set features a variety of picks, spatulas, scissors, and forceps. Other companies, including Medtronic (Xomed/Microfrance) and Storz, in cooperation with other leading phonosurgeons such as Sataloff, Bouchayer, and Kleinsasser have designed instrument sets. Powered tissue shavers (Figs. 9.4 and 9.5), initially developed for orthopedic surgery, then revised for sinus surgery, and now for laryngeal surgery, have a suction channel that draws the soft tissue into the tip of the rotating instrument and slices it off. The main role for shavers is currently for papilloma removal (Fig. 9.6). Ongoing refinements in increasingly fine scissors, tissue-grasping forceps, and dissecting picks continue to be seen. To dissect out or excise relatively small lesions such as an intracordal cyst or a polyp with minimal mucosal disruption, the array of fine instruments is essential. Accessory instruments such as coagulators, disposable blades, and injectors are also now available.

Lasers have been used for over 30 years to remove laryngeal tissue. They are machines that generate collimated, monochromatic emission of energy directed at a target. Each type of laser generates a specific wavelength, which has different effects on tissue. The CO_2 laser was the first and still most commonly used laser for laryngeal surgery, because its energy can be passed in a straight beam to the larynx. The wavelength of energy is absorbed by the water-rich vocal folds and can be used to incise, vaporize, and coagulate tissue.

Some controversy exists regarding the appropriateness of use of the laser for procedures requiring exquisite refinement, precision, and control. The primary concern

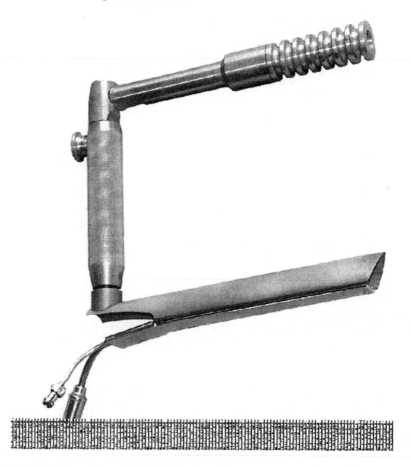

Figure 9.1. The glottiscope. (From Zeitels, S. M. [2000]. Phonomicrosurgery I: principles and equipment. *Otolaryngology Clinics of North America, 33,* 1047–1062.)

has been that the thermal injury in laser use extends beyond the target area and can damage adjacent tissue. Full knowledge of the concept of power density is mandatory for a surgeon using a laser. Some advocate using iced saline on the vocal folds before using the laser. Another concern has been the belief by some that healing time is longer after laser surgery than "cold knife" techniques. Benninger (2000) and Hormann et al. (Hormann, Baker-Schreyer, Keilmann, & Biermann, 1999) reported studies in which results of laser vs. "cold knife" excisions were compared. There were no significant differences between the outcomes. Abitbol (2000) has demonstrated that a laser, in the proper hands, is equivalent to "cold-knife" excision.

CONCEPTS OF MICROPHONOSURGERY

The basis for operative technique stems from understanding the gross and fine structure of the larynx. Hirano (1981) first described the "cover-body" anatomy of the vocal fold, and this led to modeling of how this structure oscillates (see Chapter 3 for full discussion). Gray and his colleagues (Chan, Gray, & Titze, 2001; Gray, Titze, Alipour,

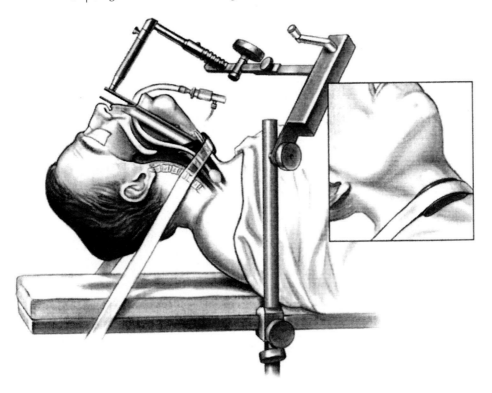

Figure 9.2. The patient in extension–flexion position is maintained in elevated vector suspension by the Boston University Gallows (Pilling Co., Fort Washington, PA). A ridged tubular extender is attached to the universal modular glottiscope handle to facilitate application of the vector force. One-inch silk tape and a soft laryngeal cushion are used to apply external counter-pressure. (From Zeitels, S. M. [2000]. Phonomicrosurgery I: principles and equipment. *Otolaryngology Clinics of North America, 33,* 1047–1062.)

& Hammond, 1999a; Gray, Titze, Alipour, & Hammond, 1999b; Gray, Titze, Chan, & Hammond, 1999) are responsible for further delineating many of the vocal fold components (elastin, collagens, laminin, hyaluronic acid), their location within the lamina, as well as their properties within the layered structure of the vocal fold. The complex detail of the epithelial attachment to the superficial lamina was described, as well as the effects of aging, vocal and surgical trauma, and pathological conditions. This work has impacted on the practice of surgical excision and on the goals of research, specifically tissue regeneration.

Preoperative considerations include accurate diagnosis, the patient's general health status, the patient's desire and need for improved voice, timing that takes into account postoperative needs for proper care and optimal healing, and informed consent. A recommendation for surgery comes only after thorough examination, consideration being given to appropriate conservative approaches, and the diagnosis being as definitively confirmed as possible. Intraoperative goals include minimal normal tissue disruption, maximum preservation of the lamina layered structure, and promotion of rapid healing. These goals can be met by using state-of-the-art knowledge and techniques of laryngeal visualization, incision placement, dissection, and wound healing.

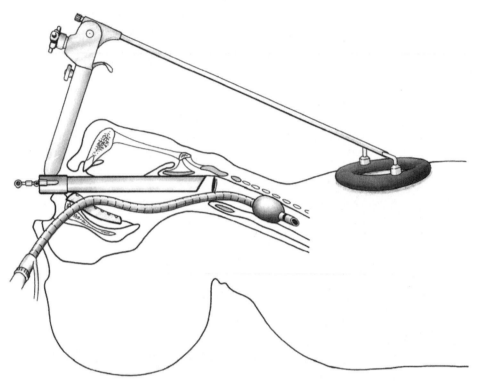

Figure 9.3. Laryngoscope placement for surgery. (From Kleinsasser, O. [1990]. *Microlaryngoscopy and Endolaryngeal Microsurgery.* [Third ed.] Philadelphia: Hanley & Belfus, Inc.)

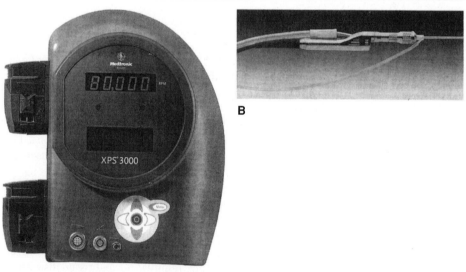

Figure 9.4. The XPS 3000 Powered ENT System (Medtronic Xomed, Jacksonville, FL). **A.** Motor. **B.** Handpiece. From Dyce, O. H., Tufano, R. P., & Flint, P. W. (2003). Powered instrumentation in laryngeal surgery. *Operative Techniques in Otolaryngology-Head and Neck Surgery, 14,* 12–17.

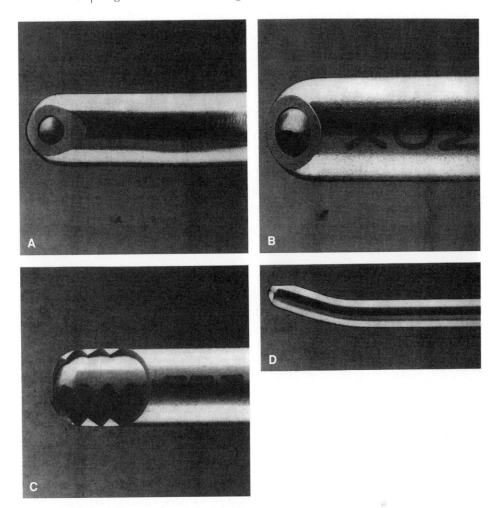

Figure 9.5. **A.** The 3.5-mm round blade cutting surface. **B.** The 4.0-mm round blade cutting surface. **C.** The 4.0-mm tricut blade cutting surface. **D.** Profile view of the 4.0-mm round blade, demonstrating the tip angulation (Medtronic Xomed, Jacksonville, FL). From Dyce, O. H., Tufano, R. P., & Flint, P. W. (2003). Powered instrumentation in laryngeal surgery. *Operative Techniques in Otolaryngology-Head and Neck Surgery, 14,* 12–17.

After obtaining exposure, the vocal folds are inspected for any other abnormalities not appreciated by stroboscopy. Concurrent subglottic scars, infra-lesion or lateral small sulci, or micro-webs are often found. Infusion of saline is very useful to inflate the epithelium from the ligament. This not only gives information about the depth of adherence but also provides additional buffer margin for dissection. With laser use, this additional volume can serve to dissipate the laser-generated heat. Care must be taken to visualize exactly where the incisions are to be made.

Creating a straight edge and preservation of the subepithelial stroma are needed to prevent tethering of the new epithelium to the fibrous ligament and allow for mucosal wave motion.

Postoperative care is extremely vital to the final surgical outcome. Medications such as antibiotics, antireflux medications (proton pump inhibitors), mucolytics, cough

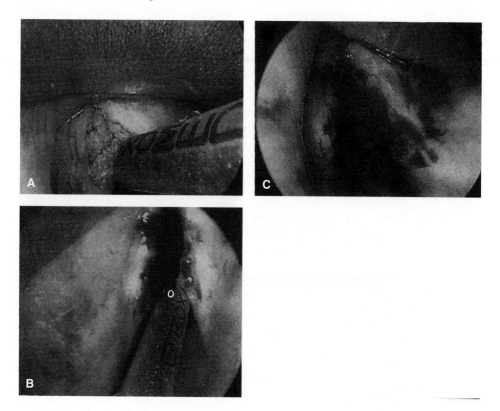

Figure 9.6. **A.** Endoscopic view with a Dedo laryngoscope. **B.** Access to posteriorly based lesions **C.** Endoscopic view after resection. From Dyce, O. H., Tufano, R. P., & Flint, P. W. (2003). Powered instrumentation in laryngeal surgery. *Operative Techniques in Otolaryngology-Head and Neck Surgery, 14,* 12–17.

suppressants, and steroids may be prescribed for a short postoperative period according to the surgeon's practice. Although there is general agreement concerning the need for some period of voice rest, the duration is still debated. Some advocate no need for any period of voice rest, others advocate fairly lengthy periods of silence, and most fall between those two extremes. Our approach is individualized and adapted to the patient. It is based on the extensiveness of the surgery, knowledge of the patient's typical presurgical voice use patterns, and the patient's ability to comply with instructions. Most typically patients are instructed to maintain complete voice rest for a period of 3 days to a week. Furthermore, all patients are instructed to avoid laughing, crying, coughing, and throat clearing. We see the patient for repeat stroboscopy 4 to 5 days postoperatively before allowing increased voice use. Depending on our findings on visualization of the surgical site, we determine how much talking the patient should be instructed to do. The patient is instructed in a gradual return to normal voice use, using a modified vocal rest approach. Care after surgery for professional voice users is a particularly important and difficult time. Once again, very specific and firm instructions have to be given but must be adapted to the individual. Cooperation between the otolaryngologist and the voice clinician is vital in both the preoperative and postoperative care of the surgical patient (see Chapter 10). Adherence by the patient to the preoperative and postoperative instructions should result in a voice restored to normal function. That is the ultimate goal.

NON-NEOPLASTIC VOCAL FOLD TISSUE REMOVAL

Vocal Fold Nodules

Vocal nodules are not typically treated by surgery. The initial treatment of choice is voice therapy. In fact, if the nodular-appearing lesions do not regress with behavioral care, then the clinical diagnosis should be re-examined. Almost all nodules in children disappear spontaneously by the end of adolescence. Surgery is indicated only in extreme cases in which the effects of the voice abnormality on the child are serious and voice therapy has not been effective. In cases of long-standing poor vocal hygiene, there may be a more mature fibrous component of the nodule and surgical removal may be needed, but again only when voice therapy has not been effective.

In adherence to the concepts previously mentioned, when nodules are surgically removed, only the excessive tissue should be ablated. The postsurgical result should be a vocal fold with a minimal surgical wound (Fig. 9.7). Forceps are used to grasp just

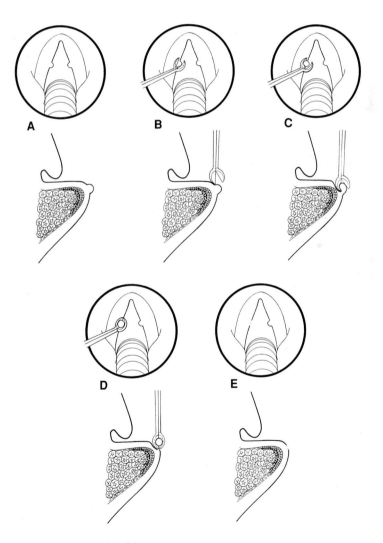

Figure 9.7. Surgery for vocal fold nodules.

the nodule, and then the vocal fold is trimmed using scissors. The wound will be small with superficial lamina exposed, but new epithelium will grow and cover this defect. If deeper structures are exposed or excessive tissue removed, then healing will be slower, and scar tissue may develop that will interfere with normal vocal fold vibration.

Vocal Fold Polyps

Small unilateral polyps usually do not respond to medical or behavioral treatments and require surgical removal. Again, only excessive mass should be removed; care should be taken not to excise healthy tissue. Small polyps are removed by incision, dissection, and trimming with scissors. The result should be a normal contour of the vocal fold (Fig. 9.8) with minimal epithelial defect.

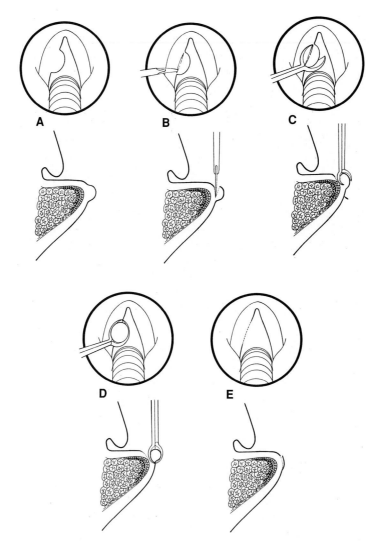

Figure 9.8. Surgery for vocal fold polyps.

In the case of polypoid degeneration, after an incision is made in the upper margin of the vocal fold edge, the mucosa is retracted medially to expose the myxoid stroma. Gentle teasing of this jelly-like material to remove excess is performed. Suctioning of the material may lead to excessive loss of lamina volume and subsequent scarring or tethering to the ligament. The mucosal edge is redraped onto the superior surface, and the excess mucosa is conservatively trimmed. The edges of mucosa may be left to rest together, or be "spot welded" with laser, or sutured to try to get better primary closure and quicker healing (Woo, Casper, Griffin, Colton, & Brewer, 1995). Steroids may be infiltrated into the wound.

Removal of hemorrhagic polyps may be easier with CO_2 laser, but the power density should be kept at a minimum. Excessive energy or an unfocused laser can lead to blanching of the lamina propria and vocal scarring. Abitbol (2000) advocates using iced-saline gauze on the vocal folds to minimize the chance of thermal injury.

Mucoceles and Pseudocysts

These lesions are exophytic fluid-filled lesions, typically small, and found along the medial margin of the vocal fold. Removal is the treatment of choice. The technique is similar to removal of polyps with maintenance of an adequate amount of lamina and mucosal cover. These are not true cysts, and therefore minimal tissue removal is needed.

Sulcus

Vocal fold sulcus is a depression along the margin of the vocal fold. This depression can extend to the vocal ligament and result in poor vibratory capability. Surgical repair of sulcus presents a difficult challenge for the surgeon. The depressed mucosa must be removed, which then exposes the deep layer of the lamina propria or vocal ligament The goal is to re-establish a mucosal wave and, of course, to avoid reparative scar and stiffness. Several surgical techniques, described below, have been proposed, and each has its proponents, but none are certain of success. In some instances there may be a need for a second procedure to medialize the fold to obtain glottic closure. Scarring and re-adherence of mucosal tissue to the underlying layers are both possible sequelae of surgery that result in stiffness of the vocal fold and dysphonia.

Sulcus removal (Hirano, 1975) involves making a mucosal incision along the upper edge of the sulcus. The stiff tissue around the sulcus is elevated from the underlying normal tissue and removed (Fig. 9.9). The mucosal edges are then approximated and held in place by means of fibrin glue or suturing.

Pontes (1993) described a novel approach to this difficult problem. The "mucosal slicing technique" is based on the idea of scar rearrangement. With the larynx exposed in standard fashion, a mucosal incision is made superior to the sulcus. The tissue involving the sulcus is elevated from the deeper vocal ligament. The elevated mucosa is then vertically sliced at several locations and for differing lengths. The wound is then left to heal secondarily. The postoperative rehabilitation may take months and involves aggressive vocal therapy (Fig. 9.10).

Epidermoid Cyst

A true cyst within the vocal fold requires complete surgical removal. In dissecting the cyst, care must be taken to observe and remove any tracts that may connect the cyst to the surface epithelium. The incision, in general, should be as small as possible to allow

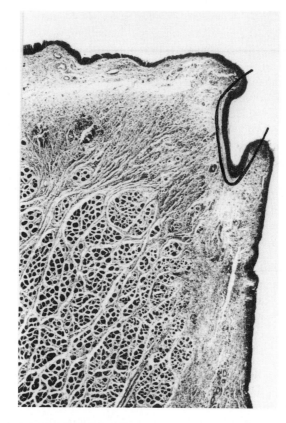

Figure 9.9. Histological picture of sulcus vocalis.

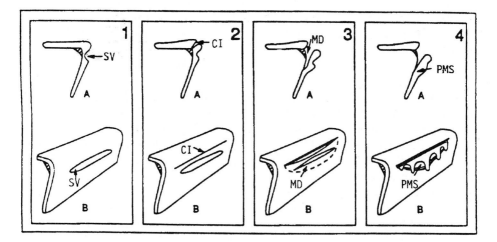

Figure 9.10. Schematic of direct vocal fold mucosa surgery. **A.** Vocal fold frontal view. **B.** Vocal fold medial view. **Panel 1:** Schematic of sulcus vocalis (SV). **Panel 2:** Cranial incision (CI). **Panel 3:** Detachment of the mucosa (DM). **Panel 4:** Positioning of the mucosa slices (PMS).

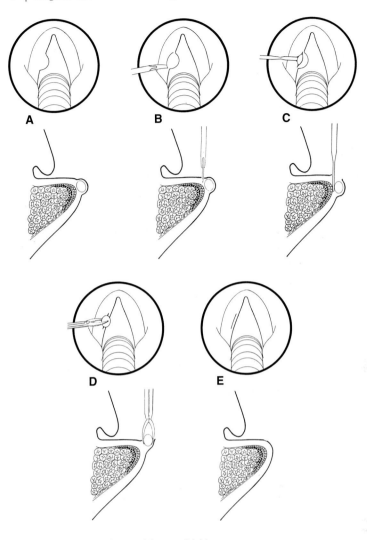

Figure 9.11. Surgery for epidermoid cyst of the vocal fold.

cyst removal. Lateral incisions preserve the vibrating edge of the vocal fold, because the dissection is within the lamina. The mucosal incision also may be made over the cyst if it is located medially. The cyst is carefully elevated from the underlying structures and removed. The mucosal edges are re-opposed and may be left to heal or be sutured. Injection of steroid is recommended by some in an attempt to reduce scar formation (Fig. 9.11).

Granuloma

These lesions most often arise at the vocal process and can be bilateral. The causes include laryngopharyngeal reflux disease (LPR), intubation, and poor vocal hygiene. Granulomas should first be treated aggressively with vocal hygiene programs and anti-reflux therapy. Proton-pump inhibitor use is very effective. Recurring cases also may benefit from a Botox (Allergan, Irvine, CA) injection to weaken the adductor force at the level of the vocal process.

When nonsurgical modalities do not prove effective or the granulomas are very large, causing respiratory distress, they need to be treated surgically. Surgery is best conducted under general anesthesia. Jet ventilation, regular intubation with a small endotracheal tube, or apneic technique all are useful to get exposure of the posterior glottis. Jet ventilation is a technique in which a fine jet of gas oxygen, nitrogen, or appropriate combination is directed into the trachea, replacing the need for an endotracheal tube. The major portion of the granuloma is first removed with the use of scissors and forceps, leaving the perichondrium covered. Steroid can be injected into this base. Whereas use of CO_2 laser has been advocated in the past, the risk of thermal injury to the perichondrium with recurring lesion formation is significant.

Epithelial Hyperplasia, Dysplasia, and Keratosis

Thickened epithelium can occur because of repeated trauma. This can take the form of physical, chemical, or even thermal trauma. Chronic vocal misuse, smoking, and chronic inhalant chemical exposure all can cause epithelial pathological conditions. Microscopic examination will aid in determining whether the diseased tissue is benign thickening, pre-cancerous, or cancer. The indications for surgical removal of diseased tissue are to re-establish a vibrating, straight vocal fold margin and provide a specimen to the pathologist to see whether any additional treatment is needed. Removal of the causative agents occasionally may result in a reduction or even disappearance of hyperplastic and dysplastic epithelium. To provide a clean, complete specimen, infusion followed by "cold" removal technique is ideal. Inclusion of the basement membrane in the specimen is essential for correct diagnosis. CO_2 laser can be used for "planing" down exophytic lesions, but again, care must be taken to not cause thermal injury (Fig. 9.12).

Laryngeal Papilloma

The most frequently occurring benign neoplasm of the larynx is papilloma. Both adults and children can be affected and require numerous surgical procedures because of the high recurrence rate. The juvenile form often is more aggressive in growth and has a much more frequent impact on the airway. When papillomas extend into the trachea, they may cause obstruction as they proliferate. Surgical excision is required, and the morbidity associated with such surgery is very complex, with implications for respiratory problems in addition to voice problems.

Surgery consists of removal of these surface lesions. The CO_2 laser for papilloma vaporization was widely accepted and is still often used. "Cold knife" removal is also possible and has been aided by use of the infiltration technique noted earlier and advancements in the design of surgical instruments. Proponents of this technique cite its benefits as: more control of the depth of injury, quicker postoperative healing, and less time expense. The recent introduction of laryngeal "shavers" offers a "cold" technique with more rapid removal of lesions. An inner rotating blade trims the tissue that is drawn into the tip of the outer sheath and suctioned up the blade and into the tubing.

Scarring of the vocal folds is not an unusual sequela of the multiple surgical excisions that are often required. Anterior webs and false-true vocal fold webs also may occur

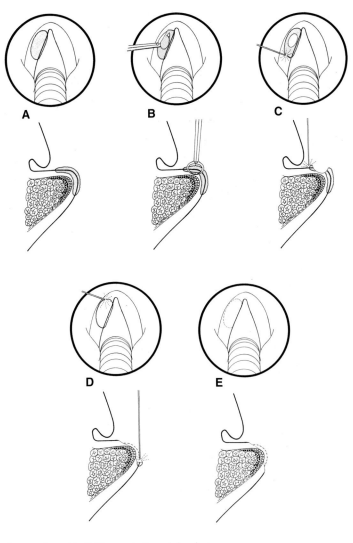

Figure 9.12. Surgery for epithelial hyperplasia and dysplasia.

and are difficult to treat. Prevention of these complications is paramount. Staging the removal of extensive and bilateral papilloma to avoid webbing is encouraged.

As with any disease that is difficult to treat, nonsurgical therapies also have been tried but have not proved universally effective, including indole-3-carbinol, ribavirin, alfa-interferon, and photo-dynamic therapies. Injection of cidofovir into the papilloma may significantly suppress papilloma growth and reduce the frequency of surgeries. The use of cidofovir is not without the potential of long-term risks.

Glottal Carcinoma

The location and the extent of glottal carcinoma dictate whether surgery can be successful in effecting a cure. Details of tumor staging and specific pathological conditions of glottic carcinoma are beyond the scope of this chapter. In general, small tumors

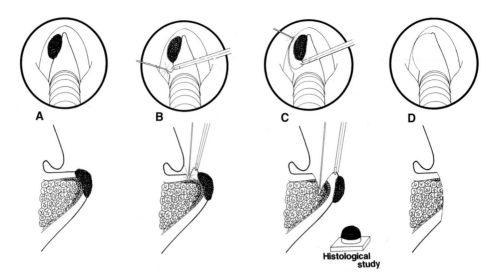

Figure 9.13. Surgery for early glottal carcinoma.

confined to the membranous vocal fold may be removed with the aid of laser for hemostasis. Care is given to excellent exposure, careful mapping of the extent of disease, particularly below the vocal fold, anteriorly, and in the ventricle. Use of rigid angled telescopes provides this capability. Infusion technique also provides information about the depth of the lesion and vocal ligament involvement.

Once the excision has begun, maintaining orientation of the specimen is needed so margins can be determined. To obtain a margin around the tumor, part and sometimes all of the thyroarytenoid muscle must be taken. In this case, cancer removal takes priority over vocal result. With large tissue loss, incomplete closure or areas of nonvibrating tissue can result (Fig. 9.13). Additional surgeries can be offered to rehabilitate the voice, and some of these techniques are discussed later in this chapter.

Some glottic carcinoma also can be treated successfully with radiation therapy alone. Voice outcomes for patients treated by surgery versus radiation therapy have been studied and are comparable.

SURGERIES TO MODIFY VOCAL FOLD POSITION, SHAPE, OR TENSION

Vocal Fold Medialization

The most common laryngeal framework surgery is vocal fold medialization. Medialization is desired when a glottic gap exists and laryngeal function is compromised. One or both vocal folds may be medialized, depending on the need. Indications include unilateral vocal fold immobility, vocal fold atrophy, or bowing caused by aging, scarring, or neurological disease. The two main classes of techniques for membranous vocal fold medialization are injection of material into the vocal fold or implantation of material into the larynx by an external approach. Movement of the membranous fold to close the glottis often yields improvement. Additional manipulation by arytenoid rotation and position adjustment in the immobile arytenoid may provide even greater benefit by closing a posterior glottic gap. In a survey by Rosen in 1998, 70% of respondents only performed medialization thyroplasty. Although it is technically more difficult, arytenoid adduction may be needed to achieve the best functional result.

Injection Technique

Injection of material into the membranous vocal fold is often done to correct an incompetent glottis (i.e., the inability to close the glottis). There are other indications, however, for vocal fold injection that do not have medialization as their goal. Among these are steroid, collagen, or fat injected as treatment for scar and Botox as treatment for adductor spasmodic dysphonia.

Numerous materials have been used in the attempt to "plump up" a paralyzed or otherwise incompetent vocal fold. The intent of such a procedure is to provide glottic closure, thereby improving vocal function and in some instances also decreasing aspiration. Teflon, autologous fat, collagens (Zyderm, Zyplast/Collagen Corp., Palo Alto, CA), acellular dermis (Cymetra/LifeCell, Branchburg, NJ), fascia, and more recently, hydroxyapatite (Radiance/BioForm, San Mateo, CA) and hyaluronic acid all have been used for medialization. Overwhelming evidence of long-term granuloma formation and substance migration associated with Teflon has placed that substance in disfavor and disuse. The other materials (collagen, fat, Cymetra) have been shown to have volume loss in animal studies or by clinical follow-up. Different methods of preparing autologous fat have been tried. Less traumatic harvesting, washing with different media, and gentler delivery of the fat all have been tried with unpredictable success. Radiance is a recently available material that was found to neither dissipate nor be absorbed. Long-term outcome with Radiance in humans is not yet known but our experience suggests some resorption occurs. Hyaluronic acid is now being used, but, again, long-term studies have not been done. The ideal goal of injecting a substance with viscosity similar to that found in normal vocal folds that would theoretically not only fill space but also provide vibratory behavior and would not resorb is still a goal.

The techniques for intrafold injection include transoral injection using either indirect laryngeal rigid mirror examination and monitoring by flexible endoscopy (Fig. 9.14), or with a direct laryngoscope, usually under general anesthesia (Fig. 9.15). Transcutaneous injection through the cricothyroid space (Fig. 9.16) also can be done, again monitoring by indirect or direct visualization.

When injection is done in the office by an indirect transoral method, the mucosa of the pharynx and larynx is anesthetized with Cetacaine (Cetylite Industries, Pennsauken, NJ) or lidocaine solution. The internal branches of the bilateral superior laryngeal nerves also may be anesthetized. The trachea can be instilled with lidocaine as well. Injection is performed while the patient sits with the mouth open and the tongue pulled forward. A curved laryngeal needle is used to administer the substance into the fold, and its effect is monitored with visual and auditory methods as the injection proceeds.

Injection using a direct laryngoscope is performed with local mucosal anesthesia with sedation or under general anesthesia. The patient is placed in a supine position. The larynx is exposed with the use of a direct laryngoscope and viewed under an operating microscope. Injection is performed by means of a specially designed injection set such as the Arnold-Bruening (Pierre, SD) Teflon injection set (also useful for fat). Other materials can be injected through a butterfly needle held by a forceps.

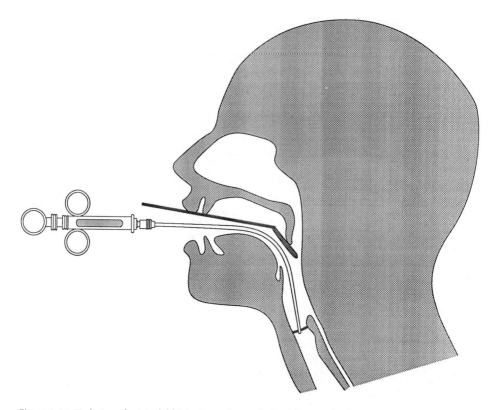

Figure 9.14. Technique for intrafold injection using an indirect laryngeal mirror.

For transcutaneous injection, the nasal, pharyngeal, and laryngeal mucosa is anesthetized with lidocaine. A fiberscope is inserted through the nose to expose the larynx. It is coupled to a video camera, and the fiberscopic image of the larynx is viewed on a television monitor screen. Local anesthesia is administered through the cervical skin at the cricothyroid space. The needle for intrafold injection is inserted into the larynx through the cricothyroid space, and its location is monitored by moving it back and forth medially. The effect of injection is monitored by visual and auditory methods during the procedure.

The target location for the injected material depends on the material and the goal of the injection. Collagen can be injected near the surface within scar tissue to try to "soften" the scar by inducing collagenase activity, or it can be injected deep into the thyroarytenoid (TA) muscle for medialization.

Radiance used for medialization should be injected lateral to the TA muscle. Fat and collagen for medialization should be placed into the body of the TA muscle. Collagen, fat, and hyaluronic acid for scar elevation and superficial lamina reconstitution should be injected into the deep lamina.

Implantation

The basic principle of augmentation is to insert the material to be used medial to the thyroid cartilage at the level of the vocal folds, thus pushing the vocal folds medially (Fig. 9.17). This is often referred to as type I, referring to Isshiki's classification

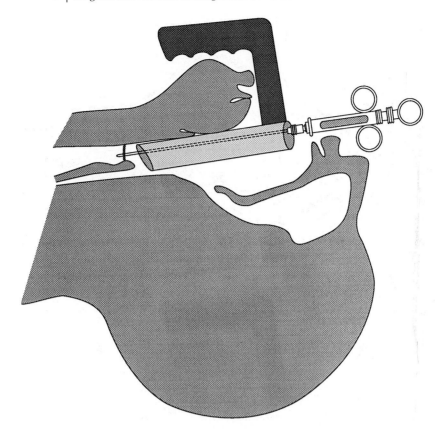

Figure 9.15. Intrafold injection under a direct laryngoscope.

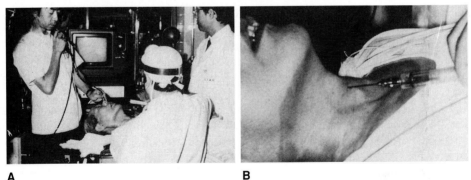

A   **B**

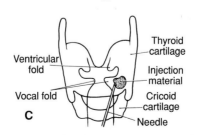

C

Thyroid cartilage
Ventricular fold
Injection material
Vocal fold
Cricoid cartilage
Needle

Figure 9.16. Transcutaneous intrafold injection. **A.** An entire view during the procedure. **B.** A view of the patient's neck. **C.** Schematic presentation of the technique.

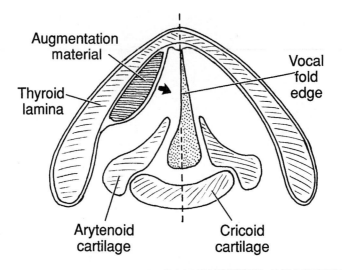

Figure 9.17. Schematic presentation of the principle of surgical augmentation developed by Meurman (1952) and modified by others.

of framework procedures. Many materials have been tried and continue to be used, including commercially available kits with premanufactured implants.

A silicone block (Silastic/Dow, Midland, MI) is commonly employed as the augmentation material. This was popularized by Netterville (1993), who describes how to individually carve the block into the ideal dimensions and how to best insert it. Of all the implant materials, this is the cheapest but does require some skill and experience in getting the best shape. Cartilage autograft from the upper part of the thyroid cartilage or nasal septum or rib cartilage also can be used. Another popular choice is Gore-Tex (Gore, Newark, DE) as the implant (McCulloch & Hoffman, 1998). Advocates state that no carving is needed, and the ribbon of material can be layered into the glottis and placement adjusted as needed to give better voice quality.

The surgery is performed under local anesthesia with sedation. A shoulder roll is used to help extend the neck. After infiltrating with local anesthetic and preparing the neck, a horizontal skin incision is made over the lower aspect of the thyroid cartilage and extended to the side in need of correction. The strap muscles are divided in the midline and the thyroid cartilage exposed. A window is created by removal of a block of cartilage approximately 4 × 10 mm. A drill may need to be used in cases of ossification. The upper surface of the vocal fold is normally situated at the midlevel of the anterior angle of the thyroid cartilage. The posterior end of the membranous vocal fold is usually located at the anteroposterior midpoint of the thyroid lamina. Therefore, the augmentation material should be placed in the lower and anterior quadrant of the thyroid lamina. The inner perichondrium is then exposed.

The augmentation material is located lateral to the vocal fold. Some advocate preservation of the inner perichondrium to prevent the prosthesis from working its way into the glottis or to prevent significant muscle atrophy or scarring. Others believe that without incising the perichondrium, the medialization will be more limited. The size and location of the material are adjusted by aurally monitoring the patient's voice during the procedure. Simultaneous visual monitoring with the use of a fiberscope attached to a monitor is also useful. Once the material is located in the right place, it is sutured to the thyroid cartilage to prevent postsurgical migration.

Silastic, Gore-Tex, and cartilage require some three-dimensional consideration when being placed. Commercially available kits without the need to carve or adjust the shape are available. The Montgomery Thyroplasty Implant System (Boston Medical Products, Westborough, MA) with polymer implant and the VoCoM hydroxyapatite implant set (Gyrus ENT, Bartlett, TN) are each designed for ease of placement. The Montgomery comes with a series of shim sizes for the male larynx and the female larynx. The VoCoM set also has a series of available sizes as well as locking shims to adjust the location within the created window.

These pre-made kits offer some advantages, such as the ability to try various implant sizes and perhaps save time; they are relatively expensive and limit the versatility of the custom-carved or placed materials. If the created window in the thyroid cartilage is just superior or not level to the desired level of the vocal fold, a carved shim can be made offset to be oriented to the level of the vocal fold. In such instances, the pre-made shims would not be able to be ideally situated.

Arytenoid Adduction

The basic principle of this technique (Fig. 9.18) is to rotate the arytenoid cartilage by traction of the muscular process in the direction of the adductor muscles, adducting the tip of the vocal process to the midline (Isshiki, Tanabe, Ishizaka, & Board, 1977).

The surgery is conducted under local anesthesia with sedation. A cervical skin incision is made starting at the midline and extending to the anterior border of the sternocleidomastoid (SCM). The strap muscles are divided in the midline, and the posterior edge of the thyroid lamina is exposed on the affected side by removal of

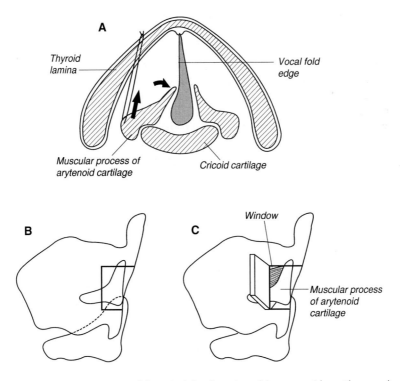

Figure 9.18. Schematic presentation of the principle of rotation of the arytenoids cartilage, as developed by Isshiki (1977).

the inferior constrictor. The muscular process of the arytenoid cartilage is exposed by either dislocating the cricothyroid joint and removing the inferior thyroid cornu or by removing a 1-cm window of the posterior ala without disturbing the joint. A Prolenc (Ethicon, Piscataway, NJ) suture is placed through the muscular process and the attachment verified by a pull while simultaneously watching the glottis through a flexible scope on a monitor. The desired vector of retraction is parallel to the pull of the lateral cricoarytenoid (LCA), thus rotating the vocal process medially. Holes are made in the anterior inferior thyroid ala just off the midline, and the sutures pass anteriorly through these holes. When the best voice is obtained by pulling and rotating the vocal process, the thread is tied. As with the implant placement, the surgeon must continually assess whether the desired glottic configuration has been achieved and be willing to make adjustments. Additional sutures with other pull vectors may be needed.

A second method of medializing the arytenoid is by placement of a large silastic prosthesis through the thyroplasty cartilage window into the paraglottic space (Hong, Kim, & Kim, 2001). Theoretical potential downsides to this technique are TA muscular atrophy and interference with nerve regeneration.

Cricoarytenoid Fixation

In addition to rotation of the arytenoid with suture fixation, direct fixation of the arytenoid cartilage may provide more precise height adjustment to the vocal fold and help reestablish more comparable tension. During the surgery, the arytenoid is approached in a similar fashion to the adduction procedure. The cricoarytenoid joint is opened, and the arytenoid is suture fixed in the optimal location to the cricoid cartilage.

Vocal Fold Lateralization

Vocal fold lateralization is indicated in the treatment of bilateral vocal fold immobility attributable to either paralysis or bilateral ankylosis of the cricoarytenoid joints. Not every patient with these conditions requires surgery, but it is indicated for patients with dyspnea who do not want a tracheotomy tube. Its purpose is to improve the airway sometimes at the expense of making the voice worse. However, when conservation of voice is part of the surgical plan, a phonosurgical approach often can help to minimize effects on the voice.

There are several techniques to lateralize the vocal fold. One of the earlier techniques was the lateral fixation by external approach. This "open" lateralization is described as being done with general anesthesia. A suture is placed in the arytenoid cartilage and is drawn laterally as the glottis is inspected. Postoperative aspiration, breathy dysphonia, and infection are risks. With the introduction of the CO_2 laser arytenoidectomy, the lateral fixation technique has fallen out of favor. Ossoff (Ossoff et al., 1984), using a CO_2 laser, removed one arytenoid cartilage and the attachment to the vocal ligament and found that the airway was improved, with acceptable voice and swallow results. The principle of arytenoidectomy is to remove the arytenoid cartilage and widen the posterior glottis (Fig. 9.19). The posterior glottis, or the intercartilaginous portion of the glottis, accounts for approximately 60% of the entire glottal area. Therefore, a widening of the posterior glottis is very effective in improving the adequacy of the airway. Initially, there is a large posterior chink due to the absence of the arytenoids. With wound healing, however, this space does diminish to where the voice is generally good and no aspiration occurs.

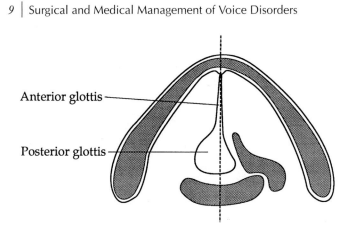

Figure 9.19. Schematic presentation of the principle of arytenoidectomy.

Kashima (1991) has advocated a lateral cordotomy with the laser. In this technique, the false vocal fold is removed and then the posterior vocal fold is incised to a depth of the ipsilateral perichondrium. Although this sounds as though the voice result would be disabling, he reports on airway improvement and maintenance of good voice in most patients.

Others have modified these techniques. Linder (1992) used fibrin glue to seal the vocal mucosal flap to lateralize it. Ejnell (1993) used an endoscopically guided, transcutaneous suture to hold the vocal fold laterally. Botox has also been used in the post-resection period to prevent muscle contracture and a scarred, closed glottis.

Thyroarytenoid myectomy constitutes a lateralizing procedure and also has been described for treatment of spasmodic dysphonia. This can be done endoscopically with a laser or by a thyroplasty approach.

VOCAL FOLD SURGERY TO ADJUST LENGTH AND TENSION

Data regarding the long-term functional results of vocal fold tensing, lengthening, or shortening are not available. We have included descriptions of these surgeries, although it appears that they have not met with resounding success and are perhaps little used at this time.

The major purpose of vocal fold tensing surgery is to raise the vocal pitch. Indications for such surgery may include (a) excessively low pitch in females caused by an androgen or by pregnancy; (b) the low vocal pitch of the "sex-transferred" female; and (c) senile, flaccid vocal folds. Surgical techniques to tense the vocal folds have been developed by Isshiki (1977); LeJeune, Guice, and Samuels (1983); and Tucker (1985). Zeitels (1999) described a unilateral tensing as an adjuvant procedure in correction of the paralyzed vocal fold. Two major surgical techniques accomplish vocal fold tensing: cricothyroid approximation and anterior commissure advancement.

The basic principle of cricothyroid approximation is to create a permanent approximation of the cricoid arch to the thyroid cartilage anteriorly (Fig. 9.20), simulating the function of the cricothyroid muscle (Isshiki et al., 1977). Recall that contraction of the cricothyroid muscle results in the approximation of the cartilages and that in

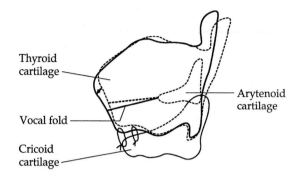

Figure 9.20. Schematic presentation of the principle of cricothyroid approximation, as developed by Isshiki.

so doing the vocal folds are lengthened and tensed. Both the decreased mass of the folds and the increased tension under which they are held result in a faster vibratory rate, and thus a higher pitch is produced. Zeitels has advocated performing this on the paralytic side when a patient undergoes medialization thyroplasty (1999). This provides additional tension and may enhance voice results. The surgery is best conducted under local anesthesia so that the pitch of the voice can be monitored during the procedure. However, if the patient is unable to tolerate the procedure, general anesthesia is given. After horizontal cervical skin incision, the thyroid and cricoid cartilages are exposed. They are approximated anteriorly by means of non-resorbable sutures (see Fig. 9.20). Stretching of the vocal fold can be visually monitored with the use of a fiberscope.

The basic principle of anterior commissure advancement is to stretch the vocal folds by advancing the anterior commissure anteriorly relative to the arytenoid cartilages (LeJeune, Guice, & Samuels, 1983).

The surgery may best be performed under local anesthesia, but general anesthesia is employed when the patient cannot tolerate the procedure. After a horizontal cervical skin incision, the thyroid cartilage is exposed. A vertical cartilage flap is made in the midportion of the thyroid cartilage. The flap may be inferiorly based, superiorly based, or sectioned both superiorly and inferiorly. The flap is advanced and stabilized in place by inserting a shim of tantalum posterior to the flap (Fig. 9.21). When local anesthesia

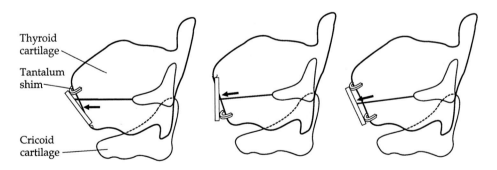

Figure 9.21. Schematic presentation of the principle of anterior commissure advancement, as developed by LeJeune, Guice, and Samuels (1983) and Tucker (1985).

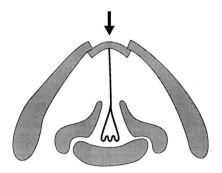

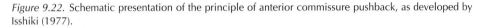

Figure 9.22. Schematic presentation of the principle of anterior commissure pushback, as developed by Isshiki (1977).

is employed, changes in vocal pitch are aurally monitored during surgery. Vocal fold stretching can be visually monitored by means of a fiberscope. The major purpose of vocal fold slackening surgery is to reduce the tension of the vocal folds (Isshiki et al., 1977). Vocal pitch can be lowered as tension is reduced. This procedure has been tried also in patients with adductor spasmodic dysphonia as a means of reducing tension (Tucker, 1989; Isshiki, Haji, Yamamoto, & Mahieu, 2001).

In this surgery, the anterior commissure is moved closer to the arytenoid cartilage. The surgery can be performed under local anesthesia, so auditory monitoring of voice change is available. A vertical cartilage flap is made in the midportion of the thyroid cartilage and pushed back and secured (Fig. 9.22). The anterior commissure is thus moved closer to the arytenoid cartilage.

SURGERY TO ALTER LARYNGEAL NEUROMUSCULAR FUNCTION

Neuromuscular Surgery for Vocal Fold Paralysis

The ideal treatment for vocal fold paralysis would be to restore normal innervation of all laryngeal muscles. This is, however, not possible in cases of axonotmesis and neurotmesis. That the recurrent laryngeal nerve contains both adductor and abductor fibers creates one of the major problems in the neurosurgical treatment of vocal fold paralysis. Simple nerve anastomosis or nerve graft of the recurrent laryngeal nerve causes misdirected reinnervation, as shown in Figure 9.23. Some neurons that originally innervated one of the adductor muscles now may innervate the abductor muscles,

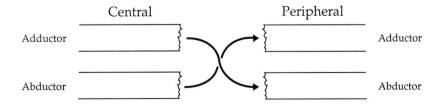

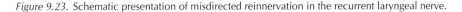

Figure 9.23. Schematic presentation of misdirected reinnervation in the recurrent laryngeal nerve.

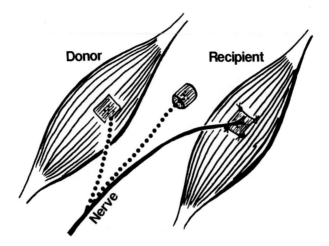

Figure 9.24. Nerve–muscle pedicle procedure.

whereas some neurons that were originally for abductor innervation now act to innervate the adductor muscles, causing a disturbance in vocal fold mobility (Hiroto, Hirano, & Tomita, 1968; Siribodhi, Sundmaker, Atkins, & Bonner, 1963).

Experimental and clinical attempts have been made to avoid the problems resulting from misdirection of regenerated nerve fibers. Among these is a nerve–muscle pedicle procedure (Fig. 9.24) wherein a muscle pedicle (along with its nerve) obtained from the ansa hypoglossi nerve that innervates the omohyoid, sternothyroid muscles (Tucker, 1978; Tucker & Rusnov, 1981) is chosen as the donor. In cases of bilateral abductor paralysis in which the vocal folds are fixed near the midline, causing dyspnea, the nerve–muscle pedicle is implanted into the LCA muscle. This technique has not met with wide acceptance or success.

Other surgical approaches for bilateral paralysis have been reported and include anastomosis of the split phrenic nerve to the posterior cricoarytenoid (PCA) or to the nerve branch innervating the PCA muscle (Crumley, 1983) and anastomosis of the split vagus nerve to the nerve branch of the PCA (Miehlke & Arnold, 1982).

Recurrent Laryngeal Nerve Section for Spasmodic Dysphonia

Dedo first reported unilateral section of the recurrent laryngeal nerve (RLN) for spasmodic dysphonia (Dedo, 1976). The procedure and its various modifications were then carried out by many laryngologists. The immediate postsurgical results were reported to be highly successful and appreciated by many patients (Dedo, 1976). However, the long-term results showed conflicting results, with many reports of symptom recurrence (Aronson & DeSanto, 1981; Aronson & DeSanto, 1983) In 1991, Netterville (1996) modified the procedure with a more distal lysis and, in a follow-up report, noted that most were without spasms but with breathy dysphonia. Although some few surgeons continue to perform the procedure today, most have abandoned it because of the too-frequent return of symptoms despite continued paralysis of the vocal fold caused by the sectioning procedure. Selective bilateral denervation of the TA muscles for adductor dysphonia has been reported (Berke, 1999). The distal nerve ends are microsutured to the ansa cervicalis to prevent aberrant reinnervation by the recurrent nerve. Initial results appear good. However, with the introduction and effectiveness of Botox injection as a treatment modality, albeit not a cure, the recurrent laryngeal nerve surgeries are not common. (See discussion later in this chapter under "Medical Management.")

SURGICAL RECONSTRUCTION FOR PARTIAL LOSS OR DEFORMITY OF LARYNX

Surgical removal of lesions and medialization surgery to correct the glottis with an immobile vocal fold are the most common laryngeal surgeries. Less frequent and often much more complicated surgeries involve surgical correction of tissue loss and deformity. These laryngeal problems can be congenital or acquired through surgical or other trauma. Creativity and careful planning are essential in reaching the optimal result. Several stages may be necessary, such as tissue transfer or stent placement and removal. A surgical treatment plan must be individualized, but a few examples will be covered.

Anterior Glottic Webs, Stenosis

Anterior glottal webs can be a rare congenital malformation or is caused by trauma, including surgical trauma. The web can be thin or thick, small or involving most of the membranous vocal edge. Two major surgical techniques may be used for its removal: endolaryngeal surgery and external approach thyrotomy. There has been a trend toward endoscopic treatment as instrumentation has improved.

With the vocal folds exposed by direct laryngoscopy under general anesthesia, the web is sectioned at the midline or partly removed. A CO_2 laser may be used for this purpose (Fig. 9.25), but "cold" scissor division also can be done. After removal of the web, a silastic plate is placed in the glottis to prevent postsurgical reunion of the vocal folds. To do this, suture is passed through a rounded, trimmed piece of silastic sheeting. A 14-gauge needle is passed transcutaneously into the larynx. One end of the thread is passed down the laryngoscope and out the needle to the skin. The needle is withdrawn and re-introduced into the larynx, and the second limb of the thread is passed through the glottiscope and out through the needle. Both ends are tied over a soft piece of silastic

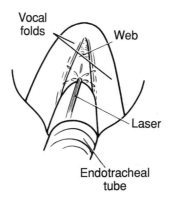

Figure 9.25. Endolaryngeal surgery for anterior glottal web.

or plastic on the anterior neck skin. Lichtenberger (2002) has made a specialized endolaryngeal needle. This allows transcutaneous sutures to be placed from the lumen side toward the skin.

The silicone plate is removed endolaryngeally 1 to 2 weeks after surgery. This can be done by cutting the external suture and retrieving the plate with a flexible bronchoscope or curved indirect laryngoscopy forceps.

The silastic sheet also can be sewn in place within the larynx using Prolene suture. To prevent reforming the web, the silastic can be placed along the length of one of the vocal folds. The silastic, however, does need to be retrieved under general anesthesia, but this affords another opportunity to inspect the glottis and remove any granulation that may have grown around the implant.

An alternative to stenting after web or scar division is application of mitomycin-C to prevent reformation of the lesion (Unal, 2004).

Posterior Glottic Stenosis

Posterior glottic stenosis may be caused by a web or scar, typically between the arytenoid cartilages. Prolonged intubation in the intensive care unit (ICU) setting may lead to arytenoid fibrosis, interarytenoid scarring, or webbing. A laser can be used to divide the web, but mucosa should be preserved as much as possible. Microflaps of mucosa are lifted, the submucosal scar removed, and the mucosa returned in place. Stents also can be placed, but a second procedure is needed for removal. Additional procedures to establish an adequate airway include the lateralization procedures described earlier.

An external approach can be used for thick and more extensive webs. A midline cervical incision is made followed by splitting the strap muscles to expose the thyroid cartilage. The midline cartilage is then divided. Endoscopic monitoring is desired to ensure that on entering the larynx, the web is divided evenly and in the center. The attachment of the vocal fold to the cartilage is rechecked and, if not secure, can be sutured to the cartilage. The wound is sutured closed in layers.

More difficult-to-treat problems involve greater tissue loss of the larynx because of burns, cancer surgery, or trauma.

Surgical ingenuity is important. Mucosa from the surrounding laryngeal region can be rotated or advanced into place. Rib cartilage grafts in addition to silastic or Gore-Tex shims can be useful for medializing the thickened, scarred hemilarynx.

MEDICAL MANAGEMENT

Although certain disease states of the larynx result in conditions that are irreversible and need to be addressed surgically, most people who have voice problems are managed without surgery. Medical management plays a large role in the treatment of many conditions. This section addresses those disease states that typically require the medical and pharmacologic expertise of the otolaryngologist.

Infection

Viral laryngitis is the most common type of laryngeal infection. The disease is self-limited but may last 5 to 10 days. Findings may consist of laryngeal edema, inflammation, thickened mucus, and decreased vibratory behavior of the vocal folds. Coughing caused by laryngeal irritation is also often a symptom.

Bacterial infection of the larynx is often confused with infection of viral origin. Laryngitis also may be attributable to allergies or bacterial infections elsewhere in the head and neck region, such as sinusitis. Antibiotics are frequently prescribed for patients who present with upper respiratory symptoms. Bacterial epiglottitis has become exceedingly rare but supraglottitis still occurs and presents as sore throat and voice changes. Depending on the clinical picture, admission for airway observation or intubation and intravenous antibiotics may be needed. Tracheotomy is rarely needed.

Fungal laryngitis also occurs, particularly in the setting of the asthmatic, diabetic, or immunocompromised patient. Chronic steroid inhaler use can cause fungal infections. On examination, the larynx has whitish material along the margin. The pharynx also may be involved and have whitish-yellow patches. These are best treated with the oral antifungal agents, particularly Diflucan (Pfizer, New York, NY), for up to 3 weeks. The pulmonologist should be informed of the infection to see whether the medication or the delivery of the medication can be changed.

Systemic Disease

Numerous systemic diseases may have effects on the voice. These may be from the disease itself or from the treatment or medications for that disease. For example, cardiac disease may lead to voice problems caused by medications that reduce body water volume. Although frustrating for the patient, they must be reminded of the importance of taking these medications unless another is available that does not have the same side effects. Sarcoidosis, amyloidosis, and Wegener's granulomatosis all can have diffuse involvement with thickening of the laryngeal tissue in characteristic patterns. The voice may have improvement as systemic treatment is instituted. Metastatic neoplastic disease also may involve the larynx, including breast or renal cell carcinoma or lymphomas. These are uncommon lesions.

Arthritis is a systemic disease that also can affect the cricoarytenoid joints, causing ankylosis and immobility. Rheumatoid nodules can occur in the membranous vocal folds, causing voice problems. A well-known endocrine abnormality affecting the voice is hypothyroidism. Typically, water retention accompanies this condition, and the vocal folds thus become edematous and the pitch of the voice lowers with the increased mass. Diabetes is a disease that can affect the larynx in several ways. Wound healing is impaired, and diabetics are more susceptible to glottic scarring from intubation. Dehydration or water loss may contribute to voice problems. Sjögren's syndrome, lupus, and other autoimmune disorders may have dysphonia as a symptom.

Allergy

Patients often comment that their voice problem is "allergy-related." However, few studies have looked at the direct organ effect of allergies. How much immunoglobulin E (IgE)–mediated histamine release occurs in the larynx is not clear. Likely, the effect on voice is secondary to other organs being affected by allergies, such as the nose and lower airways. Before prescribing medications, an extensive exploration should be done to try to determine what in the patient's environment may be the cause. Some of the most common allergens are year-round—molds, animal dander, and dust mite. Allergy testing is warranted to determine the triggers and aid in deciding a medical treatment plan. Antihistamines may help the voice by improving the health of the other organs, may help the larynx itself, but may harm the larynx by causing dryness. Topical nasal steroids and immunotherapy, however, are very effective for allergic rhinitis and do not adversely affect the vocal folds. As noted earlier, many patients with allergies also take numerous medications, including inhaled steroids. Long-term use of these inhalants can cause laryngeal and voice problems.

Laryngopharyngeal Reflux

Over the past decade, this disease has received much attention as a frequent cause of laryngeal disease. Only half of patients have symptoms of "heartburn." Lesions associated with reflux include epithelial growths, generalized inflammation of the folds, and laryngeal cancer. On endoscopy, the posterior larynx is erythematous and edematous, and thick mucus abounds.

Diagnostic testing is not always mandatory, and empiric treatment is reasonable in most circumstances. Barium swallow, upper gastrointestinal (GI) series, and esophagogastroduodenoscopy often cannot detect reflux disease that affects the upper aerodigestive tract. Koufman (1996) has promoted the term "laryngopharyngeal" rather than "gastroesophageal" to reflect that the two are different clinical entities. Dual pH probe monitoring is the current "gold standard" to detect reflux occurring at the level of the posterior larynx. It is also possible that non–acid-related enzymatic reflux occurs, causing inflammation. Recommended behavioral changes include wearing loose-fitting clothing, eating frequent small meals, not eating 2 to 3 hours before bedtime, and elevating the headboard 6″. Dietary restrictions such as alcohol and caffeine avoidance and avoidance of spicy foods are also recommended. When obesity is present, dietary restrictions for weight loss are important.

Medication is often prescribed, particularly around the time of any surgical intervention. Over-the-counter medications include antacids that are taken after meals to neutralize acids and acid suppressants including H-2 blockers such as cimetidine, famotidine, nizatidine, or ranitidine. Prokinetic agents that increase gastric emptying and increase lower esophageal pressures can be used. Proton pump inhibitors are a far more effective class of medications (omeprazole, lansoprazole, rabeprozole, pantoprazole). These are best taken 30 minutes before a meal and typically only once daily.

Noxious Inhalants

Smoking of tobacco or illegal substances is irritating to the exposed mucosa. Smoking cessation is very difficult and has been most successful when attempts are coupled with support groups and taking medications such as Zyban (GlaxoSmithKline, Research Triangle Park, NC) or Wellbutrin (GlaxoSmithKline). Nicotine gum and patches have failed to help most smokers to stop. Nonsmokers who are exposed to tobacco smoke have eye and respiratory tract irritation (U.S. Department of Health and Human Services, 1986) and increased risk of cancer.

Neurological Conditions

Spasmodic dysphonia (SD) is a neurological condition affecting the larynx. The cause is not known. Most patients have a strained, strangled, and choppy voice quality. Extensive studies have been performed on this condition, including electromyogram (EMG), confirming this as a form of focal dystonia. There are two types: adductor and abductor (Aronson, Brown, Litin, & Pearson, 1968). The adductor type is marked by irregular hyperadduction of the vocal folds, which disrupts voicing. Abductor dysphonia is characterized by whispered segments typically following the production of an unvoiced consonant. Indeed, it has been described as a disruption in the ability of the vocal folds to close. A mixed pattern, referred to by some as a third type of SD, is present in some patients with one form predominating.

Treatment consists of periodic injections of botulinum toxin (Botox) into the affected muscle group(s). Botox is thought to act by blocking neurotransmitter release at the neuromuscular junction, thus causing muscle weakness/paralysis. The most common type of Botox is "A," but many other subtypes have been described. Resistance because of antibody formation to the toxin has been shown in relatively few individuals. Botox B (Myobloc, Solstice Neurosciences, Inc., Malvern, PA), however, can then be used. The therapeutic amount is individualized and based on the historical duration of benefit and degree of side effects. The technique of Botox injection is the same as described earlier in the chapter. Teflon-coated needles are typically used so an EMG can be done to confirm placement. Transoral or transcutaneous methods can be used. After injection, there is a 1- to 3-day delay in the clinical effect that at first is breathiness. After 7 to 14 days, the voice strength returns without the spasms. The usual duration of benefit is 3 to 4 months until symptoms return as neural sprouting occurs and new neuromuscular junctions are formed. Over time, as a patient receives many injections, fibrosis occurs, making needle insertion more difficult.

For adductor spasmodic dysphonia, the Botox is injected into the TA or LCA. Most injections are given bilaterally in dosages of 2.0 units/side as a starting point. The amount may be reduced in future injections if the breathy period is prolonged or any significant aspiration occurs.

Treatment of patients with abductor SD with Botox injection is more difficult. The PCA muscle is approached either transcutaneously by rotating the thyroid cartilage or by passing the needle from anterior to posterior through the thyroid lamina. The latter is more difficult because of ossification of the cartilage. Placement is verified by having the patient sniff while recording the EMG. Removal of a posterior segment of thyroid cartilage may improve access for PCA injections.

Other Neurological Diseases

VOCAL TREMOR

Tremor is characterized by a rhythmic oscillation of the voice. It is not uncommon to note the presence of some tremor associated with SD. However, some patients present only with tremor. Although Botox treatment for tremor is not as effective as it is for SD, we have numerous patients who find the injection of Botox to be helpful. They experience a reduction in severity of tremor, an improvement in intelligibility, and less effort involved in speaking. They tend to follow a similar pattern of return of symptoms within a number of months as do the SD patients. Medications have not been found to be helpful.

PARKINSON'S DISEASE

This is a well-known, progressively deteriorating neurologic disease marked by tremor, rigidity, and bradykinesia. The voice may be an early site of deterioration, with decreased intensity and a muffled quality. A more complete discussion of this disease is found elsewhere in this text, as is the behavioral speech treatment. Although the clinical status of the patient as seen in movement characteristics is often improved with a variety of medications, these drugs have no beneficial effects on voice or speech (Larson, Ramig, & Scherer, 1994).

MYASTHENIA GRAVIS

Pyridostigmine (Mestinon, ICN Pharmaceuticals, Costa Mesa, CA) is used to control the symptoms of muscle weakness in myasthenia gravis (Ravits, 1988). Numerous other drugs are used in similar ways in the treatment of the many progressively debilitating neurological diseases, but their effects on voice and speech have not been noted to be marked, although they have not been well studied.

SUMMARY

In the first section of this chapter, a review of phonosurgical techniques currently in use for the treatment of voice problems was presented. Phonosurgical techniques are divided into four categories: (a) removal of pathological tissue; (b) correction of the position, shape, or tension of the vocal folds; (c) surgery to restore laryngeal neuro-muscular function; and (d) reconstruction for a partial loss or deformity of the larynx. A brief description of the techniques currently used by otolaryngologists was given to aid the reader in understanding the advantages and disadvantages of the techniques.

In the second section of this chapter, some of the techniques used in the medical management of voice problems were reviewed. Many of these techniques involve the use of drugs for the relief of symptoms, as well as for treating the original cause(s) of the voice problem. Allergies, asthma, and the drugs used in their treatment are often implicated as a cause of voice problems. Counseling and behavioral modification techniques to encourage the patient to change habits (smoking, drinking), lifestyle, or environment are presented in Chapter 10.

Chapter 10

Vocal Rehabilitation

GOAL OF VOICE THERAPY

The specific goal of voice therapy varies from patient to patient. Nevertheless, in general, the goal of voice therapy is to restore the best voice possible, a voice that will be functional for purposes of employment and general communication. The patient must be the final arbiter of what constitutes acceptable voice. However, it is important for both the patient and the clinician to recognize that restoring voice to the way it previously sounded or to some idealized goal may not be possible. When irreversible alterations have occurred in laryngeal structure or physiology, the voice may never return to what it once had been. This realization is particularly traumatic for persons who have relied heavily on their vocal skills for their livelihood or as their primary source of pleasure.

CONCEPT OF NORMAL VOICE

An accepted definition of normal voice does not exist. There are no established standards, and no boundaries of accepted norms have been set. Attempting to set such standards might be likened to defining what constitutes normal appearance. Voice, like appearance, comes in so many varieties. Cultural, environmental, and individual factors contribute to the determination of what is designated normal. And voice, again like appearance, does not remain constant. It changes throughout the lifespan; it changes in reaction to emotion; it changes in response to environment; it reflects the state of health of the body and of the mind. Having a single definition that would encompass all of the ways that a normal voice can sound would be difficult if not impossible. Normal is not a single state but rather exists on a continuum.

Some normative data have been gathered about specific acoustic vocal parameters (see Chapter 14). Usually these data provide ranges within which voices that have been judged as normal have been found to fall. Often even these data are suspect, because investigators remind us that both intrasubject and intersubject variability may be very large (Kent, Kent, & Rosenbek, 1987). Attempting to define the abnormal may be easier. The voice that is so reduced in volume that normal-hearing listeners have difficulty hearing it is abnormal. The voice that is so different in pitch level as to be incongruent with the age or sex of the speaker may be judged to be abnormal. The voice that lacks the flexibility to alter pitch or loudness or that has a quality that calls attention to itself in an unpleasant manner or that is so loud that we are aware of it whether we choose to be or not suggests something outside our internalized norms.

The lack of a definition of normal voice creates problems in setting therapeutic goals and in describing abnormality and its degree of severity. There is no complete and objective template against which to measure and compare it. This is one of the major obstacles in clinical research: collection of objective, quantifiable data. If a voice improves, how can we measure that improvement? With what can we compare it? Which of the vocal attributes have contributed to its improvement? How much better is it? Is it normal? Is it normal for that patient?

This last question raises another aspect of the concept of normalcy of voice; that is, how did a particular patient's voice sound before it became disordered? Usually the only voice known to the clinician and available for any measurement is the disordered voice. This can create problems if at a given point during therapy the clinician judges a patient's voice to be quite acceptable but the patient continues to be unhappy, claiming it is different from the remembered normal voice. The opposite may occur if the clinician continues to seek a better voice when the patient reports that the voice being produced sounds right and normal.

THE UNDERLYING BASES OF VOCAL REHABILITATION

Voice therapy must be rooted in and derived from an understanding of laryngeal anatomy and phonatory physiology. One must understand what is wrong to know how to fix it. When there is a hole in a bucket, understanding the effect of that hole, not only that the hole is there, is important. That understanding may lead to more than a single approach to fixing the problem. Understanding how the hole developed may be important to prevent it from recurring despite its having been fixed once.

Accurate diagnosis is critical to treatment planning. The diagnosis should provide the voice therapist with the information necessary to plan a course of treatment. However, patients are often referred for voice therapy with minimal diagnostic information. When that is the case, requests should be directed to the otolaryngologist for as detailed information as is available. Voice symptoms and signs in combination with information derived from a complete history and voice assessment must be compatible with the referral diagnosis. Communication between the speech–language pathologist and the referring laryngologist will be helpful in clarifying terminology and observations, as well as in developing a treatment plan.

The relationship between the person and the voice must be understood and incorporated into the therapy program. This is true for all voice patients regardless of whether the voice problem suggests any element of psychogenic origin. Emotionality, stress, and anxiety may be components of many voice problems, in terms of both their causes and the reactions they engender. Individual reactions to voice problems may very well determine the response to treatment and the patient's ability to follow a therapy plan.

Freed from constraints imposed by organic lesions, stress factors, or abusive habits, the larynx will usually function well. Thus, it is often possible to eliminate the constraint through voice therapy and thereby correct the voice problem. One need not teach patients every aspect of voice production, as though they had never done it correctly before.

GUIDELINES FOR VOICE THERAPY

A simplified explanation of normal vocal physiology and of the patient's specific deviance from it can be critical to the patient's response to therapy. For most patients, the idea of voice therapy is unfamiliar. They do not understand how, after many years of speaking without difficulty, they can now be speaking "improperly." They have little appreciation for the connection between various vocal behaviors and their own particular problem. What they really would like is for the doctor to prescribe some type of medication that, taken three times a day, would cure the problem. Instead, they learn that they must assume some responsibility for dealing with the problem. To do so, they must begin by gaining some knowledge. Without an understanding of the nature of the problem, the patient's approach to therapy often will be highly skeptical.

Throughout therapy, encourage the patient to verbalize perceptions of how the voice sounds and feels. This provides information for the clinician, but more importantly, it sensitizes the patient to the voice and increases self-awareness. It encourages a process of self-discovery that is exciting and motivating for the patient as changes are perceived. For the clinician, the patient's verbalizations provide information about how the patient views the problem, how tuned in to the problem the patient is, and perhaps help to shape the therapy plan.

The use of both auditory and visual feedback during therapy can be extremely helpful. Auditory feedback can be provided by the judicious use of audio recordings, using good-quality equipment. The availability of instrumentation or easily accessible computer software programs that provide realtime visual and auditory feedback has expanded rapidly. If the clinician is skilled in the use of video fiberoptic laryngoscopy and has access to such equipment, and if the patient tolerates the procedure well, visual feedback during the therapy process (Bastian, 1987; 1985) can be put to good use. The patient is taught to identify certain desirable or undesirable laryngeal behaviors and has the benefit of the visual image to assist in shaping laryngeal activity. Spectrograms, electroglottograms, and other printouts of acoustic or physiological data can be used for demonstration and explanation but do not lend themselves as easily to direct therapeutic use. Biofeedback using surface electrodes over laryngeal muscles has been reported with inconclusive results (Prosek, Montgomery, Walden, & Schwartz, 1978; Stemple, Weider, Whitehead, & Komray, 1980). Because this method, as currently used, is incapable of differentiating between the activity of those muscles that need to be active and those that should be relaxed, and because we have no data to specify how much activity is normal and how much is hyperfunctional for any given muscle during phonation, the meaning of electromyographic biofeedback is uncertain.

Another form of feedback is the use of instruments that monitor a behavior and supply a signal when a preset level of that behavior has been surpassed. For example, the Voice Intensity Controller (VIC) described by Holbrook, Rolnick, and Bailey (1974) is a small unit capable of being worn by a patient to monitor vocal intensity. A small throat microphone is affixed to the neck, an earphone is worn in the ear, and the unit fits into a pocket. The permissible intensity is preset. When that level is exceeded, a tone is emitted in the earphone. The use of this feedback device has been found to be very effective in modifying vocal loudness in a short time (Holbrook, Rolnick, & Bailey, 1974). However, these instruments are often difficult to obtain and are costly. Another device to monitor loudness is available from LinguiSystems (East Moline, IL). An inexpensive sound level meter can be purchased at Radio Shack (Cat. No. 33-2055).

Visual feedback is provided by the Voice Light and Voice Intensity Indicator, available from Wintronix (P.O. Box 514, Blue Springs, MO 64014).

Therapy should move gradually from one step or activity to the next. Give the patient adequate time to practice a technique and to master it. Familiarity with a technique and a sense of having learned it provides a sense of accomplishment for the patient. Furthermore, if the behavior is but one phase of a progression, the patient needs to have a solid foundation on which to build. A fine line exists here between overdoing a good thing and moving on too quickly. To help make this transition, begin to introduce a new technique while continuing to incorporate practice on those already learned. Also, give a technique a chance to work. The clinician must not allow the patient's anxiety and desire for instant results to affect clinical judgment. In the initial stages of therapy, often one must experiment with techniques and approaches. The patient should be made aware of this process to avoid feelings of uncertainty and confusion.

The clinician should always model therapy tasks for the patient. We often ask patients to produce sounds or engage in activities that might seem strange to them. Moreover, we ask them to do so in the presence of another person, the clinician. This raises the patient's level of self-consciousness significantly. To minimize such feelings, as well as to demonstrate clearly what the patient is being asked to do, the clinician must demonstrate therapeutic tasks. When a task is demonstrated, it must be done just as it is wished that the patient do it. If the request is for the patient to produce the loudest "hey" possible, it will not be effective to have the clinician model it quietly. Because verbally explaining or describing a vocal behavior is often difficult, modeling it takes on greater importance. A demonstration, like the proverbial picture, is worth a thousand words.

Recording therapy sessions in whole or in part is important. Doing so provides a record of the patient's voice and of the therapy session. Memory for voice is very fleeting, and both the clinician and the patient may readily forget what the voice sounded like at a given point. When therapy seems to be taking longer than the patient expected, or when it appears that little progress has been made, the playing of an earlier recording may be very helpful in providing some perspective. Another valuable use for recorded sessions is as home practice material. Patients often report that without the clinician's model or their own from a previous time, they are not sure that they are practicing correctly. The recorded session (be it tape, CD, or digital minidisks) provides the structure they need.

Patients must be carefully instructed in what to practice, for how long, and how often. Have the patient demonstrate the exercise or activity to be practiced before leaving the therapy session. Because talking is an activity that is so pervasive yet so rarely attended to by most speakers, we have found it effective to recommend frequent practice sessions of limited duration. This approach seems to help the patient focus on the voice frequently. Furthermore, there is usually some follow-up or generalization of practice for a period of time immediately after it has been done. Frequent practice periods capitalize on this "overflow effect" because it occurs more frequently.

The prognostic statement made at the initiation of a program of vocal rehabilitation must be viewed as an educated guess about the outcome of therapy. It must be realistic but must not be etched in stone. It should be modified appropriately as therapy progresses. The variety of factors that will enter into the development of a prognostic statement are discussed later in this chapter.

Not all patients are appropriate candidates for a voice therapy approach, for reasons other than the nature of the pathological condition present. A patient must recognize that a problem is present and must be willing to undertake a therapy program and to follow the regimen. Some find it extremely difficult to abandon harmful habits because of lifestyle, employment, or personality factors. Even when explicitly directed to do so, smokers may be unable to stop or even to significantly reduce this habit. The irritation created by continued smoking may be sufficient to maintain a condition and sabotage any positive effects that can be brought about through changed phonatory behavior. The therapeutic process is complex, and patient behavior may unwittingly pose a major hindrance to progress. Despite apparent cooperation, the patient may be exhibiting a variety of behaviors described by McFarlane, Fujiki, and Brinton (1984) as exemplifying the "reluctant client."

PROGNOSTIC CONSIDERATIONS

Many factors enter into the consideration of a prognosis. Because voice therapy requires full patient participation, predicting its anticipated outcome often is difficult. In determining whether a patient is an appropriate candidate for a voice therapy approach and arriving at a prognosis, the clinician should consider the following factors: First, the patient must recognize that there is a problem. People possess internal references about how they should feel, what is normal for them, and what they should sound like. A voice that sounds abnormal to us may not sound particularly deviant to the person with that voice. Similarly, although aware that the voice is not normal, the person may not find it objectionable or in need of "fixing." Second, the patient must be willing to follow a therapy plan including regular practice periods as required. This is difficult for those seeking a quick cure for which they do not have to assume responsibility. Third, the patient must have a willingness to give up traumatic habits and to alter or eliminate some voice use, at least temporarily. This is easier said than done for most people. Changing manner and amount of talking involves changes in lifestyle, in everyday habits, and even, it may seem, in personality. Fourth, psychiatric problems, if present, may interfere with the ability to modify vocal behavior. A voice problem may be a manifestation of a psychiatric problem. Amelioration of the voice problem may be possible temporarily, but it will not deal with the larger, underlying problem (recall the case of R.W. in Chapter 8). Fifth, the patient's voice disorder must be amenable to change through a voice therapy approach. For some voice problems, surgical or medical management may be the first or sole step. For other patients, the nature of the disorder may preclude any real possibility of success through voice therapy. The patient and the speech–language pathologist must be able to recognize the limitations of voice therapy. Sixth, appropriateness of the patient's expectations must be considered. If a person has an essentially normal voice but wishes to sound like a favorite role model or celebrity, voice therapy is not indicated. Seventh, one must give full consideration to the patient's laryngeal condition and general health status. Some patients are insistent on attaining full return of premorbid voice. The nature of the disorder and the resultant laryngeal changes may be such that this expectation is unrealistic. The vocal folds may be damaged to the extent that normal phonation is not possible. Patients may have other health problems that may limit their ability to participate in voice therapy or may place constraints on their ability to control phonatory behavior. Finally, the speech–language pathologist must have an adequate understanding of the problem, feel competent in handling it, and be able to establish a good relationship with the patient.

VOICE THERAPY IN THE MANAGEMENT OF CHANGES IN LARYNGEAL TISSUE OR STRUCTURE

Vocal rehabilitation may play a primary role, as either the sole treatment modality of choice or simultaneously with other treatment, or a secondary role, as a follow-up treatment after a primary approach has been performed.

When Is Voice Therapy Alone Appropriate?

A paucity of hard data exists, unfortunately, to support a position on this question. Theoretical constructs and clinical experience are the primary bases on which therapeutic judgments are made. Increasing efficacy data have been emerging.

VOCAL FOLD NODULES

Perhaps the most agreement exists about the treatment of vocal fold nodules. Prominent authorities in the treatment of voice, in the fields of both otolaryngology and speech–language pathology, generally agree that the initial treatment of choice for symptomatic vocal nodules in adults is voice therapy (Aronson, 1990; Bastian, 1986; Boone & McFarlane, 1988; Gould, 1987; Sataloff, 1987a; 1987c; 1987b; Vaughan, 1982) (see also Chapter 8 of this book). The option for surgical intervention is not compromised or eliminated by the more conservative approach of at least a 6- to 8-week period of voice therapy. Some authorities make a distinction between early nodules, which appear to be soft and reddish, and nodules that have been present for months or years and are large, hard, and white. Voice therapy as the initial treatment is recommended for the former, and surgical removal followed by a period of voice therapy is most commonly recommended for the latter (Arnold, 1980; Boone et al., 1988; Case, 1984). Sataloff (1987b) states that even nodules that are large and fibrotic may disappear, regress, or become asymptomatic through a course of voice therapy. If partial regression of pathological conditions occurs, any surgery required may be less extensive. Other authors suggest that decisions regarding choice of treatment should be made on an individual basis but that vocal reeducation must be part of any treatment protocol (Moore, Hicks, & Abbott, 1985). Once again, remember that a trial period of voice therapy does not in any way compromise the option for surgery. Prater and Swift (1984) point out that voice therapy is more cost-effective than surgery, results in less time lost from work, and is nontraumatic. Furthermore, the learning that takes place during the therapy program will serve to eliminate vocal misuse and will be readily transferable to postoperative voice use should surgery become necessary. Vocal nodules may well recur if phonotrauma is not eliminated through a vocal rehabilitation program. Although this "therapy first" approach to treatment of vocal fold nodules has become accepted, many questions and concerns remain. Differentiation of nodules from cysts, polyps, and reactive lesions based on current assessment techniques remains problematic. Patients often report vocal improvement through therapy despite the continued presence of lesions, albeit perhaps reduced in size. Thus, making generalizations with certainty is difficult.

Less agreement exists about the need for and value of any treatment for vocal nodules in children. Vaughan (1982) reports that vocal nodules in children resolve spontaneously in early adolescence and therefore usually require no treatment. Hirano, however, recognizes that the vocal symptoms resulting from vocal nodules can potentially create significant emotional problems for a child, in which case voice therapy is advocated. Most speech–language pathologists also believe that youngsters with vocal fold nodules can be effectively helped to eliminate vocally harmful behaviors, and thereby the nodules themselves, with voice therapy (Boone et al., 1988; Johnson, 1983; Teter, 1976; Wilson, 1987). Many further argue that the psychosocial effects of aberrant voice on a young child can be quite significant and advocate voice therapy for this reason as well. Surgical removal of vocal nodules in children is contraindicated (Arnold, 1980; 1985; DeWeese & Saunders, 1982).

The controversy about the role of the speech–language pathologist in the treatment of voice disorders in children has been discussed by Sander (1989) (against) and Kahane and Mayo (1989) (for). Whereas Sander claims that young children experience resolution of voice problems at puberty without the benefit of any treatment, Kahane and Mayo cite that adult vocal deviations are frequently traceable to patterns set in childhood (Cooper, 1973; Pahn, 1966) and, further, that the incidence of voice disorders in school children in the middle school grades (6th through 9th grades) may be higher than has previously been reported (Warr-Leeper, McShea, & Leeper, 1979). Kahane and Mayo present a compelling argument for the development of prevention programs and cite the positive result of such a program reported by Nilson and Schneiderman (1983).

VOCAL POLYPS

Vocal fold polyps are often thought to be the result of vocal trauma, sometimes caused by a single or intense period of trauma during which small blood vessels rupture. They are also thought by some to be amenable to a voice therapy approach, particularly the sessile, or broad-based, polyps. As with vocal nodules, opinions about the preferred mode of treatment are mixed, but also, as is the case with nodules, little is lost when a period of voice therapy is the initial treatment provided.

When Should Voice Therapy Be Combined With Other Treatment?

CONTACT ULCERS AND GRANULOMA

Contact ulcers and granulomas had been thought to result from a specific type of vocally abusive phonation. However, various studies provide additional insight into the underlying pathophysiology of contact ulcers (Cherry & Margulies, 1968; Chodosh, 1977; Delahunty & Cherry, 1968; Delahunty, 1972; Ward, Zwitman, Hanson, & Berci, 1980). Ward and Berci (1982) cite the chronic irritation caused by hiatal hernia and by gastroesophageal reflux as the basic problem, which in turn causes chronic coughing and harsh and frequent throat clearing. Granulomatous lesions typically occur on the posterior, cartilaginous vocal processes. These structures are close to the upper esophageal sphincter, and thus are likely to be irritated by refluxed material. The vocal processes also adduct forcefully during coughing and throat clearing. According to Ward and Berci, the initial irritation, and the patient's subsequent responses to it, precipitate contact ulcer and granuloma formation. These abusive behaviors, coughing and throat clearing, were thought to initiate contact ulcer and granuloma formation. Response to medical treatment as reported by Hallewell and Cole (Hallewell & Cole, 1970) was very successful in 21 of 22 cases. Chronic nonspecific laryngitis, pharyngitis, and pachydermia laryngis are included in the family of problems with this underlying pathophysiology. Voice therapy is appropriate as one part of the treatment regimen to eliminate laryngeally damaging behaviors, particularly those that involve contact between the vocal processes or affected areas. However, appropriate medical evaluation of and treatment for possible gastroesophageal reflux disease (GERD) also need to be part of the total treatment protocol. Surgical or medical treatment without the other components of care is frequently unsuccessful in the long term, because the condition recurs.

Koufman et al. emphasize the potentially destructive nature of GERD on the larynx, leading to problems that may be very serious, including cancer (Koufman, 1995; Koufman, Wiener, Wu, & Castell, 1988). These authors question the viability of using traditional diagnostic radiologic techniques to assess GERD, stating that "barium esophagography has both poor specificity and sensitivity, and its reliability is questionable" (Koufman, 1995; Koufman et al., 1988). They advocate the use of 24-hour pH probe monitoring of the esophagus and pharynx as a more reliable means for detecting when reflux is occurring. Although 69% of the patients studied had no reflux-like symptoms, Koufman et al. found that 75% had abnormal pH studies. Most had reflux as determined by the pH probe at night, but many (71%) had reflux while upright. When treated with a standard antireflux regimen (i.e., medication, dietary restrictions, head elevation during sleep, and behavioral adjustments), approximately 66% of the patients had resolution of their symptoms. In a much larger study, Koufman (1991) reported on 225 patients with suspected GERD. Eighty-eight percent of the patients underwent a 24-hour pH monitoring study, with 62% of those demonstrating abnormal studies. Of these, 30% demonstrated reflux into the pharynx. Abnormal pH probe findings were reported for 71% of the patients with carcinoma, 78% of those with stenosis, 60% of those with reflux laryngitis, 58% of those with complaints of a lump in the throat (globus), 45% with dysphagia, and 52% of patients with a chronic cough. Thus, reflux may be associated with a variety of problems affecting the larynx, not all of which produce voice symptoms.

POLYPOID CHANGES

Polypoid changes of the vocal folds (Reinke's edema) are highly related to long-term, excessive smoking and to age (Hirano, Kurita, Matsuo, & Nagata, 1980). Although a component of vocal misuse also may be present and may aggravate the condition, these lesions are generally not caused by abuse and are not responsive to voice therapy. However, many patients benefit from a course of voice therapy after surgical excision of the lesion.

OTHER PATHOLOGY

Numerous other laryngeal lesions are not caused by vocal trauma and require medical and surgical intervention. However, vocally harmful habits may result as the patient attempts to compensate for a poorly functioning mechanism. Those habits may persist beyond resolution of the pathological condition, and a period of voice therapy may be required. A specific group of patients that would be included in this category are those with papillomas, requiring frequent surgical removal over a period of years. The condition of the mucosal cover of the vocal folds after numerous surgeries will be a most important factor in determining the quality of voice that will be possible.

Goals of Voice Therapy

When voice therapy is undertaken as the treatment modality of choice in the presence of mucosal and voice changes, the primary goals are, of course, to restore the mucosa to a healthy condition and to regain clear and full vocal function. Subgoals include identification and elimination of all harmful behaviors through the reduction of laryngeal tensions, institution of a vocal hygiene program, environmental manipulation, easy voice production, and establishment of improved vocal habits. Other goals may include identification of patient needs that require other forms of attention and appropriate referral.

When voice therapy is an adjunct or secondary treatment modality, the goals depend largely on the laryngeal status of the patient. The primary goal may be to restore healthy function and return of good voice, or it may be to help the patient find the best voice of which she is capable. The limits on that voice may be imposed by permanent changes in the mucosa or the structural integrity of the larynx. Subgoals, in addition to those noted above, may include helping the patient to accept a changed voice, exploration of the adequacy of the voice for all necessary speaking situations, and suggesting environmental adjustments as necessary.

Nature of Therapeutic Intervention

Vocal rehabilitation must address a variety of factors. Patients are often called on to make significant changes in the manner in which they produce voice, the various ways in which they use voice (e.g., singing, lecturing, etc.), and the environments in which they may use voice. These changes are all very closely linked to how individuals see themselves and how they interact with others. Recognition of the highly sensitive nature of the therapeutic process and the impact that it may have on the patient cannot be overemphasized.

VOICE THERAPY IN THE MANAGEMENT OF TRAUMATIC/MISUSE PROBLEMS

When Is Voice Therapy Alone Appropriate?

Voice therapy is almost always the treatment modality of choice for voice problems stemming from behaviors that have been identified as misuse or traumatic to the laryngeal mechanism. However, our experience has been that these patients, who may have negative laryngological examinations or minimal signs of laryngeal irritation, frequently receive up to 3 months or more of medical treatment before referral to a speech–language pathologist for voice evaluation. Patients in these categories may be treated with antibiotics, antihistamines, decongestants, tranquilizers, and even corticosteroids, or may be sent home with some fairly nonspecific advice about relaxing or reducing voice use. Because of the effects on laryngeal mucosa of some medications, the actual voice symptoms may worsen over the course of the treatment, rather than improve (see Chapter 4). Recognition of the problem is critical to obtaining effective treatment.

Some patients may not be appropriate candidates for a voice therapy approach because of social/emotional problems beyond the scope of practice of the speech–language pathologist. However, it is within the speech–language pathologist's expertise to recognize such conditions and to make recommendations for or to arrange appropriate referral. Patients who do not recognize that a problem exists or who are incapable of or unwilling to change habits or lifestyle will be poor candidates for therapy.

Goals of Voice Therapy

The primary therapeutic goals are to identify and eliminate behaviors that constitute misuse or abuse and to replace them with acceptable patterns of voice production. Full return of normal voice is anticipated, especially when there is no evidence of mucosal or other tissue change. Subgoals in the treatment of vocal trauma and misuse might include reduction of laryngeal tensions, decrease of vocal loudness, decrease in amount of talking, adjusting environmental factors, and others. For those voice problems that appear to be psychogenic in nature, a goal of therapy may be to help the patient understand the dynamics that initiated and sustained the voice problem.

Nature of Therapeutic Intervention

As stated in the previous section, therapy directed toward the elimination of vocally harmful behavior requires that the patient change habits of voice production. Those habits, even if not of very long standing, nevertheless may be quite tenacious. In addition to altering the way in which voice is produced, it may be necessary for the patient to make some sacrifices in the ways the voice is used. The changes that need to be made may be imposed by the therapy process, rather than as limitations caused by the problem itself. For example, the patient who enjoys singing in a church choir may need to forego that activity at least temporarily. The college professor who has never used amplification despite having to lecture to very large classes in large rooms with poor acoustics may need to do so. These are difficult changes for people to make. The therapeutic process may involve discussion of personal and interpersonal concerns that require understanding, the ability to listen well, and a nonjudgmental attitude. It is also essential for the clinician to be able to provide support and encouragement in helping a patient to accept a changed or restored voice.

VOICE THERAPY IN THE MANAGEMENT OF NEUROLOGICAL PROBLEMS

Voice problems are but one of the dysarthric components of disability that may accompany certain neuromuscular disorders. With the possible exceptions of unilateral vocal fold paralysis (usually peripheral nerve damage) and spasmodic dysphonia (cause still questioned), it is unusual for the voice disorder to be the primary disability. The earliest symptoms of a neurological condition may be exhibited in changes or aberrations of phonation. However, in progressively debilitating neuromuscular diseases, the worsening of motor behavior and increased limitations in many areas of function may become relatively more handicapping to the person. The speech–language pathologist may well be involved with these patients in working on phonatory problems and also the related disabilities of dysarthria (articulation and resonation), apraxia, aphasia, and dysphagia, as they exist. A therapy protocol focusing on the voice has been developed and shown to be effective for patients with Parkinson's disease and the Parkinson plus syndrome (Countryman, Ramig, & Pawlas, 1994; Ramig, Bonitati, Lemke, & Horii,

1994; Ramig & Scherer, 1992). (See "Voice Therapy Techniques" later in this chapter for further discussion.)

There is still some controversy concerning the role of voice therapy in the management of unilateral vocal fold paralysis. Data to support the efficacy of vocal rehabilitation are limited. When the cause of the paralysis is idiopathic, the literature suggests that either spontaneous recovery or increased compensatory movement of the healthy fold occurs (Tucker, 1980). The major portion of such recovery is believed to take place within 6 months of onset, although there are reports of recovery for up to a year post-onset (Ward & Berci, 1982a). When voice therapy is undertaken during that period, to what can we attribute improved vocal function—to the therapy or to spontaneous recovery of function, or perhaps to a combination of the two? We do not have the data to answer this question. Several phonosurgical approaches designed to improve vocal function are available. In general, these procedures are designed to augment or position the paralyzed fold in such a manner that the intact fold can achieve contact with it during phonation, thereby minimizing air loss and improving vocal volume.

Injection of Teflon (as described by Dr. Kelley in Chapter 9) had in the past been effective in many individuals who failed to show spontaneous recovery of vocal fold function or voice (Hammarberg, Fritzell, & Schiratzki, 1984; Lewy, 1993; Reich & Lerman, 1978; Tucker, 1980). However, problems of over-injection, effects on surrounding tissues, and concern about long-term stability (positioning) of the injected material have led to a decrease in its popularity (Rubin, 1965), although some authors believe that with care these problems can be minimized (Dedo, 1988, 1992). Augmentation with autologous fat (Jiang, Titze, Wexler, & Gray, 1994; Wexler, Jiang, Gray, & Titze, 1989) also has been tried with some success, though repeat procedures may be necessary because of reabsorption of the injected material (Ford, Bless, & Loftus, 1992; Ford, Martin, & Warner, 1984). Other materials that have been used to augment the fixed vocal fold include collagen and fascia (Ford, Staskowski, & Bless, 1995; Duke, Salmon, Blalock, Postma, & Koufman, 2001).

Another widely used surgical procedure for vocal fold paralysis (see Chapter 9) is a type I thyroplasty. This procedure was described by Isshiki et al. (1974) and involves fixing an implantable material, such as silastic or, more recently, Gore Tex, lateral to the paralyzed vocal fold through a window made in the thyroid cartilage. The implant serves as a wedge to move the paralyzed fold closer to the midline. Another procedure, called arytenoid adduction was described by Isshiki, Tanabe, and Sawada in 1978 and has become increasing popular. It is designed to reduce large posterior chinks or gaps between the paralyzed and intact folds by surgically rotating the affected arytenoid's vocal process into the midline.

Our own studies comparing surgical and voice therapy treatment of patients with a unilateral vocal fold paralysis have shown that both approaches can be effective in improving the voice. Thirty-nine patients were studied, all with unilateral vocal fold paralysis or paresis. Twenty-one patients received surgical treatment (either Teflon injection or thyroplasty), and 18 received voice therapy as their major treatment. Both treatment groups showed improvement in voice quality and changes in several measures of vocal fold function. These measurements are shown in Figure 10.1. Note that the surgery patients tended to have higher pretreatment mean, peak, and leakage airflow rates, suggesting greater severity of glottal incompetence than the therapy group. Leakage flow reflects glottal incompetence, and both treatment approaches reduced the magnitude of leakage flow. Not shown in the figure are open quotient data for both

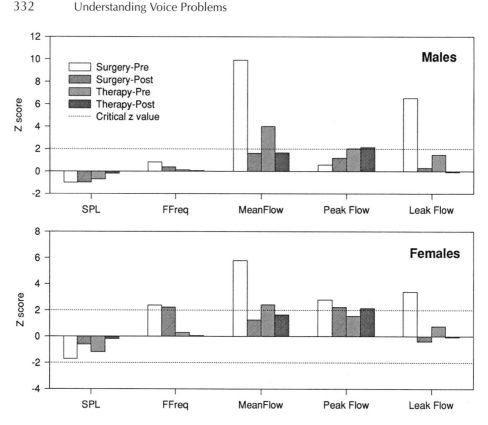

Figure 10.1. Z scores for a group of patients with unilateral vocal fold paralysis on selected voice measurements made before and after treatment. There were 15 males and 6 females in the surgery group and 6 males and 12 females in the therapy group. The dotted line represents the critical value of Z to exceed normal limits at the 0.05 level. Normal data were obtained from Holmberg, Hillman, and Perkell (1988) for 25 males and 20 females producing phonations at normal loudness and frequency levels.

groups. For patients in the surgery group, the open quotient was much greater before treatment than after treatment (0.67 vs. 0.54, males and females pooled). For patients in the therapy group, the open quotient was also greater before treatment than after treatment (0.61 vs. 0.56). These results mean that the vocal folds were open a greater proportion of the time during the vibratory cycles before treatment for both groups but that those who underwent surgery had preoperative open quotients larger than those patients who received therapy. After surgery, the open quotient decreased, suggesting greater vocal fold adduction.

The issue of voice therapy procedures recommended for treatment of unilateral vocal fold paralysis are discussed later in the section "Unresolved Issues and Myths."

Another area of continued concern regarding the benefit of voice therapy is that of spasmodic dysphonia. Controversy continues about the cause of this puzzling condition, as well as about its treatment. Historically, the strain/struggle voice of the patient with spasmodic dysphonia was first thought to be entirely psychologically based (Arnold, 1959). This view has been modified at least to the extent that most authors now believe that more than a single cause may exist but that a neurological basis for the disorder exists in most cases. The need for very thorough differential diagnosis is also well accepted to differentiate spasmodic dysphonia from other neurogenically based disorders and from those of psychogenic origin. A trial of voice therapy is often recommended to determine whether relief can be obtained through that approach. Indeed, a trial of voice therapy is often diagnostically useful. Although voice therapy is generally not an effective treatment modality for significantly modifying the symptoms of true spasmodic dysphonia, it has been shown to increase the interval between Botox injections (Murry & Woodson, 1995). Furthermore, voice therapy can be helpful in educating patients about the disorder: what they can expect and how to manage the variable vocal function they will experience.

Goals of Voice Therapy

Voice therapy can offer no cures when neuromotor disability is involved. However, through voice therapy, patients may be able to learn to produce the best voice possible and to exert a degree of voluntary control over the production of voice that may allow them to remain communicatively functional in occupational and social settings (Ramig et al., 1994; Rosenfield, 1987) for a longer time than might have been anticipated. The speech–language pathologist can also be helpful in assessing the effects of medications on the patient's voice and speech production. If functional verbal communication is not a viable option, direct voice therapy becomes inappropriate, and the goal then must be to provide the patient with a means of nonverbal communication. Teaching how to optimize voice production and communication within the limits imposed by the disability can be productive.

Nature of Therapeutic Intervention

The manner in which voice is produced may receive very direct attention, particularly in cases of vocal fold paralysis and sometimes of spasmodic dysphonia. Very direct work on loudness, pitch range, flexibility, and vocal stamina is the hallmark of voice therapy with parkinsonian patients (see "Voice Therapy Techniques" later in this chapter). Attention may be directed to suprasegmental factors such as breath groups, prosody, rate, and marking for stress and inflection in work with other neurologically based disorders. Patients may have adopted particular patterns of voice use in an attempt to compensate for alterations in control of the voice. Some of these compensatory behaviors may be helpful, but others may not. Adjustment in communication patterns and behaviors are often imposed on the individual by the nature of the disability. For example, the inability to increase loudness will restrict the environments in which the person can communicate effectively. In some instances, manipulation of environmental factors may be of some assistance. Hanson and Metter (1980) describe the use of a small, wearable, delayed auditory feedback (DAF) device in the treatment of a patient with progressive supranuclear palsy and severe hypokinetic dysarthria. They report that the patient, who was noted to have weak vocal intensity, demonstrated an increase of vocal intensity with the introduction of 100 msec DAF in both reading and counting aloud conditions, and that this increase was maintained in follow-up testing after a 3-month period of daily use of the device. Desired changes were also noted in a reduction of speech rate and increased speech intelligibility.

The therapeutic process may be difficult for neurologically impaired patients with progressive disorders and also for their voice clinicians because of the constraints of the underlying disorder and the gradual but inexorable deterioration in the patient's condition. It is incumbent on the clinician to recognize the limitations of the therapeutic approach and not to promise what cannot be delivered but to make every effort to help the patient arrive at the best means of communication possible for as long as possible.

THERAPY FOR SPECIAL VOICE PROBLEMS

A number of voice problems that do not readily fit the above categories but that may appropriately require a period of vocal rehabilitation are covered in this section.

The Transsexual Voice

"It is important for the clinician to acquire an understanding of the life experiences of transgendered clients in order to provide thoughtful, effective therapy" (Freidenberg, 2002, p. 1). Freidenberg presents a complete tutorial on working with this population of patients, including much information on therapeutic approaches.

The voice problem most immediately associated with a gender reassignment is that of inappropriate pitch. In the case of change from a female to male, this problem is usually resolved through the use of male hormones, which cause an increase in laryngeal mass and thus lower fundamental frequency. However, no drugs are available to reduce the mass of the vocal folds, so that a male-to-female change is not accompanied by elevation of pitch secondary to hormone therapy. The incongruity of a masculine voice in a woman can present a significant psychological barrier. Therapeutic attempts to elevate speaking fundamental frequency should be undertaken with care, recognizing the physiological limits of the larynx. The use of breathy phonation can be helpful in giving the illusion of a higher pitch without the risk of inviting laryngeal trauma.

However, in addition to differences in pitch between the male and female voice, there are differences in other speech patterns, habits, and mannerisms. This has been demonstrated experimentally by Coleman (1971, 1973, 1976), who found that female voices are still recognized as female even when the pitch difference between male and female voice is removed. Some of the difference between male and female voice lies in vowel quality, in that the relative sizes of the oral and pharyngeal cavities are different in the two sexes. Other differences include those of stress, inflection, timing, and even choice and use of words and conversational style. Changes in these areas will go far in feminizing a voice even in the presence of a low speaking fundamental frequency. The actress Lauren Bacall presents a good model of someone whose voice is low in pitch and yet whose style is entirely feminine. A program of voice therapy designed to make the man-to-woman change should include careful study of this and other models of feminine low-pitched speech. The goal of therapy should be to make those changes that will be effective in changing the overall image, rather than to work on artificial changes, such as pitch change, that may never become natural and that in fact may court laryngeal problems.

The pitch of the voice is only one of many aspects of communication that differentiates and distinguishes the sexes. Because we do not advocate artificial elevation of pitch that can be potentially damaging, we recommend that some of the following areas be targeted for change.

1. Slight increase in breathiness of voice
2. Using the concept of vocal effort, a lighter and softer voice may be encouraged by reducing vocal effort

3. Increased use of pitch variability rather than loudness to mark inflection and stress, and to alter rhythm of speech
4. Target nonphonatory areas such as conversational topics, conversational style, pragmatic aspects of communication. In some instances, listening to other voices may provide the patient with insights into particular vocal characteristics that are more or less appealing.

Voice Problems Due to Endocrine Disorders or Hormone Imbalance

HYPOTHYROIDISM

Hypothyroidism is a condition that can occur at any age. The symptoms may develop gradually over a lengthy period. As a result, their effect may not be recognized until a critical level of symptomatology has been reached. Change in the voice may be one such symptom. Typically, the voice of the patient with hypothyroidism is hoarse and has gradually lowered in pitch because of increased mass (edema) of the vocal folds. Therefore, the diagnostician must be alert to this as a possible diagnosis when vocal fold edema is noted and does not appear to be related to factors of vocal abuse. Referral back to the physician for appropriate testing should be pursued, and voice therapy is not indicated.

VIRILIZATION

This term is used to refer to the increase in size and mass of the vocal folds that occurs in women as the result of excessive secretion of the androgenic hormones or because of ingestion of androgen-containing hormones in treatment of menopausal symptoms or other problems. Damste (1967) described these changes and also showed them to be irreversible frequently. Voice therapy is contraindicated.

MENSTRUATION, PREGNANCY, AND BIRTH CONTROL PILL USE

Most of the voice-related negative effects of hormonal changes associated with the menstrual cycle occur in the pre- or early menstrual days. Excess loading of the vocal folds with fluid changes their mass and thus may affect vibratory behavior. This is usually not problematic for the average speaker but may present a problem for the professional singer. Submucosal hemorrhages in the larynx are not uncommon. Diuretics should be avoided because they do not free the protein-bound submucosal fluid (Sataloff, 1987b) and may have irritating drying effects on airway tissues. Voice therapy should be limited to counseling/information/vocal hygiene instruction. The clinician should be aware of the possibility of some subtle voice changes in female patients during these times.

Pregnancy also may result in change in the voice. During pregnancy the woman's endocrinological state undergoes great change. If a change in voice occurs, it is usually irreversible (Sataloff, 1987b). No available drugs counteract the normal physiological effects of either the menstrual period or pregnancy, and voice therapy is of no value in these cases. Voice clinicians must be aware, however, that such changes may be reported by patients.

A very small number of women appear to experience changes in the voice as a result of the use of birth control pills (Simkin, 1964). The quality and range of the voice may show these effects. Once again, they are usually not noted by the average speaker but may create problems for the singer. These voice changes are reversible when use of the pills is terminated.

Paradoxical Vocal Fold Motion or Vocal Fold Dysfunction

This is a disability that can easily be mistaken for asthma and treated accordingly, even to the point of tracheostomy. The primary characteristic is obstruction of the airway with vocal fold closure throughout the respiratory cycle, including inspiration. It has been referred to historically by as many as 35 names, which attests to its confusing nature and presentation (Gallivan & Andrianopoulos, 2004). A 1983 study by Christopher, Wood, Eckert, Blager, Raney, and Souhrada described five patients 14 to 68 years of age, of whom four were male and one female, who presented with paroxysms of wheezing and dyspnea and had initially been diagnosed as severe, uncontrollable asthmatics. However, the patients' symptoms failed to respond to standard therapy for asthma and, indeed, did not test positively for the expected symptoms of asthma. All patients had a chronic history of repeated "attacks," ranging from 1 to 13 years. One patient had undergone eight tracheotomy procedures. Laryngological examination during the spasm showed adduction of both true and ventricular folds during the full respiratory cycle, and patients exhibited both inspiratory and expiratory stridor. Laryngeal function was normal during asymptomatic periods. Inhalation of a mixture of helium (80%) and oxygen (20%) was found to be effective in relieving at least the acute symptoms and frequently resulted in symptom reduction even after cessation of the treatment. All patients were found to have psychological problems, and all were referred for both speech therapy and psychological counseling. Follow-up ranged from 3 to 21 months, and no patient had recurrence of the symptoms.

Other varieties of paradoxical vocal fold motion have been reported in which the vocal folds seem to behave in a manner opposite to the normal, that is, adduction is observed during deep inspiration, and there is at least slight abduction on expiration (Kellman & Leopold, 1982; Rogers & Stell, 1978). One such patient had undergone tracheotomy twice for relief of symptoms that had been diagnosed as laryngospasm. Patients were reported to show significant reduction, if not elimination, of symptoms in response to various interventions, including speech therapy, intravenous injection of diazepam or of a placebo, hypnosis, and verbal support. Although voice symptoms ranging from aphonia to weak or hoarse voice may be present, restoring the airway and eliminating recurrence of the symptoms are of primary importance. Voice therapy can be helpful in teaching these patients specific breathing techniques. Psychological treatment also may be indicated in some cases.

Although an apparently rare or underreported or misdiagnosed disability for many years, paradoxical vocal fold motion (PVFM) or vocal cord dysfunction (VCD) has been reported in increasing numbers in recent years. Bless and Swift (1995) make the claim that "PVCM is a symptom with multiple determinants." Their definition of the problem is broader than has previously been reported, and the cause is not limited to psychological problems, but includes (a) hyperreactivity of the airway; (b) neurogenic cause of either central or peripheral origin; and (c) psychological (has not been ruled out), pharmacological, or other unspecified medical problems. Treatment involves a combination of medical, behavioral, and psychological approaches. Gracco et al. (1995) reported instances of exercise-induced upper airway dysfunction in which the vocal folds were observed to adduct and fall inward during inspiration.

Diagnosis of PVFM often is difficult to make, and the disorder is frequently unrecognized. Because patients often present with some degree of respiratory distress and its hallmarks, for example, inspiratory stridor, apparent inability to inhale, sometimes momentary loss of consciousness, they are often seen in emergency rooms and immediately treated symptomatically before a diagnosis is made. The symptoms mirror those of an asthma attack or laryngospasm. Laryngospasms that wake the patient from sleep and are accompanied by a burning sensation in the throat are now usually recognized to be caused by gastroesophageal reflux and generally abate within a short time. However, they can be exceedingly frightening initially, create a panic reaction, and may result in emergency medical attention. When the correct diagnosis of PVFM is made, the treatment course is clear, and further extreme but inappropriate treatments can be avoided. For further discussion, see "Voice Therapy Techniques" later in this chapter.

VOICE THERAPY TECHNIQUES: ASSOCIATED PHYSIOLOGY AND INDICATIONS FOR USE

The manner in which a therapeutic technique is used will vary from clinician to clinician. Furthermore, with experience each clinician will develop and perfect those techniques found to be most useful and effective. Clinicians bring their own personalities and approaches to the clinical process, and the techniques that fit that style and produce a level of comfort and confidence are most likely to be adopted and well used.

It is the philosophy of this book that an understanding of laryngeal anatomy and phonatory physiology is basic to being a skilled voice clinician. Therapeutic techniques are only valid when they are used knowledgeably. The clinician must develop the knowledge base and the skill to determine what therapeutic approaches make sense for the individual patient. Indeed, a skilled clinician may make up a technique never tried before but something that makes sense for a given person, and for which there is an underlying rationale. Note the following case study.

Case Study

J.M. was a patient whose use of ventricular phonation was thought to be of psychological origin. A variety of techniques had been tried to elicit clear voice, but to no avail. The clinician then instructed her to simply blow through her fingers while holding them in front of her mouth and to feel the stream of air. At first J.M. seemed to have difficulty sustaining a smooth flow of air. However, with support and encouragement, she showed rapid improvement and a goal of blowing steadily for 5 seconds was set. When this goal was met, the clinician demonstrated the addition of a very soft, easy, high-pitched sound while continuing to feel the air flow. The patient was instructed to emulate this task but to make sure to concentrate on smooth airflow. She successfully produced acceptable voice quality with this task. Very gradually the good voice was shaped into speech, with no return of the ventricular phonation. This was a technique the clinician had never used or read about previously.

There is nothing magical in the technique. For this patient, a way had been found to allow her to release laryngeal tension and produce easy voice. In this example, as in many others that might be cited, the clinician had a working hypothesis, perhaps unspoken, relating the technique to be used to the physiological effect that is desired.

A patient may respond favorably to a number of approaches, all of which have the same goal. No single technique is always effective with all people. The clinician must understand what the patient is doing that is undesirable and then ask the question, "How can I get this patient to alter that specific behavior?"

Returning to the previous case study, the clinician knew from previous fiberoptic laryngoscopic studies of this patient that the ventricular phonation was produced with tight squeezing of the whole larynx, including supraglottal structures. Tension was apparent in respiratory function as well. The patient seemed to hold her breath during attempted phonation, releasing only when the effort to phonate was terminated and the vocal folds abducted fully. Perceptually, the voice sounded tight and strained, in addition to being very hoarse. It also seemed that this particular patient "froze" and became even more tense when asked to try any new activity that required phonation. Therefore, she was asked to carry out an activity, blowing, that does not require phonation and was therefore not threatening. The addition of feeling the stream of air captured J.M.'s attention and provided tangible, nonphonatory feedback. If J.M. continued to concentrate on this smooth, constant stream of air, phonation would begin softly and easily in perhaps a breathy manner. The introduction of tension and strain would surely interrupt or markedly change the airflow. For these various reasons, it was hypothesized that if the patient was able to carry out the instructions, there was a good chance that she would do so with good voice.

Few techniques are specific to a single voice disorder because there is so much similarity in laryngeal physiology across many disorders. For example, patients who misuse their voices and those who traumatize them to the point of creating mucosal changes may be engaging in the same form of vocal behavior from a physiological point of view. Thus, many of the same therapeutic techniques may be appropriate for both. The specific type of misuse or abuse (i.e., talking too much vs. talking too loud) will differ from patient to patient, and that issue must be addressed individually. However, the suggested means of changing those patterns may be similar across patients.

A major lack in voice research is documentation of the efficacy of therapeutic techniques and outcome data. This lack, although decried by many (Johnson, 1985; Ludlow, 1981; Moore, 1977; Perkins, 1985; Reed, 1980), is not easily corrected. Problems of terminology, of definition, of qualitative and quantitative assessment procedures, and of well-established normative standards (as discussed previously) plague the researcher who wishes to address the issue. Brewer and McCall (1974) used the fiberoptic laryngoscope to demonstrate visible changes in laryngeal physiology as patients were instructed in a therapeutic technique. Johnson (1985) reported on the efficacy of his particular program of reducing vocal abuse, which uses a highly structured behavior modification approach. Casper, Brewer, and Conture (1981) reported on computer-assisted measurement of specific intrasubject changes in laryngeal physiology, visible on fiberoptic images, that were thought to be the result of therapeutic intervention. The procedure, although workable, was fairly time consuming, and the results could be interpreted only relative to each individual's performance. Such research is helpful, but the approach does not lend itself to all voice problems. In the case study cited earlier, a new technique was used, and although in this case it proved to be effective, it would not necessarily be an appropriate or effective procedure with other cases of psychogenic dysphonia. If the research question to be answered is concerned not with specific techniques but rather with the question of whether the voice improved as a result of therapy, perhaps the patient is the best judge. Tools such as the Voice Handicap Index and the Voice-Related Quality of Life scale are steps in that direction. Standards for measuring vocal parameters that would objectively reflect improvement of voice continue to escape us.

Thus, we are left with a variety of therapy techniques whose efficacy is acclaimed by many authors. The most often used of these are discussed in this section, which not only describes how they are done but also gives at least a theoretical rationale as to why clinically they seem to be of value. The authors want to caution again that the techniques are only as good as the clinician who is making use of them. Clinicians should use them wisely but should continue to question their efficacy and search for ways to demonstrate it. It is not the intent of the authors to suggest that a single technique need be chosen and that only that technique should be used. Quite the opposite is often the case, and several techniques may be used concurrently or at different points in the therapy plan.

There is no particular meaning to be assigned to the order in which these techniques are presented. There is also no intent to make this an all-inclusive list. Indeed, most clinicians adapt procedures to fit their personal styles and develop unique ones, as do most voice coaches. The challenge is to be able to think through a problem in such a way that it is possible to devise techniques to use based on an understanding of the type of vocal behavior desired. No single technique will be equally effective with all people.

Breathy Phonation: The Confidential Voice

We have found this technique to be widely appropriate and easy for patients to learn and to use, and it has resulted in clinical success. Producing voice is a holistic activity that is usually accomplished without conscious attention to pitch, loudness, variability, or other aspects of voice production. In light of this it seems reasonable to think that a therapy technique that can function in a holistic manner to accomplish its goals should be beneficial and easy for patients to adopt. The use of breathy phonation is such a technique (Casper, 1993). The patient has only to concentrate on making the voice very breathy and in so doing accomplishes a number of other desirable goals. These include reduction of loudness, reduction of rate (no more than 5–6 syllables per breath), reduction of hyperfunction, and a beginning awareness of allowing the expiratory airflow do the work of producing sound.

Breathy voice is being recommended here as a technique to be used for a circumscribed period of time during therapy and not as the end product of therapy. The voice is described to patients as being the softest intensity they can produce, much like the voice one would use to exchange a confidence with a friend when one does not wish others nearby to hear. It is a confidential voice. It differs from whisper in that some voicing is present. The very breathy quality of the voice is its hallmark and differentiates it from a voice just reduced in intensity.

Instruction to talk in a confidential voice and the model of that voice presented by the clinician are often all that is necessary for the patient to understand and to be able to produce the voice. However, when that is not sufficient, it is often helpful to start vocalization activities with other techniques such as the sigh and the yawn/sigh. In both of these the focus is on producing easy, unimpeded airflow and breathy voicing without stress.

Several undesirable behaviors may accompany a patient's use of breathy phonation that are very easily resolved if the clinician is alert. It is not enough for the voice just to be lowered in intensity; it must be breathy. The breathiness must be marked by ease of airflow without evidence of pushing or forcing air. The phonation that is produced must be "well focused" in that pitch should not be lowered nor should mouth opening be reduced. It will not and, indeed, cannot be a resonant voice at this stage.

The patient is instructed to use this voice for all speaking and is forewarned that it will be inaudible in any noisy environment. All loud talking is thus eliminated temporarily. It is also important to instruct the patient that fewer words per breath will be possible because of the increased expenditure of air. Furthermore, because one effect of the increased airflow may be a drying of the mucosa, we suggest that the patient increase fluid intake. This technique is appropriate for patients who need to eliminate phonotrauma. It is helpful as part of a vocal hygiene program whenever a period of modified voice rest or reduction of voice use is indicated.

Verdolini-Marston and her colleagues (Verdolini-Marston, Burke, Lessac, Glaze, & Caldwell, 1995) investigated the efficacy of the confidential voice therapy technique with five female patients with vocal fold nodules. The therapy was provided by two clinicians over a 2-week period. Pretreatment and post-treatment measurements of phonatory effort, auditory perceptual ratings of voice disorder severity, and visual ratings of vocal fold characteristics seen in videostroboscopic recordings were obtained. An additional five patients with nodules constituted the control group. Many patients showed improvement after the 2-week therapy period, whereas there was little improvement of voice production in the control group. Most therapy patients had a decrease of phonatory effort and a decrease in the rated severity of dysphonia. Four of the five patients in the therapy group showed visible changes of the vocal folds. These data suggest that the confidential voice therapy approach can be effective in reducing vocal trauma and result in better voice production.

Another interesting finding from this study was the report that continued use of the therapeutic techniques after therapy had ended contributed to improved voice performance. Patient compliance and willingness to use the new form of voice production in routine voice usage appear to be predictive of long-term voice improvement.

Rationale: We have observed laryngeal physiology endoscopically as we have asked patients and normal speakers to use this confidential voice and have noted the desired effect (Casper, Colton, Brewer, & Woo, 1989). The glottis remains very slightly open, thus reducing the force of contact and of medial compression of the vocal folds. The larynx seems to remain vertically at about the resting level. There is an absence of any appearance of laryngeal tightness or squeezing, and the closed phase of the glottal cycle is reduced. In some patients, there may be a tendency to produce breathiness with a posterior glottal chink and Y appearance. This is not as desirable as incomplete glottal closure along the full length of the folds, and may be indicative of a greater than necessary degree of tension or strain in producing the phonation. In such cases, the use of visual biofeedback with the flexible endoscope in place can be very effective. Thus, with one maneuver the patient is provided with a type of voice production that eliminates trauma yet allows continued voice use, albeit different and reduced. It is a holistic approach that does not require that the act of speaking be broken down into its component parts, with each addressed separately and then put back together. We have also found it rather simple for patients to move gradually from the breathy, confidential voice to increased voicing without returning to previous habits.

After approximately 3 to 4 sessions, most patients are ready to begin reducing vocal breathiness and increasing intensity. The previous vocal hoarseness should not be present. Full voicing is re-introduced gradually for certain situations or certain amounts of time. During this time it is appropriate to introduce the concepts of vocal resonance and vocal focus. If the clear vocal quality is maintained for the next 3 weeks, therapy can be terminated or reduced in terms of frequency. Re-visualization of the larynx and other post-therapy testing (i.e., QOL) should be completed.

Sigh, Aspirate Initiation, and Easy Initiation of Phonation

These three techniques are combined under one heading because they are variations on a theme sharing a common rationale. For the sigh, the patient is instructed to produce the most relaxed, effortless, natural sigh possible. Whether voicing is present does not matter initially, but as this is practiced it is hoped that some voicing emerges naturally and easily. In a natural, spontaneous sigh, releasing some air audibly before the actual voicing begins, then producing just minimal voicing in terms of loudness and duration, and finishing the sigh with audible expiration of the rest of the breath supply, is not uncommon. The patient must not hold the breath after the inspiration. There must be a continuous flow from inhalation through exhalation; otherwise, there is a tendency to close the glottis tightly as the breath is held.

From the sigh it is easy to have the patient practice aspirate initiation of voicing, using words that begin with an /h/. This should be done in a slightly exaggerated manner so that the /h/ is held and the voicing is initiated much as in the sigh and with a breathy quality. As the patient becomes adept at this maneuver, it is possible to omit the actual production of the /h/ yet continue the effortless gliding into easy initiation of phonation.

Rationale: These techniques reduce laryngeal and vocal tract tensions, reduce the force of vocal fold contact and of medial compression, teach easy coordination of airflow and phonation, counteract traumatic habits of tension and hard glottal attack, and foster resting level laryngeal posture. They may be very helpful for patients who have difficulty in learning to use a breathy voice for general conversation and appear to need more direct step-by-step work to learn to reduce tensions. In a fiberoptic and stroboscopic study of aspirate initiation of phonation, Casper et al. (1989) observed the expected physiological characteristics just described.

Yawn/Sigh

The patient is instructed to simulate a real yawn, or if possible, to actually trigger a real yawn. The yawn is completed with a sigh, making sure to allow air to be released in a relaxed way. This is not always easy for patients to do. We tend to be socialized into hiding and stifling public yawns. It is sometimes helpful to instruct the patient to open the mouth very wide, pull the tongue back and inhale long and deeply. Initiation of voicing should be carried out with this same oral posture, with a gradual closing of the mouth as the yawn and sigh progress. Patients become aware of natural yawns and try to concentrate on how they feel when they occur spontaneously. As the patient learns the technique and can identify the tension reduction, a gradual shaping of the yawn/sigh into production of words, then phrases, and finally sentences should proceed slowly. The yawn should be gradually eliminated.

Rationale: In a true vegetative yawn, the larynx lowers dramatically (Casper et al., 1989). This change can be observed fiberoptically. The physiology of a yawn is incompatible with the excessive laryngeal tensions that many patients exhibit. Easy, natural airflow and phonation are fostered. The intent is to eliminate tight initiation and maintenance of phonation and to reduce laryngeal tensions. Individuals who have adopted hyperfunctional habits of voice production tend to have a high laryngeal posture. They often complain of pain in the extrinsic laryngeal muscles. The yawn/sigh maneuver, which lowers laryngeal posture, serves to "stretch" those muscles, providing relief from the tightness. This is a further benefit of the technique.

Post Botox Injection Therapy

After successful injection, patients often experience a brief period of breathy voice. During that time there is a natural desire to "push" the voice so as to get the most voicing possible. The thrust of voice treatment, which should be restricted to three or four sessions, is to counteract this tendency. Easy onset of phonation is taught using techniques described earlier. The patient must be taught to concentrate on the airflow, specifically the initiation and gentle maintenance of that flow. Pushing for increased loudness is discouraged. Indeed, we encourage the patient to "give in" to the soft voice and learn from it. The aspects of voicing on which they can focus are the ease of producing it (albeit quietly), the slowed rate of speech, the shorter phrase groups. The fact that the voice will get louder with time and without any effort on their part is stressed. However, we also urge them to maintain some of the new voice behaviors they have learned during the breathy period.

Trill

The trill is a sound made by the tongue tip making contact with the alveolar ridge and oscillating rapidly as sound is produced. The sound can be described as the trilled /r/ heard in many languages, including Spanish. The trill can also be made using the lips and allowing them to oscillate rapidly as voice is produced. Both of these trills also can be produced in a voiceless manner but are not beneficial to voice production that way. When used as a vocal exercise, the sound is essential, and the patient is asked to sustain the trill. This is an exercise used by many singers to "warm up" the voice. Very rapid and strong laryngeal vibrations can be felt if the fingers are placed on the larynx during production of the trill.

We have found the trill to be very useful and productive with a variety of disordered voices. We began using it with patients whose vocal folds were scarred postoperatively. The results seemed to be much better than any we had obtained with this population using other techniques. Subsequently, we have used it with patients who present with a variety of disorders, particularly of the hypofunctional type.

Patients are first instructed in production of the sustained trill at a comfortable pitch and loudness. Pitch variation is then introduced by sustaining the trilled sound at various pitches and then by gliding the trill through a range of pitches in both descending and ascending glides. We find it helpful as therapy progresses to extend the trilled sound into voicing without trill. This is done by instructing the patient to start the trill and smoothly transition into a prolonged vowel with no break in phonation or change in pitch. This can be done with a variety of vowel sounds and at various pitches as well. And finally, the sound is shaped into speech. Although we extend practice beyond the trill itself, we also instruct patients to continue practice of the trill as such, and to use it as a warm-up exercise at the start of the day and before any extended speaking. During therapy, patients are instructed to practice the trill for short periods as often as possible throughout the day. This is particularly important for patients with scarred, stiff vocal folds and may be required over a lengthy period. These exercise protocols may be done with either the lip or tongue trill. Some individuals are incapable of producing the tongue trill, and it does not warrant the use of valuable therapy time to try to teach that. It also has been our experience that some older patients may have difficulty with this task.

Rationale: The trill appears to "jump start" the vibratory behavior of the vocal folds. Production of the trill balances resonance, fosters normal laryngeal tension by equalizing the aerodynamic and the myoelastic forces, and enhances coordination of respiration/phonation/articulation (Behlau & Pontes, 1990). McGowan (1992) described some work on modeling the tongue-tip trill based on some physiological data and modeling experiments. Basically, the tongue tip acts like a springed trap door that creates pressure differences between the outside air and the cavity behind the tip constriction. These pressure differences oscillate to produce the desired effect. What happens in the cavity behind the constriction is dynamic, with oscillatory changes of air pressure and air volume velocity. There appear to be oscillations on the pharyngeal walls creating small-volume velocity changes of the air passing through them. These pharyngeal wall variations may be important also for vocal fold oscillation because they could create a greater pressure difference across the vocal folds producing oscillation. McGowan also suggests that the subglottal air pressures during the production of tongue trills may be greater than during normal phonation, again creating a greater force for vocal fold oscillation. Few research data substantiate these claims, but clinical experience suggests that the technique is a very useful one capable of eliciting improved voice in many patients. In the patient with postoperative scarring of the vocal folds, the increased stiffness of the cover interferes with vibratory behavior. The trill appears to have the potential to reduce the effect of the stiffness, probably because of the forceful but healthy vibratory behavior.

Pitch Extension Exercises

This technique focuses on extending the pitch range in patients who experience difficulty with restricted range. It should only be used with patients who do not have vocal fold pathological conditions such as nodules, polyps, cysts, hemorrhage, etc. Although restricted pitch range is a characteristic sign accompanying those conditions, the presence of the lesions acts to impede the laryngeal adjustments necessary for production of a full pitch range. When the pathological condition is resolved, those patients generally regain a full pitch range without any therapeutic attention specifically directed to that skill. Those patients for whom the pitch extension exercises seem most appropriate and effective are those whose restricted range is caused by stiffening of the vocal fold cover (as in a scar), rigidity of the entire phonatory system including vocal folds (as in some Parkinson's patients), hypofunction (as in presbyphonia), and hyperfunction or musculoskeletal tension. Make certain that this activity is done in a gentle manner free of strain. The patient is instructed in producing a sustained vowel (or the syllable /la/) at a comfortable pitch level. When that is established, the patient is instructed to sing one or two notes up the scale. How far this is extended depends on the patient's capabilities. Singing up and down these several notes, and perhaps extending the pitch range downward as well, is used as practice material to be done several times per day. The range is extended gradually as the patient demonstrates the ability to do so.

Rationale: The act of raising pitch, when done without strain, usually involves the elongation of the vocal folds, thereby thinning the mass and placing it under greater tension. Patients with scarred vocal folds usually have an area of stiffness of the cover that does not vibrate well. Stiffness is a characteristic of scar tissue. The intent of this exercise is to encourage active stretching of the folds, and thus a stretching of the scarred area as well. This, in turn, should increase the flexibility of the scarred vocal fold and improve its vibratory behavior. In persons with Parkinson's disease, this exercise is designed to counteract the tendency toward monotonic voice production as the neurological control of the entire laryngeal mechanism becomes increasingly impaired. Patients who present with presbyphonia and those with other hypofunctional voice disorders benefit from vocal activities that increase the work of the phonatory mechanism.

Chewing

The act of chewing as a therapy technique was described by Froeschels in 1952. The technique requires that the patient practice the motions of chewing in an exaggerated manner and then sequentially, over time, add voicing, random sounds, words, phrases, sentences, and conversation while gradually reducing the degree of exaggeration of the mouth movements. As the technique is described, it is very important to help the patient imitate the chewing act quite exactly. This must involve constant movement of the tongue. Exaggeration of the act requires that the mouth be open while chewing. The resulting sounds produced when the activity is carried out correctly should be very variable. If the sound produced tends to be a repetitive, unchanging "yam yam," the chewing is being done with inadequate tongue movement. It has been our experience that it is often difficult for patients to learn to do this chewing motion correctly. As with yawning, we have been socialized into chewing as unobtrusively as possible, and certainly with the mouth closed. If this technique is to be used, the clinician must be adept at, and comfortable with, modeling it for the patient. It is often helpful for the clinician to do the activity along with the patient, thereby reducing self-consciousness. The use of chewable substances can help the patient identify the components of the chewing act. It then becomes somewhat easier to carry out that activity based on recall and imagery and without the actual substance in the mouth. (It is not a good idea for the clinician to provide chewable material. Instead, the clinician should suggest that the patient bring crackers, gum, or other chewable foods to the therapy session.) Each step of chewing as a therapy approach must be mastered before the next level is introduced. Thus, the patient must learn to chew in the most exaggerated manner while producing voicing and random sounds before being asked to practice words. It is important to realize that articulatory clarity will be reduced in the early stages of using this technique, because the focus remains on the chewing motion. Use of words and phrases that begin with vowels may be the easiest to begin practice. As the patient progresses and longer utterances are introduced, the chewing motions are almost eliminated, but excess tensions associated with phonation should not be evident.

Rationale: In adopting this technique, Froeschels sought a natural vegetative movement onto which phonation could be added without changing the totality of the act and without adding tensions or other negative behaviors the patient had habituated into the speaking act. The chewing motion has a tendency to release excess tensions in the vocal tract and laryngeal area, and when done correctly encourages mouth opening and reduction of mandibular tensions. These behaviors in turn foster easy onset of phonation without making that a specific focus of attention.

Chant-Talk

The name of this technique describes a manner of speaking that is a cross between speaking and singing or, from the singer's point of view, a form of singing that is a cross between singing and speaking. We tend to think of it as having limited frequency variability while retaining the flow of song. It can be used as a therapeutic technique in a number of different ways. Most simply, the patient can be asked to chant an utterance rather than speak it. If this is effective in eliciting effortless phonation of a good quality, the technique can be extended in practice with gradual reduction of the sing-song quality of the chant. If a particular "voice placement" or "focus" is sought, this chanting can be one of a variety of ways of finding that focus. For example, using Cooper's "um-hum" technique (1973; see also the "um-hum" therapy technique described later), the patient may be asked to sustain that sound and chant the counting of numbers, or series of words or a sentence. It may be helpful for some patients to locate and identify the desired vocal sound through this chanting approach. When the sound can be produced at will, therapy moves on through chanting of syllables, words, and sentences. When that is mastered, practice turns to reducing the chanting quality while maintaining the vocal focus. All of this should take several weeks.

Rationale: The chanting of an utterance encourages an easy flow of phonation, reducing the tendency toward hard glottal attack and increased force of vocal fold contact. Voicing flows continuously rather than the start/stop characteristic of connected speech. There may be some increased proprioceptive feedback as vibrations are felt through the nose and cheek areas, thus helping the patient to reduce focus on the larynx. If the voice is produced in this manner, a reduction in laryngeal and vocal tract tensions usually occurs. Because chanting differs from talking and is usually a new way for patients to produce voice, it may be easier for them to alter voice production through this activity than to attempt to do so in speaking, wherein the habits are entrenched.

Hum and Nasal Consonants

This is another technique designed to teach easy voice production through a "natural" approach. The patient is asked to produce a hum and to be able to feel the resonance of that hum in the nose and cheeks. The pitch of the voice is generally not of direct concern, although it may seem to change as the patient searches for an easily produced, fully resonant sound. The hum is sustained, and the patient practices this until the target sound is produced without difficulty. It is often instructive to then ask the patient to fully lower and then elevate the mandible, keeping the lips closed while sustaining the hum. This results in an almost palpable forward movement of the focus of the voice, with a tickling sensation often being reported around the lips and along the alveolar ridge of the palate. One of the authors was instructed by a voice coach to "hook" the sound in the back of the throat to master this kind of voice quality. The sound used for practice was the /ng/. Bear in mind that the sound being sought is not a nasal sound but rather a sound that might best be described as the "twang" that is typical of Country Western singing (Colton & Estill, 1981). Gradually the production of these sounds is shaped into speech by first using nonsense syllables and words heavily loaded with the nasal consonants. Although the early practice of this technique may result in greater nasal resonance than is desirable, the nasality is temporary and normalizes as speech is introduced. This technique can easily be combined with the chant-talk technique.

Rationale: As described in the rationale for chant-talk, the act of humming is different from speaking and thus may not be encumbered with undesirable habituated behaviors. A hum encourages easy initiation of phonation and provides proprioceptive feedback of nasal and facial vibration, thus refocusing the patient's preoccupation with the laryngeal area. The continuant nasal consonant promotes ease of sustained phonation, and it can easily be coordinated with the idea of smooth airflow from inhalation through exhalation. The "twang" sound also elicits a mode of vocal fold vibration that produces a greater number of harmonics and thus a richer sound (Colton & Estill, 1981).

Vocal Function Exercise Program

Stemple, Glaze, and Gerdeman (1995) propose a specific program of exercises that are reported to be efficacious in the treatment of various voice disorders. Specifically, patients are instructed in four exercises and required to practice them several times a day: (a) sustaining the vowel /ee/ on the note F, above middle C for females and below middle C for males, softly and for as long as the person is capable of sustaining the voiceless /s/; (b) producing the word "knoll" starting on a high pitch and allowing the pitch to glide down while still holding on to the word; (c) the same as (b) but in reverse, starting low and gliding high; and (d) sustaining the vowel /o/ softly on the notes C, D, E, F, and G, beginning on middle C for females and an octave lower for males.

Rationale: *The authors state that many factors may be responsible for weakening, straining, and creating imbalance of the laryngeal mechanism. These exercises are believed to address these areas and provide a systematic exercise program to restore balance, strength, and ease of phonation.*

Digital Manipulation, Pressure, and Massage

Aronson (1985) has described a technique that involves direct physical manipulation and massage of the laryngeal area. The clinician must identify the tips of the hyoid bone and exert light pressure in a circular motion in that area. The clinician then moves the fingers into the thyrohyoid space and carries out the circular motion massage, moving posteriorly from the thyroid notch area. The massage is then done on the posterior borders of the thyroid cartilage. With the fingers along the superior border of the thyroid cartilage, the clinician begins to gently exert pressure in a downward manner to move the larynx down. There should be an increase in the thyrohyoid space. During these maneuvers, the patient is asked to phonate vowels. When a positive change in the voice is noted (clearer quality and lowered pitch), the focus shifts to the production of that voice with, and then without, the manipulation. This entire activity needs to be carried out with care and with recognition that some pain might result. Patients must be reassured that the pain is temporary and is like any muscular pain associated with excessive tension and its reduction through direct manipulation and massage. According to Aronson, this technique may be effective in eliciting normal voice in a single therapy session in cases of dysphonia that is caused by increased musculoskeletal tensions. However, when the condition has been of long duration, a longer course of treatment using this technique may be necessary.

Nelson Roy has recently described the use of this technique and reported data on its efficacy (Roy, 1994; Roy & Leeper, 1993; Roy, Tasko, & Harvey, 1995; Tasko, Roy, & Harvey, 1994). Roy confirms the finding that many patients are able to achieve normal voice in a single therapy session. The diagnoses of the patients so treated fall primarily into two categories: musculoskeletal tension and functional or psychogenic disorder. He states that 88% of the patients in his study population reported pain on palpation of the laryngeal area, often radiating to the ear. His description of the technique begins with palpation of the laryngeal area to determine the degree and location of tension and pain, the mobility of the larynx in the vertical dimension, and the extent of laryngeal elevation. The technique is otherwise as described.

Rationale: This technique is based on the need to reduce "cramping" in the extrinsic and intrinsic laryngeal muscles, which is believed to be the cause of dysphonia in many patients. The massaging of muscles induces relaxation, and the technique promotes a lowered laryngeal position, permitting ease of phonation, and relieves pain of muscle tension. In using this technique, the clinician must understand and be able to identify the specific disturbance of phonatory physiology exhibited by a patient. Many but not all voice patients who are classified as having a hyperfunctional voice disorder speak with the larynx in an elevated posture. Care must be taken not to exert undue effort in pushing the larynx lower than is comfortable for the patient.

Boone (1983) has described a method of digital pressure that is very different in both intent and technique from that described. Boone suggests that digital pressure be applied as a gentle inward push on the anterior aspect of the thyroid cartilage while a patient sustains a vowel. This pressure should result in lowered fundamental frequency and can be used to elicit and then habituate this lowered pitch, when that is a therapeutic goal.

Rationale: Applying pressure as described tilts the thyroid cartilage posteriorly and in so doing shortens vocal fold length and increases mass. This then results in a lowered fundamental frequency of vibration, perceived as lowered pitch. Once elicited in this manner, the lowered pitch becomes the target to be practiced and produced voluntarily.

Easy Production of Falsetto or High-Pitched Sounds

This technique is yet another that tends to shift the patient away from habituated patterns of voice use. It is especially helpful for patients who demonstrate anteroposterior laryngeal squeezing and for some who are found to be using ventricular phonation. It may require trial and error and much suggestion on the part of the clinician to facilitate the patient's ability to produce a high-pitched sound. The use of imagery can be very helpful (see "Imagery"), as can the use of animal sounds, such as the meow of a kitten or a wolf's howl. Note that there should be a continuous flow of air from inhalation through exhalation, because the patient may have the tendency to increase tension and hold the breath before initiation of voicing. When the patient learns to easily produce the high-pitched vowels at will, that sound can be sustained and the pitch gradually lowered in a glissando to the comfortable speaking level, without a change in voice quality. The patient is then asked to produce a sustained vowel at that targeted speaking pitch, maintaining the improved quality. As this is established, it can be shaped into speech. There is no attempt to specify a pitch level beyond that which is identified by the patient as comfortable and normal sounding.

Rationale: Easy production of the upper frequency range is most commonly produced by a lengthening of the vocal folds, decreasing their mass. It cannot be done using ventricular phonation, for example. Therefore, if a high-pitched sound is elicited from a patient who has been using ventricular phonation, the technique has successfully shifted the patient out of that phonatory mode. The same rationale may be applied to patients who tend to constrict the larynx in the anteroposterior dimension or to those whose aberrant voice production behaviors are psychologically based. Patients with psychogenic voice problems have "learned" a particular manner of phonation that produces their aberrant sound. If they are asked to produce sound in some novel way, they often must abandon their "learned" method and in so doing normal voice may be elicited. Thus, the change in laryngeal physiology from their particular behavior to that required for the production of the upper frequency range, if successful, may be sufficient to restore normal phonatory function, which can then be maintained as pitch is normalized.

Imagery

The use of imagery can be very helpful in describing how a particular type of sound should be produced. For example, statements of imagery such as "Make it feel as if your voice is floating effortlessly out of your throat and up into your head" can describe to the patient a way that effortless voicing might feel. Patients should be encouraged to provide their own imagery as they release tensions and change their manner of initiating phonation. The use of imagery can be combined with many of the other techniques, as it can help patients keep in mind what they are attempting to do. Imagery is often used in those techniques designated by some as "placing the voice" or finding a "focus" for the voice. It has been reported that professional singers and actors use imagery concerning their breathing, which, although often in contradiction to known physiological fact, works well for them (Hixon, 1987; Watson, Hixon, & Maher, 1987).

Rationale: *The physiology of imagery is receiving increasing attention as its use grows in the training of athletes and in fighting disease (Keaton, 1983; Ungerleider, 1986). It has been used in singing pedagogy for many years, and its effectiveness is perhaps attested to by legions of superb performers. We use it in voice therapy to help a patient understand something about how to produce voice or what quality to attempt to produce, when other types of explanations are either not possible or have not been effective. Imagery, although perhaps not physiologically correct, can describe what seems to happen in a very subjective, sensory way. No doubt a patient will remember an image used to describe the feeling of producing a certain sound long after the muscles involved are forgotten.*

Pushing, Pulling, and Isometrics

These techniques are placed together because they are used interchangeably to produce the same end result. Pushing refers to any of the many ways that patients may be encouraged to push against a wall, push down on a chair, and so on, and pulling refers to the opposite maneuvers of pulling up on a very heavy desk, pulling up on the chair one is sitting in, and the like. Isometric forms of these activities include placing the palms of the hands together at chest height and pressing them together or locking the fingers of the hands together at chest height and pulling them apart. Whichever method is used, the patient is instructed to phonate at the point of maximum pull or push. The sound produced will be a forceful grunt and should be demonstrated by the clinician. All of the varieties of these techniques are designed to force effort closure of the glottis, a form of hyperfunction of the mechanism. They often can be used with surprising success in eliciting a low-pitched phonation in cases of puberphonia and in eliciting voicing in patients who present with psychogenic aphonia. Once the patient has learned to carry out the push or pull, the same effect can be obtained by holding the breath, bearing down, and grunting. As the desired voicing is produced, the patient is instructed to sustain that sound as the force of the maneuver is gradually released. In a gradual stepwise fashion, the targeted sound is practiced with less and less need for the forceful push or pull activity.

Because these activities enforce a certain behavior on the larynx, patients with psychogenic problems also may have difficulty holding on to their typical mode of voice production. Thus, through the use of push, pull, or isometric activities, these patients may find an acceptable way to abandon their symptom and produce voice in a more typical fashion.

Rationale: *These maneuvers are designed to create effort closure of the glottis with the larynx in a lowered position. As such they are the opposite of hypofunction. Furthermore, the posture of the laryngeal mechanism is determined by the activity and dictates a particular type of vocalization. This shifts the individual from the usual manner of vocal production and introduces a behavior difficult to counteract. If tension is released before phonation, then the technique will be ineffective.*

As noted earlier, we have found these techniques to be effective in eliciting a low-pitched voice from patients with puberphonia. The vocal fold and laryngeal postures that naturally occur in the use of these techniques are incompatible with anything but a low-pitched voice, if they are being done correctly.

Although these techniques are potentially useful, there is a caveat. By their nature they induce hyperfunction and thus are potentially abusive. They should therefore be used judiciously. We have found that their effectiveness will be noted fairly quickly, if indeed they are going to be effective. Thus, prolonging their use is usually not necessary. When assigned for home practice, the amount of time involved should be clearly specified. These effort closure techniques should be used cautiously and sparingly, in recognition of their potentially abusive nature.

These procedures have been recommended by some authors for treatment of unilateral vocal fold paralysis, believing that the effort closure forces a crossing of the midline of the unaffected vocal fold to approximate the paralyzed fold. We, however, caution against the use of effort closure techniques with patients who demonstrate unilateral vocal fold paralysis. In our experience, the result of practicing these push/pull techniques appears to fatigue the mechanism. Patients report increased hoarseness and reduced volume, almost to aphonia, after a period of such practice. Further discussion of this topic is found later in this chapter under "Unresolved Issues and Myths."

Laughing, Coughing, Throat Clearing, Gargling, and Other Reflexive Acts

In the attempt to elicit voice from the aphonic patient who appears to have a normally functioning larynx, or to find a normal voice for the dysphonic patient when there are no positive laryngologic findings, the use of any of these nonspeech vocalizations can be extremely effective. Indeed, it is important for the clinician to listen for spontaneous laughing, coughing, vocalized pauses, or throat clearing during general conversation with the patient. Patients are not aware that the mechanism used for producing these sounds is the same as is used for producing the speaking voice. Thus, such sounds may be heard during conversation or even when the patient is asked to produce them. The skilled clinician can make use of that sound by shaping it into speech in a gradual manner. This technique may occasionally be startlingly effective. However, it also may be ineffective with some who will continue to use dysphonic voice or no voice in response to a direct request even though they may have produced such sounds spontaneously. Again, it takes the skill of the clinician to use all instances of good voicing to reestablish normal voice.

Rationale: These behaviors are so automatic that the patient may perform them unaware that voice is being produced. Thus, they may be produced with a much better sound than is heard in speech. Because they are not speech behaviors, their production may be free of habituated but undesirable phonatory speech behaviors. The inability to elicit an improved voice using these behaviors also may be a meaningful finding. It may suggest that the patient is somewhat resistant to "giving up" the bad voice, or perhaps there is a problem present that has not been identified. Further exploration may reveal ways to elicit voice or a cause of the problem that was not previously identified. Although throat clearing and coughing can be abusive to the laryngeal mechanism, and are thus not recommended for extensive therapeutic use, they can be used judiciously in the search for normal voicing.

"Um-Hum"

In this technique, the patient is instructed to say "um-hum," the vocalized utterance used by a listener to indicate agreement with the speaker, in a naturally spontaneous and sincere manner. There is a deceptive simplicity to this technique, and the clinician must be sure to elicit a very natural production of "um hum." This is difficult for some persons to do when it becomes a conscious and voluntary utterance. When it is captured in a natural manner, the production is then shaped by adding single words, as in "um-hum one." Gradually this is extended through the use of increasingly longer utterances until the patient is able to produce the targeted voice without needing the starting "um-hum."

Rationale: According to Cooper (1984), this simple utterance, if said as naturally as possible, results in producing a voice at the appropriate pitch level and with the correct focus for the individual. Vibration should be perceptible along the bridge and sides of the nose and down to the lips. This technique, similar to the preceding one, capitalizes on a phonatory act that is almost reflexive in nature. The fact that a nasal component is present in the consonant /m/ adds to the appropriate focusing of the voice.

Whispering

Whispering is the act of moving the articulators to form words in the presence of rapid airflow but the absence of phonation. Very little instruction is usually required to elicit whispering. A quiet, unforced whisper can be used when vocal rest or minimal voice use is part of the treatment plan. It is sometimes instructive to ask patients who habitually use excessive loudness to limit themselves to a quiet whisper for part (or parts) of each day. The pronounced contrast between the whisper and the habitual loudness level may help to focus the patient's awareness and to make reducing loudness to an acceptable level easier to accomplish.

Rationale: Despite many caveats in the literature that whispering is harmful, no experimental evidence supports that notion. Indeed, evidence suggests otherwise. This issue is addressed more completely in the section "Unresolved Issues and Myths." An unforced whisper by definition is an absence of phonation. This suggests that the vocal folds are not fully adducting and thus collision forces are reduced. Gentle airflow is present, and there should be an absence of tensions. Caution is taken to ensure that the whisper does not become excessive and strained, which is counter to the reduction of tension sought in the first place.

Respiratory Facilitation of Phonation

Paying direct attention to respiration is sometimes helpful. By focusing on the breathing, tensions that may be generalized throughout the chest as well as the larynx and vocal tract can be reduced. Patients should be instructed as simply as possible to sit at rest and allow their breathing to function normally and without conscious control. It is, after all, an autonomic nervous system function. Remember that the diaphragm is a muscle of inhalation and is active during the inspiratory cycle (Fig. 10.2). At high lung volumes, however, it may be necessary to contract the diaphragm to prevent the rapid, unwanted descent of the rib cage, producing greater than needed subglottal pressures that will produce louder and uncontrolled voice production. As shown in Figure 10.2, a number of muscles are activated during a speaking event. At high lung volumes, the muscles activated will be inspiratory, but as lung volume falls, expiratory musculature will be needed to provide the proper air pressure to drive the vocal folds. Excess muscle activity in the respiratory musculature will prevent the smooth coordination of the respiratory system and the steady maintenance of subglottal air pressure and phonation.

The clinician should observe the patient's breathing pattern at rest and, assuming that it is normal, that is, consistent with tidal breathing, instruct the patient to gently place one hand on the area of the abdomen (diaphragm) and the other on the upper chest, while continuing to breathe quietly. The patient should be able to identify slight outward movement of the abdomen (diaphragm) area on inhalation with imperceptible movement of the upper chest. The patient's attention also needs to be directed to the continuous movement in the respiratory cycle from inspiration through expiration. If the patient exhibits a breathing pattern at rest and in general conversation that seems aberrant, additional attention needs to be addressed to pulmonary function in general.

As soon as the effortless breathing has been established, the patient should be instructed to breathe in a little more deeply and to release the exhalation cycle as a sigh without changing the manner of breathing. It should be sufficient to instruct the patient to fill the body with air. Thus, the focus on breathing leads easily into incorporation of the sigh, the yawn-sigh, aspirate initiation of phonation, and so on. A nasal or humming sound produced on tidal exhalation also may be possible. Again, it is important initially to simulate tidal breathing as closely as possible, with pauses between breath groups, and an emphasis on exhalation associated with relaxation. Voice is lightly "tapped," or superimposed, on the tidal exhalation. As the patient learns to do these activities easily, the task can continue to be altered so that the inhalation stage of breathing occurs more quickly, as it does normally during speech, while the exhalation stage is lengthened. When adding the latter refinement, the patient must not introduce tensions or attempts to extend exhalation beyond the available air supply. The clinician must determine whether the work on breathing has helped the patient to also reduce or eliminate laryngeal tensions. The patient must be instructed in the generalization of the improved respiratory control to conversational speech. The clinician must remember that average conversational utterances on one continuous respiration tend to be very short, approximately 5 seconds (Boone & McFarlane, 1988), and that, therefore, nonprofessional voice users do not need to inhale as deeply as do professional voice users in singing, acting, or public speaking. The amount of therapeutic time devoted to work on breathing and, indeed, the need for any such attention, must be decided on a case-by-case basis.

Extended training in breath support and breath control is important for the professional voice user. Many activities or exercises can be designed to accomplish this, but

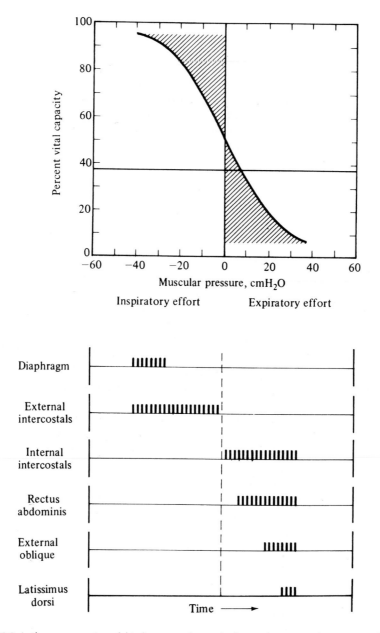

Figure 10.2. In the upper portion of this figure are shown the lung volume–muscle pressure relationships during the production of a sustained vowel. At high lung volumes, a large amount of inspiratory muscle pressure is needed to counteract the large lung pressures that are created. As lung volume decreases, less inspiratory effort is needed, until resting lung volume is reached (the point where the curve crosses the vertical line in the middle of the graph). At still lower lung volumes, expiratory muscle effort is needed to produce the necessary subglottal pressures for speech. In the panel below, a schematic of muscle activity in the diaphragm, external intercostals, internal intercostals, rectus abdominis, external oblique, and latissimus dorsi is shown in relationship to the pressure relationships shown above.

they are beyond the scope of this book. Note, however, that any such exercises must be done with an understanding of respiratory physiology and recognition of the need to build control in a gradual way, as in any activity of muscle building and training.

Rationale: The respiratory system is the power source for the voice. The systems involved in phonation are closely intertwined, and tensions in one system cannot easily be isolated from the rest. Thus, reducing respiratory tensions and assuring continuous airflow from inspiration through expiration assists in reducing laryngeal tensions and avoiding closure of the glottis before the initiation of phonation. Tidal breathing represents perhaps the least effortful, most economical breathing available to us. Using it to support vocalization, even if limited, can help reduce the overall effort level associated with voice production and facilitate elicitation of normal voice. This is not to say, however, that respiration is somehow disturbed in dysphonic speakers. Most patients, with the exception of those who have chronic respiratory problems, chronic obstructive lung disease, or neuromotor impairment of the control of respiration, tend to have normal respiration and adequate air supply for speech. This topic is discussed later in "Unresolved Issues and Myths." Singers, actors, and other professional voice users may have demands placed on voice use that require greater control of increased volumes of air. This group of voice users will need more extended training in the management of breath support and breath control than the average speaker.

Relaxation

A variety of techniques are used to teach generalized relaxation. These include progressive relaxation in which the patient is instructed to concentrate on specific parts of the body one at a time and then through imagery and suggestion to release the tensions present (Jacobson, 1938). Another part of the technique involves purposefully tensing a specific body area, followed by a release of that tension. Imagery is often used in teaching relaxation, and deep breathing exercises frequently are incorporated as well. The shoulders, upper back, and neck are very vulnerable to muscle tightening in tense individuals (Nagler, 1987). A popular activity for relaxation of these tensions has been the head roll, in which the patient is instructed to very, very slowly allow the head to be rotated 360°. However, circular rotation of any part of the spine may not be helpful to the intervertebral disks, and the following exercises are recommended instead (Nagler, 1987):

1. While holding the left elbow in the right hand, pull it over to the right side, hold, then relax. Do the same with the other arm, and repeat the sequence three times for each arm. Maintain a normal breathing pattern.
2. Place the hands, palms in, on the upper chest, with elbows out to the sides. Circle the elbows in one direction and then reverse. Repeat three times. Maintain a normal breathing pattern.
3. Raise shoulders up as high as possible, hold, then slowly release. Repeat three times while maintaining a normal breathing pattern.

Rationale: The rationale for engaging in relaxation therapy as one segment of a vocal rehabilitation program is primarily to release excess tensions in systems involved with phonation. However, it must be recognized that most of our talking is done in states other than complete relaxation. Thus, these techniques must be used in specific ways and then be incorporated into healthy patterns of phonation. Patients should be instructed in these techniques and then asked to practice them at home. In view of the restrictions placed by third-party payers on the number of voice therapy sessions that will be covered, typically it is not possible to spend much therapy time on such practice. This is also applicable to practice on breathing.

Phonating on Inhalation

The technique for creating voice in this way is just as described by the title. The patient is instructed and shown how to make sound in the reverse of the normal pattern, that is, as air is being drawn into the lungs. This is usually a fairly simple sound for most people to make. The technique has been described by many authors as useful in reversing ventricular phonation. This author has rarely found that to be true but has used the technique for other purposes. The patient is instructed to switch directly from voice produced on inhalation into voice produced on exhalation. If this technique is successful in eliciting an improved voice quality in the exhalation phase, it can then be gradually shaped into speech with a gradual reduction of the need to start with phonation on inhalation. It is also another manner in which to force change in a habituated but maladaptive phonatory pattern. We have found it useful occasionally in eliciting phonation from an otherwise aphonic or dysphonic patient who presents with normal laryngeal examination.

Another use of inspiratory speech has been described by Harrison et al. (1992) in a patient with spasmodic dysphonia. The technique of speaking on inhalation differs from that described above in that there is no attempt to transfer from the phonation produced on inhalation to similar phonation on exhalation. Rather, the focus here is on learning to use inspiratory speech to replace expiratory speech, to establish the inspiratory speech as the habitual pattern. Harrison et al. (1992) describe a patient with adductor spasmodic dysphonia who had discovered that he could produce speech during inhalation in a much more fluent and less effortful manner than his spasmodic speech. He adopted that form of speech, which was judged to be perceptually somewhat rough but intelligible and more acceptable to listeners than the strain/struggle interrupted spasmodic speech. One of the authors of the Harrison et al. paper was able to learn the inspiratory form of speech with relative ease, although the authors recognize that may not be the case for all patients. Nevertheless, it is offered as an alternative to other methods of treatment for patients with spasmodic dysphonia. Others have described use of this type of phonation for spasmodic dysphonia (Freeman, Shulman, personal communication). It is a noninvasive form of treatment that, if successfully learned, may offer consistent voice to the patient.

Rationale: *Voice produced on inhalation is said to be produced by the true vocal folds with a pulling away (abduction) of the ventricular folds (Lehmann, 1965; Williams, Farquharson, & Anthony, 1975). In our experience, this observation has been frequently confirmed by endoscopic visualization of patients engaging in this task. Thus, in patients who are using ventricular fold phonation or those who are improperly using the vocal folds, this technique is theorized to stimulate more appropriate physiology. In the pattern of inspiratory speech described by Harrison et al. (1992), the vocal folds were not fully approximated, and the authors believe that a posterior gap was present although not fully visible. Clearly this laryngeal posture differs from the abducted folds that we expect to see on inhalation without phonation. The authors suggest that contraction of the cricothyroid muscle, which begins along with the diaphragm, an involuntary action that is not likely to be accessible to voluntary control, may serve as a counter to the adductory forces of the laryngeal muscles, thereby reducing the force of vocal fold approximation and allowing for fluent speech. A second explanation offered by the authors has to*

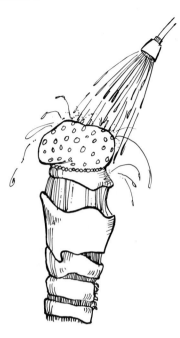

Figure 10.3. Vocal hygiene.

do with the respiratory reflexes of the larynx, which may be abnormal in persons with spasmodic dysphonia.

Vocal Hygiene

This category includes techniques that should be incorporated into most voice therapy programs. Instruction in vocal hygiene occasionally may constitute the entire rehabilitation program, but it is typically but one part of the program. In most instances of misuse of the voice, it should be a routine part of the program, and training in vocal hygiene as a preventive measure should be the final stage of voice therapy after a successful outcome has been attained (Fig. 10.3). Morrison and Rammage (1994) provide a useful listing of dos and don'ts and helpful hints about vocal hygiene. The following are components of vocal hygiene instruction.

REDUCING THE AMOUNT OF TALKING

Patients who are excessive talkers, those who have a tendency toward traumatic voice use or vocal fatigue, those who have undergone laryngeal surgery, and certainly those involved in voice therapy for conditions associated with misuse with or without tissue change should be counseled about the need to significantly curtail their voice use. This restriction may be necessary for perhaps only a specified period. This is sometimes referred to as modified vocal rest. Instructions should be as detailed as needed and should include all restrictions on voice use. If patients are able to eliminate all but essential talking, that is usually sufficient. Additional restrictions having to do with loudness of voice will tend to further reduce voice usage because of the limitations imposed by environmental noise levels. Using therapy time to work out a plan for where and when the voice will have to be used may be helpful. Other behavior modification approaches, such as charting when, where, and for how long voice is used, may help accomplish this reduction in the amount of talking. The topic of complete voice rest is discussed in greater detail in "Unresolved Issues and Myths."

REDUCING LOUDNESS

This may involve eliminating all use of the voice when the ambient noise level requires a vocal intensity level above that permitted by a soft breathy voice. Such a restriction will not allow yelling for the dog or for children playing outside or upstairs; it will not allow talking in a car, above a television or radio, above machinery or other noise in an employment setting, at a cocktail party, or in a bar with loud music playing, and so on. Such reduction of loudness is necessary when there have been mucosal changes, whether evidenced by inflammation, edema, or vocal nodules.

Some patients routinely use excessive loudness. Modification of this habituated behavior often requires intensive effort; it is not an easy pattern to alter. We all have a vocal image in our minds, which includes a loudness level. Patients who are excessively loud often do not believe that listeners will be able to hear them if they speak more softly. They must be willing to test whether this is the case by engaging in intensity reduction activities. Devices that provide visual or auditory feedback can be extremely helpful in establishing an acceptable level of loudness. A useful device known as the Voice Intensity Controller (VIC, Behavioral Controls, Inc.) is small enough to be worn by the patient and preset to beep when a specific loudness level has been exceeded. Visual feedback of loudness also can be provided with the use of the Visi-Pitch (Kay Elemetrics Corp., Lincoln Park, NJ), the Vocal Loudness Indicator (LinguiSystems, East Moline, IL), or a number of computerized programs that permit online imaging of the voice signal.

IDENTIFYING AND REDUCING OR ELIMINATING VOCAL MISUSE

All potentially vocal behaviors detrimental to laryngeal health should be identified and eliminated if possible, or at least reduced to a minimum. Exploration of such behaviors needs to be very thorough. They may include smoking of legal or illegal substances; use of certain drugs; spending large amounts of time in dry, dusty, or smoke-filled environments; exposure to airborne irritants; frequent habitual throat clearing; constant cough; excessive drinking of alcoholic beverages; as well as the traumatic behaviors of excessive talking, excessive loudness, and excessive strain, discussed elsewhere. All identified behaviors need to be discussed, and specific plans need to be made as to how they will be reduced or eliminated. Patients should be required to monitor their performance on the agreed-on plan.

ENVIRONMENTAL MANIPULATION

Whenever it seems appropriate, changes can be made in the environment to help patients function with reduced voice use or to make the environment itself more hospitable. For example, humidification can be increased by the use of room humidifiers, amplification can be used when there are demands on vocal loudness, whistles or bells can be adopted by teachers to obtain attention in place of typically loud voice use, the television volume can be muted when it is necessary to talk, and so on. Creativity is sometimes required to plan environmental changes. People may be resistant to changing their habitual modes of functioning. It is often necessary to work through this resistance and for the clinician to find ways to encourage patients to adopt the plans and give them a fair trial.

The need for adequate moisturization and humidification of the upper respiratory tract should be discussed as part of a vocal hygiene program. Conditions that may deter and interfere with good levels of environmental humidity should be explored. These might include the use of wood stoves for home heating, a work environment that is extremely dry or dust-filled (e.g., old school buildings, theaters), extensive airplane travel, and others. When such conditions exist, individual has the responsibility to take whatever remedial or compensatory actions possible, such as using room humidifiers or increasing liquid intake.

At the successful conclusion of a therapy program with voice restored to its normal state, patients should be advised about monitoring their vocal health. Because hoarseness may accompany an upper respiratory infection or may result from an evening's overuse, patients need to understand that it need not signal a recurrence of the initial problem. However, they should be advised to immediately restrict voice use and loudness and increase liquid intake. They, of course, should follow any additional course of treatment prescribed by their physician for the condition. If such hoarseness persists for more than a week, or if it persists beyond the resolution of other symptoms of upper respiratory infection, it would be advisable to return for laryngological examination.

Rationale: *The rationale for all of the above is to help patients engage in those activities and behaviors that foster laryngeal and vocal health. Several of them serve to reduce either the force or the amount of vocal fold contact, or both. In so doing, they potentially eliminate irritation of the mucosa and change. Others have to do with maintaining the healthiest possible conditions for the mechanism to work well. Prevention of recurrence is certainly a major reason for employing these vocal hygiene procedures. The history of vocal hygiene as a therapeutic technique and the meanings associated with it are discussed more fully in the MIT Encyclopedia of Communication Disorders (Casper, 2003).*

ENERGIZING THE VOICE

This technique is difficult to describe because of the abstractness of the concept. It is perhaps analogous to the car engine that is chugging along on only three spark plugs rather than all six. It is akin to the desire to "set a match" under someone who is too low keyed, too subdued and laid back. It is appropriate for use with patients who are known to have normal metabolic states and a normal ear, nose, and throat examination and who are not psychiatrically depressed. It includes (a) the use of adequate mouth opening and movement of the articulators, (b) the use of more inflection or variability of pitch, (c) the use of adequate loudness level and increased variability of loudness as appropriate to mark meaning, and (d) the use of a "well-placed" and well-supported (respiration) voice. Many methods can be used to accomplish this energization of the voice. They vary depending on the age, personality, and speaking needs of the patient. The use of scripted material from plays or other sources can be helpful, as can exercises such as practicing the role of a drill sergeant, calling out cadences, practicing in a large room, moving and using the whole body while counting, and so forth. Care must be taken so that the patient does not simply begin to shout. Whatever exercise or material is used, the patient must have specific goals that have been explained and practiced at lower levels of difficulty first. Many of these activities are often better carried out with the patient and the clinician standing some distance away from each other. Increasing mouth opening requires much work and practice. It is often helpful for the patient to practice very exaggerated movements first while receiving feedback from a mirror. The exaggeration is reduced gradually to the point where oral use is adequate. At that point, the increased mouth opening should no longer feel unusual or bizarre to the patient. In other cases, asking the patient to imagine that he or she is speaking to someone who has a hearing problem and needs, not greater loudness, but more visual cues to better read the speaker's lips, may produce the desired result. Variability in pitch and loudness can be aided by the use of instruments that provide visual feedback (Visi-Pitch, computer programs, etc.) until such time as the patient has improved auditory sensitivity to and discrimination of these parameters.

Rationale: Some patients complain about having "weak" voices that do not carry, that do not convey the desired image, and that seem to fatigue as the day goes by. In the absence of hormonal imbalance, serious psychiatric problems, laryngeal abnormality, or other organic problems, most likely that the problem lies in the way in which the person has learned to speak. These are behaviors that should be accessible to change. The activities described above address the types of speech patterns often seen in patients with these complaints and are designed to introduce changes in those patterns. Clearly, personality factors may be heavily involved, and the clinician must always keep this in mind.

VOCAL EFFORT

The concept and technique of measuring vocal effort was described in Chapter 8. It is a simple concept that can be adapted for use as a therapy technique. It requires that the patient assign a number to represent the amount of effort being expended in habitual speech. (The only stipulation is that the numbers used increase with an increase of effort.) To obtain a comparative scale for that patient, have him produce phonations at a minimum effort level, a comfortable effort level, and a maximum effort level. For example, if a patient complains of feeling that it is a strain to talk and assigns the number 17 to the degree of effort involved, but phonation with minimum effort is produced at a number 5, suggest that he talk with a degree of effort corresponding to a number 8 or 10. Patients can learn to internally monitor their effort levels and modify their behavior accordingly, thereby achieving an increased measure of control over phonation. They are able to experiment with how they produce sound to achieve a more efficient and vocally less tiring, and probably less traumatic, mode of phonation. Yet another benefit of this technique is the ease with which progress can be tracked. After a period of use of either reduced or increased effort (whichever was the goal), patients can again be asked to assign a number to their habitual phonations. This can be compared to the previous judgment.

Rationale: Because patients are able to estimate vocal effort and their estimates are manifested acoustically by variation in sound pressure level and fundamental frequency (Colton & Brown, 1973; Wright & Colton, 1972a, 1972b), using that ability in a therapeutic manner is quite appropriate. This approach accomplishes its desired goals in a holistic manner without fragmenting the various components of producing voice. It is also a technique that is easy for patients to understand and to retain in memory, thereby increasing the likelihood that they will be able to put it to use. It does not require extensive practice and provides almost immediate reinforcement, through both a sense of accomplishment and control and awareness of the reduction in strain.

THE RESONANT VOICE—LMRVT

Resonant voice therapy is based on techniques used to improve voice production in actors and singers (Cooper, 1973; Lessac, 1987). It is a form of sound production that is based on "sensations on the alveolar ridge and other facial plates during phonation."

It appears to result from a tuning of F1 to individual components of the glottal tone (Raphael & Scherer, 1987) or it may be a change in the source spectrum. It is produced with a slightly abducted vocal fold posture; thus, it should not be harmful. A variety of exercises can be used to teach the technique, although some patients may require some time to learn the desired sound.

Verdoloni (2004) has proposed a structured therapy program, Lessac Madsen Resonant Voice Therapy (LMRVT), for patients with hyper- or hypoadducted voice disorders that is designed to teach the resonant voice.

Tone placement and "flow phonation" are the main tools of the resonant therapy program (Lessac, 1987). Patients with dysphonic voices often report feeling the voice vibrating in the throat. In the resonant therapy program, sensory processing is also stressed as the patient is taught to produce a more forward placement so that the sensations of voice production can be felt in the palate, tongue, and lips. The configuration of the vocal folds is noted to be in a barely separated posture. This configuration is said to maximize the ratio of voice output intensity to the intensity of vocal fold impact pressure (Berry et al., 2001). In other words, it results in the production of the most voice with the least effort. The structured program involves eight sessions over an 8-week period.

Verdolini-Marston, Burke, Lessac, Glaze, and Caldwell (1995) compared the resonant therapy technique with the confidential voice therapy technique described earlier in this chapter. Measures of phonatory effort, auditory-perceptual ratings of severity of dysphonia, and visual impressions of the appearance of the vocal folds were obtained from 13 patients with vocal fold nodules. Three patients constituted the resonant therapy group, and five patients were part of the confidential therapy group. In addition, five patients received no therapy (control group). The results showed that both therapy programs improved the voice. Phonatory effort was reduced in both groups, with little change in the control group. Two of the five patients in the confidential therapy group showed improvement on ratings of the severity of dysphonia, whereas all three patients showed improvement in the resonant therapy group. Four of the five patients in the confidential therapy group showed visual changes in appearance of the nodule as viewed stroboscopically whereas two of the three patients in the resonant therapy groups showed similar changes. Few changes were seen on any of the measures studied for patients in the control group.

The authors of this study also reported that patient compliance was predictive of voice improvement, more so than the type of therapy program. Although preliminary, these results suggest that the resonant voice therapy approach is viable for the treatment of vocal fold nodules and perhaps similar lesions.

Rationale: *It has been reported (Verdolini & Titze, 1995; Verdolini-Marston et al., 1995) that this type of phonation results in limited vocal fold adduction as compared with "pressed voice." It is theorized, therefore, that the impact forces of the vocal folds as they adduct are also reduced. Such an effect is desirable when attempting to change hyperfunctional voice behaviors. Despite the reduced adductory forces, the voice remains strong.*

Voice Therapy for Patients With Parkinson's Disease

Traditional speech therapy has been provided for patients with Parkinson's disease for many years and with less than resounding success. That therapy focused on rate of speech and on the dysarthric components as they affect articulation. However, several authors have reported therapeutic success by targeting phonation (Johnson & Pring,

1990; Ramig, Mead, Scherer, Horii, Larson & Kohler, 1988; Robertson & Thompson, 1984; Scott & Caird, 1983). Building on these beginnings, Ramig and her colleagues have developed and shown the efficacy of a very specific therapy protocol (Ramig, 1995; Ramig et al., 1994; Ramig & Scherer, 1992; Smith et al., 1994), called the Lee Silverman Voice Treatment program (LSVT). Although this program focuses entirely on phonation, improvement in clarity of articulation, rate, and overall intelligibility has been documented. Countryman, Ramig, and Pawlas (1994) studied the efficacy of this program with three patients diagnosed with Parkinson's plus syndromes. Patients so diagnosed often have more severely debilitating symptomatology and more rapidly progressive decline of function than those with idiopathic parkinsonism. Nevertheless, all three patients showed improvement in overall speech intelligibility, functional communication, and voice deficits. All three patients maintained some carryover above pretreatment levels at 6 months post-treatment.

The LSVT is designed as an intensive program of four individual sessions per week for 1 month, during which loudness, maximum phonatory effort, high therapeutic effort, and voice awareness are targeted. The methods used include some of the techniques already described in this chapter as well as others, as follows: maximum duration sustained loud phonation; maximum frequency range (sustained highest and lowest pitches); posture; and maximal loudness. Patients receive immediate reinforcement from their productions. The method is simple, making it possible for patients to practice at home and to remember to incorporate the new learning into all speech events. Patients are advised to "think loud, think shout."

Rationale: *Vocal fold bowing and incomplete glottal closure are characteristic of the phonatory behavior of parkinsonian patients, as is reduction in respiratory support. Some of the exercises are designed to increase vocal fold adduction. The high effort and stress on "maximum" performance are necessary to override the rigidity and hypokinesia of Parkinson's disease. The intensity of the therapy maintains consistency of the high effort over the course of a month. It is reinforcing for the patient, because progress is seen, thereby motivating him to continue to put forth the effort maximizing habituation and generalization of the improved voice and speech. The single primary focus on loud voice is maintained to make it easier for these neurologically compromised patients to hold that thought in memory and make it operational.*

Voice Therapy for Patients With Paradoxical Vocal Fold Movement (PVFM) Vocal Fold Dysfunction (VFD)

Treatment for this condition was first described in the 1970s and 80s. The condition often requires the teamwork of otolaryngologists, pulmonologists, psychologists, and speech–language pathologists. The latter are primarily responsible for treatment. Our experience has been that an explanation to the patient, parent, or significant other of the nature of the problem is one of the most important initial therapeutic steps. It is difficult otherwise for them to understand or accept the need to see a speech–language pathologist. This explanation should include the way in which the vocal folds work in coordination with breathing.

As described by Florence Blager (Martin, Blager, Gay, & Wood, 1987), a therapy protocol that has been found to be effective with many patients who display PVFM involves the following steps:

1. Inhalation through the nose with lips closed
2. Relaxed tongue posture

3. Prolonged audible exhalation through pursed lips or on the production of sustained /s/

4. Diaphragmatic breathing with emphasis on exhalation

Rationale: These activities focus the patient's attention on a breathing technique, thus reducing the tendency to panic and increase tension. The patient is taught a technique over which she has control, which replaces the panic of feeling out of control. Nasal rather than oral inhalation increases full glottal abduction, and attention to exhalation helps relax the system. The various steps must be practiced many times so as to be almost automatically brought into play at the first sign of difficulty. If the patient is able to trigger the "attack," it is desirable to do that in practice and immediately reverse it through the use of these techniques. Because these "attacks" are often brought on by stress or exercise, it is important to have the patient move fairly slowly at first through the process of (a) awareness of early symptoms, (b) cessation of ongoing activity, (c) initiation of breathing exercise, and (d) restoration of normal breathing. Several minutes of rest are then helpful before resuming the activity or getting the stress under control. The goal of therapy is to be able to abort the "attack" without the need for the cessation of the activity and finally to eliminate the symptom. A number of variations of the therapeutic scheme have been reported (see Gallivan & Andrianopoulos, 2004).

Voice Therapy for the Patient With Presbyphonia

These are treatment approaches for those often described as the well elderly, people usually over 65 years of age who are in generally good health (in that they are not suffering from any progressive neurological problems), do not have severe emphysema or significant hearing loss, can participate in general physical conditioning activities, and have no laryngeal pathological conditions.

The approaches to treatment with these patients can be similar to the therapy program described for parkinsonian patients but adapted to the needs of this population. Therapy need not be intensive, although patient practice and involvement in the treatment requires full effort. The concept of vocal effort can be incorporated into the therapy, as can other techniques that "push" the system and are effective for hypofunctional voice disorders. Posture is an important consideration, and respiratory support may need some attention. Our experience also has been that encouraging these individuals to become involved in a program of fitness conditioning or regular exercise, including some aerobic activities, is beneficial to the voice.

Rationale: Biological aging is different from chronological aging. Some individuals who are age 65 or older are healthy, active, and seem younger than their years, whereas others of the same age may show very obvious signs of aging. These differences are also revealed in the voice (Ramig & Ringel, 1983). The voice described as presbyphonic is usually lacking in stability, as evidenced by increased aperiodicity and pitch breaks, reduced intensity, and a "muffled" quality lacking in resonance. The laryngeal or stroboscopic findings usually reveal glottic incompetence (often a bowed pattern), reduced amplitude of excursion, and reduced mucosal wave. All of the activities described above should potentially "push" the system to greater performance, thereby increasing glottal competence and improving all other functions. Surgical approaches to the treatment of this condition were described in the previous chapter.

Phonoscopic Approach to Treatment Probing and Treatment

Over the last several years, increasing numbers of voice clinicians have been able to take advantage of endoscopic instruments in their assessment and treatment of dysphonic patients observing the structures of the larynx at the same time voice is produced. (Hence the term *phonoscopic*, or observation of phonation.) Aspects of such an examination, the need for voice clinicians to be proficient in the use of endoscopic tools and to be skilled in the interpretation of laryngeal images, diagnostic probing, and wide sampling of phonatory behavior are all discussed in greater detail in the chapters on examination and testing earlier in this text. During treatment, visual information, in addition to the sound and "feel" of voicing, becomes part of the feedback to patients regarding the appropriateness, or lack thereof, of various behaviors. Not surprisingly, the capability to combine visual and auditory information in these ways represents a significant inclusion in our clinical toolbox. Leonard and Kendall (2001) have described in detail a rationale for, and the utility of, the "phonoscopic" approach to both evaluation and treatment in voice disorders. It is applicable to most dysphonic patients, regardless of pathological condition, and adds both precision and economy to our treatment efforts.

CRITERIA FOR TERMINATION OF THERAPY

When undertaking any treatment plan, considering possible outcomes and how they are to be handled is necessary. In the current climate of accountability and stress on outcomes of treatment, documentation of the therapy process, beginning with the evaluation and all test data, is essential in helping to determine and to support the decision to continue or to terminate therapy. If comparison of the data indicates positive changes that can logically be attributed to the therapy although the desired endpoint has not been reached, one may make a good case for continuation of the treatment plan. Furthermore, awareness of such progress can be effectively used to motivate the patient and inspire an added measure of confidence—confidence the patient has in the clinician and self-confidence the patient gains based on the progress made. If the data are negative, revealing essentially no change, the door is opened for discussion of possible reasons, and support is lent to the need for additional testing, examination, or in some instances, termination of therapy. The following sections set forth some criteria for the termination of therapy.

Elimination or Reduction of Vocally Asymptomatic Tissue Changes

For some patients, a significant reduction in the size, extent, or severity of mucosal pathological conditions may lead to essentially normal voice. We have known of patients who, although totally asymptomatic for voice problems, were found (during routine ear, nose, and throat examination) to have vocal fold nodules. These patients were not only vocally asymptomatic at the time of the examination but denied experiencing any change in voice in the past. It appears that certain small lesions may be so situated as to have minimal effect on glottal closure or on mucosal vibratory behavior, leaving the voice perceptually unchanged. This may be the case with a patient who has reached a stage in therapy at which the voice is normal-sounding and a complete vocal range has been restored despite the continued presence of some mucosal pathological conditions. In the first example, voice therapy may take the form of a single session in which vocal hygiene concepts are taught. In the second example, vocal hygiene should be taught before termination of treatment to prevent a recurrence or worsening of the laryngeal condition. The patient who experiences full resolution and elimination of signs of pathological conditions and return of good voice is obviously also a candidate for termination of voice therapy.

Improved Voice of a Quality Acceptable to Patient

In clinical practice, a patient may experience a degree of improvement that is looked on by the clinician as only a point along the road to the "best" voice but that is accepted by the patient as being totally adequate. This may be a form of resistance to therapy or it may be related to the expense incurred in continuation of the therapy, or it may reflect the patient's view and expectation quite precisely. At some point, the clinician must raise the self-directed question, "Whose needs am I interested in fulfilling, mine or this patient's?"

Many situations occur in which restoration of normal voice is not a realistic goal. For those patients, the attainment of an acceptable voice should signal the consideration of termination of therapy.

Elimination of Physical Symptoms of Pain, Discomfort, and Fatigue

Patients sometimes complain of pain, discomfort, and fatigue associated with voice production more vigorously than they do of voice symptoms such as hoarseness and pitch breaks. Indeed, the voice symptoms may be fairly minimal perceptually. Thus, for such patients, the relief of pain, discomfort, and fatigue associated with phonation is the goal, and attainment of that goal may be the proper time to terminate therapy. Incidentally, when these symptoms are relieved, patients have usually changed phonatory behavior in ways that are also reflected in improved voice production.

Habituation of Changed Vocal Behaviors With No Return of Symptoms

When a patient has fully adopted the desired vocal behaviors and no longer complains of any of the initial phonatory problems that brought him or her to treatment, therapy should be terminated.

Lack of Improvement After an Appropriate Therapy Trial

Voice therapy is generally not a long-term process. Some improvement should be perceptually discernible with most voice patients after a month of therapy, assuming at least one session per week and a patient who complies with the therapeutic protocol. If that is not the case, the clinician should review the case thoroughly. Every attempt should be made to resist adopting the facile excuse that the patient is resistant to therapy and is not practicing. Indeed, that may sometimes be the case, but it is incumbent on the clinician to fully explore all other possibilities as well. These may include an erroneous initial diagnosis, an inappropriate therapeutic approach, the presence of psychological factors that do not allow the patient to abandon a symptom, environmental or medical factors helping to maintain a problem that have not been identified or dealt with, or the presence of a condition that is not responsive to a voice therapy approach. Possible actions to be taken would include consultation with the referring physician, referral to a voice laboratory for additional testing, reassessment and alteration of the therapy approach, and referral for additional consultations (neurological, psychiatric, etc.). It may well be that after all of the appropriate steps have been taken a decision to terminate therapy may be the correct one.

UNRESOLVED ISSUES AND MYTHS

Clavicular Breathing: The Cause of Voice Problems?

After many years of experience in examining and working with voice-disordered patients, we are struck by the absence of clavicular breathing as a symptom or a sign. This is especially so in view of the frequent mention of this breathing pattern in many texts. Moreover, despite the claims, there is an absence of data to support this notion.

Clavicular breathing may be present in patients whose respiratory function is compromised as a result of chronic obstructive airway disease, other disease states, or neurological impairment. It also may be apparent in persons who are anxious and extremely tense. It is difficult to understand what the nature of the pathophysiology would be for an otherwise healthy individual to develop true clavicular breathing.

It is often the case, indeed it happens almost universally, that when people are asked to take a deep breath during examination, they will lift the shoulders and give a good example of clavicular breathing. However, if the patient's breathing pattern is carefully observed (without comment) during general conversation and at rest, we would submit that clavicular breathing will rarely be seen. That is not to say that a patient's manner of voice production does not affect respiratory function or is not affected by it. It is difficult to isolate excess tension only to the larynx and supraglottal vocal tract. Increased generalized thoracic tensions, thus, might be a part of the total voice production behavior, disrupting effective respiratory support for phonation. This should not be interpreted, however, as a basic respiratory problem or abnormality.

Talking From the Diaphragm

"Talking from the diaphragm" seems to have become a phrase known to all regardless of whether any understanding of its meaning is attached to its utterance. It no doubt stems from singing pedagogy and early elocution training. If taken literally, it is physiologically impossible. However, it seems to be understood to mean that exhalation may be controlled in some way by the diaphragm. Physiologically, we know that the diaphragm is the primary muscle of inspiration, acting to enlarge the thoracic cavity in the vertical dimension. It is not an active muscle of expiration. When it is important to fully enlarge the thoracic cavity to be able to fill the lungs, then it would seem to be of value to spend time working on "diaphragmatic breathing." In addition, it has been shown that the diaphragm is active during the initial expiratory phase of respiration when phonation is begun on high lung volumes (Hixon, 1987). Professional voice users should be well trained in respiratory control. However, the average speaker is rarely called on to have that degree of control. The normal speaker adjusts inspiration (speed and amount) and expiration (rate) to the demands of the utterance (Bless & Miller, 1972). Daniloff, Schuckers, and Feth (1980) state that speakers tend to breathe deeper when the utterance ahead is a long one, and less deeply when the anticipated utterance is short. In soft speech, the average duration of expiratory airflow is reported to be 2.4 to 3.5 seconds, as compared with the well-trained singer's ability to phonate loudly for more than 15 to 20 seconds (Daniloff et al., 1980). At high (or low) lung volumes, greater muscular control of respiration needs to be exercised. However, for normal speech activity, great diaphragmatic breaths are not required.

A great deal more emphasis has been placed on "teaching" or "correcting" breathing than is usually necessary in working with the voice-disordered patient who is not a professional voice user. Occasionally, as has been noted here several times, attention to easy and relaxed breathing can be helpful in reducing tensions and diverting focus from the larynx. We would suggest that more attention should be paid to the ways in which the speaker uses the air supply.

For example, does the person release a lot of the available air supply before initiating phonation? Or does he keep talking after the easily available air supply has been exhausted, and in so doing increase tension? Or does she tend to stop in mid-sentence without releasing the air supply or replenishing it before starting up again? Is there a tendency to hold the breath before starting to talk? Direct work on such behaviors will help to indirectly change respiratory behavior and improve smooth respiratory/phonatory coordination.

Ventricular Phonation: Diagnosis or Description?

The term "dysphonia plica ventricularis," or dysphonia resulting from ventricular fold phonation, was very often given as the diagnosis of a voice disorder, before we had ready access to improved laryngeal imaging. We suggest that ventricular phonation is really a description based on visual observation, through indirect, flexible fiberoptic or stroboscopic laryngoscopy, of greater than expected approximation of the ventricular folds during phonation. The descriptive term does not reveal the underlying cause of the behavior. The name given to this problem implies that the ventricular folds are the actual source of sound, which would suggest that the true vocal folds are not fully adducting. However, we have observed full true vocal fold adduction in the presence of compression of the ventricular folds, suggesting perhaps that the ventricular folds, rather than being the source of sound, may produce a damping effect on the sound emitted at the true vocal fold level or a restraining effect on the vibratory behavior of the true vocal folds. We have also observed ventricular fold vibratory behavior in some instances. Often the medialization of the ventricular folds obscures visualization of the true vocal folds, making it difficult to determine their movement characteristics. When the true vocal folds are not adducting, it appears that the ventricular fold activity is a compensatory behavior and may actually result in the best voice a person is capable of producing. One must, however, attempt to determine the reason for the impairment of true vocal fold adduction.

Caution should be exercised in diagnosing ventricular phonation based on indirect mirror examination alone. The positioning of the oropharyngeal structures required for indirect laryngoscopy, with the tongue held firmly in a fully protruded posture, may result in laryngeal adjustments that may not be typical for that person during conversational speech. Flexible fiberoptic laryngoscopic examination allows for habitual phonatory physiology to be observed.

Much is yet to be learned about the physiology, acoustics, and causes of ventricular phonation. When the observation of excessive ventricular fold activity is made, it is necessary to continue the process of differential diagnosis in an attempt to uncover its cause. Therapeutically we have found that ventricular phonation as a maladaptive hyperfunctional laryngeal gesture often associated with psychogenic origin is rather easily reversed. However, when the true vocal folds are incapable of adduction, ventricular phonation appears to be a compensatory mechanism that is very resistant to change through behavioral therapy.

Unilateral Vocal Fold Paralysis: Does It Cross the Midline?

For many years, the compensatory behavior involved in the restoration of good voice in the presence of unilateral vocal fold paralysis has been considered a crossing beyond the midline of the uninvolved fold to make contact with the paralyzed fold. As a result, the goal of therapeutic procedures that have been espoused for use with this population has been a strengthening of the normal vocal fold through activities of forceful closure of the glottis. Scant data have supported the crossover effect in the presence of unilateral vocal fold paralysis. The question also must be raised as to whether return of voice has been in some instances inappropriately credited to the therapy program when the patient has, in fact, experienced spontaneous return of function (as is often the case with an idiopathic paralysis). Or perhaps the therapy hastened or assisted the return of function. Answers to these speculations are unavailable. And, indeed, some patients, despite continued paralysis, have experienced return of good voice. How? What makes the difference between those who experience return of voice in the presence of paralysis and those whose voices continue to be aberrant?

Although the notion of the crossover effect is appealing, we have been impressed by the lack of its occurrence in many patients we have examined using flexible fiberoptic endoscopy (Casper, Colton, & Brewer, 1985), regardless of whether they exhibited return of voice. We explored whether the crossover could be elicited through various voice therapy maneuvers and failed to observe its occurrence in the few patients we studied. Schematic representations based on information obtained from high-speed films of the behavior of the vocal folds in the presence of unilateral paralysis have shown that the glottis remains open, with the normal vocal fold approaching the midline but not crossing it, whereas the affected fold has a motion described as being like a "flag flapping in the wind" (Hirano, Kakita, Kawasaki, & Matsushita, 1977). More recently, using the rigid stroboscope, which permits an enlarged image, we have become aware of instances that appeared to show a crossover effect of the intact vocal fold. Further investigation of this effect is needed to determine whether in fact the vocal fold crosses the midline, whether there is a shifting of the entire larynx, how this is accomplished and learned by some individuals but apparently unavailable to others, and many other questions.

Paralysis of the vocal fold not only results in its inability to be moved by contraction of the affected muscle(s) but also in changes of its level and shape. These parameters— the level, tension, thickness, and eventual position relative to midline—of a paralyzed vocal fold are determined by a variety of factors, including muscle fibrosis and contractures (Ballenger, 1985). These effects must be better understood to be factored into an understanding of the variability of vocal performance in the presence of paralysis. Note also that the term "paralysis" may refer to a condition in which there is known or suspected injury to a laryngeal nerve, but is also used frequently to describe a vocal fold that may be fixed because of other factors, such as scarring from an intubation injury. In some cases, innervation to the fold may remain intact. Possible differences in fold position and function between an immobile fold and one that is paralyzed because of a nerve injury have not been thoroughly elaborated. Similarly, we do not fully understand the effects of residual electrical activity in a fold that is paralyzed. Even if the fold is not moving, different degrees of residual electrical activity could possibly influence its function or position.

Some authors (Yamaguchi, Yotsukura, Sata, Watanabe, Hirose, & Kobayashi, 1993) report good success with pushing exercises to achieve greater glottal closure. In our own experience, we have not been impressed by the results obtained in voice therapy using effort closure techniques. Indeed, many patients have reported such exercises to be fatiguing to the voice and seeming to result in poorer vocal performance for a time during and after their execution. In view of these many concerns, we feel constrained not to recommend the routine use of such exercises in these cases. Other techniques have been incidentally reported to be effective in producing clearer and less breathy voice. Among these is the use of a high pitch. When the superior branch of the recurrent laryngeal nerve is intact and functional, stretching and thinning of the affected vocal fold still occur because of the action of the cricothyroid muscle. This action has a component of adduction and results in greater approximation of the folds and increased tension in the lax paralyzed fold. The problem with this technique is that the effect and the improved voice quality that it allows are not transferrable to a modal register phonation at an acceptable frequency level for general communication.

Often patients with unilateral paralysis attempt to compensate for the loss of the ability to increase loudness level by increasing subglottic pressure and phonatory effort. The effect that this particular compensatory behavior has is to worsen the voice and make the patient fatigued with the effort of talking. In such instances, therapy designed to reduce effort and increase tension and pressures can result in improved phonation. Methods of treating unilateral vocal fold paralysis through the use of phonosurgical techniques were described in Chapter 9.

The Myth of Optimum Pitch

The concept of an optimum pitch dates back to at least 1940, when it was described by Fairbanks (1960). It has been defined variously as (a) that pitch at which the voice has good quality and maximum intensity with the least effort; (b) that pitch at which there is a "vocal swell"; and (c) a biologically determined ideal pitch for an individual, determined by the anatomical and physiological characteristics of individual larynges. The methods for its determination also have varied somewhat, and include

1. Listening for that pitch at which the quality of the voice is best and intensity is the greatest
2. Counting the number of musical notes in a person's full range (optimum pitch will be that which is 25% of the way up from the bottom of the range)
3. Using the same technique as in (2) above and going up one third of the way from the bottom of the range
4. Having the patient say "um-hum" naturally, with the lips closed and a rising inflection, while feeling the oronasopharyngeal surfaces for the most resonant frequency
5. Finding the pitch at which the sustained phonation of the vowel /ah/ is the longest and loudest
6. Finding the lowest pitch a person can produce and counting at least four notes up the scale
7. Listening for the pitch of the sigh of a yawn/sigh maneuver, which is said to represent a person's optimal pitch

Experimental attempts have been made to explore the claims made about optimum pitch. In 1958, Thurman measured intensity at the various frequencies as subjects hummed a scale. Only 11% of the highest intensity levels occurred within the range of frequencies that might be considered to be appropriate for an adult's optimum pitch. A number of other investigators have examined frequency–intensity relationships (Coleman, Mabis, & Hinson, 1977; Damste, 1970; Komiyama, Watanabe, & Ryu, 1984) and have reported maximum intensity occurring approximately 70% up from the subject's lowest sustainable frequency (not the 25%–30% claimed for optimum pitch). Vocal efficiency, another tenet of optimum pitch, can be measured as the ratio of the total output (acoustic) power over the total input (aerodynamic) power at the glottis. Van den Berg (1956), using a catheter between the vocal folds to obtain a direct measure of subglottal pressure and an esophageal catheter for an indirect measure, found a positive relationship between subglottal pressure and sound pressure level (SPL). He converted the SPL into speech power in watts to measure laryngeal efficiency at various frequencies and intensities. If optimum pitch exists, the expectation would be that an increased output power would be obtained for the same level of input power at a given frequency. This did not occur. Using slightly different methodology, Isshiki (1964) reported results similar to van den Berg's. House (1959) demonstrated an important contribution of the vocal tract when he reported that a perceptible change in overall intensity occurred when a vocal harmonic coincided with the center of a vocal tract resonance. The so-called "vocal swell" thus does not appear to be related to the concept of laryngeal efficiency. Another line of questioning was pursued by Stone (1983) when he questioned the perceptibility of the intensity change that was claimed to mark the optimum pitch. He found that the intensity changes between 100 and 200 Hz, the range in which optimum pitch would be expected to fall for adult males, were very minimal and thus imperceptible. Similar to previous reports, Stone also found greatest intensity for half of his subjects to occur at frequencies well above the level at which optimum pitch would be anticipated. And still further, using the Fairbanks method for measuring optimum pitch, Stone reported that in 23 of 30 trials the "optimal pitch" fell above the speaker's modal pitch. Minifie (1984) reported that the efficiency of the power conversion increased with intensity rather than with frequency. This author could find no evidence to support the concept of an optimal pitch as being most efficient.

All of the studies cited thus far used normal-speaking subjects. However, Ludlow, Connor, and Coulter (1984) explored the viability of the optimum pitch concept in patients with laryngeal pathological conditions. Their results suggested that vocal function is best at the frequencies in the upper 50% of the speaking range for normal speakers, but not for those with laryngeal pathological conditions. They interpreted their findings to mean that a set of lawful relationships exists between several measures of phonatory function and frequency in normal speakers, which are disturbed in the presence of pathological conditions. Pathological conditions compromise phonatory function, limiting it to a particular range in frequencies. Thus, in pathological states the disturbance of the lawful relationships is meaningful rather than the existence of a particular fundamental frequency range at which phonation can be expected with least effort.

These data all seem to substantially reject the notion of an optimum pitch, at least as currently defined. Finally, be wary of subjective perceptions of pitch level. Murry (1978) demonstrated that judgments of pitch in dysphonic voices may be confounded by other voice signal parameters, such as loudness, effort, and voice quality. He found a reduction in phonational range in patients with laryngeal paralysis but did not find speaking fundamental frequency in dysphonic patients to be significantly lower than in the normal-speaking population. In Chapter 5, we reported that a prominent perceptual characteristic of voice in Huntington's chorea was low pitch. However, actual measurements of fundamental frequency in this population showed it to be within the normal range. Wilson, Wellen, and Kimbarow (1983) demonstrated that trained listeners were not better than untrained listeners in judgments of perceived fundamental frequency (pitch) of children's voices and that neither group could identify differences of less than 20 Hz at better than chance level. Raising pitch level may appear to reduce breathiness or hoarseness, but this happens at the expense of, not for the benefit of, the larynx. The extra effort put forth by the patient may serve to override some of the vocal symptoms. Reduction of loudness is physiologically a much sounder approach. It seems quite logical that even an optimum pitch, if there were one, could be used in improper, abusive ways.

The philosophical approach of this book is that if phonatory physiology is normalized, the voice that emerges will be at an appropriate pitch level for that individual. Therefore, approaching the rehabilitation of disordered voice by attempting to impose an arbitrary pitch level seems inappropriate, perhaps incorrect, and often unproductive.

Whispering: Is It Harmful?

Some authors believe that whispering should be avoided during periods of voice rest or as a therapeutic technique because they claim that it results in vocal fold adduction that is undesirable, or that extreme glottal friction characterizes the whisper, which is also undesirable. Do available experimental data support these contentions? A number of investigations of laryngeal configurations during whisper (Hamlet, 1972; Monoson & Zemlin, 1984; Pressman, 1942; Pressman & Kelemen, 1955; Solomon, McCall, Trosset, & Gray, 1989; Zemlin, 1988) have described a variety of configurations, including (a) lack of complete adduction along the full length of the glottis, (b) an inverted V shape, (c) a bowed appearance, (d) a Y shape with a posterior chink, (e) a bimodal (anterior and posterior) chink, (f) a parallel configuration with some adduction, and (g) toeing in of the vocal processes. Various reasons have been suggested for these differences in glottal configuration. Some have suggested that the glottal shape is a function of the effort involved in the whisper, others suggest it has to do with the type of whisper (quiet versus forceful whisper), and yet others claim a relationship to the phonetic context.

Monoson and Zemlin (1984) compared laryngeal appearance (high-speed films), electromyograms, acoustic, and airflow data for four conditions: quiet whisper, forced whisper, breathy phonation, and conversational phonation. Glottal configurations varied to some extent among the conditions and were believed to be at least partially determined by the effort level involved. Vibratory behavior was absent in both whisper conditions and present in both breathy and conversational phonation. Airflow was greatest in forced whispering, which was felt to be attributable in part to an increase in activity of the expiratory muscles in that condition. The data do not support the thesis that whispering is an abusive behavior. However, the increases in expiratory muscle activity and in airflow attributed to the forced whisper suggest an increase in effort and perhaps in tension.

Solomon et al. (1989) reported on a study of laryngeal configurations for two types of whispering (high effort and low effort) in 10 speakers using consonant–vowel units and running speech. The laryngeal configurations were visualized with a fiberoptic bronchoscope and videotaped for analysis. Significant individual variability was reported. Intrasubject inconsistency also was noted, although most subjects exhibited a preferred configuration. A medium-sized glottal opening was described for most subjects, with a large glottal size occurring more frequently in the high-effort whisper than in the low-effort whisper. Although some constriction of supraglottal structures was reported, it apparently occurred less than half of the time, even in high-effort whispering. The glottal configurations described by these authors were primarily of two types: a straight edge, parallel configuration or a toeing in of the vocal processes.

How such approximation of the vocal folds occurs during whisper is still not clear, although these authors report observation of more contact during running speech than in the production of consonant–vowel units. Four of the 10 subjects displayed the straight margin configuration of the glottis, and these same subjects did not approximate the vocal folds. These authors suggest that the determination regarding the use of whisper as a therapeutic technique or during periods of vocal rest should be made on an individual basis, depending on the type of glottal configuration assumed for whisper by that patient. The efficacy of whispering as a therapeutic approach was not addressed in this study. Hufnagle and Hufnagle (1988) reported that patients demonstrated improved voice quality after a period of whispering, suggesting therefore that the behavior is not harmful and, indeed, may be helpful.

Sufficient evidence is not yet available to state unequivocally that whispering is not harmful. However, our clinical intuition suggests that it may be helpful for some patients, with a few caveats. Because the high-effort forced whisper tends to suggest increased tension and effort somewhere in the system, and because tension and force are precisely the behaviors that most patients need to reduce or eliminate, it seems to us that the use of the forced whisper could be counterproductive. The patient also must recognize that whispering may have a drying effect on the mucosa of the vocal folds, which should be counteracted by an increase of fluid intake.

In short, the available evidence about whisper is not nearly as frightening as some of the strongly stated admonitions against its use. However, much remains to be learned about the mechanism of whispering. The amount of force in medial compression of the folds when they appear to make contact during whispering has not been addressed and remains an open question, as does the degree of expiratory muscle effort involved.

PREVENTION OF VOICE PROBLEMS

We can discuss the prevention of voice problems by addressing both primary prevention—preventing the occurrence of the problem in the first place—and secondary prevention—preventing the recurrence of a problem. In the category of primary prevention, an understanding of the deleterious effects of cigarette smoking has been effective in convincing many people to change their habits and eliminate smoking. Throughout American society, steps have been taken to minimize the spread of the effects of inhaling environmental cigarette smoke by establishing prohibitions against smoking in theaters, planes, certain sections of restaurants, and other places of public gathering. Much more needs to be done, however, because in absolute numbers, the population of smokers has not decreased significantly. The evidence linking smoking with laryngeal cancer, heart disease, and numerous other medical problems is impressive.

Greater strides need to be made in recognizing the adverse effects on the airway of certain noxious gases. However, in the absence of widespread information, it behooves professionals to suggest safeguards that individuals may take when knowingly exposed to a variety of potentially harmful agents. Such safeguards include wearing appropriate protective masks, avoidance of unnecessary exposure, and introducing air-purifying systems or improved ventilation.

Education is the primary need in decreasing vocal misuse. We know that cheerleading constitutes a very stressful, abusive use of the voice that often results in mucosal damage. However, this knowledge seems not to have penetrated the cheerleading world so that training in voice use and voice conservation might be provided. Other abusive activities could be similarly identified. Some, such as rock singing in the presence of highly amplified sound, may not be amenable to change. Despite, or perhaps because of, laryngeal pathological conditions such as nodules or polyps, some rock singers have a "sound" uniquely theirs that would not have been possible without abuse.

Another group of people who would benefit from increased education about the voice are choir singers. Many have untrained voices and abuse them with regularity but without awareness. Choir directors frequently have limited backgrounds in vocal pedagogy and are thus ill equipped to train their choirs in healthy habits of singing and voice use. This becomes increasingly critical when the choir is composed of or includes prepubertal children.

Primary prevention through education needs to be increased in the public schools so that children learn to recognize beginning signs of vocal problems and are trained in voice conservation. In addition to education of the children, all school personnel should have a greater understanding of vocal misuse, its harmful effects, and ways to avoid or eliminate it. Such education not only would be helpful to them in managing their own voice production but also would make them more capable of identifying the problem in children. Such a program, which had impressive results, is described by Nilson and Schneiderman (1983). Their program was directed at 2nd and 3rd grade students and their teachers and included discussion of the vocal mechanism and voice production, voice qualities both normal and abnormal, and learning to identify vocal abuse. Both the children and the teachers were found to have gained and retained significant knowledge about the voice, and when the children who had been part of the program were retested for voice, no new cases of dysphonia were identified. A primary prevention plan has been proposed by Flynn (1983), and Marge (1984) has addressed prevention of voice disorders as one area under the broader topic of prevention of communication disorders.

Secondary prevention, for those who have experienced even a single episode of vocal disturbance that required treatment, is essential. Laryngologists who successfully treat a patient with a preventable problem must either take the time to clearly instruct the patient in a program of vocal hygiene or refer that patient to a speech–language pathologist for such education and counseling. Indeed, failure to do so might leave the door open for medical-legal problems.

MALPRACTICE

In the current litigious climate, all those who treat patients with voice problems, including speech–language pathologists, must recognize how they may be vulnerable to malpractice actions and take appropriate steps to safeguard themselves. Instances of persons with voice problems bringing suit against otolaryngologists or speech–language pathologists and of speech–language pathologists being called on to testify as "expert witnesses" in suits brought against others have already occurred. During the years 1980 to 1985, a 10% increase in claims against speech–language pathologists occurred (Kooper & Sullivan, 1986).

Prime candidates to bring such suits are persons who claim that the treatment provided, surgical or otherwise, created or resulted in a permanent condition no better or worse than the original problem, and that they had not been advised of the possibility of that outcome. Others might claim damages for a missed diagnosis that resulted in unnecessary treatment or delayed initiation of appropriate treatment. The extent of liability for a disabling condition appears to be directly related to the severity of the injury as measured by its duration (Kooper & Sullivan, 1986). Thus, if a voice disorder is present and is not expected to abate or change over the person's lifespan, its severity will be judged to be greater if the patient is 25 years old than if she is 85. The extent of liability will be related to the perception of the degree of severity of the problem.

Very complete, dated records must be maintained on each patient. Such records should contain the results of all testing and examination, case history material, statements of diagnosis, or a listing of the differential diagnosis if full exploration has not been completed, a treatment plan, statements of prognosis specific to planned treatment modalities, and a record of all contacts with the patient or about the patient. Furthermore, whenever surgical intervention is planned, a recorded sample of the patient's voice should be a part of the record. A second recording should be made postoperatively, with additional recordings made periodically as changes in voice occur. The speech–language pathologist should make audio recordings of the patient's voice at the time of the initial visit and periodically after that.

Those who work with voice-disordered patients, when called on to testify in court as an expert witness, must establish their expertise. They must be knowledgeable and articulate about phonatory physiology, as well as about testing and treatment procedures, the nature of voice disorders, and the emotional ramifications of disturbed communication skills or loss of the source of a livelihood. The primary question to which they will be expected to respond deals with the acceptability of the treatment that was provided in the case. This does not require that the witness agree with the course of treatment, as long as it is an accepted form of treatment for the problem.

SUMMARY

Vocal rehabilitation in its broadest sense is discussed in this chapter. Concepts, principles, and guidelines basic to vocal rehabilitation receive attention, then specific therapeutic techniques are presented. The role of voice therapy in the treatment of voice disorders, the appropriate goals of such treatment, and the nature of the therapeutic process are proposed for the various categories of voice disorders, such as those associated with mucosal changes, those involving misuse and abuse, and those with neurological involvement. A section is devoted to discussion of some special voice problems that do not fit into these categories. The discussion of specific therapeutic techniques includes a description of how they are done, with suggestions and cautions gained from clinical practice. A rationale is presented for each technique that relates its physiological implications to the disturbed physiology typical of the voice disorders to which it is applicable. The considerations that must be taken into account in developing a prognostic statement are discussed, and some criteria for termination of therapy are suggested. The authors raise some issues in vocal rehabilitation that are based on unresolved questions and for which no substantiating data are available and question the continued use of optimum pitch as a viable concept. Discussions of the prevention of voice disorders and of malpractice concerns complete the chapter.

Chapter 11

Anatomy of the Vocal Fold Mechanism

INTRODUCTION

In the human body, structure determines function. That is, the shape and form of a structure determine the manner in which the structure will operate. Thus, it is important to understand the anatomy of a structure to understand how it works. The larynx has several important functions. Primarily, it is a respiratory organ controlling the flow of air into and out of the lower respiratory tract. Another function is to protect the lower airway from access by anything other than air, and in that regard it also has a role in deglutition. Because the focus of this book is phonation, we focus primarily on the role of the larynx as the primary sound generator.

A brief review of the anatomy of the larynx is presented in this chapter. The focus is on functional anatomy, that is, the determination of how a structure functions based on its anatomy. It is not the intent of this chapter to present full anatomical details of structures, their articulation with other structures, and their blood and nerve supply. Such details may be found in many complete anatomy texts (Dickson & Dickson, 1982; Fink & Demarest, 1978; Zemlin, 1988). Rather, it is our purpose to present those details needed to understand the structure and how it functions in voice production. This information is presented so that clinicians can rapidly review a segment of anatomy and use that information to better understand a given voice problem. It is hoped that this section will be actively used during the process of differential diagnosis and in the management plan. Anatomy need not be memorized if it is understood and if reference materials are consulted in a meaningful manner.

We begin our discussion of laryngeal anatomy from the outside and proceed to the inside; that is, we first consider the extrinsic muscles of the larynx, then move inward to the cartilages of the larynx and the intrinsic muscles. A brief overview of the internal structures and cavities of the larynx follow and, finally, we consider the body cover model of vocal fold structure and laryngeal anatomy as viewed through a flexible fiberoptic laryngoscope.

EXTRINSIC MUSCLES OF THE LARYNX

The extrinsic muscles of the larynx are those that are attached at one end to a structure within the larynx and have one or more attachments to a structure outside the larynx. It is necessary to understand that the hyoid bone, which is a rather distinct structure,

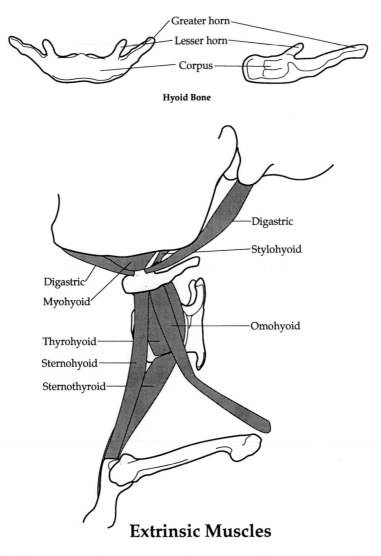

Extrinsic Muscles

Figure 11.1. Schematic representation of the hyoid bone and the extrinsic muscles of the larynx. Part of the extrinsic muscle group forms a sling to support the hyoid bone and larynx from above. These muscles can move the hyoid and larynx upward, forward, or backward. The other group of extrinsic muscles can pull the hyoid and larynx down.

is considered here to be part of the larynx. Some of its features are shown in the upper panel of Figure 11.1. All extrinsic muscles have their laryngeal attachments on the hyoid bone. The attachments outside of the larynx include many different structures, such as the mandible, the mastoid, and structures in the thorax. Recall that in anatomy the origin of a muscle refers to its least movable attachment, whereas the insertion refers to its more movable attachment.

There are eight extrinsic muscles, four that lie below the hyoid bone and four that lie above it. For those reasons, they are divided into the suprahyoid and infrahyoid groups. The muscles that constitute these two groups are listed in Table 11.1

Table 11.1. Extrinsic Muscles of the Larynx

Suprahyoid Muscles

Digastric   A two-part muscle consisting of a posterior belly and an anterior belly
  Origin   Anterior belly: originates on the lower border of the mandible near the
                      mandibular symphysis
                    Posterior belly: originates on the mastoid process
  Insertion   Anterior belly: intermediate tendon
                    Posterior belly: intermediate tendon connecting to the hyoid bone
  Function   Anterior belly: pulls hyoid bone anteriorly and slightly upward
                    Posterior belly: pulls hyoid bone posteriorly and upward

Mylohyoid   A thin muscle forming the floor of the mouth
  Origin   Along the mylohyoid line on the inner surface of the mandible
  Insertion   Most fibers meet with fibers of the opposite side at the midline raphe
  Function   Pulls hyoid bone anteriorly and slightly upward, depending on
                      position of jaw

Geniohyoid   A cylindrical muscle located above the mylohyoid muscle
  Origin   On the mental spine at the mental symphysis of the mandible
  Insertion   Anterior surface of the corpus of the hyoid bone
  Function   Pulls hyoid bone anteriorly and slightly upward

Stylohyoid   A long slender muscle located superficially to the posterior belly of the
                      digastric
  Origin   On the styloid process of the temporal bone
  Insertion   On the body of the hyoid bone
  Function   Pulls hyoid bone posteriorly and upward

Infrahyoid Muscles

Thyrohyoid   A thin muscle that lies deep to the omohyoid
  Origin   From the oblique line on the thyroid lamina
  Insertion   On the lower border of the greater horn of the hyoid bone
  Function   Decreases distance between thyroid and hyoid, especially anteriorly

Sternothyroid   A long, thin muscle on the anterior side of the neck
  Origin   Posterior surface of the manubrium of the sternum and the first costal
                      cartilage
  Insertion   On the oblique line of the thyroid
  Function   Pulls down on the thyroid cartilage

Sternohyoid   A thin muscle lying on anterior side of the neck
  Origin   On the posterior surface of the manubrium of the sternum and end of
                      the clavicle
  Insertion   On the lower border of the body of the hyoid bone
  Function   Pulls down on the hyoid bone

Omohyoid   A long, narrow, two-part muscle on the anterior and lateral surfaces of
                      the neck
  Origin   Inferior belly: along the upper surface of the scapula
                    Superior belly: intermediate tendon
  Insertion   Inferior belly: intermediate tendon
                    Superior belly: the border of the great horn of the hyoid bone
  Function   Both divisions pull down on the hyoid, although the superior belly has
                      a more pronounced effect in this direction than the inferior belly

---

and shown in Figure 11.1. The morphological characteristics of these muscles and the intrinsic laryngeal muscles are presented in useful tables by Kahane (2004, p. 16).

Suprahyoid Group

In Figure 11.1, note how the suprahyoid group forms a sling supporting the hyoid bone and, secondarily, the larynx. The anterior part of the sling is formed by portions of the digastric (anterior belly), the geniohyoid, and the mylohyoid muscles. When contracted, this group of muscles pulls the hyoid bone (and thus the larynx) forward. These muscles are active during the production of a front vowel or a consonant that requires a high front tongue position. The posterior belly of the digastric and the stylohyoid form the rear part of the sling. Their contraction pulls the hyoid posteriorly. Note that the angle of pull is steep for this muscle group, whereas the angle of pull of the anterior muscle group is shallow. Thus, the action of the posterior group is to pull up on the larynx, whereas the anterior muscle group exerts a pull on the hyoid bone that is more forward than upward. In fact, if the jaw is lowered, it is possible that the anterior group could lower the larynx slightly.

Infrahyoid

This group is made up of four muscles: the thyrohyoid, sternohyoid, omohyoid, and sternothyroid. With the exception of the thyrohyoid, the other muscles in this group have attachments from the hyoid to structures below the larynx. As a result, their contraction has the effect of pulling the larynx downward. The lowered laryngeal position results in a lengthening of the vocal tract, which has a primary effect on vocal resonance characteristics affecting the formant frequencies. A more direct effect on the voice may result from the restriction of thyroid cartilage movement that is caused by contraction of this muscle group. This restriction of movement has directly to do with vocal fold length, mass, and tension, and thereby affects vocal pitch regulation. Other muscles are also involved in pitch regulation, and they are discussed later.

The thyrohyoid muscle connects to the larynx, and its action contributes to determining the angle of the thyroid with respect to the cricoid cartilage. If the thyroid cartilage is fixed (by other muscles) so that it cannot move, then contraction of the thyrohyoid would contribute to pulling the hyoid bone down. If, however, the hyoid bone is fixed (by contraction of muscles above it), then contraction of the thyrohyoid would pull upward on the thyroid, increasing the distance between it and the cricoid cartilage (especially anteriorly). Thus, most of the effect of the thyrohyoid muscle is to rock the thyroid cartilage upward and in so doing to potentially alter length, mass, and tension of the vocal folds, thereby affecting the pitch of the voice.

Positioning of the larynx in the vertical dimension during speaking is primarily related to vowel or consonant production. Some variation of position takes place in singing, and good singers may vary the vertical position of the larynx considerably, depending on their style of singing and the music (Shipp, 1975; Shipp & Izdebski, 1975). Speakers with voice problems may have a tendency to maintain higher than normal laryngeal position. This may be indicative of excessive muscle tension (Aronson, 1985; Morrison, Rammage, Belisle, Pullan, & Nichol, 1983) in the extrinsic muscles of the larynx.

CARTILAGES OF THE LARYNX

The framework of the larynx is composed of hyaline cartilage. Cartilage is softer and more flexible than bone. Hyaline refers to the type of cells that make up the cartilage.

The cartilages of the larynx are presented in Figure 11.2. The major cartilages are the thyroid, cricoid, and arytenoid. The other cartilages are much smaller and form parts of other structures. For example, the corniculates are small cartilages attached to the arytenoid at their apices. The cuneiforms are small cartilages embedded in the muscle tissue that connects the arytenoids to the epiglottis.

Thyroid Cartilage

The thyroid cartilage is the largest cartilage of the larynx. The most anterior angle of this cartilage, commonly referred to as the Adam's apple, is a very prominent feature

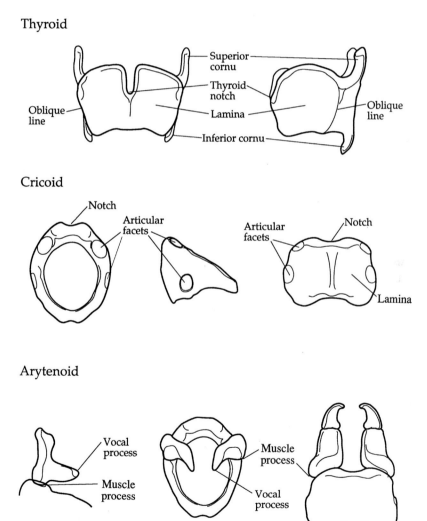

Figure 11.2. Schematic of the cartilages of the larynx.

in some men. It is shaped like a shield and can be thought of as shielding the structures inside. The thyroid is actually composed of two plates of cartilage, called lamina, joined at the midline to form an angle of approximately 80° in men and approximately 90° in women (Zemlin, 1988). The more acute angle of the thyroid together with laryngeal size accounts for the more pronounced outline of the larynx in the male neck.

Posteriorly, the thyroid cartilage has two horns or cornua. The superior horn connects the thyroid to the hyoid bone, and the inferior horn connects it to the cricoid cartilage below. Along the lateral surface of the thyroid lamina is a ridge identified as the oblique line. Here the thyrohyoid and sternothyroid muscles attach.

Cricoid Cartilage

The second largest laryngeal cartilage is the cricoid, which completely surrounds the trachea. Sometimes it is referred to as the uppermost tracheal ring, but it is quite different in configuration from the other tracheal rings. It is larger and higher posteriorly, whereas anteriorly it tapers to the cricoid arch. The thyroid cartilage articulates with the cricoid on its posterolateral surface. Two kinds of movements of the thyroid on the cricoid cartilage are permitted, as illustrated in Figure 11.3. The arytenoids articulate with the cricoid on its posterosuperior surface. The details of this articulation are important and are discussed further in the next section.

Arytenoid Cartilages

Two arytenoid cartilages are each positioned on either side of the midline on the supraposterior surface of the cricoid cartilage. The arytenoids are roughly pyramidal and have four surfaces, three angles at the base, and, of course, a single point at the apex. The basal surface is important to consider because essential musculature attaches at two of its angles.

The most anterior angle of the base of the arytenoid is referred to as the vocal process. Here the true vocal folds attach. The more lateral angle, referred to as the

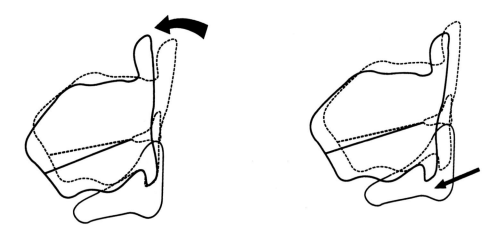

Figure 11.3. Movements permitted by the articulation of the thyroid and cricoid cartilages. A rocking motion of the thyroid on the cricoid is the major movement permitted (left panel). In addition, a slight anteroposterior movement is possible (right panel).

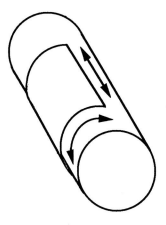

Figure 11.4. Type of movements permitted by the cricoarytenoid joint.

muscle process, is the point of attachment for the posterior cricoarytenoid and the lateral cricoarytenoid muscles.

The surface of the arytenoid that articulates with the cricoid cartilage is concave. The surface of the cricoid that meets the arytenoid is convex. These surfaces help to determine how the arytenoid will move on the surface of the cricoid. Because of the shape of these surfaces, a rotating motion is not permitted, but a rocking motion can occur (Broad, 1973; von Leden & Moore, 1961). Broad has described the permitted motions by comparing them to the movement of two matching cylinders, as shown in Figure 11.4. Two kinds of motion are permitted, a gliding motion along an anteroposterior plane and a rocking motion in a mediolateral direction. When these two motions occur together, the appearance of a rocking motion occurs either medially and anteriorly directed (if the arytenoids are moving in) or posteriorly (if the arytenoids are moving out). Depending on speed of medial movement relative to anterior movement of the arytenoids, the vocal processes may be the first point of contact during adduction of the vocal folds.

Epiglottis

The epiglottis is a leaf-shaped cartilage attached on the mesial surface of the thyroid cartilage at the juncture of the two thyroid plates. The anterior surface of the epiglottis attaches to the hyoid bone by a ligament.

The epiglottis assists in directing food and liquids into the esophagus during swallowing. During phonation, it is usually out of the way of the egressive airstream. However, it moves considerably during the production of different vowels and consonants. In some cases, it will obscure the view of the vocal folds. However, tongue position in the production of vowels such as /ee/ and /oo/ usually results in forward movement of the epiglottis, thereby allowing a good view of the vocal folds. No evidence supports the contention that the shape of the epiglottis will alter the voice. Certainly, pulling the epiglottis over the laryngeal opening will affect sound transmission and intensity level.

The epiglottis can vary considerably in shape and curvature. Usually it is slightly concave when viewed with a laryngeal mirror or fiberscope. Sometimes it may have a very pronounced omega shape. The so-called omega-shaped epiglottis appears to be found most often in immature larynges or children's larynges. However, it also may be simply a variation of normal human laryngeal anatomy.

Other Cartilages

The remaining cartilages are the corniculate and the cuneiform cartilages. The corniculates are small cone-shaped cartilages that form the apex of the arytenoid. The cuneiforms are small rod-shaped cartilages found within the aryepiglottic fold, a fold of tissue and muscle coursing from the arytenoids to the epiglottis.

INTRINSIC MUSCLES OF THE LARYNX

Muscles that have both of their attachments to structures within the larynx are called intrinsic laryngeal muscles. The five muscles, along with their origins and insertions, are shown in Table 11.2. In this review they are discussed roughly in order of their activation when a person produces voice.

Arytenoideus

The arytenoideus or interarytenoid muscle is a two-part muscle lying between the two arytenoid cartilages. One part consists of muscle fibers that course in a horizontal direction. The effect of these fibers is to pull the bases of the two arytenoids toward each other, thus adducting them. The other part consists of fibers that course from the base of one arytenoid to the apex of the other arytenoid. The effect of these fibers is to pull the tips of the arytenoids together. Together, the two parts adduct the arytenoids and close off the extreme posterior airway. Although the time when these muscles are activated depends on the speech task, in general, activity in the arytenoideus occurs anywhere from 0.5 to 0.3 seconds before sound is produced.

Lateral Cricoarytenoid

The lateral cricoarytenoid muscle is a paired muscle coursing from the sides and upper surface of the cricoid cartilage to the muscle process of the arytenoid. The effect of this muscle is to pull the muscle process anteriorly, rocking the arytenoid medially and adducting the vocal folds themselves. Time of activation may be approximately 0.1 second after activity in the arytenoideus.

These two muscles (arytenoideus and lateral cricoarytenoid) function together to adduct the vocal folds. It is not necessary to completely adduct the folds for phonation to commence. Rather, there need only be sufficient adduction to impose an obstruction to the flow of air coming from the lungs, for phonation to begin.

Posterior Cricoarytenoid

This is the only intrinsic muscle that abducts the vocal folds. From its origin on the posterior lamina of the cricoid, the muscle fibers converge to insert on the muscle process. Contraction of the muscle will pull the muscle process posteriorly, thus opening the vocal folds.

The posterior cricoarytenoid is active at the end of phonation to open the folds. However, it is also active during speech, because many speech sounds require an absence of vocal fold vibration (e.g., the stop consonants /p/, /t/, and /k/; the fricative consonants

Table 11.2. Intrinsic Muscles of the Larynx

Arytenoideus	An unpaired muscle consisting of fibers oriented in two directions, oblique and transverse
Origin	Oblique fibers originate at the base of one arytenoids and course to the apex of the other arytenoids. Transverse fibers originate along the lateral margin of one arytenoids and course to the lateral margin of the other arytenoids.
Insertion	Arytenoid of opposite side
Function	Adducts arytenoids, thus closing the cartilaginous glottis
Lateral Cricoarytenoid	A fan-shaped muscle lying along the upper surface of the cricoid cartilage
Origin	On the upper border of the cricoid
Insertion	Anterior surface of the muscular process of the arytenoid
Function	Adducts the vocal processes of the arytenoids, thus closing the membranous glottis
Posterior Cricoarytenoid	A fan-shaped muscle located on the posterior surface of the cricoid
Origin	On the posterior lamina of the cricoid
Insertion	Posterior surface of the muscular process of the arytenoid
Function	Abducts the arytenoids, thus opening the glottis
Cricothyroid	A fan-shaped muscle located between the cricoid and thyroid cartilages, consisting of two divisions, pars oblique and pars recta. These divisions refer to the different orientation of the fibers.
Origin	Arch of the cricoid
Insertion	Inner inferior margin of the thyroid
Function	Decreases the space between the thyroid and cricoid, thus increasing the distance between the thyroid and arytenoids cartilages; increasing the length of the vocal folds, decreasing their mass, and increasing their tension; and increasing vocal pitch
Thyroarytenoid	A bundle of muscle fibers making up the true vocal folds
Origin	Anteriorly, from the posterior surface of the thyroid at its angle
Insertion	Along the lateral base of the arytenoids from the vocal process to the muscle process
Function	Decreases the distance between the thyroid and arytenoids cartilages, shortening the vocal folds, increasing their mass, decreasing their tension, and decreasing vocal pitch

/s/ and /sh/, etc.). Thus, a short burst of activity in the posterior cricoarytenoid quickly abducts the vocal folds enough to stop their vibration.

Cricothyroid

The origin of the cricothyroid muscle is along the upper surface of the sides of the cricoid cartilage. Its insertion is along the lower border of the thyroid cartilage. It is considered to be the main muscle for pitch control, and its major function is to raise vocal pitch. It does so by rocking the cricoid cartilage upward or the thyroid cartilage downward, thereby increasing the distance between the thyroid cartilage and the vocal processes of the arytenoids, which are situated on the rear surface of the cricoid. The vocal folds, which are attached anteriorly on the inner surface of the thyroid cartilage and posteriorly on the vocal processes of the arytenoids, are stretched and elongated by either of these actions. Stretching the vocal folds decreases their cross-sectional area and subjects the folds to greater longitudinal tension. The decrease of area and increase of tension permit the vocal folds to vibrate at higher frequencies and thus produce the perception of higher pitch.

Decreasing the level of activity in the cricothyroid will result in a decrease of tension, resulting in a slower vibratory rate and a decrease of fundamental frequency. However, the rate of decay of muscle activity in the cricothyroid may be too slow for speech purposes. That is, it may be necessary, for linguistic purposes, to lower pitch more rapidly than would be possible by waiting for the decay of cricothyroid activity. Thus, other physiological mechanisms of frequency change may be operating to actively lower vocal pitch during speech.

Thyroarytenoid

The thyroarytenoid muscle constitutes the bulk of the vocal folds. Its contraction decreases the length of the vocal folds, increases their cross-sectional area, and decreases longitudinal tension. The action of this muscle represents one way to actively lower vocal pitch. Of course, contraction of this muscle also changes the configuration of the vocal folds themselves, thereby affecting how they will move within the vibratory cycle.

The thyroarytenoid may be divided into two muscle groups. The medial portion of the muscle is called the thyrovocalis muscle, and the more lateral portion is referred to as the thyromuscularis muscle. Some controversy exists about whether the two parts are anatomically distinct (Dickson et al., 1982). From a functional point of view, the medial portion of the thyroarytenoid (or thyrovocalis) is most active during the vibratory activity of the vocal folds and therefore may have a significant effect on phonation. The lateral (or thyromuscularis) portion may exhibit little movement during vibration, and thus its action may have minimal effect on the vibratory characteristics of the vocal folds.

DETAILED ANATOMY OF THE VOCAL FOLDS:
THE BODY COVER MODEL

Hirano (1974; 1981) has proposed a model of the vocal folds that has considerable merit in explaining the variation of human voice production. Simply stated, the vocal folds consist of three layers: (a) the outer cover, consisting of epithelium; (b) a middle layer, the lamina propria; and (c) the body. A schematic diagram of the three layers is shown in Figure 11.5

The cover of the vocal folds is composed of squamous cell epithelium. Mechanically, epithelium is very stiff, making this layer much stiffer than its neighbor, the lamina propria (Kakita, Hirano, Kawasaki, & Matsushita, 1976). It is this difference of stiffness that determines the manner in which the layers will respond to deformation

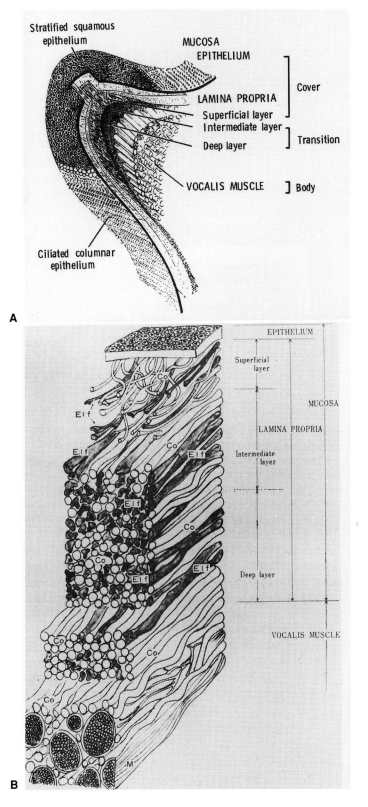

Figure 11.5. Schematic representation of the vocal fold as a body and cover. **A.** Cross-sectional representation. **B.** The kinds of fibers present in each layer.

during vibration. In some modes of vibration, the degree of coupling between the epithelium and the lamina propria is very small (as in low-frequency speech activities). In other modes of vibration, the degree of coupling between the cover, the lamina propria, and the body may be very great (as may be the case in falsetto voice). Thus, the combination of the mechanical characteristics of the three layers will ultimately determine the mode of vocal fold vibration. (See Fujimura [1981] for a good discussion of the relationships between biomechanical characteristics of the vocal folds and sound production.)

The lamina propria is actually a three-layered area lying between the cover and the body. Its superficial layer is very pliable, consisting of loose fibrous components. The intermediate layer consists primarily of elastic fibers. The deepest layer consists of collagenous fibers. Mechanically, each layer exhibits different characteristics, and variation in the composition of each of the three layers of the lamina propria alters the manner of vocal fold vibration.

The body of the vocal fold is the vocalis muscle. Although muscle cells are the primary components of muscle, blood cells, collagen cells, and inorganic material are also present. Muscle fibers themselves exhibit different mechanical characteristics when they are in the process of contracting than when they are contracted or at rest (Colton, 1988). Thus, considerable variation can occur in the mechanical characteristics of the body, depending on the amount of muscle activation, the amount of collagenous or elastic fibers present, the amount of heat generated (Cooper & Titze, 1985; Hill, 1938; Titze, 1981), and other variations caused by blood flow, oxygen consumption, and the like.

FOLDS AND CAVITIES OF THE LARYNX

Folds

The folds and cavities of the larynx are shown in Figure 11.6, sagittal and coronal cross-sections of the larynx. The major folds of interest are the true vocal folds. Superior and lateral to the true vocal folds are the false or ventricular folds. The false vocal folds do not usually vibrate in normal voice production, except perhaps at very low fundamental frequencies (50 Hz or below). They have few muscle fibers, and it is very difficult to regulate their tension, mass, and length. Occasionally they are seen to adduct partially or almost completely and obscure the true vocal folds. Only infrequently is vibration of the ventricular folds observed.

The aryepiglottic folds constitute a ring of muscle and connective tissue extending from the tips of the arytenoids to the epiglottis. In effect, they form a sphincter enclosing the entrance to the larynx. During swallowing and protective acts, the aryepiglottic folds contract to reduce the diameter of the laryngeal entrance and thus protect the airway. We have occasionally observed sphincteric movement of these folds during phonation.

Cavities

The major cavities of the larynx are (a) the supraglottal cavity, (b) the subglottal cavity, and (c) the ventricles.

The supraglottal cavity lies above the glottis or the opening between the vocal folds. Its superior boundary is the aryepiglottic sphincter. This cavity could potentially act as

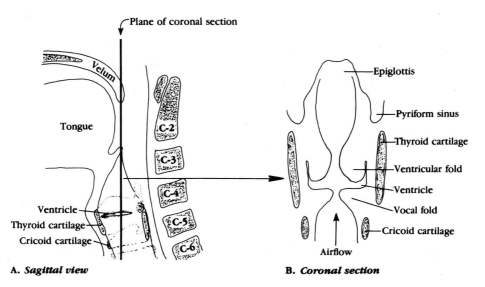

Figure 11.6. Cross-sectional representation of the larynx.

a resonator of the sound produced by the vibrating vocal folds, although it is usually considered to be part of the entire vocal tract acoustically.

The subglottal cavity lies beneath the true vocal folds. Its lower boundary is the first tracheal ring. In this cavity, pressure increases beneath the closed vocal folds until it becomes sufficient to force the vocal folds open and begin phonation.

The ventricles, often referred to as the ventricles of Morgagni, are paired cavities lying above and slightly lateral to the true vocal folds. The opening of these cavities is usually very small, and thus they seem to have little effect on the sound produced at the vocal folds. However, in some conditions encountered in singing, the opening may be sufficient to permit meaningful resonance and thus add to the glottal tone. Sundberg (1974) has shown that under certain conditions, it could resonate frequencies in the vicinity of 2,800 Hz. In most speech conditions, however, its resonant effect on sound is minimal.

LARYNGOSCOPIC VIEW OF THE LARYNX

Figure 11.7 presents a view of the larynx typically seen when observing the larynx either through a laryngeal mirror or a laryngeal endoscope (flexible or rigid). It is a common view to most otolaryngologists and to speech–language pathologists and voice scientists. The various structures that can be viewed are identified in this figure. One must know these landmarks to properly interpret images of the larynx. A good knowledge of normal anatomy and its variations is needed to correctly identify laryngeal pathological conditions. Much variability occurs in normal anatomic structures. Examples of this variability as seen fiberscopically were discussed by Casper, Brewer, and Colton (1987). The most marked structural variability occurred in the configuration of the "arytenoid complex" (arytenoids, cuneiforms, corniculates). Obvious movement differences were seen among the subjects in this area. Some subjects exhibited symmetrical movement, whereas in others the movements were asymmetrical. Asymmetry was also found in the

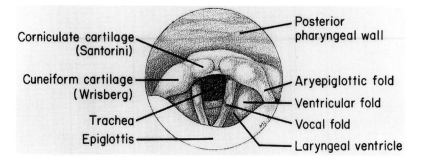

Figure 11.7. Laryngoscopic view of the larynx. This is a view typically seen during indirect mirror, fiberoptic, or stroboscopic examination of the larynx.

apparent length of the true vocal folds. Notably, the marked anteroposterior movement and twisting of the larynx, often seen in patients with voice disorders, were not observed in normal speakers. "Normal" can span a broad range of differences in both structure and function. Asymmetry is not necessarily a sign of an abnormal larynx.

SUMMARY

A brief review of the anatomy of the larynx and the vocal folds is presented. The extrinsic muscles of the larynx help to support and adjust the position of the larynx. The intrinsic muscles of the larynx attach to the various cartilages of the larynx (thyroid, cricoid, arytenoid) and serve to adjust the length, tension, and mass of the vocal folds, as well as to adduct them. A brief discussion of the cavities and folds of the larynx is presented, concluding with a presentation of the laryngoscopic view of laryngeal anatomy.

Chapter 12

Phonatory Physiology

The vibrating vocal folds are the major source of periodic sound for speech. Other periodic sound sources (e.g., flapping lips) exist, but these are minor compared with the sound produced from the vocal folds. In addition, aperiodic sound sources produce voiceless consonants. The vocal folds may be involved in the production of aperiodic sound, as, for example, in the consonant /h/.

In this chapter, we review the basic concepts of phonatory physiology. First, the conditions that must exist before sound can be produced are presented, followed by discussion of the mechanisms necessary for initiating and sustaining sound. The third and fourth sections are brief outlines of the physiological mechanisms for control of vocal pitch and intensity control by the vocal folds, respectively. Finally, a review of some of the mechanisms for control of voice quality is presented. The reader interested in further information on these topics is referred to the excellent text by Titze (1994).

GLOTTAL TONE INITIATION

Before sound can be produced from the vocal folds, several conditions must be established. First, the vocal folds must be approximated or almost approximated in the phonatory position. This position, in comparison to the inspiratory position of the vocal folds (Fig. 12.1A), is shown in Figure 12.1B. Phonation also may be initiated after completely closing the vocal folds.

One also must properly tense and elongate the vocal folds before actually producing sound. Length and tension are important determinants of the fundamental vibrating rate of the vocal folds, in ways that are discussed later under "Mechanisms of Vocal Frequency Change."

Finally, there must be airflow from the lungs. To be able to produce the required flow of air from the lungs, the lungs must contain a sufficient quantity of air. Typically, we inhale before we begin producing sound for an utterance.

Once these initial conditions have been established, phonation can start. When the vocal folds are in the phonatory position, one must close them to start vibration. If one starts with the vocal folds fully closed, it is necessary to open them to start vibration. Whatever the starting point, the process thereafter is similar and is simply described as a series of alternate openings and closings of the vocal folds. The opening and closing is regulated by the degree of tension in the vocal folds and two aerodynamic events.

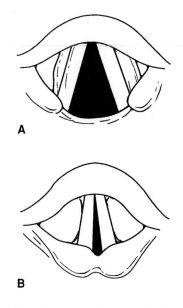

Figure 12.1. Schematic representaion of the stages of vocal fold adduction. **A.** During inspiration. **B.** At start of phonation.

The aerodynamic event important for closing the vocal folds is called the Bernoulli effect, named after a famous 18th-century Swiss physicist. Bernoulli was most interested in fluid flows, but his principles hold for gas flows as well. Simply stated, Bernoulli's second law of fluid mechanics states that the sum of the static pressures and the kinetic pressures in a gas is always equal to a constant. The constant may vary according to the temperature, pressure, or molecular structure of the gas. Within these conditions, however, when motion of the molecules changes, there is a change in the static pressure exerted by the molecules. Stating the principle another way, increased motion of gas molecules results in decreased pressure.

The Bernoulli effect is often evoked to explain how airplanes rise in the air. The undersurface of the wing of an airplane is rather flat, whereas the upper surface is markedly convex in shape. This curvature on the upper wing surface means that the air molecules passing over the top of the wing have a greater distance to travel to pass over the wing than those molecules that pass under the wing. The velocity of the molecules traveling along the surface of the upper wing must increase in order to travel the distance in the same time as the molecules traveling under the wing . In short, their kinetic "pressure" has been increased. According to Bernoulli's principle, when the kinetic pressure increases, the static pressure must decrease. Thus, there is less pressure along the upper surface of the wing. By the same token, there is greater pressure below the wing, and this greater pressure will lift the wing (and the airplane) into the sky.

The same principle holds for the vocal folds. The vocal folds impose a partial obstruction to the flow of air. The molecules traveling along the sides of the trachea, when meeting the vocal folds, must travel a greater distance around the fold to meet the molecules traveling up the center of the trachea. The molecules along the surface of the vocal folds must increase their velocity and kinetic pressure. Again, static

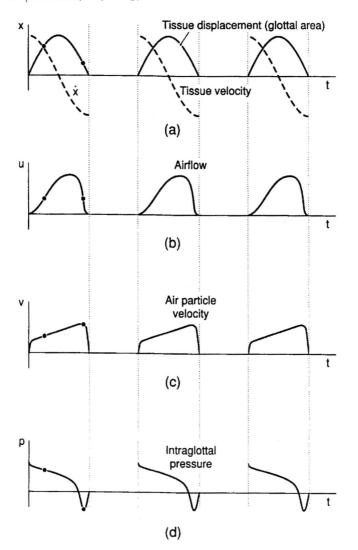

Figure 12.2. Relationships between displacement and velocity of the vocal folds, airflow, air particle velocity, and intraglottal air pressures.

pressure on the surface of the vocal folds is decreased. The vocal folds, being pliable and movable, begin to move toward the center of the trachea because of this pressure differential. Eventually, the two vocal folds meet at the midline, and airflow ceases.

The trick that needs to be performed to produce vibration is to create the Bernoulli effect when you wish to close the vocal folds and a positive pressure when you wish to open them (Titze, 1994). When the vocal folds close, a sudden decrease of airflow results (See Fig. 12.2B). When the vocal folds open, a momentary delay in the start of air flow results because of this inertia. This explains the characteristic shape of the airflow pulse through the glottis, in which the rising airflow phase is slower than the opening of the vocal folds (Fig. 12.2A and B). Air particle velocities through the glottis also show asymmetry (Fig 12.2C). Generally, these velocities increase as the vocal folds open and change direction when the airflow pulse shuts off at closure. Intraglottal air pressure is solely dependent on air particle velocity (Titze, 1994). The classic Bernoulli equation states that as kinetic energy increases, static "energy" must decrease, because the two values sum to a constant. Thus, as air particle velocity increases, intraglottal pressure decreases. Air particle directional change results in an abrupt negative change of intraglottal pressure (Fig. 12.2C and D) just when we need it to produce vocal fold closure. Positive pressure below the vocal folds forces them open.

The tension and mass of the vocal folds create a resistance to vibration. Consequently, a minimum pressure is required to force the folds into vibration. Titze (1992) calls this pressure phonation threshold pressure (PTP). PTP is dependent on the frequency of phonation and may be slightly different for males and females (and probably for children as well). PTP is also dependent on hydration levels of vocal fold tissues (Verdolini-Marston, Titze, & Druker, 1990). Intensity control is also related to PTP.

MECHANISMS OF VOCAL FREQUENCY CHANGE

The human vocal mechanism is capable of producing a wide range of frequencies, sometimes in excess of three octaves. In this section, we review some of the physiological mechanisms that determine the fundamental vibrating rate of the vocal folds.

Early in the study of phonation, individuals compared the vocal folds with vibrating strings. After all, both the vocal folds and strings had a length and a mass and were under tension. Furthermore, much was known about the determinants of frequency in strings, and the analogy appeared to be a good one.

As research on voice physiology progressed, evidence accumulated that prompted a reevaluation of the analogy between the mechanism of frequency variation by the vocal folds and by a string. Recent evidence has confirmed that the physical properties that determine the frequency of a vibrating string also determine the vibrating frequency of the vocal folds.

The vibratory frequency of a string, and of the vocal folds, is determined by its length, tension, and mass. Actually, in the case of the vocal folds, their total mass is not significant but rather the mass that is set into vibration. The amount of mass set into vibration will depend on fundamental frequency, intensity, and mode of vibration. Furthermore, the amount of mass varies as a function of the length of the string or vocal fold. The relationship of vocal fold thickness to length is similar to that observed in a rubber band. As the band is stretched, the thickness of the band decreases.

Vocal Fold Length and Fundamental Frequency

A convenient way of understanding the relationships between length, mass, and tension in a string and in the vocal folds is by graphing the parameters as a function of frequency. A plot of fundamental frequency as a function of vocal fold length is shown in Figure 12.3. In the modal register, as vocal fold length increases, frequency increases. This relationship is clearly opposite to that predicted by the classic equation for determining the frequency of a vibrating string. However, when phonation is produced in the falsetto or upper register, fundamental frequency appears to decrease as vocal fold length is increased. Subsequent research has shown that the length of the vibrating portion of the vocal folds decreases as frequency is increased. This oppositional effect, at least for modal register phonation, is why the string analogy was thought by some to be inappropriate for the control of fundamental frequency by the vocal folds. Length

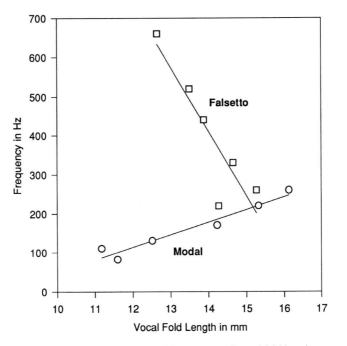

Figure 12.3. The relationship between fundamental frequency and vocal fold length.

is not the sole mechanism for control of fundamental frequency, however, either in strings or in the vocal folds.

Vocal Fold Mass and Fundamental Frequency

The mass of the vocal folds also may play a role in frequency control. Figure 12.4 shows the relationship between thickness of the vocal folds and frequency. Note that for the vocal folds, vocal frequency decreases as mass increases, a relationship similar to that for a vibrating string.

Vocal Fold Tension and Fundamental Frequency

Tension affects the vibrating frequency of a string and the vocal folds. The relationship between tension and frequency of the vocal folds is shown in Figure 12.5. As tension increases, so too does frequency. In general, the effect of tension on the vocal folds produces changes of frequency much like those in a string.

Measuring tension directly in the living human vocal fold is very difficult. Indirect evidence must be obtained from recordings of muscle activity or measurements made on dog or excised human larynges (Perlman, Titze, & Cooper, 1984; Perlman & Titze, 1988). Moreover, the variations of tension produced by muscle contraction also must be considered (Colton, 1988) when trying to understand how tension determines the fundamental frequency of phonation.

Tension becomes more important in the determination of fundamental frequency at certain areas of an individual's total phonational range. Van den Berg and Tan (1959) have shown that the largest variation of tension occurs at upper frequencies, most often

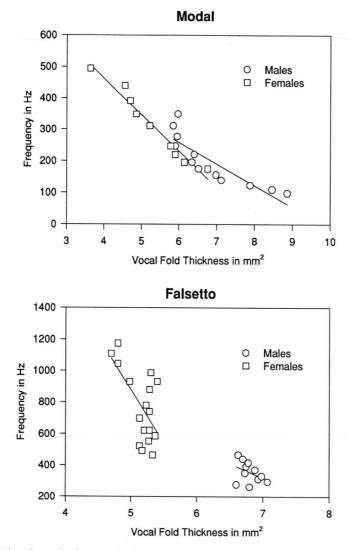

Figure 12.4. The relationship between fundamental frequency and vocal fold thickness.

those produced in the falsetto register. A small amount of tension variation occurs at frequencies typically heard in speech. Thus, although tension is an important determinant of fundamental frequency variation, it is not the only determinant. As has been shown, the mass of the vocal folds (or more accurately, their mass per unit length) has a pronounced influence on the fundamental frequency of the vibration.

Clearly, there may be several mechanisms determining fundamental frequency in the human voice. At some frequencies (usually in the modal register), overall mass may be the most important determinant (Allen & Hollien, 1973), whereas at other frequencies (usually in the falsetto register), tension may be the dominant factor. The combination of these factors ultimately determines the fundamental frequency of vocal fold vibration.

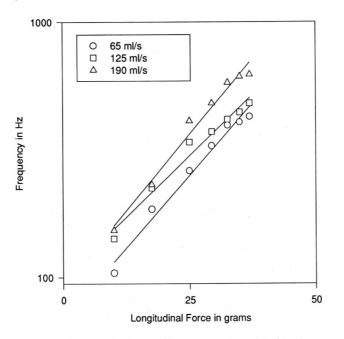

Figure 12.5. The relationship between fundamental frequency and vocal fold tension.

The data from van den Berg and Tan also show that the relationship between tension and fundamental frequency differs as airflow rates differ (Fig. 12.5). Thus, airflow appears to be another contributing factor in the physiological mechanisms of vocal frequency control. In some cases, airflow may be the major determinant of frequency, much as it is for aeolian tones. You may have walked through an open field in which telephone or electrical wires passed overhead and heard the sound the wind makes when striking the wires. This is an example of an aeolian tone whose frequency is determined by the speed of the airflow rushing across the wire. In many patients with phonatory disorders, there is excessive airflow. Although the speed of the airflow may not directly affect the fundamental frequency of the vocal folds as in an aeolian tone, it may be a sign of an inefficient mechanism being used for the variation of vocal pitch. Or the patient may be using a combination of tension, mass, and airflow that causes or contributes to the voice problem. These possibilities point to the need for information about all of these parameters with voice patients. The availability of such information may help in understanding the bases for the patient's vocal problem.

As in a string, the fundamental frequency of the vocal folds is determined by a complex interaction between length, mass, and tension. Various combinations of these parameters may produce the same fundamental frequency. However, not all combinations of length, mass, and tension may be efficient for the production of voice.

MECHANISMS OF LOUDNESS CHANGE

The human voice is capable of producing a wide range of vocal intensities, sometimes exceeding 60 dB. Additional changes of intensity result from variation in the size and shape of the vocal tract, which acts as a resonator of sound. The mechanisms for the control of vocal intensity, much as those of pitch control, involve muscular activity in combination with airflows and pressures.

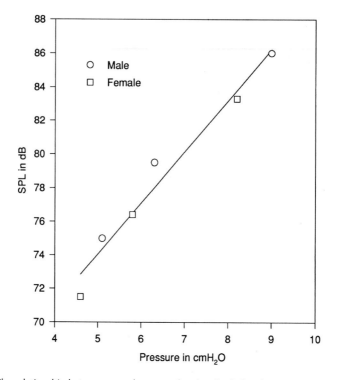

Figure 12.6. The relationship between sound pressure level and subglottal air pressure.

Vocal intensity is usually reported in decibels of sound pressure level. Because sound is basically a pressure disturbance, we expect that increased pressures beneath the vocal folds, when released by the folds, would produce a greater intensity, and indeed, experimental evidence supports this expectation (Ladefoged & McKinney, 1963). As shown in Figure 12.6, when the subglottal air pressure increases, intensity increases, although the exact relationship varies for different vowels and voice qualities.

However, the controlling mechanism of vocal intensity is not subglottal air pressure. Rather, the controlling mechanism is the degree and time of closure of the vocal folds themselves. That is, by maintaining closure of the vocal folds, there is more time to build up pressure beneath them. More intense sound results when the subglottal air pressure is sufficient to overcome the resistance of the vocal folds. Resistance is the important factor in intensity control. The more vocal fold resistance there is to opening, the greater the pressure disturbance when the resistance is overcome and the folds are forced to open. Thus, intensity is most often controlled by the vocal folds through variations of glottal resistance. Glottal resistance is defined as the ratio of the pressure divided by the flow. Measuring these two quantities will allow the calculation of resistance.

Isshiki (1964; 1965) has shown that glottal resistance is a major controlling mechanism of vocal intensities for low fundamental frequencies, that is, fundamental frequencies produced in the lower part of an individual's phonational range or in the modal register. At higher frequencies, especially frequencies produced in falsetto, glottal resistance is no longer the major factor. Rather, airflow appears to become the dominant variable in intensity variation at these high fundamental frequencies. Furthermore, the range of intensities an individual can produce in the falsetto register is much smaller

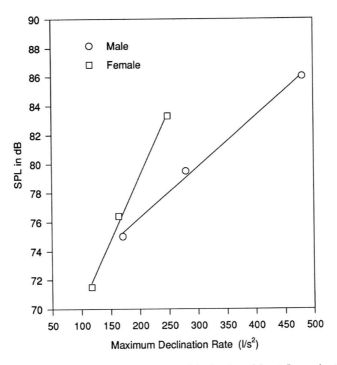

Figure 12.7. Sound pressure levels and maximum rate of declination of the airflow pulse (or the slope of the closing portion of the airflow pulse) as derived from inverse filtering.

than can be produced in the modal register (Colton, 1973). This finding suggests, or at least is in consonance with, the existence of a different controlling mechanism for intensity control in falsetto.

Another mechanism of intensity control has been described (Sundberg, Titze, & Scherer, 1993; Titze, 1994). The vocal folds produce sound when they close. The intensity (and spectra) of the sound is dependent on the velocity of closure of the vocal folds. Glottal power is directly related to the rate of change of the airflow pulse at the moment of closure (Titze & Sundberg, 1992). This rate of change of airflow at closure is often referred to as maximum declination rate or simply airflow closing slope. The relationship between the airflow closing slope of the airflow pulse and intensity is shown in Figure 12.7. Therefore, intensity control by the vocal folds may be dependent on at least two factors, glottal resistance and the rate of airflow change at the moment of closure.

For a variety of reasons, some patients have difficulty in completely closing their vocal folds. In an attempt to speak at a normal vocal intensity, these patients increase air pressure by increasing the expiratory force from the thorax–abdomen system. The patient also may attempt to increase glottal closure in an effort to increase glottal resistance and to maintain an adequate level of tension in the vocal folds. As a result of this effortful vocal behavior, greater than normal subglottal pressures are developed, and there is increased tension in the vocal folds. Because greater than normal muscle activity is involved, these conditions may create vocal fatigue as well as excessive air rushing across the vocal folds. The latter creates greater noise levels in the voice. A vicious cycle ensues, as the vocal fatigue may result in even poorer vocal fold adduction and the need for even greater effort on the patient's part, leading cyclically to poorer voice.

Another factor affects the sound pressure level (SPL) of phonation. That factor is the spectral characteristics of the tone produced by the vocal folds. It is well known that variation of the frequency composition of a tone also vary its intensity. Adding frequencies or varying the amplitude of the components of the tone affects the intensity of the complex tone. Similarly, the spectrum of the vocal folds can be varied within limits and thus alter the overall intensity of the vocal fold tone. Consequently, the vocal folds can affect the intensity of the tone by variation of the frequency components in the tone. Speed of closure of the vocal folds affects the spectral features of the glottal tone (Löfqvist, 1993).

In some patients with phonatory disorders, the spectral characteristics of the tone produced are markedly different from normal. Usually, but not always, the number of frequency components in the pathological voice is much smaller than in the normal voice. When that is the case, lower intensities would be expected to compensate for the different spectral characteristics and their effect on intensity; a patient may try to increase subglottal pressures or adductory forces, resulting in increased strain and subsequent abuse of the vocal folds.

Loudness is the perceptual correlate of intensity, but intensity is not the only physical factor that affects loudness. The pitch of the voice and its spectral composition also may affect its perceived loudness. Of course, factors such as the distance from the speaker, room acoustics, diffraction, and interference also may affect the loudness of a voice as perceived by a listener.

MECHANISMS OF QUALITY VARIATION

Voice quality is an important attribute of normal and abnormal voices. Voice quality identifies the individual and sets him or her apart from another. A change of voice quality may signal the presence of a benign problem or one that could be life threatening. Defining voice quality can be difficult and imprecise, however (Kreiman, Gerratt, & Berke, 1994; Kreiman & Gerratt, 1998; Kreiman & Gerratt, 2000).

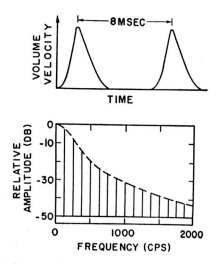

Figure 12.8. Inverse filtered airflow waveform of the vocal folds (top panel) and its corresponding frequency spectrum (bottom panel) from a phonation produced by a male subject.

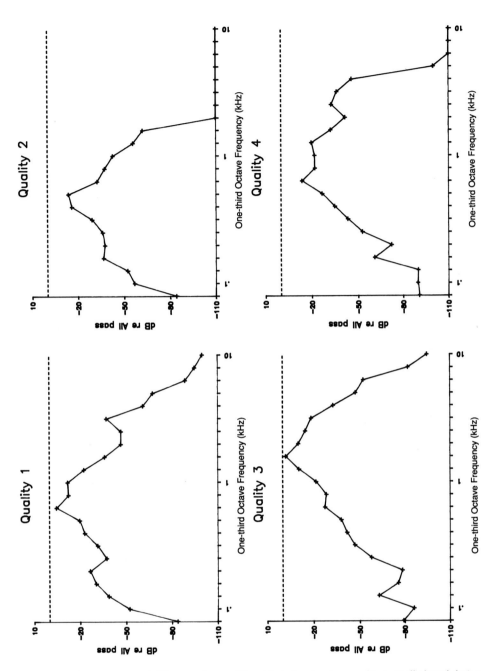

Figure 12.9. Some spectra of different voice qualities. Mode 1 refers to a quality typically heard during speech, mode 2 to a quality of a sound heard during sobbing or during the singing of a lullaby, mode 3 to a quality typically heard in Country Western singing, and mode 4 to a quality heard in operatic singing.

Many adjectives are used to describe voice quality: pleasant and unpleasant, normal and pathological. Singers, actors, professional speakers, and those who work with the voice use jargon to describe the variation of normal voice quality. Quantification of these terms either acoustically or physiologically has proved very difficult.

Acoustically, the important parameter concerned with voice quality is spectrum. Spectrum refers to the number and amplitude of the frequencies present in a complex tone, such as the vocal fold tone. Figure 12.8 presents the spectrum of a typical vocal fold tone produced during speech. However, the vocal folds can produce many different voice qualities, each with its own spectral characteristics (Fig. 12.9).

Other factors may be important in describing a voice quality acoustically. Although pitch would be expected to be one such factor, it apparently is not used in distinguishing one voice quality from another (Colton, 1987). This finding is similar to the influence of pitch in the perception of nonphonatory sounds such as complex sounds (Plomp, 1976) and noise bands (Chipman & Carey, 1975). Varying the pitch level may alter some of the details of a voice, but not its basic voice quality.

Voice quality is not determined solely by the vibratory characteristics of the vocal folds. The shape and configuration of the vocal tract are also determinants of voice quality. For example, females have slightly different vocal tract configurations than males, and as a result, female voices can still be recognized as female even when the obvious pitch difference is removed (Coleman, 1971; 1973; 1976). The overall characteristics of an individual's vocal tract, such as the length, cross-sectional area, ratio of oral to pharyngeal cavity size, and so on, also determine that individual's voice quality.

Physiological change in laryngeal and vocal tract configurations and characteristics have been observed in individuals as they produced various voice qualities (Colton & Estill, 1981; Painter, 1986; 1991). For example, in some voice qualities, the size of the pharyngeal cavity is much larger than in other voice qualities. Many of these differences appear to occur in the larynx itself, as well as in the pharynx. We have little information about the vocal tract characteristics of patients with voice disorders.

SUMMARY

In this chapter, a brief review of the mechanisms for voice production, frequency control, intensity variation, and the generation of voice quality have been reviewed. The tone produced by the vocal folds results from the complex interaction of airflow, air pressure, and muscular activity, which regulate the length, mass, and tension of the vocal folds. Variation in these parameters affects the fundamental frequency of the voice, as well as its intensity and voice quality. Measurement of these acoustic parameters of the voice will assist in the quantification of the vocal behavior and help to determine the nature of the problem. Accurate measurement of these acoustic, perceptual, or physiological parameters can play a part in understanding and treatment planning.

Chapter 13

Neuroanatomy of the Vocal Mechanism

Volitional control of the muscles of the larynx resides in the brain. However, many connecting points or stations exist within the brain, including the cortex, subcortical areas, midbrain, and medulla, which play an important role in the ultimate control of phonation. Thus, saying that phonation is controlled by the brain is much too simplistic and underemphasizes the roles various structures play in integrating information and coordinating the activity of the muscles active in phonation. In this chapter, a brief review of the neuroanatomy and neurophysiology of phonation is presented. A further and more detailed review of brain mechanisms controlling vocalization may be found in Larson (1988).

CORTICAL MECHANISMS OF PHONATORY CONTROL

The cerebral cortex is that portion of the brain responsible for the conceptualization, planning, and execution of the speech act, including phonation. Some areas of the cortex may be responsible for creating the act, others for its linguistic characteristics, and still others for the emotionality of the act. Penfield and Roberts (1959) have identified three major areas of the cortex directly responsible for vocalization. These are, in decreasing order of importance, (a) the precentral and postcentral gyrus (Rolandic area), (b) the anterior (or Broca's) area, and (c) the supplementary motor area. These areas are shown in Figure 13.1. Experiments have shown that vocalization occurs when certain spots within these areas are stimulated in both the dominant and nondominant hemispheres (Fig. 13.2). Within these areas, depending on the specific areas stimulated, vocalization can be initiated or stopped and speech can be slurred or distorted. These behaviors occur as the result of stimulation in either the dominant or the nondominant hemisphere. Speech and phonation are complex motor acts involving simultaneous activation and control of many muscles. Although the control of these motor acts occurs primarily in the cortex, control of individual muscles seems to occur at a much lower level in the brain. No evidence has been found to suggest that cortical stimulation produces a response in a single, solitary muscle. Higher brain function is concerned with idealization of the event, integration of sensory information, feedback control, and coordination of various muscles required for the motor act.

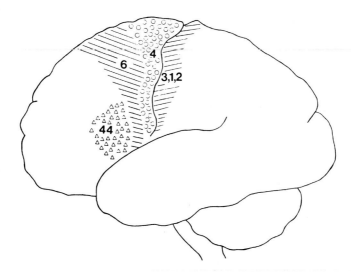

Figure 13.1. Diagram of the cortical areas involved in speech movement control. Area 4 (primary motor cortex), areas 3, 1, and 2 (somatosensory cortex), area 44 (Broca's area), and area 6 (premotor cortex and supplementary motor area).

SUBCORTICAL MECHANISMS

The motor cortex has numerous connections to the thalamus, a major portion of the diencephalon or interbrain. Other parts of the diencephalon include the hypothalamus, metathalamus, epithalamus, and subthalamus (Riklan & Levita, 1969). The third ventricle is also part of the diencephalon (Gardner, 1963). The thalamus has major pathways to the motor cortex and Broca's area (Penfield & Roberts, 1959). In addition, the thalamus has numerous connections to the cerebellum, midbrain, and other structures in the diencephalon (Fig. 13.3). Various nuclei in the thalamus project to parts of the cerebral cortex. These are shown in Figure 13.4. Note that the motor area (precentral gyrus) located anterior to the central sulcus receives much of its projection from the ventral lateral nucleus of the thalamus. Botez and Barbeau (1971) concluded that

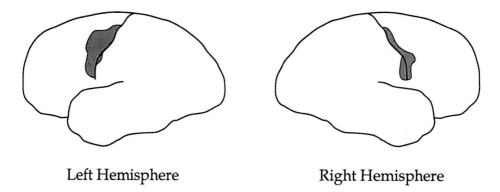

Left Hemisphere   Right Hemisphere

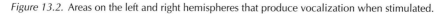

Figure 13.2. Areas on the left and right hemispheres that produce vocalization when stimulated.

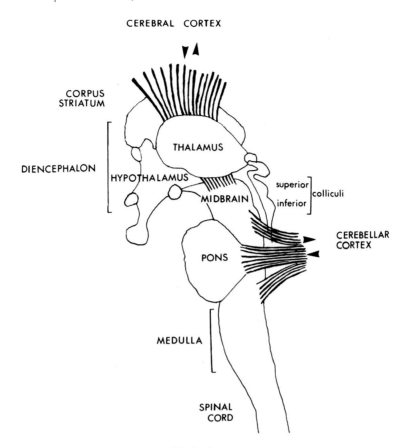

Figure 13.3. Diagrammatic representation of the brainstem.

the ventrolateral nucleus was responsible for the initiation of speech movements as well as control of loudness, pitch, rate, and articulation. Broca's area receives connections from the dorsal median and centromedian nuclei of the thalamus. (The centromedian nuclei help form the massa intermedia shown in Fig. 13.4.)

The thalamus is a most fascinating structure in the diencephalon, because it appears to act both as a relay for impulses occurring in lower areas of the brain and as an integrator of information (Riklan & Levita, 1969). Furthermore, the thalamus is involved in the maintenance of consciousness, alertness, and attention and also may integrate emotion into a complex motor act. Some of the thalamic nuclei are nonspecific and project to many areas on the cortex (Fig. 13.5). Thus, insofar as speech and voice are concerned, the thalamus plays a major role in integrating incoming sensory information, coordinating outgoing information from the cortex and other areas of the brain, and, perhaps, adding emotionality to speech and voice.

MIDBRAIN STRUCTURES

The midbrain or mesencephalon lies beneath the thalamus (House & Pansky, 1967). On the anterior surface of the midbrain are the cerebral peduncles that connect the cerebrum with the brainstem and spinal cord. On its posterior surface, four rounded

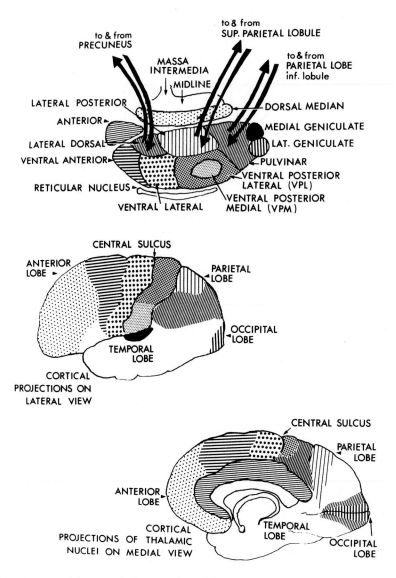

Figure 13.4. Diagram of the major thalamic nuclei and their projections.

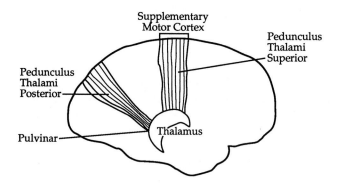

Figure 13.5. Drawing showing the connections between the pulvinar nuclei of the thalamus and the posterior speech area of the cortex. Diagram also shows the pathway between the thalamus and the superior speech cortex (supplementary motor area).

areas are called the colliculi. The superior colliculi are concerned with visual function, whereas the inferior colliculi are concerned with audition. Within the midbrain is a cavity called the cerebral aqueduct of Sylvius, which is surrounded by a thick zone of gray matter. An important area of this gray matter, dorsal to the aqueduct, is called the periaqueductal gray (PAG).

Several investigators have shown that stimulation of the dorsal and ventrolateral areas of the PAG produces activity in some laryngeal muscles (Larson, 1985; Larson & Kistler, 1986; Ortega, DeRosier, Park, & Larson, 1988). Larson (1985) has reported that some cells in the ventrolateral area stimulate muscle activity, whereas other cells suppress activity. He suggested that the PAG may be an intermediate area between the recognition of a stimulus or event and the subsequent production of the motor act. Other areas, such as the hypothalamus, amygdala, and anterior cingulate gyrus, are responsible for vocalizations but of a kind that Larson (1985) notes are species specific. Botez and Barbeau (1971) also implicated the PAG in disorders involving mutism.

Lesions in the PAG and adjacent areas have produced mutism (Adametz & O'Leary, 1959; Randall, 1964). Moreover, electrical stimulation of the PAG has produced natural-sounding vocalizations in a variety of species (Jürgens & Pratt, 1979; Kelly, Beaton, & Magoun, 1946; Yajima, Hayashi, & Yoshii, 1982). Chemical stimulation of the PAG has elicited two kinds of vocalizations in cats (Zhang, Davis, Bandler, & Carrive, 1994). One vocalization type (type A) consisted of meows, howls, and growls remarkably similar to normal feline vocalizations. The other vocalization type (type B) was described as a hiss, also found in normal feline repertoire. Type A vocalizations were all voiced with a fundamental frequency and strong harmonics. They involved activity in the cricothyroid, genioglossus, and internal oblique muscles. Type B has no voicing and no activity in the cricothyroid muscles but normal activity in the genioglossus and internal oblique muscles. Zhang and his colleagues point out that these vocalization types are very similar to voiced and unvoiced sounds produced by humans.

Zhang et al. (1994) found strong evidence for the PAG to be involved in the control of patterns of muscle activity involving muscles of respiration and vocalization and in the orofacial area. They specifically pointed out that no PAG sites were found that activated individual muscles. They concluded that the PAG contains neurons involved in the control of at least two kinds of vocalization.

BRAINSTEM

The major bilateral structures in the brainstem implicated in the neural control of phonation include the nucleus ambiguus, nucleus tractus solitarii, and nucleus parabrachialis. Yoshida, Mitsumasu, Hirano, Morimoto, and Kanaseki (1987) performed an elegant study in which they traced the connections among these structures. When they injected a tracer chemical into one nucleus ambiguus, they found evidence of the tracer throughout the contralateral nuclei, in the nuclei tractus solitarii bilaterally, in the nuclei parabrachialis, and bilaterally in the lateral and ventrolateral parts of the PAG area, with a predominance ipsilaterally. Injection of a tracer into the nucleus tractus solitarii resulted in labeled cells throughout the nucleus itself, as well as in the dorsal motor nucleus of the vagus, part of the hypoglossal nucleus, the medial portion of the nucleus gracilis, and the dorsal part of the reticular formation. Clearly, many interconnections exist bilaterally among the nucleus ambiguus, nucleus tractus solitarii, reticular formation around the nucleus ambiguus, motor roots of the vagus, and PAG area.

Zhang, Davis, Carrive, and Bandler (1992) also have implicated the nucleus retroambigualis in the control of vocalization. This "structure" is actually the caudal third of the ventral respiratory group located in the ventrolateral medulla. Neurons in this area have long been implicated in the control of respiration (von Euler, 1986); however, they also have an important role in the control of laryngeal muscles and vocalization.

CEREBELLUM

The cerebellum, a structure lying immediately posterior to the midbrain area, is strongly implicated in the control of movement. Its location is shown in Figure 13.6A. Figure 13.6B shows the cerebellum from a dorsal view after the cerebrum has been removed. The three main portions of the cerebellum are seen in this diagram: the vermis (V), the pars intermedia (PI), and the hemispheres (H). The cerebellum consists of many transverse folia, shown in Figure 13.6C, whose complex infolding vastly increases the surface area of the cerebellum in much the same way as is seen in the cerebrum. The fissura prima (FP) is a deep fissure separating the anterior and posterior lobes.

Two major areas of the cerebellum are instrumental in the control of movement (von Euler, 1986). The first, the pars intermedia, has many direct connections via midbrain nuclei with the cerebrum (Fig. 13.7A). Impulses from the motor cortex are quickly relayed from the pyramidal tracts (PT) to the PI via the nuclei pontis, lateral reticular nucleus, and inferior olive. The PI analyzes the movement patterns and quickly returns the results of its analysis to the cerebral cortex through connections through the interpositus nucleus, the ventral lateral nuclei of the thalamus, and the red nucleus. As such, the PI acts like a computer controlling a missile. It may not have given the original command to fire, but it constantly monitors the missile, taking small corrective actions whenever the missile deviates from its intended flight plan (Eccles, 1977).

The role of the cerebellar hemispheres in movement control seems to be one of planning the stages of a movement pattern. As shown in Figure 13.7B, there are few direct connections to tracts that lead to lower motoneurons, as was the case for

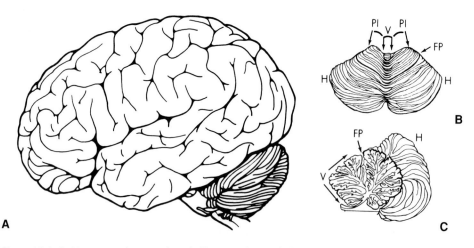

Figure 13.6. **A.** Human cerebrum and cerebellum. **B.** The cerebellum from its dorsal aspect. **C.** Midline view after sagittal section. Legend: H, hemispheres; V, vermis; PI, the pars intermedia; FP, fissura prima.

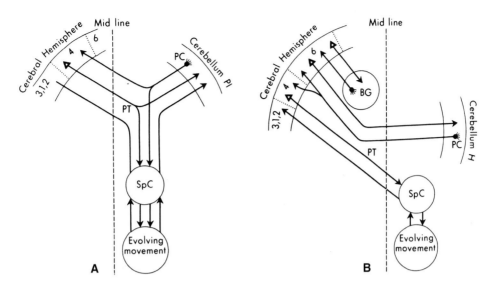

Figure 13.7. Cerebrocerebellar circuits in motor control. **A.** The main circuit starts in the motor cortex (4) and travels down the pyramidal tract (PT) to the spinal cord, with side branches via the pars intermedia (PI) to the cerebellum. Impulses from Purkinje cells (PC) in the cerebellum communicate with the motor cortex and to the spinal cord. **B.** Circuits from area 6 in the cerebrum to the cerebellar hemispheres (H). A return circuit from the Purkinje cells (PC) back to areas 4 and 6 is shown. Also shown is a circuit from area 6 to the basal ganglia (BG) and its return to the cerebrum. Spinal centers (SpC) are indicated. Evolving movement refers to the desired movement pattern of a structure.

the connections between the cerebrum and PI of the cerebellum. Rather, the connections from the motor cortex pass through the nuclei pontis and inferior olive directly to cells within the cerebellar hemispheres, and impulses from the cerebellar hemispheres pass through the nucleus dentatus to the ventral lateral nuclei of the thalamus and red nucleus back to the cerebral hemispheres, where movement is initiated. The command center, after drafting a movement plan, sends it on to the cerebellar hemispheres for revision and refinement before adopting it. According to Eccles (1977), the cerebellar hemispheres are concerned with anticipatory planning based on learning, experience, and sensory information they receive from other brain centers.

The importance of the cerebellum in the control of speech movement cannot be emphasized enough. Kornhuber (1977) believes that without it (and other midbrain areas) the cerebral cortex could not function and would be ineffective in the generation of movements. The cerebellum acts to regulate motor movement continuously and quickly, requiring some degree of preprogramming and adjustment by learning. Certainly, coordination of muscles within the larynx is necessary for phonation, as is coordination with other systems involved in speech production.

PERIPHERAL CONNECTIONS: THE VAGUS NERVE

The vagus nerve is the major nerve that supplies the larynx (and other parts of the body as well). The vagus provides sensory fibers within the larynx, as well as fibers that control all the muscles of the larynx. The cell bodies of the vagus are located in

FUNCTIONAL COMPONENTS OF PERIPHERAL NERVES

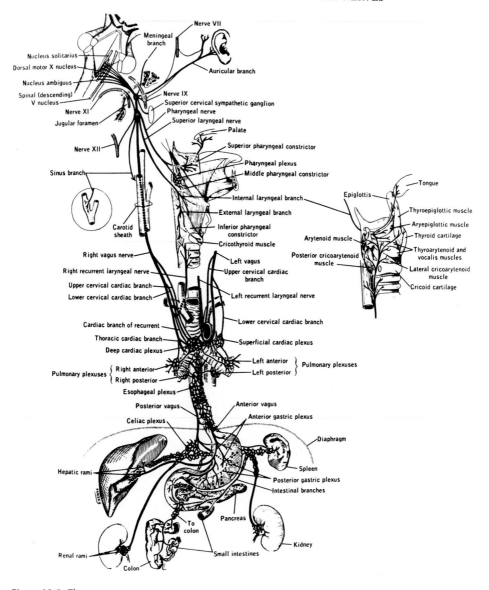

Figure 13.8. The vagus nerve.

the nucleus ambiguus. Laryngeal muscles are controlled by cells in the more caudal portions of the nucleus. The vagus emerges from the surface of the medulla between the cerebellar peduncle and the inferior olives in the midbrain. It exits the skull through the jugular foramen.

After exiting the skull, the vagus divides into many branches that serve the head, neck, thorax, and abdomen. These are shown schematically in Figure 13.8. Shortly after exiting the jugular foramen, a small filament (the meningeal filament) exits the nerve to serve the dura mater on the posterior fossa of the base of the skull. The auricular branch provides sensory fibers to the skin behind the pinna and to the posterior part of the external auditory meatus. The pharyngeal branch provides motor fibers to the muscles of the pharynx and soft palate.

The major portions of the vagus serving the larynx are the superior laryngeal and the recurrent laryngeal nerves. The superior laryngeal is the primary sensory nerve for the larynx. It arises from the inferior ganglion of the vagus and descends along the side of the pharynx behind the internal carotid artery, where it sends off two branches. The external branch descends along the side of the larynx to serve the cricothyroid muscle. The internal branch descends to an opening in the thyrohyoid membrane and enters the larynx to serve the mucous membrane of the larynx down to the true vocal folds. The recurrent laryngeal nerve follows a different course on either side of the body. On the right side, the recurrent descends in the neck to loop around the subclavian artery (just below the clavicle) and then ascends alongside the trachea to serve the remaining intrinsic muscles of the larynx. On the left side, the recurrent laryngeal nerve takes a much more circuitous route, descending into the thorax, looping around the aorta, and then ascending alongside the trachea until it reaches the larynx. It also provides motor fibers to the remaining intrinsic laryngeal muscles.

Other branches of the vagus nerve in the neck, thorax, and abdomen provide sensory innervation to various structures within these areas. These branches of the vagus are shown in Table 13.1.

The extrinsic laryngeal muscles are innervated by several nerves. The anterior belly of the digastric muscle receives its innervation from the mylohyoid branch of the inferior alveolar nerve, whereas the posterior belly is innervated by the 7th cranial nerve (the facial). The mylohyoid muscle is innervated by the mylohyoid branch of the inferior alveolar nerve, and the geniohyoid, sternohyoid, sternothyroid, and omohyoid muscles by the ansa cervicalis (C1). The thyrohyoid is innervated by ansa cervicalis (C1) through the hypoglossal nerve.

Numerous protective mechanisms are present within the respiratory tract, but the most vigorous exist in the larynx. Some are mechanical and act to close off the airway; others are expulsive and serve to force foreign substances from the airway. All are reflexive and operate under involuntary control.

Many sensory endings within the larynx collect information about the state of the larynx and respiratory tract and transmit this information through several reflex arcs as well as directly to the central nervous system. Wyke (1969; Wyke, 1967) has written extensively about these reflex control mechanisms. The complexity of these control systems and their interactions with the respiratory and other body systems make this a fascinating area of study. For example, sensory endings exist in the mucosa or lining of the larynx that respond to mechanical forces or air pressure changes within the tract. These nerve endings are capable of sending information to the central nervous system about the mechanical state of the lining of the respiratory tract. Furthermore, reflex endings exist within the joints of the various cartilages of the larynx that discharge when these joints are moved. These discharges have been shown to affect the ongoing electrical activity of some intrinsic laryngeal muscles (Wyke, 1967). Finally, the intrinsic laryngeal muscles contain specialized stretch receptors that discharge when the muscle is stretched or contracted (Wyke, 1969). The various levels of reflex mechanisms within the larynx suggest that elaborate precautions are in place to protect the airway and maintain life. From our perspective in voice pathology and its treatment, they are important to consider when trying to understand the physiology of normal and aberrant

Table 13.1. Branches of the Vagus (10th Cranial Nerve)

In the Jugular Fossa	
Meningeal	Serves dura mater in posterior fossa at the base of the skull
Auricular	Serves skin on back of outer ear (auricle) and posterior part of the external acoustic meatus
Pharyngeal	Joins with glossopharyngeal, sympathetic, and external laryngeal nerves to from pharyngeal plexus, which serve the muscles and membranes of the pharynx and muscles of the soft palate, with the exception of the tensor
In the Neck	
Superior laryngeal	
External	Supplies cricothyroid
Internal	Pierces the hypothyroid membrane to supply the mucous membrane of the larynx down to the true vocal folds
Recurrent	
Right side	Arises in front of the subclavian artery to travel upward along the trachea
Left side	Arises on the left side of the arch of the aorta
Both	Enters the larynx behind the articulation of the inferior cornu of the thyroid with the cricoid
	Serves all intrinsic muscles with the exception of the cricothyroid
Superior cardiac	Serves cardiac plexus
Inferior cardiac	Serves cardiac plexus
In the Thorax	
Anterior branchial	Sensory to the lung
Posterior bronchial	Sensory to the lung
Esophageal	Sensory to the esophagus
In the Abdomen	
Gastric	Sensory to the stomach
Celiac	Sensory to the pancreas, spleen, kidneys, suprarenal bodies, and intestine
Hepatic	Sensory to the liver

human phonation and laryngeal behavior. Wyke (1969) hypothesizes that some types of stuttering may be related to disorders of the various reflex mechanisms within the larynx.

SUMMARY

Proper control of the muscles of the larynx is critical in the production of voice. The levels of control within the central nervous system are multiple and complex. Lesions in some parts of the system, especially in the cortex and thalamus (and related structures) would be expected to have profound effects on speech and voice production. However, the fact that cortical and some subcortical controls are present bilaterally provides some measure of safety when lesions are unilateral. Indeed, cases have been reported wherein portions of the cerebral cortex were surgically removed with little lasting effect on speech and phonation. Lesions farther down in the brain might be expected to have a more singular effect on a specific muscle or set of muscles. However, innervation is still bilateral and redundant in some lower level brain areas, thus affording considerable protection of the systems involved in speech production. Once the nerves exit the skull, lesions of a nerve will have more specific effects involving, perhaps, a single muscle or small number of muscles bilaterally or unilaterally.

Chapter 14

Some Normative Data on the Voice

In this chapter, some normative data on the voice are presented. Our purpose is not to present all the available data, much of which is incomplete and confusing, but rather to provide the most meaningful data against which patient data may be compared clinically. The data reported here were gathered from a variety of sources, all of which are referenced for those seeking further information. An invaluable source for more complete data is the Baken and Orlikoff book, *Clinical Measurement of Speech and Voice* (Baken & Orlikoff, 2000). The sources of the data in the tables in this chapter are indicated by numbers in the body of the table, keyed to references below the table. The full citation for these sources appears in the reference list at the end of the book. Additional information about these measures and how they are obtained can be found in Chapter 8.

FUNDAMENTAL FREQUENCY

The measure of fundamental frequency, reflecting the vibratory rate of the vocal folds, is useful for comparing intrasubject and intersubject pitch levels. Fundamental frequency can be measured during production of sustained vowels or during a reading passage. Note, however, that fundamental frequency will vary depending on the type of speech material used. Considerable data are available on fundamental frequency, covering ages from birth to death. At many ages, however, fundamental frequency plateaus and may not change for many years. The data in Table 14.1 represent a summary of fundamental frequencies. Several studies have reported fundamental frequency at certain ages or within certain age ranges. The data in Table 14.1 represent the average of these studies. Table 14.2 presents summary data for untrained and trained speakers.

Fundamental Frequency Variation

The standard deviations of fundamental frequency, often referred to as the variability of fundamental frequency or pitch sigma, are also shown in Table 14.1. Variability is much smaller for sustained vowels than for reading passages. Fundamental frequency variability or lack thereof may be a physical measure that relates to the perception of voice monotone, a perceptual sign noted in some voice disorders.

Table 14.1. Fundamental Frequencies

Age Range	Mean F_0	Standard Deviation[a]	Range	Reference[b]
Males Reading				
7	294	2.2		1
8	297	2.0		1
10	270	2.4		1
11	227	1.5	192–268	2
14	242	3.4		1
19	117	2.1	85–155	3
Adult	132	3.3		4
20–29	120			5
30–39	112			5
40–49	107			5
50–59	118			5
60–69	112			5
70–79	132			5
80–89	146			5
Females Reading				
7	281	2.0		6
8	288	2.8		6
11	238	1.51	98–271	2
19	217	1.71	65–255	3
20–29	224	3.8	192–275	7
30–40	196	2.5	171–222	8
40–50	189	2.8	168–208	8
60–69	200	4.3	143–235	7
70+	202	4.7	170–249	7
80–94	200	2.7	183–225	9

[a] Standard deviation (SD) is expressed in semitones.
[b] Reference key:
1. Fairbanks, Wiley, & Lassman, 1949.
2. Horii, 1983.
3. Fitch & Holbrook, 1970.
4. Snidecor, 1943.
5. Hollien & Shipp, 1972; Shipp & Hollien, 1969.
6. Fairbanks, Herbert, & Hammond, 1949.
7. Stoicheff, 1981.
8. Saxman & Burk, 1967.
9. McGlone & Hollien, 1963.

Frequency Perturbation

Frequency perturbation or jitter refers to the variation of fundamental frequency present in all speakers to some degree and detected when the subject is attempting to produce a steady, sustained vowel. The frequency variations are the result of instability of the vocal folds during vibration. As such, perturbation reflects the biomechanical characteristics of the vocal folds, as well as variations of neuromuscular control. Normal speakers have a small amount of frequency perturbation, which may vary according to

Table 14.2. Mean Speaking Fundamental Frequencies for Various Age Groups

	20–35		40–55		65–85	
Age Groups	Mean	SD	Mean	SD	Mean	SD
Females						
Naive	192.00	2.00	195.00	3.40	175.00	2.40
Trained	217.00	3.60	205.00	4.10	201.00	5.20
Males						
Naive	118.00	2.60	100.00	2.60	127.00	3.10
Trained	131.00	3.10	126.00	3.90	125.00	4.00

age, physical condition, and in some cases, sex. These variables are included in Table 14.3, obtained from data reported by Casper (1983).

Maximum Phonational Range

Maximum phonational range refers to the range of frequencies, from lowest to highest, that an individual can produce. The intensity of the tone is usually not controlled, and the person may be asked to sustain the tone for approximately 1 second. Placing further demands on the production of the sound (i.e., production at a specific intensity or for a longer duration) may be expected to alter the magnitude of the range obtained. The data reported in Table 14.4 were obtained from many sources and represent the means of several studies. Note that there are no data for children.

Table 14.3. Frequency Perturbation Data

		Jitter Factor		Directional Perturbation Factor		Pitch Perturbation Quotient	
Age Range	Measure	/ee/	/oo/	/ee/	/oo/	/ee/	/oo/
Males							
20–29	Mean	0.78	0.72	70.73	69.48	0.65	0.57
	SD	0.4	0.36	11.25	14.87	0.3	0.26
40–49	Mean	0.99	0.87	74.37	72.49	0.77	0.7
	SD	0.61	0.51	10.86	14.84	0.38	0.32
60–69	Mean	0.91	0.87	67.77	69.43	0.77	0.74
	SD	0.63	0.56	15.46	14.55	0.5	0.43
Females							
20–29	Mean	0.55	0.56	46.3	47.83	0.56	0.57
	SD	0.41	0.41	19.67	19.68	0.39	0.37
40–49	Mean	0.63	0.61	53.06	51.67	0.65	0.61
	SD	0.4	0.42	16.57	19.76	0.41	0.4
60–69	Mean	0.66	0.7	49.91	48.88	0.65	0.69
	SD	0.52	0.59	19.1	18.64	0.49	0.56

Table 14.4. Maximum Phonational Range

Age Range	Low Frequency	High Frequency	Range	Reference[a]
		Males		
17–26	80	764	39.06	1
18–36	80	675	36.92	2
35–75	80	260	20.4	3
40–65	83	443	28.99	5
68–89	85	394	26.55	4
		Females		
18–38	140	1,122	36.03	2
66–93	134	571	25.09	4
35–70	136	803	30.75	5

[a] *Reference key:*
1. *Hollien and Jackson, 1973.*
2. *Hollien, Dew, and Phillips, 1971.*
3. *Canter, 1965.*
4. *Ptacek, Sander, Maloney, and Jackson, 1966.*
5. *Colton and Hollien, 1972.*

VOCAL INTENSITY

The intensity of phonation observed during speech is dependent on several factors. These include the intensity produced at the glottis, the shape of the vocal tract, the amount of lip opening, and the distance of the microphone from the lips of the speaker. Physical and emotional characteristics of the speaker also may affect vocal intensity. Thus, the data presented in Table 14.5 should be used with caution. They may be useful as an indicator of expected approximate intensity levels, but be sure to check the specific vowel/syllable used and the lip–microphone distance.

Amplitude Perturbation

During sustained vibration, the vocal folds exhibit slight variation of amplitude from one cycle to the next. This is called amplitude perturbation or shimmer. Normal speakers present a small amount of shimmer, which depends both on the vowel used and the sex of the person. Some typical shimmer values are shown in Table 14.6.

Maximum Intensity Level

Patients may vary considerably in their ability to produce loud tones. This may be a helpful diagnostic sign or a measure of change following treatment. Thus, measuring maximum intensity output may prove useful. Normal speakers usually can produce maximum outputs in excess of 110 dB; this is somewhat dependent on sex, age, the frequency at which the phonation is produced, and the measurement procedure. Table 14.7 presents a summary of maximum intensity levels for different ages and both sexes.

S/Z Ratio

The s/z ratio is a simple measure designed to examine the effect of pathological conditions on phonation. Although there is some variation among normal speakers, generally

Table 14.5. Vocal Intensity in Monosyllables and Reading Passage

Utterance Type	Loudness Level	N	Age	Mean dB	SD (dB)	Reference[a]
		Females				
/pa/						
	Soft	10	20–30	65.35	1.84	1
	Comfortable	10	20–30	70.44	1.88	1
	Loud	10	20–30	76.75	3.38	1
/pœ/						
	Soft	20	18–36	83.30[b]	3.20	2
	Comfortable	20	18–36	76.40	4.00	2
	Loud	20	18–36	71.50	4.90	2
Rainbow Passage			20–30	68.15		3
		Males				
/pa/						
	Soft	10	20–30	70.42	3.19	1
	Comfortable	10	20–30	74.69	3.08	1
	Loud	10	20–30	80.72	3.51	1
/pœ/						
	Soft	25	17–30	75.00	2.50	2
	Comfortable	25	17–30	79.50	3.30	2
	Loud	25	17–30	86.00	4.30	2
Rainbow Passage			20–30	70.42		3

[a] Reference key:
1. Stathopoulos and Sapienza, 1993. SPL was measured from a pressure transducer placed in a circumferentially exhausted face mask. Therefore, distance of the microphone to the lips of the speaker is estimated to be about 1 inch.
2. Holmberg, Hillman, and Perkell, 1988.
3. Ryan and Gelfer, 1993.
[b] Averaged over 15 syllable repetitions.

Table 14.6. Amplitude Perturbation Data

Vowel	Mean	SD
	Males	
/ah/	0.47	0.34
/ee/	0.37	0.28
/oo/	0.33	0.31
Mean	0.33	0.31
	Females	
/ah/	0.33	0.22
/ee/	0.23	0.08
/oo/	0.19	0.04
Mean	0.25	0.11

Table 14.7. Maximum Intensity Levels

Age	Mean	SD	Range	Reference[a]
		Males		
18–39	106	5.1	92–116	1
45–65	110	7.1	99–129	2
68–89	101	5.9	88–110	1
		Females		
18–38	106	3	99–112	1
40–70	101	18.2	93–115	2
66–93	99	4.5	90–104	1

[a] *Reference key:*
1. *Ptacek, Sander, Maloney, and Jackson, 1966.*
2. *Colton, Reed, Sagerman, and Chung, 1982.*

ratios greater than 1.4 are considered abnormal. Ratios around 1 are normal and expected for both children and adults of different ages (Table 14.8). The clinician is cautioned to use this measure as one of a battery of measures rather than as a single definitive measure. Numerous authors (Case, 1991; Hufnagle & Hufnagle, 1988; Mueller, Larson, & Summers, 1993; Sorensen & Parker, 1993) have raised concerns about the validity of the measure.

Maximum Phonation Duration

Maximum phonation duration is the maximum time a person can sustain a tone on one continuous expiratory breath. It supposedly is a measure of phonatory control and respiratory "support." As Kent, Kent, and Rosenbek (1987) have pointed out,

Table 14.8. S/Z Ratios

Age	Mean	Range	Reference[a]
	Males		
5	0.92	0.82–1.08	1
7	0.7	0.52–0.97	1
9	0.92	0.66–1.5	1
	Females		
5	0.83	0.50–1.14	1
7	0.78	0.51–1.10	1
9	0.91	0.75–1.26	1
Adults	0.99	0.41–2.67	2
Aged	0.76		3
	0.82		3

[a] *Reference key:*
1. *Tait, Michek, and Carpenter, 1980.*
2. *Eckel and Boone, 1981.*
3. *Young, Bless, McNeil, and Braun, 1983.*

Table 14.9. Maximum Phonation Duration

Group	Ages	Mean (sec)	SD
Males			
Young children	3–4	8.95	2.16
Children	5–12	17.74	4.14
Adults	13–65	25.89	7.41
Aged	65+	14.68	6.25
Females			
Young children	3–4	7.5	1.8
Children	5–12	14.97	3.87
Adults	13–65	21.34	5.66
Aged	65+	13.55	5.7

maximum phonation duration can be influenced by variables that have little to do with phonatory control. Important variables include age, sex, and, of course, the physical characteristics of the respiratory system. Table 14.9 presents a summary of the data reported on maximum phonation duration from many studies. This measure should be used with care because of uncertainty about its validity and stability on repeat trials (Kent, Kent, & Rosenbek, 1987).

AIRFLOW

Average Airflow Rates

Measurements of physiological parameters such as airflow and air pressure have some face validity in that vocal pathological conditions will affect their magnitude. Both airflow and air pressure are dependent on a number of factors, however, including respiratory drive, vocal fold valving, frequency, and intensity. Thus, the conditions under which these measurements are obtained must be understood and controlled to be properly interpreted.

Average airflow measures are shown in Table 14.10. Average airflow is reported in cubic centimeters per second or milliliters per second. Many researchers and clinicians have reported data on airflow for both normal speakers and those with vocal pathological conditions. Some of the data for normal-speaking subjects are reported in Table 14.10. There is some variation depending on the task the subject performs, and there is some suggestion that children have much smaller flows than adults. Females tend to have slightly lower flows than males.

Vibratory Airflow

Vibratory airflow refers to the variations of airflow during a cycle of vibration. Two major aspects of vibratory flow have been measured and are reported in Table 14.11. The first, AC flow, refers to the peak airflow during vibration. The second, minimum or DC flow, refers to any airflow that occurs when the vocal folds are supposedly closed. Both appear to be correlated with breathiness in the voice. AC flow varies both as a function of sex and of the intensity level at which the phonation is produced. Females have much lower AC flows than males, and there is a tendency for minimum or DC

Table 14.10. Average Flow Rates (mL/sec)

Age	Task	Mean	Range	N	Reference[a]
		Males			
7	/ah/	96	51–128	10	3
Adult	/ah/	119	96–141	5–36	1
	/ee/	144	89–136	30	4
	Reading	177	141–218	4	2
Adult	/pah/				
	Soft	130		10	5
	Comfortable	120		10	5
	Loud	140		10	5
		Females			
7	/ah/	72	45–115	10	3
Adult	/ah/	112	89–136	5–36	1
	/ee/	177		30	4
	Reading	191	152–170	4	2

[a] Reference key:
1. Based on data presented in Table 3.1 of Hirano, 1981a.
2. Horii and Cooke, 1978.
3. Beckett, Thoelke, and Cowan, 1971.
4. Woo, Colton, and Shangold, 1987.
5. Stathopoulos & Sapienza, 1993.

Table 14.11. Vibratory Airflows Based on Inverse Filtering of Oral Airflow Data (mL/sec)

Age Range	N	Condition[a]	AC Flow	DC Flow	Reference[b]
		Males			
17–30	25	Normal	260	120	1
	25	Soft	220	180	1
	25	Loud	490	110	1
21–30	8	Normal			2
20–31	10	Comfortable			3
69+	10	Comfortable			3
		Females			
17–30	20	Normal	140	90	1
	20	Soft	110	120	1
	20	Loud	180	90	1
21–30	8	Normal	189	75	2
20–31	10	Comfortable	140		3
69+	10	Comfortable	150		3

[a] Normal, soft, and loud refer to the loudness level at which the speakers were asked to produce the phonation.

[b] Reference key:
1. Holmberg, Hillman, and Perkell, 1988; tables AI–AVI.
2. Brodie, Colton, and Swisher, 1988.
3. Higgins and Saxman, 1993; phonation was a series of /bcep/s.

Table 14.12. Air Pressure Measurements Based on Intraoral Pressure
Estimates (cm H_2O)

Age Range	N	Condition[a]	Pressure[b]	SD	Reference[c]
		Males			
17–30	25	Normal	5.91		1
	25	Soft	4.79		1
	25	Loud	8.39		1
2–130	8	Normal	4.12	1	2
20–31	10	Comfortable	5.81	1.4	3
69+	10	Comfortable	7.99	2.73	3
		Females			
17–32	25	Normal	6.09		1
	25	Soft	4.79		1
	25	Loud	8.46		1
21–30	8	Normal	4.28	0.88	2
20–31	10	Comfortable	6.51	0.8	3
69+	10	Comfortable	6.35	1.71	3

[a] *Loudness level at which the phonation was produced. All used the indirect intraoral air pressure method for estimating lung pressure (Smitheran & Hixon, 1981).*
[b] *To convert cm H_2O for kPa, multiply cm H_2O by 10.197.*
[c] *Reference key:*
1. *Holmberg, Hillman, and Perkell, 1988.*
2. *Brodie, Colton, and Swisher, 1988.*
3. *Higgins and Saxman, 1993.*

flow to be lower for female speakers also. As intensity levels increase, so too does airflow.

Air Pressure

The amount of air pressure used in producing phonation will, in large measure, determine the intensity of the voice. In normal speakers, air pressure ranges between 4 and 5 cm H_2O for normal conversational or moderate level phonations (Table 14.12). Air pressure also affects the magnitude of airflow; thus, one must know at what pressures airflow measures have been collected. These data were derived from measurement of intraoral air pressure according to techniques described by Rothenberg (1968), Smitheran and Hixon (1981), and Rothenberg (1982). In some current literature, pressure is reported in kiloPascals (kPa). To convert pressure in cm H_2O to kPa, multiply by 10.197.

Maximum Flow Declination Rate (Closing Slope)

Maximum Flow Declination Rate (MFDR) or the closing slope of the inverse-filtered airflow waveform reflects the closing rate of the vocal folds. The faster the closing rate, the greater the amplitude in the higher frequencies. Thus, MFDR is related to vocal intensity production by the vocal folds and their spectrum. Table 14.13 presents some data from normal speakers at three intensity levels.

Table 14.13. Maximum Flow Declination Rates (or Closing Slope of the Inverse Filtered Airflow Waveform Pulse) for Normal Speakers

Syllable	N	Age	Mean	SD	Reference[a]
Males					
/pœ/					
Soft	25	17–30	171.1	71.30	1
Comfortable	25		279.6	90.40	1
Loud	25		481.1	162.60	1
/pa/					
Soft	10	20–30	218.43	100.03	2
Comfortable	10		367.78	130.20	2
Loud	10		573.16	186.22	2
Females					
/pœ/					
Soft	20	18–36	117.2	57.80	1
Comfortable	20		164.00	57.50	1
Loud	20		248.90	84.00	1
/pa/					
Soft	10	10–20	148.05	70.62	2
Comfortable	10		248.42	87.20	2
Loud	10		397.21	168.56	2

[a] Reference key:
1. Holmberg, Hillman, and Perkell, 1988.
2. Stathopoulos and Sapienza, 1993.

Forms Used in
Voice Evaluation:
Clinic and Laboratory

Syracuse Voice Center
SUNY Upstate Medical University
Department of Communication Sciences and Disorders

STANDARD PROTOCOL—FIBEROPTIC ASSESSMENT

Task	Purpose	Instructions to the Patient
1	Observe larynx at rest	Just sit quietly for a moment
2	Observe deep inspiration	I want you to take a deep breath, and release it. Then do it two more times.
3	Observe sustained vowel phonation at comfortable (modal) pitch (3 repetitions)	I'd like you to say /ee/ at a pitch that is comfortable for you and hold on to it for a few seconds. (Can be modeled). May be repeated using /oo/
4	Observe sustained vowel phonation at elevated (modal) pitch (3 repetitions)	Now I'd like you to do the same thing, hold on to that /ee/ but at a high pitch. (Can be modeled.) May be repeated using /oo/ Alternate instruction: If the patient does not elevate pitch, request the sound of a baby kitten, the squeal of a mouse, etc. It may be helpful to model these sounds.
5	Observe dynamics of pitch change	I want you to start with that high sound and let your voice glide down to a deep glissando. 3 repetitions. Now let's start at the bottom low note and let your voice glide upward, like this: model an upward glide (3 repetitions)
6	Observe speech	Please repeat each of these sentences twice. a. See the busy bees. b. We eat green beans. c. Do queens eat honey? d. Who hoots at the moon? e. Do you chew your food?
7	Observe non-phonatory behavior	I'd like you to whistle for me like this (model a few short interrupted bursts of whistle). Now I'd like you to whistle a little bit of Happy Birthday. If patient cannot whistle, a "pretend" whistle is acceptable.
8	Period of diagnostic therapy	The instructions to the patient will depend on the vocal maneuvers you wish to elicit. It is appropriate at this time to follow-up on any of the above activities if behaviors of interest were noted, or if you wish to make another attempt to teach a task. If a particular type of voice usage is of concern, for example, the high notes in singing or during lecturing, it is helpful to obtain a sample of that behavior.

Consensus Auditory-Perceptual Evaluation of Voice (CAPE-V)

Name:_____ **Date:**_____

The following parameters of voice quality will be rated on completion of the following tasks:

1. Sustained vowels/a/ and /i/ for 3-5 second duration each.
2. Sentence production:
   a. The blue spot is on the key again.
   b. How hard did he hit him?
   c. We were away a year ago.
   d. We eat eggs every Easter.
   e. My mama makes lemon muffins.
   f. Peter will keep at the peak.
3. Spontaneous speech in response to:"Tell me about your voice problem." or "Tell me how your voice is functioning."

> **Legend:** C = Consistent I = Intermittent
> MI = Mildly Deviant
> MO = Moderately Deviant
> SE = Severely Deviant

Overall Severity _____ C I ___/100
        MI   MO   SE

Roughness _____ C I ___/100
        MI   MO   SE

Breathiness _____ C I ___/100
        MI   MO   SE

Strain _____ C I ___/100
        MI   MO   SE

Pitch   Indicate nature of abnormality: _____

         _____ C I ___/100
        MI   MO   SE

Loudness Indicate nature of abnormality: _____

         _____ C I ___/100
        MI   MO   SE

         _____ C I ___/100
        MI   MO   SE

         _____ C I ___/100
        MI   MO   SE

COMMENTS ABOUT RESONANCE: NORMAL OTHER (Provide Description) _____

ADDITIONAL FEATURES (for example, diplophonia, fry, falsetto, asthenia, aphonia, pitch instability, tremor, wet/gurgly, or other relevant terms:

Clinician: _____

Voice Clinic Evaluation Results

Name [   ]   UCDMC # [   ]   Evaluation Date [   ]

Birthdate [   ]   Age [0]   Gender [   ]   Referring N [   ]

Diagnosis [   ]   Diagnosis Test [▼]

Onset
Quality [   ]   History [   ]

Fundamental Frequency Range [   ]   st.   Fundamental Freq. (Speaking) [   ] Hz [   ] (text)

Avg. Dur. [   ]   [   ] Hz   Fundamental Freq. (Reading) [   ] Hz [   ] (text)

Maximum Phonation Duration [   ]   sec. Fundamental Freq. (Counting) [   ] Hz
during vowel production   Vowel

Avg. Airflow Rate (sust. vowel) [   ] cc/sec   SPLV(dB) [0]   Duration [0] secs

Avg. Airflow Rate (not sust.) [0] cc/sec   SPLV(dB) [0]   Duration [0] secs

Syllable Repetition

                        Peak Airflow Rate [   ]   cc/sec
SPL(dB) [   ]   Glottal Resistance [   ]   dynes-sec/cm5
                       Subglottal Pressure [   ]   dynes/cm2

Other [   ]

VOICING VARIABILITY

	Rep 1	Rep 2	Rep 3	Rep 4	Rep 5
Hz					
Jitter (%)					
Shimmer (dB)					
N/H Ratio					

Pulmonary Function Screen [   ]

Pulmonary Screen Date [   ]

Impressions: [   ]

Summary: [   ]

Monitor screen showing Voice Evaluation Form used at University of California-Davis. Software program used is Microsoft Access. The program allows a user to set up a table with "fields" of data or text that are of interest. The user can also design forms and reports that will be "linked" to the table. The voice clinician adds data and narrative text in the evaluation form, shown above as it appears on the computer monitor. All information entered is then automatically stored in the table, which can be queried for clinical and research purposes. A report incorporating the information also can be generated.

UNIVERSITY OF CALIFORNIA, DAVIS

UC DAVIS MEDICAL CENTER
OTOLARYNGOLOGY AND DENTAL SERVICES
2521 STOCKTON BOULEVARD
SACRAMENTO, CALIFORNIA 95817

BERKELEY : DAVIS : IRVINE : LOS ANGELES : RIVERSIDE : SAN DIEGO : SAN FRANCISCO : SANTA BARBARA : SANTA CRUZ

VOICE DISORDERS CLINIC

Name: **Birthdate:**   10/13/1943   **UMC #:**   150 11 14   **Evaluation Date:**   6/10/2004

Diagnosis: left tvf paralysis, s/p fat injections   **Ref MD:**   M. Hambly, PCP

Brief History: Ms.   eturns for reevaluation. She reports fairly good voice over the past year, with occasional lapses in quality with greater use and seasonal allergy flare-ups. She is s/p bilateral fat injections to the tvfs in November of 2002. Previous history includes right tvf medialization with Gore-Tex implant and right arytenoid adduction due to right tvf paralysis following 4/99 cervical spine fusion.

Impressions:

Acoustic phonatory function measures, when compared to the 12/02 evaluation (one month post fat injections) suggest a decreased fundamental frequency range (at 12/02 exam, low pitch was abnormally so, and is today more normal), comparable ability to sustain sound, elevated but still low speaking fundamental frequency, and imrpoved form moderately to mildly elevated voicing variability values for jitter. Aerodynamic phonatory function measures suggest normal average airflow rates for sustained, unsustained sounds, and a syllable repetition task. Glottal resistance and subglottic pressure estimates were normal.

Laryngeal imaging with rigid endoscopy and stroboscopy reveals fixed R tvf mildly injected. L tvf is wnl in size, shape and color and moves well on abduction and adduction. On phonation, the L tvf moves to the midline and approximates the R fold, which is fixed in a near midline position. The impression is that closure is generally quite good, with occasionally a very tiny gap at the anterior commissure. IN stroboscopic mode, it is apparent that there is an asymmetry in vibratory displacement and mucosal wave characteristics from R to L (though amplitude of mucosal displacement is wnl).

Summary:

This patient is being followed in the ENT Clinic. Significant findings at this evaluation include evidence of generally good closure between the vocal folds for voicing, and phonatory function measures that are comparable and in some cases better than at last exam 12/02. Of particular interest, laryngeal function measures are wnl. Our impression is that dysphonia is primarily related, at this point, to asymmetry in vibratory characteristics of folds, rather than to excessive or early airloss. Pt. will return to see Dr. Belafsky in the fall. Conservative voice use/vocal hygiene measures are reviewed.

Rebecca Leonard, Ph.D.   Susan Goodrich, M.S.

Example of report generated by Voice Evaluation database program used at University of California-Davis. Page 1, shown here, includes narrative report.

Name:
UMC #:
Evaluation Date: 6/10/2004

Evaluation
Quality: moderately rough   Onset: 1999   Pulmonary Function Screen:

	Fundamental Frequency Range	Average Speaking Fundamental Frequency	Maximum Phonation Duration during vowel production	Airflow Mean (cc/sec.) vowel production	Airflow Peak (cc/sec.) syllable repetition	Glottal Resistance during syllable repetition (Ns/m5)	Subglottal Pressure during syllable repetition (dynes/cm2)	Voicing Variability Comfortable Io and Fo		
Normal Range	24-36 st	93-147 Hz (M) 185-282 Hz (F)	25-30 sec. (M) 15-25 sec. (F)	100-200		20-100 dy sec/cm5; low and comft. F o's	5-10dynes/cm2	< 1.0 Jitter (%) < 0.5 Shimmer (dB) < 0.2 N/H Ratio		

Evaluation Date

Evaluation Date	Fund. Freq. Range	Avg. Speaking	Max Phonation	Airflow Mean	Airflow Peak	Glottal Resistance	Subglottal	Voicing Variability		
6/10/2004	17.32 st. 132-369 Hz	146 Hz	8 sec.	190.00 at dB = 75 secs = 2.9	170.00 at 81 dB	26.26 at 81 dB	4.56 at 81 dB	1.96 % Jitter 0.29 dB Shimmer 0.26 N/H Ratio	Mean/5 repetitions at 251.8 Hz avg. intensity	
12/23/2002	22.06 st. 92-329 Hz	107 Hz	9 sec.	0.00 at dB = 0 secs = 0	at dB	at dB	at dB	3.04 % Jitter 0.32 dB Shimmer 0.12 N/H Ratio	Mean/5 repetitions at 251.2 Hz avg. intensity	
7/29/2002	33.36 st. 65-449 Hz	149.4 Hz	9 sec.	140.00 at dB = 78 secs = 2.4	22.00 at 72 dB	110.82 at 72 dB	7.28 at 72 dB	2.56 % Jitter 0.32 dB Shimmer 0.12 N/H Ratio	Mean/5 repetitions at 220.552 Hz avg. intensity	
1/24/2002	17.74 st. 131-365 Hz	148 Hz	12 sec.	226.00 at dB = 78 secs = 3.7	168.00 at 83 dB	58.33 at 83 dB	9.60 at 83 dB	2.24 % Jitter 0.24 dB Shimmer 0.12 N/H Ratio	Mean/5 repetitions at 268.6 Hz avg. intensity	

Page 2 of report includes a summary table of acoustic data, perceptual impressions, and laryngeal function studies (and pulmonary function if performed). Note that results from previous examinations are also included for easy comparison of treatment effects or changes over time. Report can be entered into patient's medical record and sent to referring professional.

Syracuse Voice Center
BoTox VOICE QUALITY RATING INVENTORY

Name: _____

Date of Injection _____   Date of Return of Symptoms: _____

Circle the number under each quality which best describes your voice.

Hoarse/Rough	1 = None	5 = Very hoarse
Breathy/Airiness	1 – None	5 = Very breathy
Choppy	1 = None	5 = Very choppy

	Hoarse/Rough					Breathy/Airy					Choppy				
Pre-Treatment	1	2	3	4	5	1	2	3	4	5	1	2	3	4	5
Post-Treatment															
Day 1	1	2	3	4	5	1	2	3	4	5	1	2	3	4	5
Day 3	1	2	3	4	5	1	2	3	4	5	1	2	3	4	5
Day 5	1	2	3	4	5	1	2	3	4	5	1	2	3	4	5
Day 7	1	2	3	4	5	1	2	3	4	5	1	2	3	4	5
Day 9	1	2	3	4	5	1	2	3	4	5	1	2	3	4	5
Day 11	1	2	3	4	5	1	2	3	4	5	1	2	3	4	5
Day13	1	2	3	4	5	1	2	3	4	5	1	2	3	4	5
Day 14	1	2	3	4	5	1	2	3	4	5	1	2	3	4	5
Week 3	1	2	3	4	5	1	2	3	4	5	1	2	3	4	5
Week 4	1	2	3	4	5	1	2	3	4	5	1	2	3	4	5
Week 5	1	2	3	4	5	1	2	3	4	5	1	2	3	4	5
Week 6	1	2	3	4	5	1	2	3	4	5	1	2	3	4	5
Week 7	1	2	3	4	5	1	2	3	4	5	1	2	3	4	5
Week 8	1	2	3	4	5	1	2	3	4	5	1	2	3	4	5
Month 3	1	2	3	4	5	1	2	3	4	5	1	2	3	4	5
Month 4	1	2	3	4	5	1	2	3	4	5	1	2	3	4	5
Month 5	1	2	3	4	5	1	2	3	4	5	1	2	3	4	5
Month 6	1	2	3	4	5	1	2	3	4	5	1	2	3	4	5
Month 7	1	2	3	4	5	1	2	3	4	5	1	2	3	4	5

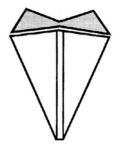

Syracuse Voice Center

Department of Otolaryngology & Communication Sciences

**GASTROESOPHAGEAL REFLUX OR
LARYNGOPHARYNGEAL REFLUX**

(GERD OR LPR)

What Is It?

In some people, stomach acids flow back into the esophagus and pharynx and can create various forms of irritation. Symptoms vary from individual to individual, with some people being very aware of them while others report little awareness. These symptoms <u>may</u> include the following: hoarseness, coughing, burning or soreness in the throat, frequent need to clear the throat, excess mucus, bad taste in the mouth, bad breath, sensation of lump in the throat, and others. Symptoms may occur during the day, or may be most pronounced in the morning or may happen at night. Nocturnal occurrences may present as a laryngeal spasm with momentary difficulty breathing and a burning sensation in the throat. This should not be confused with other forms of laryngeal spasm.

Is It Serious?

It is possible that left untreated, GERD can cause some serious complications, including coughing, bleeding in the esophagus, and difficulty swallowing. GERD has also been implicated etiologically with esophageal cancer and with laryngeal lesions. It also may produce an irritation in the larynx, resulting in hoarseness or difficulty with your voice.

What can you do about it?

The following instructions are things that you can do to obtain some relief from reflux. Your doctor should decide whether these changes will be sufficient or whether prescription strength medication (such as Zantac, Propulsid, Prilosec,

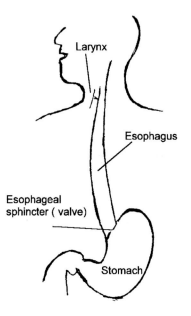

Prevacid, or similar medication) or other treatment is required. If you are given a prescription, you should take it about 30 minutes before your evening meal. If you should take the pill twice a day, take it before 30 minutes before breakfast and 30 minutes before dinner.

1. Take an over-the-counter antacid in liquid form (Gelusil, Maalox, or one of your choice) 30–40 minutes after meals and at bedtime. If symptoms are severe, take antacids every 1½–2 hours between meals. If your symptoms persist or you need to take

antacids very frequently, consult your physician concerning more appropriate treatment.

2. GERD is affected by body weight. If you are significantly overweight, loss of weight may reduce the symptoms.

3. Diet restrictions can help control the symptoms. Avoid the following, which tend to increase the acid in your stomach and also weaken the sphincter, allowing the acidic contents of your stomach to back up: coffee, tea, cola drinks (with and without caffeine); fatty foods, spicy foods, citrus fruits and tomatoes, onions, peppermint, chocolate, alcohol.

4. Chew your food thoroughly.

5. Eat smaller meals even if you have to eat more frequently.

6. Do not lie down right after eating. Do not eat for 2–4 hours before bedtime.

7. For nighttime relief, elevate the head of your bed 6–10 inches by placing blocks or bricks under the legs or by placing a wedge pillow under the mattress. Do not attempt to use additional pillows to raise your head. That will often increase abdominal pressure, making the reflux worse.

8. Avoid wearing tight-fitting clothing, particularly across the midsection of the body. Belts, girdles, and abdominal support-type belts should all be avoided.

9. Avoid bending or stooping. This includes activities such as gardening, exercises that require lifting or bending.

10.   Stress can aggravate the symptoms. Take steps to decrease stress.

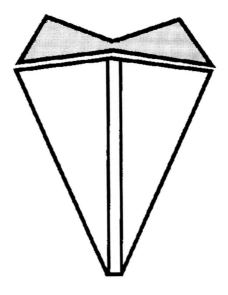

Syracuse Voice Center

SPASMODIC DYSPHONIA
(SD)

What is spasmodic dysphonia (often referred to as SD)?

It is generally believed that SD is a neurological problem—a movement disorder. It is one of the family of movement disorders called dystonias. Its effects on voice include voice stoppages, or a struggle to speak, or sudden interruption of voice along with hoarseness and voice strain. Not all people with SD will have all of these symptoms. Other dystonias may involve rapid uncontrollable blinking (blepharospasm) or other uncontrolled body movements.

How do you get it?

We do not know what causes SD. We know some things that DO NOT cause it, such as the way you use your voice, or an infection or other illness, or emotional trauma or stress. The symptoms may become worse in stressful situations, but that is true for many problems. There is no known hereditary factor.

Is there more than one type?

Yes. We usually talk about three types even though we are not completely certain that they are variations of the same problem.

Adductor spasmodic dysphonia: when the vocal folds close tightly and seem to go into spasm, interrupting the voice and making it difficult to talk.

Abductor spasmodic dysphonia: when the vocal folds suddenly open or fail to close as you are speaking so that no sound, or a very breathy sound, comes out, again interrupting the voice.

Mixed spasmodic dysphonia: both types of symptoms are noted

What is the treatment?

The most effective treatment we know at this time is injection of Botox (botulinum toxin) in extremely small amounts into the muscles that control the movement of the vocal folds. A trial of voice therapy may be indicated in very mild cases or when the diagnosis is not entirely certain. Also, a few sessions of voice therapy after the first Botox injection have been found to be helpful.

What does the Botox do?

The Botox acts to weaken the muscles into which it has been injected. This weakening then does not allow the vocal folds to either "overclose" or fail to close.

Does it cure the problem?

Unfortunately, we know of no cure for spasmodic dysphonia. However, the Botox injections alleviate the symptoms for up to 3 to 6 months on average. Then you return for the next injection. This process can continue over years and seems to be generally well tolerated.

How will I sound after the injection?

Immediately after the injection, you will not notice any change in your voice. However, over the course of the next day or 2 your voice may become soft and breathy (whispery) for a period of 7 to 10 days on average. During that period you may also need to be careful when you swallow—particularly liquids—to avoid choking a little. After that short time, you should have fairly good voice with a significant reduction of your original symptoms and no more difficulty swallowing. This period of good voice can last anywhere up to 3 to 6 months, sometimes less, sometimes more. When you notice your symptoms returning, you will need to schedule a re-injection appointment.

What are the side effects of the injection?

We mentioned that your voice would get weak and breathy and that you might choke a little when swallowing liquids. We do not know of any other side effects or long-term effects of the injections. The effect of the Botox wears off in time, as you can tell by the return of the symptoms. The Botox does not travel to or affect other parts of the body, according to current knowledge.

Where and how is the injection done?

The injection is given here at the Syracuse Voice Center as an outpatient procedure. We inject a little local anesthetic into the skin of the neck in the area of the larynx (voice box). Then, using a very thin needle, we inject the Botox into the muscles involved. We listen to and observe the activity of those muscles, using a special machine (EMG) that helps to guide us to the correct location for the injection. The entire procedure usually takes less than 5 minutes. You go home right after your treatment.

How are appointments for the injections scheduled?

When you begin to experience the return of symptoms that you find uncomfortable, please call our office to arrange an appointment for re-injection. You should not wait until the symptoms are as severe as they were originally. You may find that the appointment date you are given is several weeks away. There is a reason for that: Botox is a very expensive substance and it is very perishable. Each small bottle of Botox contains enough material to inject several people. Because it is perishable, once the bottle is opened, it must be used on that day. Whatever remains in the bottle must be discarded.

The cost to you is determined by dividing the cost of the toxin by the number of patients for whom it was used. In our attempt to keep your charges down, we group a number of patients for each Botox clinic date. We occasionally have had to change appointments when only one or two people have been scheduled so that the charge to those individuals would not be excessive. We make every effort to avoid doing that because we know the discomfort and disability involved for you when your symptoms return. Please talk to us about this if it creates a problem for you.

YOUR VOCAL HEALTH

SYRACUSE VOICE CENTER

Department of Otolaryngology & Communication Sciences

SUNY Health Science Center
Syracuse, New York

Your vocal mechanism is meant to last for your lifetime. Although it is built to do that, it cannot tolerate excess wear and tear. There are things you can do to take care of your voice.

If you have had surgery on your vocal folds, you were given instructions on how to use your voice in the immediate postsurgical period. The following suggestions apply for how you can care for your voice on a daily basis.

1. <u>Drink lots of water</u>. Your vocal folds need to be moist and the entire mechanism needs moisture to work efficiently. If you do a lot of talking or singing, always have water nearby and take frequent sips.

2. <u>Humidify the environment</u>. Make sure there is enough humidity in your environment. In your home you can use a humidifier. In old buildings with dry heat, the old method of setting out pots of water still works. Individual steam inhalers can be helpful.

3. <u>Control and limit vocal loudness</u>. Do not speak louder than the situation/environment demands. Avoid yelling, loud cheering, speaking over loud noises. Use new nonvocal methods to get attention of a group (e.g., clap your hands, blow a whistle, ring a bell, turn lights on and off). Use amplification in large or noisy places. Be aware of how you use your voice in talking over music, over the TV, communicating up and down stairs in the home, calling the dog, etc. Modify this as needed.

4. <u>Avoid excessive amounts of talking</u>. If you have to give a lecture, try to reduce voice use before and after. If you must talk a lot at work, try to reduce amount of talking outside of work. Listen more and talk less. If you will be performing in the evening, don't strain your voice during the day. Don't try to "out talk" others by increasing loudness.

5. <u>Eliminate habitual and frequent throat clearing.</u> We all must clear our throats on occasion but recognize that when you clear your throat you harshly "grind" the vocal folds together. Frequent "grinding" of that type can damage the vocal folds. It is not uncommon for people to get into the habit of clearing the throat without conscious awareness. You first need to become aware of it and then you can work on eliminating it. When you feel the need to clear your throat, try to sip some water first. If that is not effective, try to do a silent throat clearing by closing your mouth and saying the /h/ sound followed by a swallow. That sound should be silent because it is just air being blown between your vocal folds.

6. <u>Be careful about medications/drugs.</u> Decongestants and other drugs tend to release fluid from body tissues, including the vocal folds. If you must take such drugs for medical reasons, you need to try to counteract their drying effect by increasing your liquid intake. Check with your doctor about other drugs you might take that would not have such a drying effect. Do not take over-the-counter decongestants for long

periods. Alcohol is a drug and has a drying effect, as does caffeine.

7. <u>Smoking is a no-no!</u> Obviously, smoking of cigarettes or other substances is detrimental to the health of your entire respiratory system, including the upper airway. The only effective way to counter the effects of smoking is to eliminate it.

8. <u>Avoid or learn to manage stress.</u> Tension in the body affects the way the body functions. Excess tension in the larynx results in stressful voice production that can result in feelings of vocal fatigue or can actually result in swelling or damage of the vocal folds themselves.

9. <u>Give in to laryngitis.</u> When you have true laryngitis, that is, hoarseness associated with an upper respiratory infection or a laryngeal infection, the vocal folds become swollen and do not work properly. Do not try to override that or to force your voice. Use a very soft whisper or do not talk at all until the swelling resolves.

10. <u>Learn to use your voice correctly.</u> If you have frequent periods of hoarseness or feelings of vocal fatigue, you may not be using your voice properly. Appropriate voice therapy can be very effective. If you are a singer and have had no formal vocal training, it is important that you begin.

11. <u>Pay attention to how your voice sounds and feels.</u> Your voice has a unique sound that is recognized by your friends and family. If that sound changes, there is usually a reason. If the change lasts more than 5–7 days when you are otherwise well, you should see your doctor. Often it may be best to see an otolaryngologist (ear, nose, and throat doctor) who specializes in problems of the larynx.

12. <u>Symptoms of gastroesophageal reflux disease (GERD).</u> If you have sensations of heartburn, have a bad taste in your mouth, especially in the morning, have a rough voice in the morning, have greater than usual difficulty warming up your voice, have a burning sensation in your throat, etc., you may have gastroesophageal reflux disease. You should talk to your doctor about this condition and obtain appropriate treatment. GERD can have an effect on the health of your vocal folds.

Websites of Companies and Universities Mentioned in Book

Company/Institution	URL
Avaaz	http://www.avaaz.com/
F-J Electronics	http://www.f-jelectronics.dk
Glottal Enterprises	http://www.glottal.com/
GW Instruments	http://www.gwinst.com/html/frameset.html
Kay Elemetrics	http://www.kayelemetrics.com/homepage.html
Kelleher	http://www.kellehermedical.com/
Laryngograph	http://www.laryngograph.com/
Marantz	http://www.marantzpro.com/Products/PMD670.html
Pitch Intsruments	http://www.winpitch.com/
Praat	http://www.fon.hum.uva.nl/praat/
Sensimetrics	http://www.sens.com/Speechstation.htm
Visualization Software	http://www.visualizationsoftware.com/gram.html
VoceVista	http://www.vocevista.com/

Department of Otolaryngology & Communication Sciences
Upstate Medical University
Syracuse, NY 13210

Syracuse Voice Center

Stroboscopic Examination

Name of Patient _____   **Date** _____   **Tape No** _____

Chart Number: _____   **SS No.:** _____

Referring Physician _____   **DOB:** _____

History _____

_____

_____

_____

Type of Exam ▒: Rigid ▒: Flexible   Comments: _____

Exam Condition   ▒: Pre ▒: Post Treatment Number _____

Voice Measurements   Modal   High   Low   Loud

Fundamental   _____   _____   _____   _____   _____   _____
Frequency

SPL   _____   _____   _____   _____   _____   _____

Severity of	: Normal	: Mild	: Moderate	: Severe	: Aphonic
Dysphonia	(0)	(1,2,3)	(4,5,6)	(7,8,9)	(10)

Vocal Fold	Right	: Smooth (1)	: Slightly rough (2)	: Moderately rough (3)	: Extremely rough (4)
Edge	Left	: Smooth (1)	: Slightly rough (2)	: Moderately rough (3)	: Extremely rough (4)

Glottal Closure Pattern	:Complete (1)	:Anterior Chink (2)	:Posterior Chink (3)	:Hourglass (4)
	:Irregular (5)	:Bowed (6)	:Incomplete (7)	:Posterior V (8)

		Normal (1)	Increased (2)	Decreased (3)	Absent (4)
Amplitude	Right				
	Left				
Mucosal Wave	Right				
	Left				

Observations and Impressions _____

_____

_____

Diagnosis _____

Recommendations _____

Revised 1/12/2000

References

American Joint Committee for Cancer Staging and End Results Reporting (1983). Philadelphia: JB Lippincott.

Diseases of the nose, throat, ear, head and neck (1985). Philadelphia: Lea & Febiger.

Handbook of theories of aging (1999). New York: Springer.

Abitbol, J. M., & Abitbol, P. M. (2000). Surgical management of nonneoplastic vocal fold lesions: laser versus cold knife excision. *Current Opinion in Otolaryngology & Head & Neck Surgery, 8,* 514–523.

Abramson, A. L., Shikowitz, M. J., Mullooly, V. M., Steinberg, B. M., & Hyman, R. B. (1994). Variable light-dose effect on photodynamic therapy for laryngeal papillomas. *Archives of Otolaryngology & Head & Neck Surgery, 120,* 852–855.

Adametz, J., & O'Leary, J. L. (1959). Experimental mutism resulting from periaqueductal lesions in cats. *Neurology, 9,* 636–642.

Adran, G. M., Demp, F. H. l., & Marland, P. M. (1954). Laryngeal palsy. *British Journal of Radiology, 27,* 201–209.

Ahmed, A., & Tollefsbol, T. (2001). Telomeres and telomerase: basic science implications for aging. *Journal of the American Geriatric Society, 49,* 1105–1109.

Alberti, P. W. (1978). The diagnostic role of laryngeal stroboscopy. *Otolaryngology Clinics of North America, 11,* 347–354.

Alberts, B. (1999). *Molecular biology of the cell.* New York: Garland.

Allen, E. L., & Hollien, H. (1973). A laminagraphic study of pulse (vocal fry) register phonation. *Folia Phoniatrica et Logopedica, 25,* 241–250.

American Speech–Language Hearing Association (1992). Vocal tract visualization and imaging. *ASHA, 34,* 37–40.

American Speech–Language Hearing Association (1993). Preferred practice patterns for the professions of s–lp and audiologist: voice assessment. *ASHA, 11.*

Aminoff, M. J., Dedo, H. H., & Izdebski, K. (1978). Clinical aspects of spasmodic dysphonia. *Journal of Neurosurgery and Psychiatry, 41,* 461–365.

Ardran, G., Kinsbourne, M., & Rushworth, G. (1966). Dysphonia due to tremor. *Journal of Neurology, Neurosurgery and Psychiatry, 29,* 219–223.

Aring, C. D. (1965). Supranuclear (pseudobulbar) palsy. *Archives of Internal Medicine, 115,* 198–199.

Arnold, G. E. (1959). Spastic dysphonia I: changing interpretation of a persistent affliction. *Logos. 2,* 3–14.

Arnold, G. E. (1962). Vocal nodules and polyps: laryngeal tissue reaction to habitual hyperkinetic dysphonia. *Journal of Speech and Hearing Disorders, 27,* 205–217.

Arnold, G. E. (1980). Disorders of laryngeal function. In M. M. Paparella & D. Shumrick (Eds.), *Otolaryngology* (pp. 2470–2488). Philadelphia: WB Saunders.

Arnold, J. (1894). Myelocyste, Transposition von Gewebskeimen and Sympodie. *Beitr Pathol Anat Allg Pathol, 51,* 259–275.

Arnold, K. S., & Emanuel, F. W. (1979). Spectral noise levels and roughness severity ratings for vowels produced by male children. *Journal of Speech and Hearing Research, 22,* 613–626.

Aronson, A. E., (1973). Psychogenic voice disorders. Philadelphia: WB Saunders.

Aronson, A. E. (1980). *Clinical Voice Disorders: An Interdisciplinary Approach.* New York: Brian C. Decker.

Aronson, A. E. (1985). *Clinical voice disorders: an interdisciplinary approach.* New York: BC Decker.

Aronson, A. E. (1990). *Clinical voice disorders: an interdisciplinary approach.* (3rd ed.) New York: Thieme.

Aronson, A. E., Brown, J.R., Litin, E. M., & Pearson, J. S. (1968a). Spastic dysphonia. I. Voice, neurologic, and psychiatric aspects. *Journal of Speech and Hearing Disorders, 33,* 203–218.

Aronson, A. E., Brown, J. R., Litin, E. M., & Pearson, J. S. (1968b). Spastic dysphonia II. Comparison with essential (voice) tremor and other neurologic and psychogenic dysphonias. *Journal of Speech and Hearing Disorders, 33,* 219–231.

Aronson, A. E., & DeSanto, L. W. (1981). Adductor spastic dysphonia: 1½ years after recurrent laryngeal nerve resection. *Annals of Otology, Rhinology and Laryngology, 90,* 1–6.

Aronson, A. E., & DeSanto, L. W. (1983). Adductor spastic dysphonia: three years after recurrent laryngeal nerve resection. *Laryngoscope, 93,* 1–8.

Aronson, A. E., & Hartman, D. E. (1981). Adductor spastic dysphonia as a sign of essential (voice) tremor. *Journal of Speech and Hearing Disorders, 46,* 52–58.

Aronson, A. E., Peterson, H. W., & Litin, E. M. (1966). Psychiatric symptomatology in functional dysphonia and aphonia. *Journal of Speech and Hearing Disorders, 31,* 115–127.

Avidano, M. A., & Singleton, G. T. (1995). Adjuvant drug strategies in the treatment of recurrent respiratory papillomatosis. *Otolaryngol. Head Neck Surg., 112,* 197–202.

Baer, T. (1979). Vocal jitter: A neuromuscular explanation. In V.Lawrence (Ed.), *Transcripts of the Eighth Symposium: Care of the Professional Voice* (pp. 19–22). New York: The Voice Foundation.

Baer, T., Gore, J. C., Boyce, S., & Nye, P. W. (1987). Application of MRI to the analysis of speech production. *Magnetic Resonance Imaging, 5,* 1–7.

Baer, T., Gore, J. C., Gracco, L. C., & Nye, P. W. (1991). Analysis of vocal tract shape and dimensions using magnetic resonance imaging—vowels. *Journal of the Acoustical Society of America, 90,* 799–828.

Baer, T., Löfqvist, A., & McGarr, N. (1983). Laryngeal vibrations: A comparison between high-speed filming and glottographic techniques. *Journal of the Acoustical Society of America, 73,* 1304–1308.

Baken, R. J. (1987). *Clinical measurement of speech and voice.* San Diego: College Hill Press.

Baken, R. J., & Orlikoff, R. (2000). *Clinical measurement of speech and voice.* (2nd ed.) San Diego: Singular Publishing Group.

Baker, A. B. (1958), *An outline of clinical neurology.* Dubuque, IA: William Brown & Co.

Balazs, E., & Larsen, N. (2000). Hyaluronan: Aiming for perfect skin regeneration. Scarless wound healing. In H.Garg & M. Longaker (Eds.), *Scarless wound healing* (pp. 143–160). New York: Marcel Dekker Inc.

Balestrieri, F., & Watson, C. (1982). Intubation granuloma. *Otolaryngologic Clinics of North America, 15,* 567–579.

Ball, J., & Lloyd, J. (1971). Myasthenia gravis as hysteria or the sounds of silence. *Medical Journal of Australia, I,* 1018–1020.

Ballantyne, J. C., & Groves, J. (1978). *A synopsis of otolaryngology.* Bristol: John Wright and Sons Ltd.

Ballenger, J. J. (1985). Neurologic diseases of the larynx. In J. J. Ballenger (Ed.), *Diseases of the nose, throat, ear, head, and neck* (pp. 513–548). Philadelphia: Lea & Febiger.

Bamberger-Bozo, C. (1987). The Chiari II. In P. J. Vinken, G. W. Bruyn, H, L. Klawans, & N. C. Myrianthopoulos (Eds.), *Handbook of clinical neurology.* (pp. 403–412). Amsterdam: Elsevier.

Bannister, R., & Oppenheimer, D. R. (1972). Degenerative diseases of the nervous system associated with autonomic failure. *Brain, 95,* 457–474.

Barker, K. D., & Wilson, F. B. (1967). Comparative study of vocal utilization of children with hoarseness and normal voice. paper presented at the convention of the American Speech Language Hearing Association, Chicago, 1967.

Barlow, S. M., Netsell, R., & Hunker, C. J. (1986). Phonatory disorders associated with CNS lesions. In C. Cummings, J. Fredrickson, L. Harker, C. Krause, & D. Schuller (Eds), *Otolaryngology—head and neck surgery* (pp. 2087–2093). St. Louis: CV Mosby.

Barry, H. C., & Eathorne, S. W. (1994). Exercise and aging: issues for the practitioner. *Medical Clinics of North America, 78,* 357–376.

Basmajian, J. V. (1979). *Muscles alive: their functions revealed by electromyography.* Baltimore: Williams & Wilkins.

Bassich, C. J., & Ludlow, C. L. (1986). The use of perceptual methods by new clinicians for assessing voice quality. *Journal of Speech and Hearing Disorders, 51,* 125–133.

Bastian, R. W. (1985). Laryngeal biofeedback for voice modification. In V. Lawrence (Ed.), *Transcripts of the 14th symposium: care of the professional voice* (pp. 330–333), New York: Voice Foundation.

Bastian, R. W. (1986). Benign mucosal disorders, saccular disorders and neoplasms. In C. Cummings, J. Fredrickson, C. Krause, & D. Schuller (Eds.), *Otolaryngology—head and neck surgery* (pp. 1965–1987). St. Louis: Mosby.

Bastian, R. W. (1987). Laryngeal image feedback for voice disorder patients. *Journal of Voice, 1,* 279–282.

Beasley, D., & Davis, G. (1981). *Aging communication processes and disorders.* New York: Grune & Stratton.

Beckett, R. L., Thoelke, W., & Cowan, L. (1971). A normative study of air flow in children. *British Journal of Disorders of Communication, 6,* 13–17.

Beckman K. B., & Ames, B. N. (1988). Mitochondrial aging: open questions. *Annals of the New York Academy of Science, 854,* 118–127.

Behlau, M., & Pontes, P. (1990). *Principios de reabilitaçào vocal nas disfonias* (2nd ed.). Sao Paulo, Brazil: Paulista Publicaçòes Medicas.

Belafsky, P. C., Postma, G. N., Amin, M. R., & Koufman, J. A. (2002). Symptoms and findings of laryngopharyngeal reflux. *Ear Nose & Throat Journal, 81,* 10–13.

Benjamin, B. (1981). Frequency variability in the aged voice. *Journal of Gerontology, 36,* 722–726.

Benjamin, B. J. (1982). Phonological performance in gerontological speech. *Journal of Psycholinguistic Research, 11,* 159–167.

Benjamin, B. (1983). Chevalier Jackson Lecture. Congenital laryngeal webs. *Annals of Otology, Rhinology and Laryngology, 92,* 317–326.

Benjamin B. (1990). *Diagnostic laryngology: adults and children.* Philadelphia: Saunders.

Benjamin, B. J. (1997). Speech production of normally aging adults. *Seminars in Speech & Language, 18,* 135–141.

Benjamin, B., & Croxson, G. (1985). Vocal cord granulomas. *Annals of Otology, Rhinology and Laryngology, 94,* 538–541.

Benjamin, B., & Croxson, G. (1987). Vocal nodules in children. *Annals of Otology, Rhinology and Laryngology, 96,* 530–533.

Benjamin, B., & Mair, E. A. (1991). Congenital inter-arytenoid web. *Archives of Otolaryngology—Head and Neck Surgery, 117,* 1118–1122.

Benjamin, B. N., Gatenby, P. A., Kitchen, R., Harrison, H., & Cameron, K. (1988). Alpha-interferon (Wellferon) as an adjunct to standard surgical therapy in the management of recurrent respiratory papillomatosis. *Annals of Otology, Rhinology and Laryngology, 97,* 376–380.

Benjamin, B. N., Gray, S. D., & Bailey, C. M. (1993). Neonatal vocal cord paralysis. *Head and Neck, 15,* 169–172.

Benjamin, B., & Mair, E. A. (1991). Congenital inter-arytenoid web. *Archives of Otolaryngology—Head and Neck Surgery, 117,* 1118–1122.

Bennett, S. (1983). A 3-year longitudinal study of school-aged children's fundamental frequencies. *Journal of Speech Language and Hearing Research, 26,* 137–141.

Bennett, S., Bishop, S. G., & Lumpkin, S. M. (1989). Phonatory characteristics following surgical treatment of severe polypoid degeneration. *Laryngoscope, 99,* 525–532.

Benninger, M. S. (2000). Microdissection or microspot CO2 laser for limited vocal fold benign lesions: a prospective randomized trial. *Laryngoscope, 110,* 1–17.

Benninger, M. S., Ahuja, A. S., Gardner, G., & Grywalski, C. (1998). Assessing outcomes for dysphonic patients. *Journal of Voice, 12,* 540–550.

Benninger, M. S., Gardner, G., & Grywalski, C. (2001). Outcomes of botulinum toxin treatment for patients with spasmodic dysphonia. *Archives of Otolaryngology—Head and Neck Surgery, 127,* 1083–1085.

Benninger, M. S., Gillen, J. B., & Altman, J. S. (1998). Changing etiology of vocal fold immobility. *Laryngoscope, 108,* 1346–1350.

Berke, G. S., Blackwell, K. E., Gerratt, B. R., Verneil, A., Jackson, K. S., & Sercarz, J. A. (1999). Selective laryngeal adductor denervation-reinnervation: a new surgical treatment for adductor spasmodic dysphonia. *Annals of Otology, Rhinology, and Laryngology, 108,* 227–231.

Bernstein, L., & Berstein, R. S. (1985). *Interviewing, a guide for health professionals.* (4th ed.) Norwalk: Appleton-Century-Crofts.

Berry, R. J., Epstein, R., Fourcin, J., Freeman, M., & MacCurtain, F. (1982). An objective analysis of voice disorder: Part one. *British Journal of Disorders of Communication, 17,* 67–76.

Berry, R. L., Epstein, R., Freeman, M., MacCurtain, F., & Noscoe, N. (1982). An objective analysis of voice disorders: part two. *British Journal of Disorders of Communication, 17,* 77–85.

Berry, D. A., Montequin, D. W., & Tayama, N. (2001). High-speed digital imaging of the medial surface of the vocal folds. *Journal of the Acoustical Society of America, 110,* 2539–2547.

Berry, D. A., Verdolini, K., Montequin, D. W., Hess, M. M., Chan, R. W., & Titze, I. R. (2001). A quantitative output-cost ratio in voice production. *Journal of Speech, Language, and Hearing Research, 44,* 29–37.

Bever Jr, C. T. (1999). Multiple sclerosis: symptomatic treatment. *Current Treatment Options in Neurology, 1,* 221–238.

Bielekova, B., & Martin, R. (1999). Multiple sclerosis: immunotherapy. *Current Treatment Options in Neurology, 1,* 201–220.

Biever, D. M., & Bless, D. M. (1988). Posterior glottal gap in normal young adult and geriatric women. Unpublished manuscript.

Biever, D. M., & Bless, D. M. (1989). Vibratory characteristics of the vocal folds in young adult and geriatric women. *Journal of Voice, 3,* 120–131.

Bless, D. M., & Brandenburg, J. H. (1983). Stroboscopic evaluation of "functional" voice disorders. Paper presented at the middle section of the Triologic Society, Madison, WI.

Bless, D. M., Hirano, M., & Feder, R. (1987). Videostroboscopic evaluation of the larynx. *Ear, Nose, and Throat Journal, 66,* 289–296.

Bless, D. M., & Hicks, D. M. (1996). Diagnosis and measurement: assessing the who. In W. S. Brown, Jr., B. P. Vinson, & M. A. Crary (Eds.), *Organic voice disorders assessment and treatment* (pp. 119–171). San Diego: Singular Publishing Group, Inc.

Bless, D. M., Miller, J. (1972). Influence of mechanical and linguistic factors on lung volume effects during speech. Paper presented at the convention of the American Speech-Language-Hearing Association, San Francisco.

Bless, D. M., & Swift, E. (1995). Paradoxical vocal cord dysfunction: episodic laryngeal dyskinesia; one disorder, multiple causes? Paper presented at the convention of the American-Speech-Language-Hearing Association, Orlando, FL.

Bless, D., & Hirano, M. (1982). Verbal instructions: A critical variable in obtaining optimal performance for maximum phonation time. Paper presented at the convention of the American Speech Language Hearing Association, Toronto, Canada.

Bless, D., Hunker, C., & Weismer, G. (1981). Comparison of noninvasive methods to obtain chest-wall displacement and aerodynamic measures during speech. In V. Lawrence (Ed.), *Transcripts of the Tenth Symposium: Care of the Professional Voice* (pp. 43–51). New York: Voice Foundation.

Blitzer, A., & Brin, M. F. (1991). Laryngeal dystonia: a series with botulinum toxin therapy. *Annals of Otology, Rhinology and Laryngology, 100,* 85–89.

Blitzer, A., & Brin, M. F. (1992). The dystonic larynx. *Journal of Voice, 6*, 294–297.

Blitzer, A., Brin, M. F., Fahn, S., & Lovelace, R. E. (1988). Clinical and laboratory characteristics of focal laryngeal dystonia: study of 110 cases. *Laryngoscope, 98*, 636–640.

Blitzer, A., Brin, M. F., Stewart, C., Aviv, J. E., & Fahn, S. (1992). Abductor laryngeal dystonia: a series treated with botulinum toxin. *Laryngoscope, 102*, 163–167.

Blitzer, A., Lovelace, R. E., Brin, M. F., Fahn, S., & Fink, M. E. (1985). Electromyographic findings in focal laryngeal dystonia (spastic dysphonia). *Annals of Otology, Rhynology and Laryngology, 94*, 591–594.

Blitzer, A., & Sulica, L. (2001). Botulinum toxin: basic science and clinical uses in otolaryngology. *Laryngoscope, 111*, 218–226.

Block, P. (1965). Neuro-psychiatric aspects of spastic dysphonia. *Folia Phoniatrica, 17*, 301–364.

Bloch, I., & Behrman, A. (2001). Quantitative analysis of videostroboscopic images in presbylaryn-ges. *Laryngoscope, 111*, 2022–2027.

Blum, R. H. (1960). *The management of the doctor-patient relationship*. New York: McGraw-Hill.

Boone, D. R. (1977). *The voice and voice therapy*. (2nd ed.) Englewood Cliffs: Prentice Hall.

Boone, D. R. (1983). *The voice and voice therapy*. (3rd ed.) Englewood Cliffs N.J.: Prentice Hall Inc.

Boone, D. R. (1987). *Human communication and its disorders*. Englewood Cliffs: Prentice Hall.

Boone, D. R., & McFarlane, S. C. (1988). *The voice and voice therapy* (4th ed). Englewood Cliffs, NJ: Prentice-Hall.

Borden, G. J., Baer, T., & Kenney, M. K. (1985). Onset of voice in stuttered and fluent utterances. *Journal of Speech and Hearing Research, 28*, 363–372.

Botez, M. I., & Barbeau, A. (1971). Role of subcortical structures and particulary of the thalamus in the mechanisms of speech and language. *International Journal of Neurology, 8*, 300–320.

Bouchayer, M., & Cornut, G. (1984). Les vergetures des cordes vocales. *Revue de Laryngologie Otologie Rhinologie, 105*, 421–423.

Bouchayer, M., Cornut, G., Witzig, E., Loire, R., Roch, J., & Bastian R. (1985). Epidermoid cysts, sulci and mucosal bridges of the true vocal cord: A report of 157 cases. *Laryngoscope, 95*, 1087–1094.

Boukamp, P. (2001). Aging mechanisms: the role of telomere loss. *Clinical and Experimental Dermatology, 26*, 562–565.

Boutsen, F., Cannito, M. P., Taylor, M., & Bender, B. (2002). Botox treatment in adductor spasmodic dysphonia: a meta-analysis. *Journal of Speech, Language and Hearing Research, 45*, 469–481.

Bowling, A. C., & Stewart, T. M. (2003). Current complementary and alternative therapies for multiple sclerosis. *Current Treatment Options in Neurology, 5*, 55–68.

Bozymski, E. M. (1993). Pathophysiology and diagnosis of gastroesophageal reflux disease. *American Journal of Hospital Pharmacy, 50*, 456.

Bradley, R. M. (2000). Sensory receptors of the larynx. *American Journal of Medicine, 108 Suppl 4a*, 47S–50S.

Bralley, R. C., Bull, J. L., Gore, C. H., & Edgerton, M. T. (1978). Evaluation of vocal pitch in male transsexuals. *Journal of Communication Disorders, 11*, 443–449.

Brandt, J. F., Ruder, K. F., & Shipp, T. (1969). Vocal loudness and effort in continuous speech. *Journal of the Acoustical Society of America, 46*, 1543–1548.

Brantigan, C. O., Brantigam, T. A., & Joseph, N. (1982). Effects of beta blockade and beta stimulation on stage fright. *American Journal of Medicine, 72*, 88–94.

Brewer, D. W. (1975). Early diagnostic signs and symptoms of laryngeal disease. *Laryngoscope, 85*, 499–515.

Brewer, D. W., Casper, J. K., Gould, L. V., Colton, R. H., & Conture, E. G. (1983). Team evaluation of patients with voice problems. In V. Lawrence (Ed.), *Transcripts of the Twelfth Symposium: Care of the Professional Voice* (pp. 270–272). New York: Voice Foundation.

Brewer, D. W., & Gould, L. V. (1974). Pyriform sinus: functional visualization. *Annals of Otology, Rhinology and Laryngology, 83*, 720–724.

Brewer, D. W., & McCall, G. N. (1974). Visible laryngeal changes during voice therapy. *Annals of Otology, Rhinology and Laryngology, 83*, 423–427.

Brewer, D. W., Woo, P., Casper, J. K., & Colton, R. H. (1991). Unilateral recurrent laryngeal nerve paralysis: a re-examination. *Journal of Voice, 5*, 178–185.

Briant, T. D. R., Blair, R. L., Cole, P., & Singer, L. (1983). Laboratory investigation of abnormal voice. *Journal of Otolaryngology, 12*, 285–290.

Briggaman, R. A., & Wheeler, C. E., Jr. (1975). Epidermolysis bullosa dystrophica-recessive: a possible role of anchoring fibrils in the pathogenesis. *Journal of Investigative Dermatology, 65*, 203–211.

Brin, M. F., Blitzer, A., & Stewart, C. (1998). Laryngeal dystonia (spasmodic dysphonia): observations of 901 patients and treatment with botulinum toxin. *Advances in Neurology, 78*, 237–252.

Brin, M. F., Fahn, S., Blitzer, A., Ramig, L. O., & Stewart, C. (1992). Movement disorders of the larynx. In A. Blitzer, M. F. Brin, C. T. Sasaki, S. Fahn, & K. S. Harris (Eds.), *Neurologic disorders of the larynx* (pp. 248–278). New York: Thieme.

Brin, M. F., Velickovic, M., Ramig, L. O., & Fox, C. (2004). Dysphonia due to Parkinson's disease: pharmacological, surgical and behavioral management perspectives. In C. Sapienza & J. Casper (Eds.), *For clinicians by clinicians: vocal rehabilitation in medical speech-language pathology*, Austin, TX: Pro-Ed.

Broad, D. J. (1973). Phonation. In F. D. Minifie, T. J. Hixon, & W. Williams (Eds.), *Normal aspects of speech, hearing and language* (pp. 127–167). Englewood Cliffs, NJ: Prentice-Hall.

Brodie, K., Colton, R. H., & Swisher, L. (1988). Reliability of Inverse filtered and EGG measurements of vocal function. *unpublished manuscript*.

Brodnitz, F. (1976). Spastic dysphonia. *Annals of Otolaryngology, 85*, 210–214.

Brooks, S. L. (1993). Computed tomography. *Dental Clinics of North America, 37*, 575–590.

Brown, J. E., & Simonson, J. (1963). Organic voice tremor. *Neurology, 13*, 520–525.

Brown, J. R., Darley, F. L., & Aronson, A. E. (1970). Ataxic dysarthria. *International Journal of Neurology, 7*, 302–318.

Brown, W. S., Jr., & Brandt, J. F. (1971). Effects of auditory masking on vocal intensity and intraoral air pressure during sentence production. *Journal of the Acoustical Society of America, 49*, 1903–1905.

Brown, W. S., Jr., & Brandt, J. (1972). The effect of masking on vocal intensity during vocal and whispered speech. *Journal of Auditory Research, 12*, 157–161.

Brown, W. S., Jr., & Feinstein, S. H. (1977). Speaker sex identification utilizing a constant laryngeal source. *Folia Phoniatrica et Logopedica, 29*, 240–248.

Brown, W. S., Jr., Hunt, E., & Williams, W. N. (1988). Physiological differences between the trained and untrained speaking and singing voice. *Journal of Voice, 2*, 102–110.

Brown, W. S., Jr., & McGlone, R. E. (1969). Relation of intraoral air pressure to oral cavity size. *Folia Phoniatrica, 21*, 321–331.

Brown, W. S., Jr., & McGlone, R. E. (1969). Constancy of intraoral air pressure. *Folia Phoniatrica, 21*, 332–339.

Brown, W. S., Jr., & McGlone, R. E. (1974). Aerodynamic and acoustic study of stress in sentence production. *Journal of the Acoustical Society of America, 56*, 971–974.

Brown, W. S., Jr., & McGlone, R. E. (1974). Letter: Further observations of intraoral pressures during sentence production. *Journal of the Acoustical Society of America, 56*, 1916–1918.

Brown, W. S., Jr., McGlone, R. E., & Proffit, W. R. (1973). Relationship of lingual and intraoral air pressures during syllable production. *Journal of Speech & Hearing Research, 16*, 141–151.

Brown, W. S., Jr., Morris, R. J., DeGroot, T., & Murry, T. (1998). Reliability of single sample experimental designs: comfortable effort level. *Journal of Voice, 12*, 453–459.

Brown, W. S., Jr., Morris, R. J., Hicks, D. M., & Howell, E. (1993). Phonational profiles of female professional singers and nonsingers. *Journal of Voice, 7*, 219–226.

Brown, W. S., Jr., Morris, R. J., Hollien, H., & Howell, E. (1991). Speaking fundamental frequency characteristics as a function of age and professional singing. *Journal of Voice, 5*, 310–315.

Brown, W. S., Jr., Morris, R., & Michel, J. (1989). Vocal jitter in young adult and aged female voices. *Journal of Voice, 3*, 113–119.

Brown, W. S. Jr., Morris, R. J., & Murry, T. (1996). Comfortable effort level revisited. *Journal of Voice, 10*, 299–305.

Brown, W. S., Jr., Rothman, H. B., & Sapienza, C. M. (2000). Perceptual and acoustic study of professionally trained versus untrained voices. *Journal of Voice, 14*, 301–309.

Brown, W. S., Jr., & Shearer, W. M. (1970). Constancy of intraoral air pressure related to integrated pressure-time measures. *Folia Phoniatrica, 22*, 49–57.

Brown, W. S., Jr., Vinson, B. P., & Crary, M. A. (1996). *Organic voice disorders assessment and treatment*. San Diego: Singular Publishing Group, Inc.

Browne, K., & Freeling, P. (1976). *The Doctor-patient relationship*. (2nd ed.) New York: Churchill-Livingstone.

Bryant, N. J., Gracco, L. C., Sasaki, C. T., & Vining, E. (1996). MRI evaluation of vocal fold paralysis before and after type I thyroplasty. *Laryngoscope, 106*, 1386–1392.

Burch, P. R. (1981). Passive smoking and lung cancer. *British Medical Journal, 282*, 1393.

Butler, J. E., Hammond, T. H., & Gray, S. D. (2001). Gender-related differences of hyaluronic acid distribution in the human vocal fold. *Laryngoscope, 111*, 907–911.

Butler, J. P., & Mohler, J. G. (1979). Estimating a distribution's central moments: a specific tidal ventilation application. *Journal of Applied Physiology: Respiratory, Environmental and Exercise Physiology, 46*, 47–52.

Cadenas, E., & Davies, K. J. (2000). Mitochondrial free radical generation, oxidative stress, and aging. *Free Radical & Biology Medicine, 29*, 222–230.

Campisi, P., Tewfik, T. L., Pelland-Blais, E., Husein, M., & Sadeghi, N. (2000). MultiDimensional Voice Program analysis in children with vocal cord nodules. *Journal of Otolaryngology, 29*, 302–308.

Canter, G. J. (1963). Speech characteristics of patients with Parkinson's disease. I. Intensity, pitch and duration. *Journal of Speech and Hearing Disorders, 28*, 221–229.

Canter, G. J. (1965). Speech characteristics of patients with Parkinson's disease. II: Physiological support for speech. *Journal of Speech and Hearing Disorders, 30,* 44–49.

Carpenter, R. J., McDonald, T. J., & Howard, F. M. (1979). The otolaryngologic presentation of myasthenia gravis. *Laryngoscope, 89,* 922–928.

Carpenter, R. J., McDonald, T. J., & Howard, F. M. (1988). The otolaryngologic presentation of amyotrophic lateral sclerosis. *Otolaryngology, 86,* 479–484.

Carrow, E., Mauldin, M., & Shamblin, L. (1974). Deviant speech characteristics in motor neuron disease. *Archives of Otolaryngology, 100,* 212–218.

Caruso, A., & Burton, E. K. (1987). Temporal acoustic measures of dysarthria associated with amyotrophic lateral sclerosis. *Journal of Speech and Hearing Research, 30,* 80–87.

Case, J. L. (1984). *Clinical management of voice disorders.* Rockville, MD: Aspen Systems.

Case, J. L. (1991). *Clinical management of voice disorders.* (2nd ed.) Austin: Pro-ed.

Casper, J. K. (1983). *Frequency perturbation in normal speakers: a descriptive and methodological study.* Syracuse University.

Casper, J. K. (1993). Objective methods for the evaluation of vocal function. In J. Stemple (Ed.), *Voice therapy: clinical methods* (pp. 39–45). St. Louis: Mosby Yearbook.

Casper, J. K. (2001). Vocal fold paralysis, paresis and Immobility. In M. Fawcus & M. Freeman (Eds.), *Voice disorders and their management* (pp. 192–218). Whurr Publishers.

Casper, J. K. (2004). Vocal hygiene. In R. D. Kent (Ed.), *MIT encyclopedia of communication disorders,* Cambridge, MA: MIT Press.

Casper, J. K., Brewer, D. W., & Colton, R. H. (1987b). Pitfalls and problems in flexible fiberoptic videolaryngoscopy. *Journal of Voice, 1,* 347–352.

Casper, J. K., Brewer, D. W., & Colton, R. H. (1987). Variations in normal human laryngeal anatomy and physiology as viewed fiberscopically. *Journal of Voice, 1,* 180–185.

Casper, J. K., Brewer, D. W., & Conture, E. G. (1981). Speech therapy patient evaluation techniques with the fiberscope. In V. Lawrence (Ed.), *Transcripts of the Tenth Symposium: Care of the Professional Voice* (pp. 136–140). New York: The Voice Foundation.

Casper, J. K., C, Clark, W. R., Kelley, R., & Colton, R. H. (2002). Laryngeal and phonatory status after burn/inhalation injury: a long term follow-up study. *Journal of Burn Care & Rehabilitation, 23,* 235–243.

Casper, J. K., & Colton, R. H. (1992). *Clinical manual for laryngectomy and head and neck cancer rehabilitation.* San Diego: Singular Publishing Group.

Casper, J. K., & Colton, R. H. (2000). Current understanding and treatment of phonatory disorders in geriatric populations. *Current Opinion in Otolaryngology—Head and Neck Surgery, 8,* 158–164.

Casper, J. K., Colton, R. H., & Brewer, D. W. (1985). Selected therapy techniques and laryngeal physiological changes in patients with vocal fold immobility. In V. Lawrence (Ed.), *Transcripts of the Fourteenth Symposium: Care of the Professional Voice* (pp. 318–323). New York N.Y.: The Voice Foundation.

Casper, J. K., Colton, R. H., Brewer, D. W., Kelley, R., Woo, P., & Griffin, B. (1995). Nodular diversity. Paper presented at the 24th Symposium: Care of the Professional Voice, June 1995, Philadelphia, PA.

Casper, J. K., Colton, R. H., Brewer, D. W., & Woo, P. (1989). Investigation of selected voice therapy techniques. paper presented at the Eighteenth Symposium: Care of the Professional Voice, Philadelphia, PA.

Casper, J. K., Colton, R. H., Woo, P., & Brewer, D. W. (1990). Investigation of selected voice therapy techniques in a patient population. Paper presented at the Nineteenth Symposium: Care of the Professional Voice, Philadelphia, PA.

Casper, J. K., Colton, R. H., Woo, P., & Brewer, D. W. (1992). Efficacy of treatment for the post-surgically dysphonic patient. Unpublished manuscript.

Casper, J. K., Colton, R. H., Woo, P., & Brewer, D. (1992). Physiological characteristics of selected voice therapy techniques: a preliminary research note. *Voice, 1,* 131–141.

Cassisi, N. J., Sapienza, C., & Vinson, B. P. (1996). Malignant lesions of the larynx. In W. S. Brown, Jr., B. P. Vinson, & M. A.. Crary (Eds.), *Organic voice disorders assessment and treatment* (pp. 279–300). San Diego: Singular Publishing Group, Inc.

Catten, M., Gray, S. D., Hammond, T. H., Zhou, R., & Hammond, E. (1998). Analysis of cellular location and concentration in vocal fold lamina propria. *Otolaryngology—Head and Neck Surgery, 118,* 663–667.

Chagnon, F., & Stone, R. E. (1996). Nodules and Polyps. In W. S. Brown, Jr., B. P. Vinson, & M. A. Crary (Eds.), *Organic voice disorders assessment and treatment* (pp. 219–244). San Diego: Singular Publishing Group, Inc.

Chan, R. W., & Titze, I. R. (1999). Hyaluronic acid (with fibronectin) as a bioimplant for the vocal fold mucosa. In I. R. Titze (Ed.), *NCVS Status and Progress Report* (pp. 53–62). Iowa City: National Center for Voice and Speech.

Chan, R. W., Gray, S. D., & Titze, I. R. (2001). The importance of hyaluronic acid in vocal fold biomechanics. *Otolaryngology—Head and Neck Surgery, 124,* 607–614.

Cherry, J., & Margulies, S. I. (1968). Contact ulcer of the larynx. *Laryngoscope, 73*, 1937–1940.

Chevrie-Muller, C., Arabia-Guidet, C., & Pfauwadel, M. (1987). Can one recover from spasmodic dysphonia? *British Journal of Disorders of Communication, 22*, 117–128.

Cheyne, H. A., Nuss, R. C., & Hillman, R. E. (1999). Electroglottography in the pediatric population. *Archives of Otolaryngology—Head and Neck Surgery, 125*, 1105–1108.

Chiari, J. (1986). Über Veränderungen des Kleinhirns, des Pons aund Medulla oblongata in Folge von Kongenitaler Hydrocephalie des Grosshirns. *Dtsch Akad Wiss Wien, 63*, 71–116.

Childers, D. G., Alsaka, Y. A., Hicks, D. M., & Moore, G. P. (1986). Vocal fold vibrations in dysphonia: model vs measurement. *Journal of Phonetics, 14*, 429–434.

Childers, D. G., Alsaka, Y. A., Hicks, D. M., & Moore, G. P. (1987). Vocal fold vibrations: an EGG model. In T. Baer, C. Sasaki, & K. S. Harris (Eds.), *Laryngeal function in phonation and respiration* (pp. 181–202). Boston: Little Brown & Co.

Childers, D. G., Hicks, D. M., Moore, G. P., & Alsaka, Y. A. (1986). A model for vocal fold vibratory motion, contact area, and the electroglottogram. *Journal of the Acoustical Society of America, 80*, 1309–1320.

Childers, D. G., & Krishnamurthy, A. K. (1985). A critical review of electroglottography. *Critical Reviews in Biomedical Engineering, 12*.

Childers, D. G., Krishnamurthy, A. K., Naik, J. M., Larar, J. N., & Moore, G. P. (1983). Assessment of laryngeal function by simultaneous measurement of speech, electroglottography and ultra-high speed film. *Folia Phoniatrica et Logopedica, 35*, 116A.

Childers, D. G., Naik, J. M., Larar, J. N., Krishnamurthy, A. K., & Moore, G. P. (1983). Electroglottography, speech, and ultra-high speed cinematography. In I. R. Titze & R. C. Scherer (Eds.), *Vocal fold physiology: biomechanics, acoustics and phonatory control* (pp. 202–220). Denver: Denver Center for the Performing Arts.

Chipman, S. F., & Carey, S. (1975). Anatomy of a stimulus domain: The relation between multidimensional and unidimensional scaling of noise bands. *Perceptual and Motor Skills, 17*, 417–424.

Chisnall, B. (1977). Increase in house fires. *Fire Protection, 4*, 119–121.

Chodosh, P. L. (1977). Gastro-esophagealpharyngeal reflux. *Laryngoscope, 87*, 1418–1427.

Chollet, G., & Kahane, J. C. (1979). Laryngeal patterns of consonant productions in sentences observed with an impedance glottograph. In H. Hollien (Ed.), *Current Issues in the Phonetic Sciences* (pp. 119–128). Amsterdam: Netherlands: John Benjamins B. V.

Cisler, J. (1927). Sur les troubles du language article et de la phonation au cours de l'encephalite epidemique. *Archives of International Laryngology, 33*, 1054–1057.

Close, L. G., Catlin, F. I., & Cohn, A. M. (1980). Acute and chronic effects of ammonia burns on the respiratory tract. *Archives of Otolaryngology, 106*, 151–158.

Cohen, S. R. (1985). Congenital glottic webs in children: a retrospective review of 51 patients. *Annals of Otology, Rhinology and Laryngology, Supplement, 121*, 2–16.

Cohen, J. T., Bach, K. K., Postma, G. N., & Koufman, J. A. (2002). Clinical manifestations of laryngopharyngeal reflux. *Ear Nose & Throat Journal, 81*, 19–23.

Colden, D., Zeitels, S. M., Hillman, R. E., Jarboe, J., Bunting, G., & Spanou, K. (2001). Stroboscopic assessment of vocal fold keratosis and glottic cancer. *The Annals of Otology, Rhinology, and Laryngology, 110*, 293–298.

Coleman, R. F. (1971). Effect of waveform changes upon roughness perception. *Folia Phoniatrica et Logopedica, 23*, 314–322.

Coleman, R. F. (1993). Sources of variation in phonetograms. *Journal of Voice, 7*, 1–14.

Coleman, R. F., Mabis, J. H., & Hinson, J. K. (1977). Fundamental frequency-sound pressure level profiles of adult male and female voices. *Journal of Speech and Hearing Research, 20*, 197–204.

Coleman, R. F., & Wendahl, R. (1967). Vocal roughness and stimulus duration. *Speech Monographs, 34*, 85–92.

Coleman, R. O. (1971). Male and female voice quality and its relationship to vowel formant frequencies. *Journal of Speech and Hearing Research, 14*, 565–577.

Coleman, R. O. (1973). Speaker identification in the absence of inter-subject differences in glottal source characteristics. *Journal of the Acoustical Society of America, 53*, 1741–1743.

Coleman, R. O. (1976). A comparison of the contributions of two voice quality characteristics to the perception of maleness and femaleness in the voice. *Journal of Speech and Hearing Research, 19*, 168–180.

Colton, R. H. (1972). Spectral characteristics of the modal and falsetto registers. *Folia Phoniatrica et Logopedica, 24*.

Colton, R. H. (1973). Some acoustic parameters related to the perception of modal- falsetto quality. *Folia Phoniatrica et Logopedica, 25*, 302–311.

Colton, R. H. (1973). Vocal intensity in the modal and falsetto registers. *Journal of Speech and Hearing Research, 25*, 62–70.

Colton, R. H. (1984). Glottal waveform variations associated with different vocal intensity levels.

In V. Lawrence (Ed.), *Transcripts of the Thirteenth Symposium: Care of the Professional Voice* (pp. 39–47). New York N.Y.: The Voice Foundation.

Colton, R. H. (1987). The role of pitch in the discrimination of voice quality. *Journal of Voice, 1*, 240–245.

Colton, R. H. (1988). Physiological mechanisms of vocal frequency control: The role of tension. *Journal of Voice, 2*, 208–220.

Colton, R. H. (1989). Objective evaluation of voice dysfunction in the elderly. In J. C. Goldstein, H. K. Kashima, & C. F. Koopmann, Jr. (Eds.), *Geriatric otorhinolaryngology* (pp. 79–91). Toronto: Brian Decker.

Colton, R. H. (1994). Physiology of phonation. In M. S. Benninger, B. H. Jacobson, & A. F. Johnson (Eds.), *Vocal arts medicine: the care and prevention of professional voice disorders* (pp. 30–60). New York: Thieme Medical Publishers, Inc.

Colton, R. H. (1994). Disinfecting face masks. *Journal of Voice, 8*, 95.

Colton, R. H. (1996). Physiology of voice quality. In W. S. Brown, Jr., B. P. Vinson, & M. A. Crary (Eds.), *Organic voice disorders assessment and treatment* (pp. 49–88). San Diego: Singular Publishing Group, Inc.

Colton, R. H., & Brewer, D. W. (1985). Fiberoptic/vibratory relationships in patients with voice disorders. In V. Lawrence (Ed.), *Transcripts of the 14th Symposium: Care of the Professional Voice* (pp. 271–275). New York: Voice Foundation.

Colton, R. H., Brewer, D., & Rothenberg, M. (1983). *Evaluation of noninvasive methods for measuring vocal function.* Syracuse, NY: SUNY Health Science Center at Syracuse.

Colton, R. H., Brewer, D., & Rothenberg, M. (1983). Evaluating vocal function. *Journal of Otolaryngology, 12*, 291–294.

Colton, R. H., Brewer, D. W., & Rothenberg, M. (1985). Vibratory characteristics of patients with voice disorders. Unpublished manuscript.

Colton, R. H., Brewer, D. W., & Rothenberg, M. (1991). Vibratory characteristics of patients with voice disorders. Unpublished manuscript.

Colton, R. H., & Brown, W. S., Jr. (1973). Some relationships between vocal effort and intraoral air pressure. *Journal of the Acoustical Society of America, 53*, 296A.

Colton, R. H., & Casper, J. K. (1990). *Understanding voice problems: a physiological perspective for diagnosis and treatment.* Baltimore: Williams and Wilkins.

Colton, R. H., & Casper, J. K. (1996). *Understanding voice problems: a physiological perspective for diagnosis and treatment.* (2nd ed.) Baltimore: Williams & Wilkins.

Colton, R. H., Casper, J. K., Brewer, D. W., & Conture, E. G. (1989). Digital processing of laryngeal images: a preliminary report. *Journal of Voice, 3*, 132–142.

Colton, R. H., Casper, J. K., & Kelley, R. (2000). Objective classification of glottal configuration: Part 2. Paper presented at the 29th Symposium: Care of the Professional Voice, Philadelphia, June 2000.

Colton, R. H., Casper, J., Natour, Y., & Sapienza, C. M. (2002). Problems and pitfalls of laryngeal image analysis. Seminar presented at the XXV IALP World Congress, Montreal, Canada, August 2001.

Colton, R. H., Casper, J. K., Woo, P., Brewer, D., Kelley, R., & Griffin, B. (1997). Objective studies of the management of voice disorders. In *Final Report: National Institute of Deafness and Other Communication Disorders*, grant number 5RO1DC011 3108.

Colton, R. H., & Conture, E. G. (1990). Problems and pitfalls of electroglottography. *Journal of Voice, 4*, 10–24.

Colton, R. H., & Cooker, H. (1968). Perceived nasality in the speech of the deaf. *Journal of Speech and Hearing Research, 11*, 553–559.

Colton, R. H., & Estill, J. (1981). Elements of voice quality: Perceptual, acoustic and physiologic aspects. In N. Lass (Ed.), *Speech and Language: Advances in Basic Research and Practice* (pp. 311–403). New York N.Y.: Academic Press.

Colton, R. H., Estill, J., & Gerstman, L. (1981). Identification of four selected voice qualities by spectral analysis. paper presented at the Vocal Fold Physiology Conference. Madison, WI.

Colton, R. H., & Hollien, H. (1972). Phonational range in the modal and falsetto registers. *Journal of Speech and Hearing Research, 15*, 708–713.

Colton, R. H., & Hollien, H. (1973). Perceptual differentiation of the modal and falsetto registers. *Folia Phoniatrica et Logopedica, 25*, 270–280.

Colton, R. H., & Hollien, H. (1973). Physiology of vocal registers in singers and nonsingers. In J. W. Large (Ed.), *Vocal registers in singing* (pp. 105–136). The Hague: Mouton.

Colton, R. H., Reed, G., Sagerman, R., & Chung, C. (1982). An investigation of voice change after radiotherapy. In *Final Report National Cancer Institute NIH* (Bethesda Md.: National Institutes of Health.

Colton, R. H., Sagerman, R., Chung, C., Young, Y., & Reed, G. (1978). Voice change after radiotherapy. *Radiology, 127*, 821–824.

Colton, R. H., & Steinschneider, M. (1980). Acoustic relationships of Infant cries to the sudden infant death syndrome. In T. Murry & J. Murry (Eds.), *Infant communication: cry and early speech* (pp. 183–208). Houston: College Hill Press.

Colton, R. H., Steinschneider, A., Black, L., & Gleason, J. (1985). The newborn infant cry: its potential implications for development and SIDS. In B. M. Lester & C. F. Z. Boukydis (Eds.), *Infant crying theoretical and research perspectives* (pp. 119–138). New York: Plenum Press.

Colton, R. H., & Woo, P. (1995). Measuring vocal fold function. In J. S. Rubin, R. T. Sataloff, G. S. Korovin, & W. J. Gould (Eds.), *Diagnosis and treatment of voice disorders* (pp. 290–315). New York: Igaku-Shoin Medical Publishers.

Colton, R. H., Woo, P., Brewer, D. W., & Casper, J. K. (1991). Objective classification of glottal configuration. Unpublished manuscript.

Colton, R. H., Woo, P., Brewer, D. W., Griffin, B., & Casper, J. K. (1995). Stroboscopic signs associated with benign lesions of the vocal folds. *Journal of Voice, 9,* 312–325.

Conture, E. G., Colton, R. H., & Gleason, J. R. (1988). Selected temporal aspects of coordination during fluent speech of young stutterers. *Journal of Speech and Hearing Research, 31,* 640–653.

Conture, E. G., Cudahy, E., Caruso, A., Schwartz, H., Brewer, D., & Casper, J. (1981). Computer assisted measures of video taped data: A description and case study. In V. Lawrence (Ed.), *Transcripts of the Tenth Symposium: Care of the Professional Voice (Part II)* (pp. 129–135). New York: The Voice Foundation.

Cooper, D. S., Shindo, M., Hast, M. H., Sinha, U., & Rice, D. H. (1994). Dynamic properties of the posterior cricoarytenoid muscle. *Annals of Otology, Rhinology and Laryngology, 103,* 937–944.

Cooper, D., & Titze, I. (1985). Generation and dissipation of heat in vocal fold tissue. *Journal of Speech and Hearing Research, 28,* 207–215.

Cooper, D. S., & von Leden, H. (1996). The discipline of voice: an historical perspective. In W. S. Brown, Jr., B. P. Vinson, & M. A. Crary (Eds.), *Organic voice disorders assessment and treatment* (pp. 1–22). San Diego: Singular Publishing Group, Inc.

Cooper, M. (1973). *Modern techniques of vocal rehabilitation.* Springfield, IL: Charles C Thomas.

Cooper, M. (1984). Change your voice, change your life. New York: Macmillan.

Cooper, M., & Cooper, M. H. (1977). Approaches to vocal rehabilitation. Springfield, IL: Charles C. Thomas.

Corboy, J. R., Goodin, D. S., & Frohman, E. M. (2003). Disease-modifying therapies for multiple sclerosis. *Current Treatment Options in Neurology, 5,* 35–54.

Cornut, G., & Bouchayer, M. (1989). Phonosurgery for singers. *Journal of Voice, 3,* 269–276.

Cotton, R. T., & Richardson, M. A. (1981). Congenital laryngeal anomalies. *Otolaryngology Clinics of North America, 14,* 203.

Countryman, S., Ramig, W., & Pawlas, A. A. (1994). Speech and voice deficits in Parkinsonian plus syndromes: Can they be treated? *Journal of Medical Speech Language Pathology, 2,* 211–225.

Courey, M. S., Garrett, C. G., Billante, C. R., Stone, R. E., Portell, M. D., Smith, T. L., et al. (2000). Outcomes assessment following treatment of spasmodic dysphonia with botulinum toxin. *Annals of Otology, Rhinology, and Laryngology, 109,* 819–822.

Courey, M. S., & Ossoff, R. H. (1996). Lesions of the Lamina Propria. In W. S. Brown, Jr., B. P. Vinson, & M. A. Crary (Eds.), *Organic voice disorders assessment and treatment* (pp. 245–260). San Diego: Singular Publishing Group, Inc.

Courey, M. S., Shohet, J. A., Scott, M. A., & Ossoff, R. H. (1996). Immunohistochemical characterization of benign laryngeal lesions. *Annals of Otology, Rhinology, and Laryngology, 105,* 525–531.

Coyle, S. M., Weinrich, B. D., & Stemple, J. C. (2001). Shifts in relative prevalence of laryngeal pathology in a treatment-seeking population. *Journal of Voice, 15,* 424–440.

Crapo, R. O. (1981). Smoke inhalation injuries. *JAMA, 246,* 1694–1696.

Crary, M. A., & Glowaski, A. (1996). Vocal Fold Immobility. In W. S. Brown, Jr., B. P. Vinson, & M. A. Crary (Eds.), *Organic voice disorders assessment and treatment* (pp. 301–322). San Diego: Singular Publishing Group, Inc.

Critchley, M. (1949). Observations on essential (heredofamilial) tremor. *Brain, 72,* 9–139.

Crumley, R. L. (1983). Phrenic nerve graft for bilateral vocal cord paralysis. *Laryngoscope, 93,* 425–428.

Cudmore, R. E., & Vivori, E. (1981). Inhalation injury to the respiratory tract of children. *Progress in Pediatric Surgery, 14,* 173–188.

Cummings, C. W. (1986). Bilateral vocal cord paralysis/ankylosis. In C. Cummings, L. Harker, C. S. Krause, & D. Schuller (Eds.), *Otolaryngology—Head and Neck Surgery* (pp. 2181–2189). St. Louis: CV Mosby.

Damste, P. H. (1967). Voice change in adult women caused by virilizing agents. *Journal of Speech and Hearing Disorders, 32,* 126–132.

Damste, P. H. (1970). The phonetogram. *Practica Oto-Rhino-Laryngologica, 32,* 185–187.

Damste, P. H., Hollien, H., Moore, G. P., & Murry, T. (1968). An X-ray study of vocal fold length. *Folia Phoniatrica et Logopedica, 20.*

Daniloff, R., Schuckers, G., & Feth, L. (1980). *The physiology of speech and hearing.* Englewood Cliffs: Prentice-Hall.

Darley, F. L., Aronson, A. E., & Brown, J. R. (1969a). Clusters of deviant speech dimensions in the dysarthrias. *Journal of Speech and Hearing Research, 12,* 462–496.

Darley, F. L., Aronson, A. E., & Brown, J. R. (1969b). Differential diagnostic patterns of dysarthria. *Journal of Speech and Hearing Disorders, 12,* 246–269.

Darley, F. L., Aronson A. E., & Brown J. R. (1975). *Motor speech disorders.* Philadelphia: WB Saunders.

Darley, F. L., Brown, J. R., & Goldstein, N. P. (1972). Dysarthria in multiple sclerosis. *Journal of Speech and Hearing Research,* 15, 229–245.

Darley, F. L., & Spriesterbach, D. C. (1978). *Diagnostic methods in speech pathology.* (2nd ed.) New York: Harper & Row.

Davis, P. J., Boone, D. R., Carroll, R. L., Darvenzia, P., & Harrison, G. A. (1988). Adductor spastic dysphonia: heterogenicity of physiologic and phonatory characteristics. *Annals of Otology, Rhinology and Laryngology,* 97, 179–185.

Davis, S. B. (1981). Acoustic characteristics of normal and pathological voices. In C. L. Ludlow & M. Hart (Eds.), *Proceedings of the Conference on the Assessment of Vocal Pathology* (pp. 97–115). Rockville MD: American Speech-Language-Hearing Assoc.

Daya, H., Hosni, A., Bejar-Solar, I., Evans, J. N., & Bailey, C. M. (2000). Pediatric vocal fold paralysis: a long-term retrospective study. *Archives of Otolaryngology—Head & Neck Surgery,* 126, 21–25.

de Gaudemar, I., Roudaire, M., Francois, M., & Narcy, P. (1996). Outcome of laryngeal paralysis in neonates: a long term retrospective study of 113 cases. *International Journal of Pediatric Otorhinolaryngology,* 34, 101–110.

Dean, W. (1999). The neuroendocrine theory of aging: Part I. Vitamin research products [On-line]. Available: http://www.vrp.com/art/144.asp?c=1055356261365&g=Ward%20Dean&k=/srch/warddean.asp&m=/vstyle.css

Dean, W., Ahmarani, C., Bettez, M., & Heuer, R. J. (2001). The adjustable laryngeal implant. *Journal of Voice,* 15, 141–150.

Dean, W. (2003). Neuroendocrine theory of aging Part II. vitamin research products [On-line]. Available: http://www.vrp.com/art/257.asp?c=1055356261365&g=Ward%20Dean&k=/srch/warddean.asp&m=/vstyle.css

Deary, I. J., Wilson, J. A., Carding, P. N., & MacKenzie, K. (2003). VoiSS. A patient-derived Voice Symptom Scale. *Journal of Psychosomatic Research,* 54, 483–489.

Dedo, H. H. (1976). Recurrent laryngeal nerve section for spastic dysphonia. *Annals of Otology, Rhinology and Laryngology,* 85, 451–459.

Dedo, H. H. (1988). Avoidance and treatment of complications of Teflon injection of the vocal cord. *Journal of Voice,* 2, 90–92.

Dedo, H. H. (1992). Injection and removal of Teflon for unilateral vocal cord paralysis.

Annals of Otology, Rhinology and Laryngology, 101, 81–86.

Dedo, H. H., & Izdebski, K. (1981). Surgical treatment of spasmodic dysphonia. *Contemporary Surgery,* 18, 75–90.

Dedo, H. H., & Izdebski, K. (1983). Intermediate results of 306 recurrent laryngeal nerve sections for spastic dysphonia. *Annals of Otology, Rhinology and Laryngology,* 92, 9–15.

Dedo, H. H., Townsend, J., & Izdebski, K. (1978). Current evidence for the organic etiology of spastic dysphonia. *Otolaryngology,* 86, 875–880.

Dejonckere, P. H. (1984). Pathogenesis of voice disorders in childhood. *Acta Oto-rhino-laryngologica belgica,* 38, 307–314.

Dejonckere, P. H., & Lebacq, J. (1984). Regulatory mechanisms of the phasic respiratory activity in cricothyroid muscle. *Acta Oto-rhino-laryngologica belgica,* 38, 579–585.

Dejonckere, P. H., & Lebacq, J. (1985). Electroglottography and vocal nodules: an attempt to quantify the shape of the signal. *Folia Phoniatrica et Logopedica,* 37, 195–200.

Dejonckere, P. H., Wieneke, G. H., Bloemenkamp, D., & Lebacq, J. (1996). Fo/perturbation and Fo/loudness dynamics in voices of normal children, with and without education in singing. *International Journal of Pediatric Oto-Rhino-Laryngology,* 35, 107–115.

Delahunty, J. E., (1972). Acid laryngitis. *Journal of Laryngology,* 86, 335–342.

Delahunty, J. E., & Cherry, J. (1968). Experimentally produced vocal cord granulomas. *Laryngoscope,* 73, 1941–1947.

Deveney, C. W., Benner, K., & Cohen, J. (1993). Gastroesophageal reflux and laryngeal disease. *Archives of Surgery,* 128, 1021–5; discussion 1026–7.

DeWeese, D. D., & Saunders, W. H. (1982). *Textbook of otolaryngology* (6th ed.) St. Louis: Mosby.

Dickson, D. R., & Dickson, W. M. (1982). *Anatomical and physiological bases of speech.* Boston: Little, Brown & Co.

Diehl, C. F. (1960). Voice and personality: an Evaluation. In D. A. Barbara (Ed.), *Psychological and psychiatric aspects of speech and hearing* (pp. 171–203). Springfield, IL: Charles C. Thomas.

Dikkers, F. G., & Nikkels, P. G. (1995). Benign lesions of the vocal folds: histopathology and phonotrauma. *The Annals of Otology, Rhinology, and Laryngology,* 104, 698–703.

Dilman, V., & Dean, W. (1992). *The neuroendocrine theory of aging.* Pensacola: The Center for Bio-Gerontology.

Djojosubroto, M. W., Choi, Y. S., Lee, H. W., & Rudolph, K. L. (2003). Telomeres and telomerase in aging, regeneration and cancer. *Molecular Cell,* 15, 164–175.

Doherty, E. T., & Hollien, H. (1978). Multiple factor speaker identification of normal and distorted speech. *Journal of Phonetics, 6,* 1–8.

Dordain, M., & Dordain, G. (1972). L'epreuve du /a/ tenu au course des tremblements de la voix (tremblement idiopathique et dyskinesie volitionnelle, leurs rapports avec la dysphonie spasmodique). *Revue de Laryngologic, 93,* 167–182.

Dowling, P. C., Blumberg, B. M., & Cook, S. D. (1987). Guillain-Barre Syndrome. In P. J. Vinken, G. W. Bruyn, H. L. Klawans, & W. B. Matthews (Eds.), *Handbook of clinical neurology* (pp. 239–262). Amsterdam: Elsevier.

Dromey, C., Stathopoulos, E. T., & Sapienza, C. M. (1992). Glottal airflow and electroglottographic measures of vocal function at multiple intensities. *Journal of Voice, 6,* 44–54.

Duke, S. G., Salmon, J., Blalock, P. D., Postma, G. N., & Koufman, J. A. (2001). Fascia augmentation of the vocal fold: graft yield in the canine and preliminary clinical experience. *Laryngoscope, 111,* 759–764.

Dursun, G., Sataloff, R. T., Spiegel, J. R., Mandel, S., Heuer, R. J., & Rosen, D. C. (1996). Superior laryngeal nerve paresis and paralysis. *Journal of Voice, 10,* 206–211.

Duvoisin, R. (1976). Parkinsonism. *Clinical Symposia, 28,* 1–29.

Dworkin, J. P., & Hartman, D. E. (1979). Progressive speech deterioration and dysphagia in amyotrophic lateral sclerosis: case report. *Archives of Physical Medicine and Rehabilitation, 60,* 423–425.

Dworkin, J. P., Meleca, R., Abkarian, G. G., Stackpole, S., Aref, A., & Garfield, I. (1999). Phonation subsystem outcomes following radiation therapy for T1 glottic carcinoma: a prospective voice laboratory investigation. *Journal of Medical Speech and Language Pathology, 7,* 181–193.

Dyer, R. F., & Esch, V. H. (1976). Polyvinyl chloride toxicity in fires. *JAMA, 235,* 393–397.

Eccles, J. C. (1977). *The understanding of the brain.* New York NY: McGraw Hill Book Co.

Eckel, F. C., & Boone, D. R. (1981). The s/z ratio as an indicator of laryngeal pathology. *Journal of Speech and Hearing Disorders, 46,* 147–149.

Ehrlich, P. (2000). Collagen considerations in scarring and regenerative repair. In H. Garg & M. Longaker (Eds.), *Scarless wound healing* (pp. 99–113). New York: Marcel Dekker Inc.

Ejnell, H., & Tisell, L. E. (1993). Acute temporary laterofixation for treatment of bilateral vocal cord paralyses after surgery for advanced thyroid carcinoma. *World Journal of Surgery, 17,* 277–281.

Elias, M. E., Sataloff, R. T., Rosen, D. C., Heuer, R. J., & Spiegel, J. R. (1997). Normal strobovideo-laryngoscopy: variability in healthy singers. *Journal of Voice, 11,* 104–107.

Emami, A. J., Morrison, M., Rammage, L., & Bosch, D. (1999). Treatment of laryngeal contact ulcers and granulomas: a 12–year retrospective analysis. *Journal of Voice, 13,* 612–617.

Emanuel, F., & Sansone, F. (1969). Some spectral features of normal "and simulated 'rough' vowels." *Folia Phoniatrica, 21,* 401–415.

Erim, Z., Beg, M. F., Burker, D. T., & De Luca, C. J. (1999). Effects of aging on motor-unit control properties. *Journal of Neurophysiology, 82,* 2081–2091.

Faaborg-Anderson, K. (1957). Electromyographic investigation of intrinsic muscles in humans: an investigation of subjects with normally movable vocal cords and patients with vocal cord paresis. *Acta Physiologica Scandinavica, 41 (suppl 140),* 1–148.

Faaborg-Anderson, K., & Sonninen, A. (1960). The function of the extrinsic laryngeal muscles at different pitch. *Acta Oto-laryngologica (Stockholm), 51,* 50–54.

Faaborg-Anderson, K., & Vennard, W. (1964). Electromyography of extrinsic laryngeal muscles during phonation of different vowels. *Annals of Otology, Rhinology and Laryngology, 73,* 248–254.

Fairbanks, G. F. (1960). *Voice and articulation drillbook.* (2nd ed.) New York: Harper & Row.

Fant, G. (1970). *Acoustic theory of speech production.* The Hague: Mouton.

Farmakides, M. N., & Boone, D. R. (1960). Speech problems of patients with multiple sclerosis. *Journal of Speech and Hearing Disorders, 25,* 385–390.

Faure, M., & Muller, A. (1992). Stroboscopy. *Journal of Voice, 6,* 139–148.

Feder, R. (1986). On standardizing the laryngeal examination. *Archives of Otolaryngology—Head and Neck Surgery, 112,* 145.

Feder, R. J., & Michell, M. J. (1984). Hyperfunctional, hyperacidic and intubation granulomas. *Archives of Otolaryngology, 110,* 582–584.

Ferguson, C. F. (1970). Congenital abnormalities of the infant larynx. *Otolaryngologic Clinics of North America, 3,* 2.

Fex, S. (1970). Judging the movements of vocal cords in laryngeal paralysis. *Acta Otolaryngologica Supplement (Stockholm), 263,* 82–83.

Finitzo-Hieber, T., Freeman, F. J., Gerling, I. J., Dobson, L., & Shaefer, S. D. (1962). Auditory brainstem response abnormalities in adductor spasmodic dysphonia. *American Journal of Otolaryngology, 3,* 26–30.

Finizia, C., Dotevall, H., Lundstrom, E., & Lindstrom, J. (1999). Acoustic and perceptual evaluation of voice and speech quality: a study of patients with laryngeal cancer treated with laryngectomy vs. irradiation. *Archives of Otolaryngology—Head and Neck Surgery, 125,* 157–163.

Fink, B. R., & Demarest, R. J. (1978). *Laryngeal biomechanics,* Cambridge: Harvard University Press.

Finnegan, D. F., (1984). Maximum phonation time for children with normal voices. *Journal of Communication Disorders, 17,* 309–317.

Finnegan, D. E. (1985). Maximum phonation time for children with normal voices. *Folia Phoniatrica et Logopedica, 37,* 209–215.

Fisher, C. R., Jr., & Veronneau, S. J. (2000). Herbal preparations: a primer for the aeromedical physician. *Aviation, Space, and Environmental Medicine, 71,* 45–60.

Fisher, K. V., Telser, A., Phillips, J. E., & Yeates, D. B. (2001). Regulation of vocal fold transepithelial water fluxes. *Journal of Applied Physiology, 91,* 1401–1411.

Fitz-Hugh, G. S., Smith, D. E., & Chiong, A. T. (1958). Pathology of three hundred clinically benign lesions of the vocal cords. *Laryngoscope, 68,* 855–875.

Flatau, T. S., & Gutzman, H. (1908). Die singstimme des schulkindes. *Archives of Laryngology and Rhinology, 20,* 327–348.

Flynn, P. T. (1983). Speech-language pathologists and primary prevention: from ideas to action. *Language Speech Hearing Services in Schools, 14,* 99–104.

Folkins, J. W. (1978). Lower lip displacement during voluntary activation of individual labial muscles. *Archives of Oral Biology, 23,* 189–193.

Ford, C. N. (1996). Laryngeal Papilloma. In W. S. Brown, Jr., B. P. Vinson, & M. A. Crary (Eds.), *Organic voice disorders assessment and treatment* (pp. 261–270). San Diego: Singular Publishing Group, Inc.

Ford, C. N., Bless, D. M., & Loftus, J. M. (1992). Role of injectable collagen in the treatment of glottic insufficiency: a study of 119 patients. *Annals of Otology, Rhinology and Laryngology, 101,* 237–247.

Ford, C. N., Bless, D. M., & Patel, N. Y. (1992). Botulinum toxin treatment of spasmodic dysphonia: techniques, indications, efficacy. *Journal of Voice, 6,* 370–376.

Ford, C. N., Inagi, K., Khidr, A., Bless, D. M., & Gilchrist, K. W. (1996). Sulcus vocalis: a rational analytical approach to diagnosis and management. *Annals of Otology, Rhinology, & Laryngology, 105,* 189–200.

Ford, C. N., Martin, D. W., & Warner, T. F. (1984). Injectable collagen in laryngeal rehabilitation. *Laryngoscope, 94,* 513.

Ford, C. N., Staskowski, P. A., & Bless, D. M. (1995). Autologous collagen vocal fold injection: a preliminary clinical study. *Laryngoscope, 105,* 944–948.

Ford, C. N., Unger, J. M., Zundel, R. S., & Bless, D. M. (1995). Magnetic resonance imaging (MRI) assessment of vocal fold medialization surgery. *Laryngoscope, 105,* 498–504.

Franco, R. A., & Zeitels, S. M. (2003). Surgery for laryngeal cancer. In J. S. Rubin, R. T. Sataloff, & G. S. Korovin (Eds.), *Diagnosis and treatment of voice disorders* (2nd ed., pp. 679–700). Clifton Park, NY: Thomson Delmar Learning.

Frangez, I., Gale, N., & Luzar, B. (1997). The interpretation of leukoplakia in laryngeal pathology. *Acta Otolaryngology Supplement, 527,* 142–144.

Freidenberg, C. B. (2002). Working with male-to-female transgendered clients: clinical considerations. *Contemporary Issues in Communication Sciences and Disorders, 29,* 43–58.

Freud, E. D. (1962). Functions and dysfunctions of the ventricular folds. *Journal of Speech and Hearing Disorders, 27,* 334–340.

Fritzell, B., & Fant, G. (1986). Voice acoustics and dysphonia. *Journal of Phonetics, 14 (Suppl),* 345–347.

Fritzell, B., Feuer, E., Haglund, S., Knutsson, E., & Schiratzki, H. (1982). Experiences with recurrent laryngeal nerve section for spastic dysphonia. *Folia Phoniatrica, 34,* 160–167.

Froeschels, E. (1952). Chewing method as therapy. *Archives of Otolaryngology, 56,* 427–434.

Fujimura, O. (1981) Body-cover theory of the vocal fold and its phonetic implications. In K. Stevens & M. Hirano (Eds.). *Vocal fold physiology* (pp. 271–288). Tokyo: University of Tokyo Press.

Fujiu, M., Hibi, S. R., & Hirano, M. (1988). An improved technique for measurement of the relative noise level using a sound spectrograph. *Foli Phoniatrica, 40,* 53–57.

Fulton, J., & Dow, R. (1937). The cerebellum: a summary of functional localization. *Yale Journal of Biology and Medicine, 10,* 89–119.

Fung, K., Yoo, J., Leeper, H. A., Bogue, B., Hawkins, S., Hammond, J. A., et al. (2001). Effects of head and neck radiation therapy on vocal function. *Journal of Otolaryngology, 30,* 133–139.

Gallivan, G. J., & Andrianopoulos, M. V. (2004). Dysphonia due to paradoxical vocal fold movement/episodic laryngospasm. In C. Sapienza & J. Casper (Eds.), *For clinicians by clinicians: vocal rehabilitation in medical speech-language pathology* Austin, TX: Pro-Ed.

Gardner, E. (1963). *Fundamentals of neurology.* Philadelphia: Saunders.

Garfinkle, T., & Kimmelman, C. (1982). Neurologic disorders: amyotrophic lateral sclerosis, myasthenia gravis, multiple sclerosis and poliomyelitis. *American Journal of Otolaryngology, 3,* 204–212.

Garrett, K., & Healey, E. (1987). An acoustic analysis of fluctuations in the voices of normal adult speakers across three times of day. *Journal of the Acoustical Society of America, 82,* 58–62.

Gates, G., & Montalbo, P. J. (1987). The effect of low-dose b-blockade on performance anxiety in singers. *Journal of Voice, 1,* 105–108.

Gates, G. A., Saegert, J., Wilson, N., Johnson, L., Shepard, A., & Hearne, E. A. (1985). The effect of beta blockage on singing performance. *Annals of Otology, Rhinology and Laryngology, 94,* 570–574.

Gaynor, E. B. (1991). Otolaryngologic manifestations of gastroesophageal reflux. *American Journal of Gastroenterology, 86,* 801–808.

Genack, S. H., Woo, P., Colton, R. H., & Goyette, D. (1993). Partial thyroarytenoid myectomy: an animal study investigating a proposed new treatment for adductor spasmodic dysphonia. *Otolaryngology—Head and Neck Surgery, 108,* 256–264.

Gereau, S. A., LeBlanc, E. M., & Ruben, R. J. (1995). Congenital anomalies of the larynx. In R. J. Rubin, R. T. Sataloff, G. S. Korovin, & W. J. Gould (Eds.), *Diagnosis and treatment of voice disorders* (pp. 34–54). Tokyo: Igaku-Shoin.

Gerratt, B. R., & Hanson, D. (1987). Glottographic measures of laryngeal function in individuals with abnormal motor control. In T.Baer, C. H. Sasaki, & K. Harris (Eds.), *Laryngeal function in phonation and respiration* (pp. 521–532). Boston: College Hill Press.

Gerratt, B. R., Hanson, D. G., & Berke, G. S. (1988). Laryngeal configuration associated with glottography. *American Journal of Otolaryngology, 9,* 173–179.

Gerratt, B. R., Hanson, D. G., Berke, G. S., & Precoda, K. (1991). Photoglottography: A clinical synopsis. *Journal of Voice, 5,* 98–105.

Gerratt, B. R., Hanson, D. G., Hunt, S. M. J., & Karin, R. (1985). Glottographic measurement of laryngeal paralysis. paper presented at the convention of the American Speech Language Hearing Association, Washington DC.

Gerratt, B. R., & Kreiman, J. (2001). Measuring vocal quality with speech synthesis. *Journal of the Acoustical Society of America, 110,* 2560–2566.

Giger, H. L. (1984). The value of phonetogram studies in clinical work. In V. Lawrence (Ed.), *Transcripts of the Thirteenth Symposium: Care of the Professional Voice* (pp. 367–370). New York NY: The Voice Foundation.

Gliklich, R. E., Glovsky, R. M., & Montgomery, W. W. (1999). Validation of a voice outcome survey for unilateral vocal cord paralysis. *Otolaryngology—Head & Neck Surgery, 120,* 153–158.

Golden, G. S. (1977). Tourette syndrome: the pediatric perspective. *American Journal of Disorders in Childhood, 131,* 531–534.

Goldstein, J. C. (1989). Preface. In J. C. Goldstein, H. K. Kashima, & C. F. Koopmann (Eds.), *Geriatric otorhinolaryngology.* Toronto: B.C. Decker.

Gould, W. J. (1987). Surgery in professional singers. *Ear, Nose, Throat Journal, 66,* 327–332.

Gorham, M. M., Morris, R. J., Brown, W. S., & Huntley, R. A. (1996). Intraoral air pressure of alaryngeal speakers during a no-air insufflation maneuver. *Journal of Communication Disorders, 29,* 141–155.

Gracco, C., & Kahane, J. C. (1989). Age-related changes in the vestibular folds of the human larynx: a histomorphometric study. *Journal of Voice, 3,* 204–212.

Gracco, C., Jones-Bryant, N., Fahey, J., DeStephens, R., & Naito, W. (1995). Videoendoscopic and cardiopulmonary measures of exercise induced upper airway dysfunction. Paper presented at the 24th symposium of the Voice Foundation, Care of the Professional Voice, Philadelphia.

Gramming, P. (1988). The phonetogram: an experimental and clinical study. In *Ph.D. Dissertation Lund University,* Malmo, Sweden: Malmo General Hospital.

Gramming, P., & Akerlund, L. (1988). Non-organic dysphonia. II. Phonetograms for normal and pathological voices. *Acta Oto-Laryngologica, 106,* 468–476.

Gray, S. (1991). Basement membrane zone injury in vocal nodules. In J. Gauffin & B. Hammarberg (Eds.), *Vocal fold physiology: acoustic, perceptual, and physiological aspects of voice mechanisms* (pp. 21–28). San Diego: Singular Publishing Group.

Gray, S. D., Hirano, M., & Sato, K. (1993). Molecular and cellular structure of vocal fold tissue. In I. R. Titze (Ed.), *Vocal fold physiology: frontiers in basic science* (pp. 1–36). San Diego: Singular Publishing Group.

Gray, S. D., Pignatari, S. S., & Harding, P. (1994). Morphologic ultrastructure of anchoring fibers in normal vocal fold basement membrane zone. *Journal of Voice, 8,* 48–52.

Gray, S. D., Hammond, E., & Hanson, D. F. (1995). Benign pathologic responses of the larynx. *Annals of Otology, Rhinology and Laryngology, 104,* 13–18.

Gray, S. D., Titze, I. R., Alipour, F., & Hammond, T. H. (1999). Vocal fold extracellular matrix and its biomechanical influence part i: the fibrous proteins. In I. R. Titze (Ed.), *NCVS status and progress report* (pp. 1–10). Iowa City: National Center for Voice and Speech.

Gray, S. D., Titze, I. R., Alipour, F., & Hammond, T. H. (1999). Vocal fold extracellular matrix and its biomechanical influences part ii: the interstitial proteins. In I. R. Titze (Ed.), *NCVS status and progress report* (pp. 11–20). Iowa City: National Center for Voice and Speech.

Gray, S. D., Titze, I. R., Alipour, F., & Hammond, T. H. (2000). Biomechanical and histologic observations of vocal fold fibrous proteins. *Annals of Otology, Rhinology & Laryngology, 109,* 77–85.

Gray, S. D., Titze, I. R., Chan, R., & Hammond, T. H. (1999). Vocal fold proteoglycans and their influence on biomechanics. *Laryngoscope, 109,* 845–854.

Gray, S. D., Titze, I., & Lusk, R. P. (1987). Electron microscopy of hyperphonated canine vocal cords. *Journal of Voice, 1,* 109–115.

Griffin, B., Woo, P., Colton, R., Casper, J., & Brewer, D. (1995). Physiological characteristics of the supported singing voice: a preliminary study. *Journal of Voice, 9,* 45–56.

Grob, D. (1961). Myasthenia gravis. *Archives of Internal Medicine, 108,* 615–638.

Guidi, A. M., Bannister, R., & Gibson, W. P. R. (1981). Laryngeal electromyography in multiple system atrophy with autonomic failure. *Journal of Neurology, Neurosurgery, and Psychiatry, 44,* 49–53.

Guillain-Barré Syndrome Study Group, (1985). Plasmapheresis and acute Guillain-Barré syndrome. *Neurology, 35,* 1096–1104.

Haji, T., Horiguchi, S., Baer, T., & Gould, W. J. (1986). Frequency and amplitude perturbation analysis of electroglottograph during sustained phonation. *Journal of the Acoustical Society of America, 80,* 58–62.

Haji, T., Horiguchi, S., Baer, T., & Gould, W. J. (1986). Perturbation analysis of electroglottograph during sustained phonation. *Folia Phoniatrica et Logopedica, 38,* 290A.

Hallewell, J., & Cole, T. B. (1970). Isolated head and neck symptoms due to hiatus hernia. *Archives of Otolaryngology, 92,* 499–501.

Halstead, L. A. (1999). Role of gastroesophageal reflux in pediatric upper airway disorders. *Otolaryngology—Head and Neck Surgery, 120,* 208–214.

Hamlet, S. L., (1972). Vocal fold articulatory activity during whispered speech. *Archives of Otolaryngology, 95,* 211–312.

Hamlet, S. L. (1981). Ultrasound assessment of phonatory function. In C. L. Ludlow & M. Hart (Eds.), *Proceedings of the Conference on the Assessment of Vocal Pathology* (pp. 128–140). Rockville MD: American Speech-Language-Hearing Assoc.

Hammarberg, B., Fritzell, B., Gauffin, J., & Sundberg, J. (1986). Acoustic and perceptual analysis of vocal dysfunction. *Journal of Phonetics, 14,* 533–548.

Hammarberg, B., Fritzell, B., & Schiratzki, H. (1984). Teflon injection in 16 patients with para-

lytic dysphonia: perceptual and acoustic evaluations. *Journal of Speech and Hearing Disorders, 49,* 72–82.

Hammond, E. C. (1966). Smoking in relation to the death rate of 1 million men and women. *National Cancer Institute Monographs, 19,* 127–204.

Hammond, T. H., Gray, S. D., Butler, J., Zhou, R., & Hammond, E. (1998). Age- and gender-related elastin distribution changes in human vocal folds. *Otolaryngology and Head and Neck Surgery, 119,* 314–322.

Hammond, T. H., Gray, S. D., & Butler, J. E. (2000). Age- and gender-related collagen distribution in human vocal folds. *The Annals of Otology, Rhinology, and Laryngology, 109,* 913–920.

Hammond, T. H., Zhou, R., Hammond, E. H., Pawlak, A., & Gray, S. D. (1997). The intermediate layer: a morphologic study of the elastin and hyaluronic acid constituents of normal human vocal folds. *Journal of Voice, 11,* 59–66.

Hanson, D. G., Gerratt, B. R., & Berke, G. S. (1990). Frequency, intensity, and target matching effects on photoglottographic measures of open quotient and speed quotient. *Journal of Speech and Hearing Research, 33,* 45–50.

Hanson, D. G., Gerratt, B. R., Karin, R. R., & Berke, G. S. (1988). Glottographic measures of vocal fold vibration: An examination of laryngeal paralysis. *Laryngoscope, 98,* 541–549.

Hanson, D. G., Gerratt, B. R., & Ward, P. H. (1983). Glottographic measurement of vocal dysfunction: A preliminary report. *Annals of Otology, Rhinology and Laryngology, 92,* 413–420.

Hanson, D. G., Gerratt, B. R., & Ward, P. H. (1984). Cineradiographic observations of laryngeal function in Parkinson's disease. *Laryngoscope, 94,* 348–353.

Hanson, D. G., Ludlow, C., & Bassich, C. (1983). Vocal fold paresis in Shy-Drager syndrome. *Annals of Otology, Rhinology and Laryngology, 92,* 85–90.

Hanson, D. G., Ward, P. H., Gerratt, B. R., Berci, G., & Berke, G. S. (1989). Diagnosis of neuromuscular impairment. In J. C. Goldstein, H. K. Kashima, & C. F. Koopmann (Eds.), *Geriatric otorhinolaryngology* (pp. 71–78). Toronto: Decker.

Hanson, W., & Emanuel, F. W. (1979). Spectral noise and vocal roughness relationships in adults with laryngeal pathology. *Journal of Communication Disorders, 12,* 113–124.

Hanson, W. R., & Metter, E. J. (1980). DAF as instrumental treatment for dysarthria in progressive supranuclear palsy. *Journal of Speech and Hearing Disorders, 45,* 268–276.

Harden, J. R., & Looney, N. A. (1984). Duration of sustained phonation in kindergarten children. *International Journal of Pediatric Otorhinolaryngology, 7,* 11–19.

Harman, D. (1992). Free radical theory of aging. *Mutation Research*, 275, 257–266.

Harman, D. (1998). Aging: phenomena and theories. *Annals of the New York Academy of Science*, 854, 1–7.

Harman, D. (2001). Aging: overview. *Annals of the New York Academy of Science*, 928, 1–21.

Harrison, G. A., Davis, P. J., Troughear, R, H., & Winkworth, A. L. (1992). Inspiratory speech as a management option for spastic dysphonia—case study. *Annals of Otology, Rhinology and Laryngology*, 101, 375–382.

Hartelius, L., Buder, E., & Strand, E. A. (1997). Long-term phonatory instability in individuals with multiple sclerosis. *Journal of Speech and Hearing Research*, 40, 1056–1072.

Hartelius, L., Nord, L., & Buder, E. (1995). Acoustic analysis of dysarthria associated with multiple sclerosis. *Clinical Linguistics & Phonetics*, 9, 95–120.

Hartman, D. E. (1979). The perceptual identity and characteristics of aging in normal male adult speakers. *Journal of Communication Disorders*, 12, 53–61.

Hartman, D. E. (1979). Perceptual and acoustic characteristics of esophageal speech. In R. L. Keith & F. L. Darley (Eds.), *Laryngectomee rehabilitation* (pp. 87–106). Houston: College Hill Press.

Hartman, D. E. (1984). Neurogenic dysphonia. *Annales d'Oto-Laryngologie et de Chirurgie Cervico-Faciale*, 93, 57–64.

Hartman, D. E., Abbs, J. H., & Vishwanat, B. (1984). Multidimensional analysis of idiopathic spastic (spasmodic) dysphonia. *Presented at Clinical Dysarthria Conference*.

Hartman, D. E., & Abbs, J. H. (1988). Dysarthrias of movement disorders. *Advances in Neurology*, 49, 289–306.

Hartman, D. E., Abbs, J. H., & Vishwanat, B. (1988). Clinical investigations of adductor spastic dysphonia. *Annals of Otology, Rhinology and Laryngology*, 97, 247–252.

Hartman, D. E., & Aronson, A. E. (1981). Clinical investigations of intermittent breathy dysphonia. *Journal of Speech and Hearing Disorders*, 46, 428–432.

Hartman, D. E., & Aronson, A. E. (1991). Neurologic aspects of spasmodic dysphonia. *Journal of Otolaryngology*, 20, 148.

Hartman, D. E., Daily, W. W., & Morin, K. N. (1989). A case of superior laryngeal nerve paresis and psychogenic dysphonia. *Journal of Speech and Hearing Disorders*, 54, 526–529.

Hartman, D. E., & Danhauer, J. (1976). Perceptual features of speech for males in four perceived age decades. *Journal of Acoustical Society of America*, 59, 713–715.

Hartman, D. E., Overholt, S. J., & Vishwanat, B. (1982). A case of vocal cord nodules masking essential (voice) tremor. *Acta Oto-Laryngologica*, 108, 52–53.

Hartman, D. E., & Vishwanat, B. (1984). Spastic dysphonia and essential (voice) tremor treated with primidone. *Archives of Otolaryngology*, 110, 394–397.

Hartnick, C. J. (2002). Validation of a pediatric voice quality-of-life instrument: the pediatric voice outcome survey. *Archives of Otolaryngology—Head and Neck Surgery*, 128, 919–922.

Hayflick, L. (1973). The biology of human aging. *American Journal of Medical Science*, 265, 432–445.

Heaver, L. (1959). Spastic dysphonia: II. Psychiatric considerations. *Logos*, 2, 15–24.

Hecker, M. H., & Kreul, E. J. (1971). Descriptions of the speech of patients with cancer of the vocal folds Part I: measures of fundamental frequency. *Journal of the Acoustical Society of America*, 49, 1275–1282.

Henschen, T. L., & Burton, N. G. (1978). Treatment of spastic dysphonia by EMG biofeedback. *Biofeedback and Self Regulation*, 3, 91–96.

Herrington-Hall, B. L., Lee, L., Stemple, J. C., Niemi, K. R., & McHone, M. M. (1988). Description of laryngeal pathologies by age, sex and occupation in a treatment-seeking sample. *Journal of Speech and Hearing Disorders*, 53, 57–64.

Hersen, M., & Turner, S. M. (1985). *Diagnostic interviewing*. New York: Plenum Press.

Heylen, L., Wuyts, F. L., Mertens, F., De Bodt, M., Pattyn, J., Croux, C. et al. (1998). Evaluation of the vocal performance of children using a voice range profile index. *Journal of Speech, Language, and Hearing Research*, 41, 232–238.

Heylen, L., Wuyts, F. L., Mertens, F., De Bodt, M., Pattyn, J., & Van de Heyning, P. H. (1996). Comparison of the results of the frequency and the intensity data of the BSGVD with phonetogram characteristics. *Acta Oto-Rhino-Laryngologica Belgica*, 50, 353–360.

Heylen, L., Wuyts, F. L., Mertens, F., De Bodt, M., & Van de Heyning, P. H. (2002). Normative voice range profiles of male and female professional voice users. *Journal of Voice*, 16, 1–7.

Heylen, L. G., Wuyts, F. L., Mertens, F. W., & Pattyn, J. E. (1996). Phonetography in voice diagnoses. *Acta Oto-Rhino-Laryngologica Belgica*, 50, 299-308.

Hibi, S. R., Bless, D. M., Hirano, M., & Yoshida, T. (1988). Distortions of videofiberscopy imaging: reconstruction and correction. *Journal of Voice*, 2, 168–175.

Hicks, D. M., & Bless, D. M. (1996). Principles of Treatment. In W. S. Brown, Jr., B. P. Vinson, & M. A. Crary (Eds.), *Organic voice disorders assessment and treatment* (pp. 172–192). San Diego: Singular Publishing Group, Inc.

Hicks, D. M., Larar, J. N., Moore, G. P., & Childers, D. G. (1985). Electroglottography for assessing laryngeal function. *Institute for Advanced Study of the Communication Processes Bulletin, 1,* 41–50.

Higgins, M. B., & Saxman, J. H. (1993). Inverse-filtered air flow and EGG measures for sustained vowels and syllables. *Journal of Voice, 7,* 47–53.

Hill, A. V. (1938). The heat of shortening and the dynamic constants of muscle. *Proceedings of the Royal Society, 126,* 136–195.

Hillman, R. E., Holmberg, E. B., Perkell, J. S., Walsh, M., & Vaughan, C. (1989). Objective assessment of vocal hyperfunction: an experimental framework and initial results. *Journal of Speech and Hearing Research, 32,* 373–392.

Hillman, R. E., & Weinberg, B. (1981). A new procedure for venting a reflectionless tube. *Journal of the Acoustical Society of America, 69,* 1449–1451.

Hirano, M. (1974). Morphological structure of the vocal cord as a vibrator and its variations. *Folia Phoniatrica et Logopedica, 26,* 89–94.

Hirano, M. (1975). Phonosurgery: basic and clinical applications. *Otologia, 21,* 239–242.

Hirano, M. (1981). *Clinical examination of voice.* Wein Austria: Springer-Verlag.

Hirano, M. (1981). Structure of the vocal fold in normal and disease states: anatomical and physical studies. In C. Ludlow & M. Hart (Eds.), *Proceedings of the Conference on the Assessment of Vocal Pathology* (pp. 11–30). Rockville MD: American Speech-Language-Hearing Association.

Hirano, M. (1985). Cover-body theory of vocal fold vibration. In R. Daniloff (Ed.), *Speech science* (pp. 1–34). San Diego: College Hill Press.

Hirano, M., & Bless, D. M. (1993). *Videostroboscopic examination of the larynx.* San Diego: Singular Publishing Group.

Hirano, M., Feder, R., & Bless, D. M. (1983). Clinical evaluation of patients with voice disorders: stroboscopic evaluation. paper presented at the convention of the American Speech Language Hearing Association, 1–25. Cincinnati, OH.

Hirano, M., Kakita, Y., Kawasaki, H., Gould, W. J., & Lambiase, A. (1981). Data from high-speed motion picture studies. In K. N. Stevens & M. Hirano (Eds.), *Vocal fold physiology* (pp. 85–91). Tokyo: University of Tokyo Press.

Hirano, M., Kakita, Y., Kawasaki, H., & Matsushita, H. (1977). *Vocal cord vibration: behavior of the layer-structured vibrator in normal and pathological conditions.* [16 mm film, also available on videotape]. New York: Voice Foundation.

Hirano, M., Koike, Y., & von Leden, H. (1968). Maximum phonation time and air usage during phonation. *Folia Phoniatrica, 20,* 185–201.

Hirano, M., Kurita, S., Matsuo, K., & Nagata, K. (1980). Laryngeal tissue reaction to stress. In V. Lawrence (Ed.), *Transcripts of the 9th symposium: care of the professional voice* (pp. 10–20). New York: Voice Foundation.

Hirano, M., Kurita, S., & Nakashima, T. (1983). Growth, development and aging of human vocal folds. In D. Bless (Ed.), *Vocal fold physiology contemporary research and clinical issues* (pp. 22–43). San Diego: College Hill Press.

Hirano, M., Kurita, S., & Sakaguchi, S. (1989). Ageing of the vibratory tissue of human vocal folds. *Acta Oto-Laryngologica, 107,* 428–433.

Hirano, M., Yoshida, Y., & Matsushita, H. (1974). An apparatus for ultra-high-speed cinematography of vocal folds. *Annales d'Oto-Laryngologie et de Chirurgie Cervico-Faciale, 83,* 12–18.

Hirano, M., Yoshida, T., Tanaka, S., & Hibi, S. (1990). Sulcus vocalis: functional aspects. *Annals of Otology, Rhinology and Laryngology, 99,* 679–683.

Hirose, H. (1988). High speed digital imaging of vocal fold vibration. *Acta Oto-Laryngologica, Suppl 458,* 151–158.

Hirose, H., Kiritani, S., & Imagawa, H. (1987). High speed digital image analysis of laryngeal behavior in running speech. *Annual Bulletin RILP, 21,* 25–40.

Hirose, H., Kiritani, S., & Imagawa, H. (1988). High speed digital image analysis of laryngeal behavior in running speech. In O. Fujimura (Ed.), *Vocal fold physiology: voice production, mechanisms and function* (pp. 335–345), New York: Raven Press.

Hirose, H., Kiritani, S., & Imagawa, H. (1991). High-speed digital imaging of vocal fold vibration and its application for analysis of hoarseness. In J. A. Cooper (Ed.), *Assessment of Speech and Voice Production: Research and Clinical Applications* (pp. 146–149). Bethesda: U.S. Dept of Health and Human Services.

Hirose, H., Kiritani, S., & Imagawa, H. (1991). Clinical application of high-speed digital imaging of vocal fold vibration. In J. Gauffin & B. Hammarberg (Eds.), *Vocal fold physiology: acoustic, perceptual and physiological aspects of voice mechanisms* (pp. 213–216). San Diego: Singular Publishing Group.

Hiroto, I., Hirano, M., & Tomita, H. (1968). Electromyographic investigation of human vocal cord paralysis. *Annals of Otology, Rhinology and Laryngology, 77,* 296–304.

Hirschi, S. D., Gray, S. D., & Thibeault, S. L. (2002). Fibronectin: an interesting vocal fold protein. *Journal of Voice, 16,* 310–316.

Hixon, T. (1987). *Respiratory function in speech and song.* Boston: Little, Brown & Co.

Hixon, T. J., & Smitheran, J. R. (1982). A reply to Rothenberg. *Journal of Speech and Hearing Disorders, 47,* 220–223.

Hodge, F. S., Colton, R. H., & Kelley, R. T. (2001). Vocal intensity characteristics in normal and elderly speakers. *Journal of Voice*, *15*, 503–511.

Hoehn, M. M., & Yahr, M. D. (1967). Parkinsonism: onset, progression and mortality. *Neurology*, *17*, 427–442.

Hoffman, H. T., Overholt, E., Karnell, M., & McCulloch, T. M. (2001). Vocal process granuloma. *Head and Neck*, *23*, 1061–1074.

Hogikyan, N. D., & Rosen, C. A. (2002). A review of outcome measurements for voice disorders. *Otolaryngology—Head and Neck Surgery*, *126*, 562–572.

Hogikyan, N. D., & Sethuraman, G. (1999). Validation of an instrument to measure voice-related quality of life (V-RQOL). *Journal of Voice*, *13*, 557–569.

Hogikyan, N. D., Wodchis, W. P., Spak, C., & Kileny, P. R. (2001). Longitudinal effects of botulinum toxin injections on voice-related quality of life (V-RQOL) for patients with adductory spasmodic dysphonia. *Journal of Voice*, *15*, 576–586.

Hogikyan, N. D., Wodchis, W. P., Terrell, J. E., Bradford, C. R., & Esclamado, R. M. (2000). Voice-related quality of life (V-RQOL) following type I thyroplasty for unilateral vocal fold paralysis. *Journal of Voice*, *14*, 378–386.

Holbrook, A., Rolnick, M. I., & Bailey, C. W. (1974). Treatment of vocal abuse disorders using a vocal intensity controller. *Journal of Speech and Hearing Disorders*, *39*, 298–303.

Hollien, H. (1960). Vocal pitch variation related to changes in vocal fold length. *Journal of Speech and Hearing Research*, *3*, 150–156.

Hollien, H. (1962). The relationship of vocal fold thickness to absolute fundamental frequency of phonation. *Proceedings of the 4th International Congress of Phonetic Sciences*, 173–177.

Hollien, H. (1962). The relationship of vocal fold length to vocal pitch for female subjects. In L. Croatto & C. Croatto-Martinoli (Eds.), *Proceedings of the XII International Speech and Voice Therapy Conference* (pp. 38–43). Padua Italy: A. Magarotto.

Hollien, H. (1962). Vocal fold thickness and fundamental frequency of phonation. *Journal of Speech and Hearing Research*, *5*, 237–243.

Hollien, H. (1964). Laryngeal research by means of laminagraphy. *Archives of Otolaryngology*, *80*, 303–308.

Hollien, H. (1972). Three major vocal registers: a proposal. In A. Rigault (Ed.), *Proceedings of the Seventh International Congress of Phonetic Sciences* (pp. 320–331). The Hague: Mouton.

Hollien, H. (1975). On vocal registers. *Journal of Phonetics*, *2*, 125–143.

Hollien, H. (1977). The Registers and ranges of the voice. In M. Cooper & M. H. Cooper (Eds.), *Approaches to vocal rehabilitation*. Springfield, IL: Charles C. Thomas.

Hollien, H. (1980). Vocal indicators of psychological stress. *Annals of the New York Academy of Science*, *347*, 47–72.

Hollien, H. (1986). Inferring laryngeal characteristics from phonatory output. In C. Cummings, L. Fredickson, L. Harker, & D. Schuller (Eds.), *Otolaryngology—head and neck surgery* (pp. 1828–1838). St. Louis: Mosby.

Hollien, H. (1987). 'Old voices': What do we really know about them. *Journal of Voice*, *1*, 2–17.

Hollien, H. (1993). That golden voice—talent or training? *Journal of Voice*, *7*, 195–205.

Hollien, H., Brown, W. S., Jr., & Hollien, K. (1971). Vocal fold length associated with modal, falsetto and varying intensity phonations. *Folia Phoniatrica et Logopedica*, *23*, 66–78.

Hollien, H., Coleman, R., & Moore, G. P. (1968). Stroboscopic laminagraphy of the larynx during phonation. *Acta Oto-Laryngologica*, *65*, 209–215.

Hollien, H., & Colton, R. H. (1969). Four laminagraphic studies of vocal fold thickness. *Folia Phoniatrica et Logopedica*, *21*, 179–198.

Hollien, H., & Copeland, R. H. (1965). Speaking fundamental frequency (SFF) characteristics of mongoloid girls. *Journal of Speech and Hearing Disorders*, *30*, 344–349.

Hollien, H., & Curtis, J. (1960). A laminagraphic study of vocal pitch. *Journal of Speech and Hearing Research*, *3*, 361–371.

Hollien, H., & Curtis, J. (1962). Elevation and tilting of vocal folds as a function of vocal pitch. *Folia Phoniatrica et Logopedica*, *14*, 23–36.

Hollien, H., Curtis, J. F., & Coleman, R. F. (1968). Investigation of laryngeal phenomena by stroboscopic laminagraphy. *Medical Research and Engineering*, *7*, 24–27.

Hollien, H., Damste, H., & Murry, T. (1969). Vocal fold length during vocal fry phonation. *Folia Phoniatrica et Logopedica*, *21*, 257–265.

Hollien, H., Dew, D., & Phillips, P. (1971). Phonational frequency ranges of adults. *Journal of Speech and Hearing Research*, *14*, 755–760.

Hollien, H., Geison, L., & Hicks, J. (1987). Voice stress evaluators and lie detection. *Journal of Forensic Sciences*, *32*, 405–418.

Hollien, H., Gelfer, M. P., & Carlson, T. (1991). Listening preferences for voice types as a function of age. *Journal of Communication Disorders*, *24*, 157–171.

Hollien, H., Girard, G. T., & Coleman, R. F. (1977). Vocal fold vibratory patterns of pulse register phonation. *Folia Phoniatrica et Logopedica*, *29*, 200–205.

Hollien, H., Green, R., & Massey, K. (1994). Longitudinal research on adolescent voice change in males. *Journal of the Acoustical Society of America, 96,* 2646–2654.

Hollien, H., Hollien, P. A., & Dejong, G. (1997). Effects of three parameters on speaking fundamental frequency. *Journal of the Acoustical Society of America, 102,* 2984–2992.

Hollien, H., & Jackson, B. (1973). Normative data on the speaking fundamental frequency characteristics of young adult males. *Journal of Phonetics, 19,* 117–120.

Hollien, H., & Majewski, W. (1977). Speaker identification by long-term spectra under normal and distorted speech conditions. *Journal of the Acoustical Society of America, 62,* 975–980.

Hollien, H., & Malcik, E. (1962). Adolescent voice change in southern negro males. *Speech Monographs, 29,* 53–58.

Hollien, H., & Malcik, E. (1967). Evaluation of cross-sectional studies of adolescent voice change in males. *Speech Monographs, 34,* 80–84.

Hollien, H., Malcik, E., & Hollien, B. (1965). Adolescent voice change in southern white males. *Speech Monographs, 32,* 87–90.

Hollien, H., Mendes-Schwartz, A. P., & Nielsen, K. (2000). Perceptual confusions of high-pitched sung vowels. *Journal of Voice, 14,* 287–298.

Hollien, H., & Michel, J. (1968). Vocal fry as a phonational register. *Journal of Speech and Hearing Research, 11,* 600–604.

Hollien, H., Michel, J., & Doherty, E. T. (1973). A method of analyzing vocal jitter in sustained phonation. *Journal of Phonetics, 1,* 85–91.

Hollien, H., & Moore, G. P. (1960). Measurements of the vocal folds during changes in pitch. *Journal of Speech and Hearing Research, 3,* 157–165.

Hollien, H., Moore, G. P., Wendahl, R., & Michel, J. (1966). On the nature of vocal fry. *Journal of Speech and Hearing Research, 9,* 245–247.

Hollien, H., & Paul, P. (1969). A second evaluation of the speaking fundamental frequency characteristics of post-adolescent girls. *Language and Speech, 12,* 119–124.

Hollien, H., & Shipp, T. (1972). Speaking fundamental frequency and chronologic age in males. *Journal of Speech and Hearing Research, 15,* 155–165.

Hollien, H., & Wendahl, R. (1968). Perceptual study of vocal fry. *Journal of the Acoustical Society of America, 43,* 506–509.

Hollinger, P., & Brown, W. T. (1967). Congenital webs, cysts, laryngoceles, and other anomalies of the larynx. *Annals of Otology, Rhinology and Laryngology, 76,* 744–752.

Holmberg, E. B., Hillman, R. E., & Perkell, J. S. (1988). Glottal airflow and transglottal air pressure measurements for male and female speakers in soft, normal and loud voice. *Journal of the Acoustical Society of America, 84,* 511–529.

Hong, K. H., Kim, H. K., & Kim, Y. H. (2001). The role of the pars recta and pars oblique of cricothyroid muscle in speech production. *Journal of Voice, 15,* 512–513.

Hong, K. H., Kim, J. H., & Kim, H. K. (2001). Anterior and posterior medialization (APM) thyroplasty. *Laryngoscope, 111,* 1406–1412.

Hong, K. H., Ye, M., Kim, Y. M., Kevorkian, K. F., Kreiman, J., & Berke, G. S. (1998). Functional differences between the two bellies of the cricothyroid muscle. *Otolaryngology—Head and Neck Surgery, 118,* 714–722.

Honjo, I., & Isshiki, N. (1980). Laryngoscopic and voice characteristics of aged persons. *Archives of Otolaryngology, 106,* 149–150.

Horii, Y. (1979). Fundamental frequency perturbation observed in sustained phonation. *Journal of Speech and Hearing Research, 22,* 5–19.

Horii, Y. (1980). Vocal shimmer in sustained phonation. *Journal of Speech and Hearing Research, 23,* 202–209.

Horii, Y. (1982). Jitter and shimmer differences among sustained vowels. *Journal of Speech and Hearing Research, 25,* 12–14.

Horii, Y. & Cooke, P. A. (1978). Some airflow, volume and duration characteristics of oral reading. *Journal of Speech and Hearing Research, 21,* 470–481.

Hormann, K., Baker-Schreyer, A., Keilmann, A., & Biermann, G. (1999). Functional results after CO_2 laser surgery compared with conventional phonosurgery. *Journal of Laryngology and Otology, 113,* 140–144.

Houben, G. B., Buekers, R., & Kingma, H. (1992). Characterization of the electroglottographic waveform: a primary study to investigate vocal fold functioning. *Folia Phoniatrica et Logopedica, 44,* 269–281.

House, A. S. (1959). Note on optimal vocal frequency. *Journal of Speech and Hearing Research, 2,* 55–60.

House, E. L., & Pansky, B. (1967). *A functional approach to neuroanatomy.* New York: McGraw Hill Book Co.

Hufnagle, J. (1982). Acoustic analysis of fundamental frequencies of voices of children with and without vocal nodules. *Perceptual Motor Skills, 55,* 427–432.

Hufnagle, J., & Hufnagle, K. (1988). S/Z ratio in dysphonic children with and without vocal cord nodules. *Language Speech Hearing Services in Schools, 19,* 418–422.

Hunt, J. L., Agee, R. N., & Pruitt, B. A. (1975). Fiberoptic bronchoscopy in acute inhalation injury. *Journal of Trauma, 15,* 641–648.

Huntley, R., Hollien, H., & Shipp, T. (1987). Influences of listener characteristics on perceived age estimations. *Journal of Voice, 1*, 49–52.

Ignotz, R. A. (1986). Transforming growth factor-B stimulates the expression of fibronectin and collagen and their incorporation into the extracellular matrix. *J Biological Chemistry, 261*, 4337–4345.

Inagi, K., Ford, C. N., Bless, D. M., & Heisey, D. (1996). Analysis of factors affecting botulinum toxin results in spasmodic dysphonia. *Journal of Voice, 10*, 306–313.

Iozzo, R. V. (1997). The family of the small leucine-rich proteoglycans: key regulators of matrix assembly and cellular growth. *Critical Reviews in Biochemistry and Molecular Biology, 32*, 141–174.

Irwin, R. J., & Mills, A. W. (1965). Matching loudness and vocal level: an experiment requiring no apparatus. *British Journal of Psychology, 56*, 143–146.

Ishii, K., Yamashita, K., Akita, M., & Hirose, H. (2000). Age-related development of the arrangement of connective tissue fibers in the lamina propria of the human vocal fold. Annals of Otology, Rhinology and Laryngology, *109*, 1055–1064.

Isshiki, N. (1964). Regulatory mechanism of voice intensity regulation. *Journal of Speech and Hearing Research, 7*, 17–29.

Isshiki, N. (1965). Vocal intensity and air flow rate. *Folia Phoniatrica et Logopedica, 17*, 92–104.

Isshiki, N. (1977). *Functional surgery of the larynx with special reference to percutaneous tension of the vocal cords.* Kyoto: Maeda Press.

Isshiki, N., Haji, T., Yamamoto, Y., & Mahieu, H. (2001). Thyroplasty for adductor spasmodic dysphonia: further experiences. *Laryngoscope, 111*, 615–621.

Isshiki, N., & Ishikawa, T. (1976). Diagnostic value of tomography in unilateral vocal cord paralysis. *Laryngoscope, 86*, 1573–1578.

Isshiki, N., Kitajima, K., Kojima, M., & Harita, Y. (1978). Turbulent noise in dysphonia. *Folia Phoniatrica, 30*, 214–224.

Isshiki, N., Morita, H., Okamura, H., & Hiramoto, M. (1974). Thyroplasty as a new phono–surgical technique. *Acta Oto-Laryngologica, 78*, 451–457.

Isshiki, N., Tanabe, M., Ishizaka, K., & Board, C. (1977). Clinical significance of asymmetrical tension of the vocal cords. *Annals of Otology, Rhinology and Laryngology, 86*, 1–9.

Isshiki, N., Tanabe, M., & Sawada, M. (1978). Arytenoid adduction for unilateral vocal cord paralysis. *Archives of Otolaryngology—Head and Neck Surgery, 104*, 555–558.

Isshiki, N., & von Leden, H. S. (1964). Hoarseness: aerodynamic studies. *Archives of Otolaryngology, 80*, 206–213.

Ivers, R. R., & Goldstein, N. P. (1963). Multiple sclerosis: a current appraisal of symptoms and signs. *Proceedings of the Staff Meetings of the Mayo Clinic, 38*, 457–466.

Iwata, S., Esaki, T., Iwami, K., & Mimura, Y. (1976). Air flow studies in the patients with laryngeal diseases during phonation. *Journal of the Naguya Cy University Medical Association, 26*, 398–406.

Iwata, S., von Leden, H. S., & Williams, D. (1972). Air flow measurement during phonation. *Journal of Communication Disorders, 5*, 67–79.

Izdebski, K. (1981). Magnetic sound recording in laryngology. *American Journal of Otolaryngology, 2*, 48–53.

Izdebski, K. (1983). Practical techniques of office voice recording. *Otolaryngology—Head and Neck Surgery, 91*, 638–642.

Izdebski, K. (1984). Overpressure and breathiness in spastic dysphonia. *Acta Otolaryngologica (Stockholm), 97*, 373–378.

Izdebski, K. (1992). Symptomatology of adductor spasmodic dysphonia: a physiologic model. *Journal of Voice, 6*, 306–319.

Izdebski, K., Dedo, H. H., & Shipp, T. (1981). Postoperative and follow-up studies of spastic dysphonia patients treated by recurrent nerve section. *Otolaryngology—Head and Neck Surgery, 89*, 96–101.

Jackson, C. L. (1941). Vocal nodules. *Transactions American Laryngological Association, 63*, 185–193.

Jacobson, E. (1938). *Progressive relaxation* (2nd ed.). Chicago: University of Chicago Press.

Jacobson, B. H., Johnson, A., Grywalski, C., Jacobson, G., Benninger, M., & Newman, G. (1997). The Voice Handicap Index (VHI): development and validation. *American Journal of Speech-Language Pathology, 6*, 66–70.

Jako, G. J. (1972). Laser surgery of the vocal cords: an experimental study with carbon dioxide lasers on dogs. *Laryngoscope, 82*, 2204–2216.

Janzen, V. D., Rae, R. E., & Hudson, A. J. (1988). Otolaryngologic manifestations of amyotrophic lateral sclerosis. *Journal of Otolaryngology, 17*, 41–42.

James, I. M., Pearson, R. M., Griffith, D. N. M., & Newburg, P. (1977). Effect of osprenolol on stage fright in musicians. *Lancet, 2*, 952–954.

Jarema, A. D., Kennedy, J. L., & Shoulson, I. (1985). *Acoustic and aerodynamic measurements of hyperkinetic dysarthria in Huntington's disease.* Paper presented at the convention of the American-Speech-Language-Hearing Association, Washington, DC.

Javkin, H. R., Antonanzas-Barros, H., & Maddieson, I. (1987). Digital inverse filtering for linguistic research. *Journal of Speech and Hearing Research, 30*, 122–129.

Jensen, J. R. (1960). *A study of certain motor-speech aspects of the speech of multiple sclerotic patients.* Unpublished doctoral dissertation, University of Wisconsin, Madison.

Jentzsch, H., Unger, E., & Sasama, R. (1981). Elecktroglottographische verlaufskontrollen bei patienten mit funktionellen stim mstorungen. *Folia Phoniatrica et Logopedica, 33,* 234–241.

Jiang, J., Lin, E., Wang, J., & Hanson, D. G. (1999). Glottographic measures before and after levodopa treatment in Parkinson's disease. *Laryngoscope, 109,* 1287–1294.

Jiang, J. J., Titze, I. R., Wexler, D. B., & Gray, S. D. (1994). Fundamental frequency and amplitude perturbation in reconstructed canine vocal folds. *Annals of Otology, Rhinology and Laryngology, 103,* 145–148.

Johns, M. E., & Rood, S. R. (1987). *Vocal cord paralysis: diagnosis and management.* Washington: American Academy of Otolaryngology-Head & Neck Surgery Foundation, Inc.

Johnson, J. A., & Pring, T. R. (1990). Speech therapy and Parkinson's disease: a review and further data. *British Journal of Disorders of Communication, 25,* 183–194.

Johnson, T. S. (1983). Treatment of vocal abuse in children. In Perkins, W. H. (Ed.), *Current therapy of communication disorders: voice disorders* (pp. 3–11). New York: Thieme.

Johnson, T. S. (1985). Voice disorders: the measurement of clinical progress. In Costello, J. (Ed.), *Speech disorders in adults: recent advances* (pp. 127–154). San Diego: College Hill Press.

Jürgens, U., & Pratt, R. (1979). Role of the periaqueductal grey in vocal expression of emotion. *Brain Research, 167,* 367–378.

Kahane, J., & Mayo, R. (1989). The need for aggressive pursuit of healthy childhood voices. *Language Speech Hearing Services in Schools, 20,* 102–107.

Kahane, J. C. (1981). Anatomic and physiologic changes in the aging peripheral speech mechanism. In D. Beasley & G. Davis (Eds.), *Aging communication processes and disorders* (pp. 22–45). New York: Grune & Stratton.

Kahane, J. C. (1981). A survey of age-related changes in the connective tissues of the human adult larynx. In D. M. Bless & J. H. Abbs (Eds.), *Vocal fold physiology: contemporary research and clinical issues* (pp. 44–49). San Diego: College Hill Press.

Kahane, J. C. (1982). Growth of the human prepubertal and pubertal larynx. *Journal of Speech and Hearing Research, 25,* 446–455.

Kahane, J. C. (1987). Connective tissue changes in the larynx and their effects on voice. *Journal of Voice, 1,* 27–30.

Kahane, J. C. (2004). Anatomy of the human larynx. In R. D. Kent (Ed.), *MIT encyclopedia of communication disorders* (pp. 13–20). Cambridge: The MIT Press.

Kahn, H. A. (1966). The Dorn study of smoking and mortality among US veterans: A report of eight 1/2 years of observation. *National Cancer Institute Monographs, 19,* 1–125.

Kakita, Y., Hirano, M., Kawasaki, H., & Matsushita, H. (1976). Schematical presentation of vibration of the vocal cords as a layer-structured vibrator: normal larynges. *Japanese Journal of Otolaryngology, 79,* 1333–1340.

Kalach, N., Gumpert, L., Contencin, P., & Dupont, C. (2000). Dual-probe pH monitoring for the assessment of gastroesophageal reflux in the course of chronic hoarseness in children. *Turkish Journal of Pediatrics, 42,* 186–191.

Kallen, L. A. (1932). Laryngostroboscopy in the practice of otolaryngology. *Archives of Otolaryngology, 16,* 791–807.

Kammermeier, M. A. (1969). A comparison of phonatory phenomena among groups of neurologically impaired speakers. Unpublished doctoral dissertation, University of Minnesota.

Karnell, M. P. (1991). Laryngeal perturbation analysis: Minimum length of analysis window. *Journal of Speech and Hearing Research, 34,* 544–548.

Karnell, M. P., Hall, K. D., & Landahl, K. L. (1995). Comparison of fundamental frequency and perturbation measurements among three analysis systems. *Journal of Voice, 9,* 383–393.

Karnell, M. P., Li, L., & Panje, W. R. (1991). Glottal opening in patients with vocal fold tissue changes. *Journal of Voice, 5,* 239–246.

Karnell, M. P., Scherer, R. S., & Fischer, L. B. (1991). Comparison of acoustic voice perturbation measures among three independent voice laboratories. *Journal of Speech and Hearing Research, 34,* 781–790.

Kashima, H. K. (1991). Bilateral vocal fold motion impairment—Pathophysiology and management by transverse cordotomy. *Annals of Otology, Rhinology and Laryngology, 100,* 717–721.

Kasuya, H., Ogawa, S., Mashima, K., & Ebihara, S. (1986). Normalized noise energy as an acoustic measure to evaluate pathologic voice. *Journal of the Acoustical Society of America, 80,* 1329–1334.

Kaszniak, A. W., Garron, D. C., Fox, J. H., Bergen, D., & Huckman, M. (1979). Cerebral atrophy, EEG slowing, age, education, and cognitive functioning in suspected dementia. *Neurology, 29,* 1273–1279.

Kawasaki, H., Kuratomi, K., & Mitsumasu, T. (1983). Cysts of the larynx: a 10-year review of 94 patients. *Auris Nasus Larynx, 10 Suppl,* S47–S52.

Keaton, A. L. (1983). The physiology of imagery. In V. Lawrence (Ed.), *Transcripts of the*

12th symposium: care of the professional voice (Part II, pp. 281–283). New York: Voice Foundation.

Kellman, R. M., & Leopold, D. A. (1982). Paradoxical vocal cord motion: an important cause of stridor. Laryngoscope, 92, 58–60.

Kelly, A. H., Beaton, L. E., & Magoun, H. W. (1946). A midbrain mechanism for facio-vocal activity. Journal of Neurophysiology, 9, 181–189.

Kempster, G. B. (1984). A multidimensional analysis of vocal quality in two dysphonic groups [doctoral dissertation]. Evanston, IL: Northwestern University.

Kent, R. D. (1976). Anatomical and neuromuscular maturation of the speech mechanism: evidence from acoustic studies. Journal of Speech and Hearing Research, 19, 421–447.

Kent, R. D., Kent, J., & Rosenbek, J. (1987). Maximum performance tests of speech production. Journal of Speech and Hearing Research, 52, 367–387.

Kent, R. D., Kim, H., Weismer, G., Kent, J. F., Rosenbek, J. C., Brooks, B. R., et al. (1994). Laryngeal dysfunction in neurological disease: Amyotrophic lateral sclerosis, Parkinson disease, and stroke. Journal of Medical Speech and Language Pathology, 2, 157–175.

Kent, R. D., & Netsell, R. (1975). A case study of an ataxic dysarthric cineradiographic and spectrographic observations. Journal of Speech and Hearing Disorders, 40, 115–134.

Kent, R. D., Netsell, R., & Abbs, J. H. (1979). Acoustic characteristics of dysarthria associated with cerebellar disease. Journal of Speech and Hearing Research, 22, 627–648.

Kent, R. D., Sufit, R. L., Rosenbek, J. C., Kent, J. F., Weismer, G., Martin, R. E., & Brooks, B. R. (1991). Speech deterioration in amyotrophic lateral sclerosis: a case study. Journal of Speech and Hearing Research, 34, 1269–1275.

Kersing, W. (1986). Vocal musculature, Aging and Developmental Aspects. Vocal Fold Histopathology: A Symposium, pp. 11–16.

Kim, K. M., Kakita, Y., & Hirano, M. (1982). Sound spectrographic analysis of the voice of patients with recurrent laryngeal nerve paralysis. Folia Phoniatrica, 34, 124–133.

King, J. B., Ramig, L. O., Lemke, J. H., & Horii, Y. (1994). Parkinson's disease: longitudinal changes in acoustic parameters of phonation. Journal of Medical Speech Language Pathology, 2, 29–42.

Kinney, J. P., Kado, R. T., & Royner, L. D. (1972). A simple encoder for labeling events recorded on analogue tape. Medical and Biological Engineering, 10, 431–432.

Kipling, D., & Faragher, R. G. (1999). Telomeres: ageing hard or hardly ageing? Nature, 398, 191, 193.

Kiritani, S., Imagawa, H., & Hirose, H. (1986). Simultaneous high–speed digital recording of vocal fold vibration, speech and EGG. Annual Bulletin RILP, 20, 11–15.

Kitajima, K. (1981). Quantitative evaluation of the noise level in the pathologic voice. Folia Phoniatrica et Logopedica, 33, 115–124.

Kitzing, P. (1985). Stroboscopy- a pertinent laryngological examination. Journal of Otolaryngology, 14, 151–157.

Kitzing, P., & Löfqvist, A. (1978). Clinical application of combined electro- and photoglottography. Proceedings of the 17th Congress of Logopedics and Phoniatrics, Copenhagen.

Klingholz, F., & Martin, F. (1985). Quantitative spectral evaluation of shimmer and jitter. Journal of Speech and Hearing Research, 28, 169–174.

Koike, Y. (1967a). Experimental studies on vocal attack. Practica Otologica Kyoto, 60, 663–688.

Koike, Y. (1967b). Applications of some acoustic measures for the evaluation of laryngeal dysfunction. Journal of the Acoustical Society of America, 42, 1209.

Koike, Y., & Hirano, M. (1968). Significance of the vocal velocity index. Folia Phoniatrica, 20, 285–296.

Kojima, H., Gould, W. J., & Lambiase, A. (1979). Computer analysis of hoarseness. Journal of the Acoustical Society of America, 65, S67.

Kojima, H., Gould, W. J., Lambiase, A., & Isshiki, N. (1980). Computer analysis of hoarseness. Acta Oto-Laryngologica, 89, 547–554.

Koller, W. C., Busenbark, K., & Miner, K. (1994). The relationship of essential tremor to other movement disorders: report on 678 patients. Annals of Neurology, 35, 717–723.

Komiyama, S., Watanabe, H., & Ryu, S. (1984). Phonetographic relationship between pitch and intensity of the human voice. Folia Phoniatrica, 36, 1–7.

Konig, W. F., & von Leden, H. (1961). The peripheral nervous system of the human larynx. II. The thyroarytenoid (vocalis) muscle. Archives of Otolaryngology, 74, 153–163.

Kooper, R., & Sullivan, C. A. (1986). Professional liability: management and prevention. In K. G. Butler (Ed.), Prospering in private practice (pp. 59–80). Rockville, MD: Aspen Systems.

Kornhuber, H. H. (1977). A reconsideration of the cortical and subcortical mechanisms involved in speech and aphasia. In J. E. Desmedt (Ed.), Progress in clinical neurophysiology (pp. 28–35). Basel SZ: Karger.

Kotby, M. N., & Haugen, L. K. (1970). The mechanics of laryngeal function. Acta Otolaryngologica (Stockholm), 70, 203–211.

Kotby, M. N., Nassar, A. M., Seif, E. I., Helal, E. H., & Saleh, M. M. (1988). Ultrastructural features of vocal fold nodules and polyps. Acta Otolaryngology, 105, 477–482.

Koufman, J. A. (1986). Laryngoplasty for vocal cord medialization: an alternative to teflon. *Laryngoscope, 96*, 726–731.

Koufman, J. A. (1991). The otolaryngologic manifestations of gastroesophageal reflux disease (GERD): a clinical investigation of 225 patients using ambulatory 24-hour pH monitoring and an experimental investigation of the role of acid and pepsin in the development of laryngeal injury. *Laryngoscope, 101*, 1–78.

Koufman, J. A. (1995). Gastroesophageal reflux and voice disorders. In J. S. Rubin, R. T. Sataloff, G. Korovin, & W. J. Gould (Eds.), Diagnosis and treatment of voice disorders (pp. 161–175). New York: Igaku-Shoin.

Koufman, J. A., & Blalock, P. D. (1991). Functional voice disorders. *Otolaryngologic Clinics of North America, 24*, 1059–1073.

Koufman, J. A., Postma, G. N., Cummins, M. M., & Blalock, P. D. (2000). Vocal fold paresis. *Otolaryngology—Head and Neck Surgery, 122*, 537–541.

Koufman, J. A., Sataloff, R. T., & Toohill, R. (1996). Laryngopharyngeal reflux: Consensus conference report. *Journal of Voice, 10*, 215–216.

Koufman, J. A., Wiener, G. J., Wu, W. C., & Castell, D. O. (1988). Reflux laryngitis and its sequelae: the diagnostic role of ambulatory 24-hour pH monitoring. *Journal of Voice, 2*, 78–90.

Kowald, A. (2001). The mitochondrial theory of aging. *Biol. Signals Recept., 10*, 162–175.

Kreiman, J., Gerratt, B. R., & Berke, G. S. (1994). The multidimensional nature of pathologic vocal quality. *Journal of the Acoustical Society of America, 96*, 1291–1302.

Kreiman, J., & Gerratt, B. (2000). Measuring vocal quality. In R. D. Kent & M. Ball (Eds.), *Voice quality measurement* (pp. 73–101). San Diego: Singular Publishing Group.

Kunze, L. H. (1964). Evaluation of methods of estimating sub-glottal air pressure. *Journal of Speech and Hearing Research, 7*, 151–164.

Kuroki, K. (1969). Subglottic pressure of normal and pathological larynges. *Otologia, 15*, 54–74.

Kurtzke, J. F., Beebe, G. W., Nagler, B., Auth, T. L., & Kurland, L. T. (1972). Studies on the natural history of multiple sclerosis. *Acta Neurologica Scandinavia, 48*, 19–46.

Ladefoged, P., & McKinney, N. P. (1963). Loudness, sound pressure and subglottal pressure in speech. *Journal of the Acoustical Society of America, 35*, 454–460.

Laitman, J., & Crelin, E. S. (1980). Developmental change in the upper respiratory system of human infants. *Perinatology/Neonatology, 4*, 15–22.

Lane, H. L., Catania, A. C., & Stevens, S. S. (1961). Voice level: Autophonic scale, perceived loudness and effects of sidetone. *Journal of the Acoustical Society of America, 33*, 160–167.

Lang, A. E., & Marsden, C. D. (1983). Spasmodic dysphonia in Gilles de la Tourette's disease. *Archives of Neurology, 40*, 51–52.

Langworthy, O. R., & Hesser, F. H. (1940). Syndrome of pseudobulbar palsy: an anatomic and physiologic analysis. *Archives of Internal Medicine, 65*, 106–121.

Larson, C. (1985). The midbrain periaqueductal gray: A brainstem structure involved in vocalization. *Journal of Speech and Hearing Research, 28*, 241–249.

Larson, C. R. (1988). Brain mechanisms involved in the control of vocalization. *Journal of Voice, 2*, 301–311.

Larson, C. R., & Kistler, M. K. (1986). The relationship of periaqueductal gray neurons to vocalization and laryngeal EMG in the behaving monkey. *Experimental Brain Research, 63*, 596–606.

Larson, C. R., Sutton, D., & Lindeman, R. C. (1978). Cerebellar regulation of phonation in rhesus monkey (Macaca mulatta). *Experimental Brain Research, 33*, 1.

Larson, K. K., Ramig, L. O., & Scherer, R. C. (1994). Acoustic and glottographic voice analysis during drug-related fluctuations in Parkinson disease. *Journal of Medical Speech and Language Pathology, 2*, 227–239.

Larsson, T., & Sjogren, T. (1960). Essential tremor. A clinical and genetic population study. *Acta Psychiatry Neurology (Scand), 36 (Suppl 144)*, 1–176.

Laurent, T. C., Laurent, U. B., & Fraser, J. R. (1995). Functions of hyaluronan. *Annals of the Rheumatic Diseases, 54*, 429–432.

Lavy, J. A., Wood, G., Rubin, J. S., & Harries, M. (2000). Dysphonia associated with inhaled steroids. *Journal of Voice, 14*, 581–588.

Lawrence, V. L. (1987). Common medications with laryngeal effects. *Ear, Nose, and Throat Journal, 66*, 318–322.

Leanderson, R., Meyerson, B. A., & Persson, A. (1972). Lip muscle function in Parkinsonian dysarthria. *Acta Oto-laryngologica (Stockholm), 74*, 350–357.

Leboldus, G. M., Savoury, L. W., Carr, T. J., & Nicholson, R. L. (1986). Magnetic resonance imaging: a review of basic principles and potential use in otolaryngology. *Journal of Otolaryngology, 15*, 273–278.

Lebrun, Y., Devreux, F., Rousseau, J., & Darimont, P. (1982). Tremulous speech. *Folia Phoniatrica, 34*, 134–142.

Lechtenberg, R., & Gilman, S. (1978). Speech disorders in cerebellar disease. *Annals of Neurology, 3*, 285–290.

Lee, K. J. (1973). *The otolaryngology boards.* New York: Medical Exam Publishing.

Leeper, H. A., Jr. (1976). Voice initiation characteristics of normal of children and children with vocal nodules: a preliminary investigation. *Journal of Communication Disorders, 9,* 83–94.

Leeper, H. A., Parsa, V., Jamieson, D. G., & Heeneman, H. (2002). Acoustical aspects of vocal function following radiotherapy for early T1a laryngeal cancer. *Journal of Voice, 16,* 289–302.

Lehmann, Q. H. (1965). Reverse phonation: a new maneuver for examining the larynx. *Radiology, 84,* 215–222.

LeJeune, F. E., Guice, C. E., & Samuels, P. M. (1983). Early experiences with vocal ligament tightening. *Annals of Otology, Rhinology and Laryngology, 92,* 475–477.

Leonard, R., & Kendall, K. (2001). Phonoscopy—a valuable tool for otolaryngologists and speech-language pathologists in the management of dysphonic patients. *Laryngoscope, 111,* 1760–1766.

Leonard, R. J., & Ringel, R. L. (1979). Vocal shadowing under conditions of normal and altered laryngeal sensation. *Journal of Speech and Hearing Research, 22,* 794–817.

Lessac, A. (1987). *The use and training of the human voice: a practical approach to speech and voice dynamics.* New York: Drama Book Publishers.

Lester, B. M. (1985). Introduction: there's more to crying than meets the ear. In B. M. Lester & C. F. Boukydis (Eds.), *Infant crying: theoretical and research perspectives* (pp. 1–28). New York: Plenum Press.

Levine, L., Hatlali, J. M., & Zaggy, M. (1985). Myasthenia gravis presenting as intermittent laryngeal paralysis. In V. Lawrence (Ed.), *Transcripts of the 14th symposium: care of the professional voice* (pp. 348–351). New York: Voice Foundation.

Leventhal, B. G., Kashima, H. K., Mounts, P., Thurmond, L., Chapman, S., Buckley, S. et al. (1991). Long-term response of recurrent respiratory papillomatosis to treatment with lymphoblastoid interferon alfa-N1. Papilloma Study Group. *New England Journal of Medicine, 325,* 613–617.

Lewis, K., Casteel, R., & McMahon, J. (1982). Duration of sustained /a/ related to number of trials. *Folia Phoniatrica et Logopedica, 34,* 41–48.

Lewy, R. B. (1993). Teflon injection: pointers and pitfalls. *Annals of Otology, Rhinology and Laryngology, 102,* 283–284.

Lichtenberger, G. (2002). Reversible lateralization of the paralyzed vocal cord without tracheostomy. *Annals of Otology, Rhinology, and Laryngology, 111,* 21–26.

Liden, S., & Gottfries, C. (1974). Beta-blocking agents in the treatment of catecholamine-induced symptoms in musicians. *Lancet, 2,* 529.

Lieberman, M., Malmgren, L., Woo, P., & Colton, R. H. (1986). The effect of tracheostomy on posterior cricoarytenoid muscle. *Laryngoscope, 96,* 1073–1082.

Lieberman, P. (1961). Perturbations in vocal pitch. *Journal of the Acoustical Society of America, 33,* 597–603.

Lieberman, P. (1963). Some acoustic measures of the fundamental periodicity of normal and pathologic larynges. *Journal of the Acoustical Society of America, 35,* 344–353.

Lieberman, P. (1968). Vocal cord motion in man. *Annals of the New York Academy of Sciences, 155,* 28–38.

Lin, E., Jiang, J., Hone, S., & Hanson, D. G. (1999). Photoglottographic measures in Parkinson's disease. *Journal of Voice, 13,* 25–35.

Lin, P., Stern, J. C., & Gould, W. J. (1991). Risk factors and management of vocal cord hemorrhages: an experience with 44 cases. *Journal of Voice, 5,* 74–77.

Linder, A., & Lindholm, C. E. (1992). Vocal fold lateralization using carbon dioxide laser and fibrin glue. *Journal of Laryngology and Otology, 106,* 226–230.

Lindestad, P. A., & Hertegard, S. (1994). Spindle-shaped glottal insufficiency with and without sulcus vocalis: A retrospective study. *Annals of Otology, Rhinology and Laryngology, 103,* 547–553.

Lindestad, P., & Persson, A. (1994). Quantitative analysis of EMG interference patterns in patients with laryngeal paresis. *Acta Oto-laryngologica (Stockholm), 114,* 91–97.

Linebaugh, C. (1979). The dysarthrias of Shy-Drager syndrome. *Journal of Speech and Hearing Disorders, 44,* 55–60.

Linville, S. E. (1987a). Acoustic-perceptual studies of aging voice in women. *Journal of Voice, 1,* 44–48.

Linville, S. E. (1987b). Maximum phonational frequency range capabilities of women's voices with advancing age. *Folia Phoniatrica, 39,* 297–301.

Linville, S. E. (1988). Intraspeaker variability in fundamental frequency stability: An age related phenomenon? *Journal of the Acoustical Society of America, 83,* 741–745.

Linville, S. E. (1992). Glottal gap configurations in two age groups of women. *Journal of Speech and Hearing Research, 35,* 1209–1215.

Linville, S. E. (2001). *Vocal Aging.* San Diego: Singular.

Linville, S. E., & Fisher, H. (1985). Acoustic characteristics of women's voices with advancing age. *Journal of Gerontology, 40,* 324–330.

Linville, S. E., & Fisher, H. (1985). Acoustic characteristics of perceived versus actual aging: controlled phonation by adult females. *Journal of the Acoustical Society of America, 78,* 40–48.

Linville, S. E., & Korabic, E. (1986). Elderly listener's estimates of vocal age in adult females.

Journal of the Acoustical Society of America, 80, 692–694.

Linville, S. E., Korabic, E. W., & Rosera, M. (1990). Intraproduction variability in jitter measures from elderly speakers. *Journal of Voice, 4*, 45–51.

Linville, S. E., & Rens, J. (2001). Vocal tract resonance analysis of aging voice using long–term average spectra. *Journal of Voice, 15*, 323–330.

Linville, S. E., Skarin, B. D., & Fornatto, E. (1989). The interrelationship of measures related to vocal function, speech rate, and laryngeal appearance in elderly women. *Journal of Speech and Hearing Research, 32*, 323–330.

Logemann, J. A., Fisher, H. B., Boshes, B., & Blonsky, E. R. (1978). Frequency and cooccurrence of vocal tract dysfunctions in the speech of a large sample of Parkinson patients. *Journal of Speech and Hearing Disorders, 42*, 47–57.

Longridge, N. S. (1987). Bilateral vocal cord paralysis in Shy-Drager syndrome. *Journal of Otolaryngology, 16*, 146–148.

Loire, R., Bouchayer, M., Cornut, G., & Bastian, R. W. (1988). Pathology of benign vocal fold lesions. *Ear, Nose, and Throat Journal, 67*, 357–362.

Lou, J. S., & Jankovic, J. (1991). Essential tremor: clinical correlates in 350 patients. *Neurology, 41*, 234–238.

Lowenthal, D. T., Kirschner, D. A., Scarpace, N. T., Pollock, M., & Graves, J. (1994). Effects of exercise on age and disease [review]. *Southern Medical Journal, 87*, S5–12.

Lowenthal, G. (1958). The treatment of polypoid laryngitis. *Laryngoscope, 68*, 1094–1104.

Löfqvist, A. (1993). Aerodynamic measurements of vocal function. In A. Blitzer, M. F. Brin, C. T. Sasaki, S. Fahn, & K. S. Harris (Eds.), *Neurologic disorders of the larynx* (pp. 98–107). New York: Thiem Medical Publishers, Inc.

Luchsinger, R., & Arnold, G. E. (1965). *Voice speech language clinical communicology: its physiology and pathology.* Belmont, CA: Wadsworth Publishing Co.

Lucier, G. E., Daynes, J., & Sessle, B. J. (1978). Laryngeal reflex regulation: peripheral and central neural analyses. *Experimental Neurology, 62*, 200–213.

Ludlow, C. (1981). Research needs for the assessment of phonatory function. In C. Ludlow & M. Hart (Eds.), Proceedings of the conference on vocal assessment of vocal pathology (pp. 3–8). Rockville, MD: American Speech-Language-Hearing Association.

Ludlow, C. L. (1990). Treatment of speech and voice disorders with botulinum toxin. *Journal of the American Medical Association, 264*, 2671–2675.

Ludlow, C. L. (1995). Management of the spasmodic dysphonias. In J. S. Rubin, R. T. Sataloff, G. S.

Korovin, & W. J. Gould (Eds.), *Diagnosis and treatment of voice disorders* (pp. 436–454). New York: Igaku-Shoin.

Ludlow, C. L., Connor, N. P., & Coulter, D. (1984). A preliminary investigation into the validity of an optimum frequency for phonatory functioning in patients with laryngeal pathology. In V. Lawrence (Ed.), Transcripts of the 12th symposium: care of the professional voice (pp. 155–168). New York: Voice Foundation.

Ludlow, C. L., Coulter, D., & Gentges, F. (1983). Differential sensitivity of frequency perturbation to laryngeal neoplasms and neuropathologies. In D. Bless & J. Abbs (Eds.), *Vocal fold physiology: contemporary research and clinical issues* (pp. 381–392). San Diego: College Hill Press.

Ludlow, C. L., Schulz, G. M., & Naunton, R. F. (1988). The effects of diazepam on intrinsic laryngeal muscle activation during respiration and speech. *Journal of Voice, 2*, 70–77.

Lufkin, R. B., & Hanafee, W. N. (1985). Application of surface coils to MR anatomy of the larynx. *American Journal of Nuclear Resonance, 6*, 491–497.

Luschei, E. S., Ramig, L. O., Baker, K. L., & Smith, M. E. (1999). Discharge characteristics of laryngeal single motor units during phonation in young and older adults and in persons with Parkinson's disease. *Journal of Neurophysiology, 81*, 2131–2139.

MacArthur, C. J., Kearns, G. H., & Healy, G. B. (1994). Voice quality after laryngotracheal reconstruction. *Archives of Otolaryngology—Head and Neck Surgery, 120*, 641–647.

MacCurtain, F., & Fourcin, A. J. (1982). Applications of the electroglottograph wave form display. In V. Lawrence (Ed.), *Transcripts of the Tenth Symposium: Care of the Professional Voice* (pp. 51–57). New York NY: The Voice Foundation.

Magriples, U., & Laitman, J. T. (1987). Developmental change in the position of the fetal human larynx. *American Journal of Physiology and Anthropology, 72*, 463–472.

Majewski, W., Hollien, H., & Zalewski, W. (1972). Speaking fundamental frequency of Polish adult males. *Phonetica, 25*, 119–125.

Mao, V. H., Abaza, M., Spiegel, J. R., Mandel, S., Hawkshaw, M., Heuer, R. J., et al. (2001). Laryngeal myasthenia gravis: report of 40 cases. *Journal of Voice, 15*, 122–130.

Marge, M. (1984). The prevention of communication disorders. *ASHA, 26*, 29–37.

Markel, N. N. (1965). The reliability of coding paralanguage: Pitch, loudness, and tempo. *Journal of Verbal Learning and Verbal Behavior, 4*, 306–308.

Markel, N. N., Meisels, M., & Houck, J. (1964). Judging personality from voice quality. *Journal of Abnormal Social Psychology, 69*, 458–463.

Martin, F. G. (1983). Drugs and the voice. In V. Lawrence (Ed.), *Transcripts of the Twelfth Symposium: Care of the Professional Voice (Part I)* (pp. 124–132). New York: The Voice Foundation.

Martin, F. G. (1984). The influence of drugs on voice (Part II). In V. Lawrence (Ed.), *Transcripts of the Thirteenth Symposium: Care of the Professional Voice Part II* (pp. 191–201). New York: The Voice Foundation.

Martin, F. G. (1988). Tutorial: Drugs and vocal function. *Journal of Voice, 2,* 338–344.

Martin, R., Blager, F., Gay, M., & Wood, R. (1987). Paradoxic vocal cord motion in presumed asthmatics. *Seminars in Respiratory Medicine, 9,* 332–337.

Martinez-Martin, P., & Bermejo-Pareja, F. (1988). Rating scales in Parkinson's disease. In J. Jankovic & E. Tolosa (Eds.), *Parkinson's disease and movement disorders* (pp. 235–240). Baltimore: Urban & Schwarzenberg.

Martins-Green, M. (1997). The dynamics of Cell-ECM interactions with implications for tissue engineering. In R. Lanza, R. Langer, & W. Chick (Eds.), *Principles of tissue engineering* (New York: RG Landes Company.

Maxwell, S., & Locke, J. (1969). Voice in myasthenia gravis. *Laryngoscope, 79,* 1902–1906.

McAllister, A., Sederholm, E., Sundberg, J., & Gramming, P. (1994). Relations between voice range profiles and physiological and perceptual voice characteristics in ten-year-old children. *Journal of Voice, 8,* 230–239.

McAllister, A., & Sundberg, J. (1998). Data on subglottal pressure and SPL at varied vocal loudness and pitch in 8- to 11-year-old children. *Journal of Voice, 12,* 166–174.

McClean, M. D. (1987). Surface EMG recordings of the perioral reflexes: preliminary observations on stutterers and non stutterers. *Journal of Speech and Hearing Research, 30,* 283–287.

McCulloch, T. M., & Hoffman, H. T. (1998). Medialization laryngoplasty with expanded polytetrafluoroethylene: surgical technique and preliminary results. *Annals of Otology, Rhinology, and Laryngology, 107,* 427–432.

McFarlane, S. C., Fujiki, M., & Brinton, B. (1984). *Coping with communicative handicaps: resources for the practicing clinician.* San Diego: College Hill Press.

McGlone, R. E., & Hollien, H. (1963). Vocal pitch characteristics of aged women. *Journal of Speech and Hearing Research, 6,* 164–170.

McGlone, R. E., & Hollien, H. (1964). An analysis of certain pitch characteristics of advanced age women. *Journal of Speech and Hearing Research, 6,* 164–170.

McGlone, R. E., & Hollien, H. (1969). Identification of the "shift" between vocal registers. *Journal of the Acoustical Society of America, 46,* 1033–1036.

McGlone, R. E., Richmond, W. H., & Bosma, J. F. (1966). A physiological model for investigation of the fundamental frequency of phonation. *Folia Phoniatrica et Logopedica, 18,* 109–116.

McGowan, R. S. (1992). Tongue-tip trills and vocal-tract wall compliance. *Journal of the Acoustical Society of America, 91,* 2903–2910.

Merritt, H. H. (1975). *A textbook of neurology* (5th ed.). Philadelphia: Lea & Febiger.

Merritt, H. H. (1979). *A textbook of neurology* (6th ed.). Philadelphia: Lea & Febiger.

Merson, R. M., & Ginsberg, A. P. (1979). Spasmodic dysphonia: abductor type. A clinical report of acoustic aerodynamic and perceptual characteristics. *Laryngoscope, 89,* 129–139.

Metz, D. E., Whitehead, R. L., & Peterson, D. H. (1980). An optical illumination system for high speed laryngeal cinematography. *Journal of the Acoustical Society of America, 67,* 719–720.

Michaels, L. (1984). *Pathology of the larynx.* New York: Springer-Verlag.

Michel, J. F., Hollien, H., & Moore, G. P. (1966). Speaking fundamental frequency characteristics of 15, 16 and 17 year-old girls. *Language and Speech, 9,* 46–51.

Michel, J. F., & Hollien, H. (1968). Perceptual differentiation of vocal fry and harshness. *Journal of Speech and Hearing Research, 11,* 439–443.

Miehlke, V. A., & Arnold, R. (1982). Chirurgie des Nervus Recurrense-ein Ausblick. In J. Berendes, R. Link, & F. Zollner (Eds.), *Hals-Nasen-Ohren-Heilkunde in Praxis and Klinik (Band 4 Teil 1)* (pp. 1–24). Stuttgart: Thieme Verlag.

Milczuk, H. A., Smith, J. D., & Everts, E. C. (2000). Congenital laryngeal webs: surgical management and clinical embryology. *International Journal of Pediatric Otorhinolaryngology, 52,* 1–9.

Miles, B., & Hollien, H. (1990). Whiter belting? *Journal of Voice, 4,* 64–70.

Millar, J. H. D. (1971). *Multiple sclerosis: a disease acquired in childhood.* Springfield: Charles C. Thomas.

Miller, J. E., & Mathews, M. V. (1963). Investigation of the glottal waveshape by automatic inverse filtering. *Journal of the Acoustical Society of America, 35,* 1876.

Miller, R. P., Gray, S. D., Cotton, R. T., & Myer, C. M. (1988). Airway reconstruction following laryngotracheal thermal trauma. *Laryngoscope, 98,* 826–829.

Milutinovic, Z., & Vasiljevic, J. (1992). Contribution to the understanding of the etiology of vocal fold cysts: a functional and histologic study. *Laryngoscope, 102,* 568–571.

Minifie, F. D. (1984). Against the clinical use of optimal pitch. In V. Lawrence (Ed.), *Transcripts of the 12th symposium: care of the professional voice* (Part II, pp. 148–154). New York: Voice Foundation.

Mitchell, G. (1993). Update on multiple sclerosis therapy [review]. *Medical Clinics of North America, 77,* 231–249.

Moll, K. L., & Peterson, G. E. (1969). Speaker and listener judgments of vowel levels. *Phonetica, 19,* 104–117.

Monday, L. A. (1983). Clinical evaluation of functional dysphonia. *Journal of Otolaryngology, 12,* 307–310.

Monoson, P., & Zemlin, W. R. (1984). Quantitative study of whisper. *Folia Phoniatrica, 36,* 53–65.

Montague, J. C., Brown, W. S., Jr., & Hollien, H. (1974). Vocal fundamental frequency characteristics of institutionalized Down's syndrome children. *American Journal of Mental Deficiency, 78,* 414–418.

Montague, J. C., Hollien, H., Hollien, P. A., & Wold, D. C. (1978). Perceived pitch and fundamental frequency comparisons of institutionalized Down's syndrome children. *Folia Phoniatrica et Logopedica, 30,* 245–256.

Moore, G. P. (1937). A short history of laryngeal investigation. *Quarterly Journal of Speech, 23,* 531–564.

Moore, G. P. (1975). Ultra high speed photography in laryngeal research. *Canadian Journal of Otolaryngology, 4,* 793–799.

Moore, G. P. (1977). Have the major issues in voice disorders been answered by research in speech science? A 50-year retrospective. *Journal of Speech and Hearing Disorders, 42,* 152–160.

Moore, G. P. (1986). Voice disorders. In G. H. Shames & E. H. Wiig (Eds.), *Human communication disorders: an introduction* (pp. 183–241). Columbus, OH: Charles E. Merrill.

Moore, G. P. (1996). The anatomy of the vocal mechanism. In W. S. Brown, Jr., B. P. Vinson, & M. A. Crary (Eds.), *Organic voice disorders assessment and treatment* (pp. 23–48). San Diego: Singular Publishing Group, Inc.

Moore, G. P., & Childers, D. G. (1984). Glottal area (real size) related to voice production. In V. Lawrence (Ed.), *Transcripts of the Twelfth Symposium: Care of the Professional Voice* (pp. 92–96). New York NY: The Voice Foundation.

Moore, G. P., Hicks, D. M., & Abbot, T. B. (1985). Defects of speech and language. In J. J. Ballenger (Ed.), *Diseases of the nose, throat, ear, head, and neck* (pp. 692–731). Philadelphia: Lea & Febiger.

Moore, G. P., & von Leden, H. S. (1958). Dynamic variations of the vibratory pattern in the normal larynx. *Folia Phoniatrica et Logopedica, 10,* 205–238.

Moore, G. P., White, F., & von Leden, H. S. (1962). Ultra high speed photography in laryngeal physiology. *Journal of Speech and Hearing Disorders, 27,* 165–171.

Morris, R. J., & Brown, W. S., Jr. (1987). Age related voice measures among adult women. *Journal of Voice, 1.*

Morris, R. J., & Brown, W. S., Jr. (1994). Age-related differences in speech intensity among adult females. *Folia Phoniatrica et Logopedica, 46,* 64–69.

Morris, R. J., & Brown, W. S., Jr. (1994). Age-related differences in speech variability among women. *Journal of Communication Disorders, 27,* 49–64.

Morris, R. J., Brown, W. S., Jr., Hicks, D. M., & Howell, E. (1995). Phonational profiles of male trained singers and nonsingers. *Journal of Voice, 9,* 142–148.

Morris, R. J., & Brown, W. S., Jr. (1996). Comparison of various automatic means for measuring mean fundamental frequency. *Journal of Voice, 10,* 159–165.

Morrison, M., & Rammage, L. (1994). *The management of voice disorders.* San Diego: Singular Publishing Group.

Morrison, M. D., & Rammage, L. A. (1993). Muscle misuse voice disorders: description and classification. *Acta Oto-Laryngologica, 113,* 428–434.

Morrison, M. D., & Rammage, L. A., Belisle, G. M., Pullan, C. B., & Nichol, H. (1983). Muscular tension dysphonia. *Journal of Otolaryngology, 12,* 302–306.

Mueller, P. B., Larson, G. W., & Summers, P. A. (1993). Additional data on s/z ratios in kindergarten children. *Language Speech Hearing Services in Schools, 24,* 177–178.

Mueller, P. B., Sweeney, R. J., & Baribeau, L. J. (1984). Acoustic and morphologic study of the senescent voice. *Ear, Nose, and Throat Journal, 63,* 292–295.

Muller, F., O'Rahilly, R., & Tucker, J. A. (1985). The human larynx at the end of the embryonic period proper. 2. The laryngeal cavity and the innervation of its lining. *Annals of Otology, Rhinology and Laryngology, 94,* 607–617.

Murphy, G., & Docherty, A. J. (1992). The matrix metalloproteinases and their inhibitors. *American Journal of Respiratory Cell and Molecular Biology, 7,* 120–125.

Murry, T. (1971). Subglottal pressure and airflow measures during vocal fry phonation. *Journal of Speech and Hearing Research, 14,* 544–551.

Murry, T. (1978). Speaking fundamental frequency characteristics associated with voice pathologies. *Journal of Speech and Hearing Disorders, 43,* 374–379.

Murry, T., Bone, R., & von Essen, C. (1974). Changes in voice production during radiotherapy for laryngeal cancer. *Journal of Speech and Hearing Disorders, 39*, 194–201.

Murry, T., & Brown, W. S., Jr. (1971). Regulation of vocal intensity during vocal fry phonation. *Journal of the Acoustical Society of America, 49*.

Murry, T., & Brown, W. S., Jr. (1971). Subglottal air pressure during two types of vocal activity: vocal fry and modal phonation. *Folia Phoniatrica et Logopedica, 23*, 440–449.

Murry, T., & Brown, W. S., Jr. (1975). Intraoral air pressure variability in esophageal speakers. *Folia Phoniatrica, 27*, 237–249.

Murry, T., Brown, W. S., Jr., & Morris, R. J. (1995). Patterns of fundamental frequency for three types of voice samples. *Journal of Voice, 9*, 282–289.

Murry, T., Brown, W. S., Jr., & Rothman, H. (1987). Judgments of vocal quality and preference: acoustic interpretations. *Journal of Voice, 1*, 252–257.

Murry, T., & Rosen, C. A. (2000). Outcome measurements and quality of life in voice disorders. *Otolaryngol. Clin. North Am., 33*, 905–916.

Murry, T., & Woodson, G. E. (1995). Combined-modality treatment of adductor spasmodic dysphonia with Botulinum toxin and voice therapy. *Journal of Voice, 9*, 460–465.

Murry, T., & Woodson, G. E. (1996). Spasmodic dysphonia. In W. S. Brown, Jr., B. P. Vinson, & M. A. Crary (Eds.), *Organic voice disorders assessment and treatment* (pp. 345–362). San Diego: Singular Publishing Group, Inc.

Mysak, E. D. (1959). Pitch and duration characteristics of older males. *Journal of Speech and Hearing Research, 2*, 46–54.

Mysak, E., & Hanley, T. (1959). Vocal aging. *Geriatrics, 14*, 652–656.

Nagler, W. (1987). *Dr. Nagler's body maintenance and repair book.* New York: Simon and Schuster.

Neely, J. L., & Rosen, C. (2000). Vocal fold hemorrhage associated with Coumadin therapy in an opera singer. *Journal of Voice, 14*, 272–277.

Neiman, G. S., & Edeson, B. (1981). Procedural aspects of eliciting maximum phonation time. *Folia Phoniatrica et Logopedica, 33*, 285–293.

Netterville, J. L., Koriwchak, M. J., Winkle, M., Courey, M. S., & Ossoff, R. H. (1996). Vocal fold paralysis following the anterior approach to the cervical spine. *Annals of Otology, Rhinology and Laryngology, 105*, 85–91.

Netterville, J. L., Stone, R. E., Luken, E. S., Civantos, F. J., & Ossoff, R. H. (1993). Silastic medialization and arytenoid adduction: the Vanderbilt experience. A review of 116 phonosurgical procedures. *Annals of Otology, Rhinology, and Laryngology., 102*, 413–424.

Newman, R. A., & Emanuel, F. W. (1991). Pitch effects on vowel roughness and spectral noise

for subjects in four musical voice classifications. *Journal of Speech and Hearing Research, 34*, 753–760.

Nielsen, V. M., Hojslet, P. E., & Karlsmose, M. (1986). Surgical treatment of Reinke's oedema (long-term results). *Journal of Laryngology and Otology, 100*, 187–190.

Nilson, H., & Schneiderman, C. R. (1983). Classroom program for the prevention of vocal abuse in elementary school children. *Language Speech Hearing Services in Schools, 14*, 172–178.

Noffsinger, D., Olsen, W. O., Carhart, R., Hart, C. W., & Sahgal, V. (1972). Auditory and vestibular aberrations in multiple sclerosis. *Acta Otolaryngologica (Stockholm), Suppl 303*, 1–63.

Olson, N. R. (1991). Laryngopharyngeal manifestations of gastroesophageal reflux disease. *Otolaryngologic Clinics of North America, 24*, 1201–1213.

Omori, K., Kacker, A., Slavit, D. H., & Blaugrund, S. M. (1996). Quantitative videostroboscopic measurement of glottal gap and vocal function: an analysis of thyroplasty type I. *Annals of Otology, Rhinology, and Laryngology, 105*, 280–285.

Omori, K., Slavit, D. H., Matos, C., Kojima, H., Kacker, A., & Blaugrund, S. M. (1997). Vocal fold atrophy—quantitative glottic measurement and vocal function. *Annals of Otology, Rhinology and Laryngology, 106*, 544–551.

Orlikoff, R. F. (1990). The atherosclerotic voice. *Ear Nose Throat J., 69*, 833–837.

Ortega, J. D., DeRosier, E., Park, S., & Larson, C. (1988). Brainstem mechanisms of laryngeal control as revealed by microstimulation studies. In O. Fujimura (Ed.), *Vocal fold physiology: voice production, mechanisms and function* (pp. 19–28). New York N.Y.: Raven Press.

Ossoff, R. H., Sisson, G. A., Duncavage, J. A., Moselle, H. I., Andrews, P. E., & McMillan, W. G. (1984). Endoscopic laser arytenoidectomy for the treatment of bilateral vocal cord paralysis. *Laryngoscope, 94*, 1293–1297.

Pabon, J. P. J. (1991). Objective acoustic voice-quality parameters in the computer phonetogram. *Journal of Voice, 5*, 203–216.

Padberg, G. W., & Bruyn, G. W. (1986). Chorea—differential diagnosis. In P. J. Vinken, G. W. Bruyn, & H. L. Klawans (Eds.), *Handbook of clinical neurology* (pp. 549–564). Amsterdam: Elsevier.

Pahn, J. (1966). Zur entwicklungund behandlung funktioneller singstimmerkrankugen. *Folia Phoniatrica, 18*, 117–130.

Painter, C. (1986). The laryngeal vestibule and voice quality. *Archives of Otolaryngology, 243*, 329–337.

Painter, C. (1988). Electroglottogram waveform types. *Archives of Oto-Rhino-Laryngology, 245*, 116–121.

Painter, C. (1991). The laryngeal vestibule, voice quality and paralinguistic markers. *European Archives of Oto-Rhino-Laryngology, 248*, 452–458.

Papp, P. (1983). *The process of change*. New York: Guilford Press.

Parnes, S. M. (1988). Laryngeal electromyography. *ENTechnology*, 48–51.

Parnes, S. M., Lavarato, A. B., & Myers, E. N. (1978). Study of spastic dysphonia using videofiberoptic laryngoscopy. *Annals of Otology, Rhinology and Laryngology, 87*, 322–326.

Parnes, S. M., & Satya-Murti, S. (1985). Predictive value of laryngeal electromyography in patients with vocal cord paralysis of neurogenic origin. *Laryngoscopy, 95*, 1323–1326.

Parsons-Winterter, P., & Sage, E. (1997). Regulation of cell behaviour by extracellular proteins. In R. Lanza & W. Chick (Eds.), *Principles of tissue engineering*. New York: RG Landes Company.

Pasic, T. R. (1996). Laryngeal ulcers. In W. S. Brown, Jr., B. P. Vinson, & M. A. Crary (Eds.), *Organic voice disorders assessment and treatment* (pp. 271–278). San Diego: Singular Publishing Group, Inc.

Pawlak, A. S., Hammond, T., Hammond, E., & Gray, S. D. (1996). Immunocytochemical study of proteoglycans in vocal folds. *Annals of Otology, Rhinology, and Laryngology, 105*, 6–11.

Peacher, G. (1947). Contact ulcer of the larynx I. history. *Journal of Speech and Hearing Disorders, 12*, 67.

Peacher, G., & Holinger, O. (1947). Contact ulcer of the larynx: II. The role of re-education. *Archives of Otolaryngology, 46*, 617–621.

Penfield, W., & Roberts, L. (1959). *Speech and brain mechanisms*. Princeton N.J.: Princeton University Press.

Pereira, J. G., Cervantes, O., Abrahao, M., Parenta Settanni, F. A., & Carrara, D. A. (2002). Noise-to-harmonics ratio as an acoustic measure of voice disorders in boys. *Journal of Voice, 16*, 28–31.

Perez, K. S., Ramig, L. O., Smith, M. E., & Dromey, C. (1994). The Parkinson larynx: tremor and videostroboscopic findings. *NCVS Status and Progress Report, 7*, 33–39.

Perie, S., St Guily, J. L., & Sebille, A. (1999). Comparison of perinatal and adult multi-innervation in human laryngeal muscle fibers. *Annals of Otology, Rhinology and Laryngology, 108*, 683–688.

Perie, S., Agbulut, O., St Guily, J. L., & Butler-Browne, G. S. (2000). Myosin heavy chain expression in human laryngeal muscle fibers: a biochemical study. *Annals of Otology, Rhinology and Laryngology, 109*, 216–220.

Perkins, W. (1971). *Speech pathology: an applied behavioral science*. St Louis: C.V. Mosby.

Perkins, W. H. (1983). Quantification of vocal behavior: a foundation for clinical management of voice. In D. M. Bless & J. Abbs (Eds.), *Vocal Fold Physiology: Contemporary Research and Clinical Issues* (pp. 425–431). San Diego: College-Hill Press.

Perkins, W. H. (1985). Assessment and treatment of voice disorders: state of the art. In Costello, J. (Ed.), *Speech disorders in adults: recent advances* (pp. 79–112). San Diego: College Hill Press.

Perlman, A. L., & Titze, I. R. (1988). Development of an in vitro technique for measuring elastic properties of vocal fold tissue. *Journal of Speech and Hearing Research, 31*, 288–298.

Perlman, A. L., Titze, I. R., & Cooper, D. S. (1984). Elasticity of canine vocal fold tissue. *Journal of Speech and Hearing Research, 27*, 212–219.

Piekarski, J. D. (1992). Imaging of the larynx. *Current Opinion in Radiology, 4*, 123–126.

Pinto, N. B., & Titze, I. R. (1960). Unification of perturbation measures in speech signals. *Journal of the Acoustical Society of America, 87*, 1278–1289.

Plomp, R. (1976). *Aspects of tone sensation*. New York: Academic Press.

Poburka, B. J. (1999). A new stroboscopy rating form. *Journal of Voice, 13*, 403–413.

Pontes, P., & Behlau, M. (1993). Treatment of sulcus vocalis: Auditory perceptual and acoustical analysis of the slicing mucosa surgical technique. *Journal of Voice, 7*, 365–376.

Prater, R. J., & Swift, R. W. (1984), *Manual of voice therapy*, Boston: Little, Brown.

Pressman, J. J. (1942). Physiology of vocal cords in phonation and respiration. *Archives of Otolaryngology, 35*, 355–398.

Pressman, J. J., & Kelemen, G. (1955). Physiology of the larynx. *Physiological Reviews, 35*, 506–554.

Prosek, R. A., Montgomery, A., Walden, B., & Schwartz, D. (1978). EMG feedback in the treatment of hyperfunctional voice disorders. *Journal of Speech and Hearing Disorders, 43*, 282–294.

Ptacek, P., & Sander, E. (1966). Age recognition from voice. *Journal of Speech and Hearing Research, 9*.

Ptacek, P. H., Sander, E., Maloney, W., & Jackson, C. C. (1966). Phonatory and related changes with advanced age. *Journal of Speech and Hearing Research, 9*, 353–360.

Rabuzzi, D., & McCall, G. N. (1972). Spasmodic dysphonia: a clinical perspective. *Transactions of the American Academy of Ophthalmology and Otolaryngology, 76*, 724–728.

Ramig, L. A. (1983). Effects of physiological aging on vowel spectral noise. *Journal of Gerontology, 38*, 223–225.

Ramig, L. A. (1986). Aging speech: Physiological and sociological aspects. *Language and Communication, 6*, 25–34.

Ramig, L. O. (1996). Neurological disorders of the voice. In W. S. Brown, Jr., B. P. Vinson, & M. A. Crary (Eds.), *Organic voice disorders assessment and treatment* (pp. 323–344). San Diego: Singular Publishing Group, Inc.

Ramig, L. A., & Gould, W. J. (1986). Speech characteristics in Parkinson's disease. *Neurologic Consultant, 4*, 1–8.

Ramig, L. O., Gray, S., Baker, K., Corbin-Lewis, K., Buder, E., Luschei, E. et al. (2001). The aging voice: a review, treatment data and familial and genetic perspectives. *Folia Phoniatr. Logop., 53*, 252–265.

Ramig, L. A., & Ringel, R. (1983). Effects of physiological aging on selected acoustic characteristics of voice. *Journal of Speech and Hearing Research, 26*, 22–30.

Ramig, L. A., Scherer, R. C., Klasner, E. R., Titze, I. R., & Horii, Y. (1990). Acoustic analysis of voice in amyotrophic lateral sclerosis: a longitudinal case study. *Journal of Speech and Hearing Disorders, 55*, 2–14.

Ramig, L. A., Scherer, R. C., Titze, I. R., & Ringel, S. P. (1988). Acoustic analysis of voices of patients with neurologic disease: rationale and preliminary data. *Annals of Otology, Rhinology and Laryngology, 97*, 164–172.

Ramig, L. O. (1995). Speech therapy for patients with Parkinson's disease. In W. C. Koller & G. Paulson (Eds.), *Therapy of Parkinson's disease.* (pp. 539–550). New York: Marcel Dekker.

Ramig, L. O., Bonitati, C. M., Lemke, J. H., & Horii, Y. (1994). Voice treatment for patients with Parkinson disease: development of an approach and preliminary efficacy data. *Journal of Medical Speech Language Pathology, 2*, 191–209.

Ramig, L. O., Mead, C., Scherer, R., Horii, Y., Larson, K., & Kohler, D. (1988). Voice therapy and Parkinson's disease: a longitudinal study of efficacy. Paper presented at the Clinical Dysarthria Conference, San Diego.

Ramig, L. O., & Scherer, R. C. (1992). Speech therapy for neurologic disorders of the larynx. In A. Blitzer, M. F. Brin, C. T. Sasaki, S. Fahn, & K. S. Harris (Eds.), *Neurologic disorders of the larynx* (pp. 163–181). New York: Thieme.

Randall, W. L. (1964). The behavior of cats (Felis catus) with lesions in the caudal midbrain region. *Behavior, 23*, 107–139.

Raphael, B. N., & Scherer, R. (1987). Voice modifications of stage actors: acoustic analyses. *Journal of Voice, 1*, 83–87.

Rasinger, G. A., Neuwirth-Riedi, K., & Kment, G. (1986). Erst ergebnisse digitaler Videobildanalyseverfahren zur Auswertung von endoskopischen. *Laryngo- Rhino- Otologic (Stuggart), 65*, 333–335.

Rastatter, M. P., & Hyman, M. (1982). Maximum phoneme duration of /s/ and /z/ by children with vocal nodules. *Language Speech Hearing Services in Schools, 13*, 197–199.

Ravits, J. (1988). Myasthenia gravis. a well-understood neuromuscular disorder. *Postgraduate Medicine, 83*, 219–223.

Reed, C. G. (1980). Voice therapy: a need for research. *Journal of Speech and Hearing Disorders, 45*, 157–169.

Reich, A. R., & Lerman, J. W. (1978). Teflon laryngoplasty: an acoustical and perceptual study. *Journal of Speech and Hearing Disorders, 43*, 496–505.

Reich, A. R., Mason, J. A., & Polen, S. B. (1986). Task administration variables affecting phonation time measures in 3rd grade girls with normal voice quality. *Language Speech Hearing Services in Schools, 17*, 262–269.

Reik, T. (1948). *Listening with the third ear.* New York: Farrar, Strauss & Giroux.

Reiser, D. E., & Schroder, A. K. (1980). *Patient interviewing, the human dimension.* Baltimore: Williams & Wilkins.

Riklan, M., & Levita, E. (1969). *Subcortical correlates of human behavior.* Baltimore: Williams and Wilkins Co.

Ringel, R. L., & Chodzko-Zajko, W. (1987). Vocal indices of biological age. *Journal of Voice, 1*, 31–37.

Robb, M. P., Goberman, A. M., & Cacace, A. T. (1997). An acoustic template of newborn infant crying. *Folia Phoniatr.Logop., 49*, 35–41.

Robb, M. P., & Goberman, A. M. (1997). Application of an acoustic cry template to evaluate at-risk newborns: preliminary findings. *Biology of the Neonate, 71*, 131–136.

Robe, E., Brumlik, J., & Moore, G. P. (1960). A study of spastic dysphonia. *Laryngoscope, 70*, 219–245.

Robertson, S., & Thompson, F. (1984). Speech therapy in Parkinson's disease: a study of the efficacy and long-term effect in intensive treatment. *British Journal of Disorders of Communication, 19*, 213–224.

Roche, A. F., & Barkla, D. H. (1965). The level of the larynx during childhood. *Annals of Otology, Rhinology and Laryngology, 74*, 645–654.

Rogers, J. H., & Stell, P. M. (1978). Paradoxical movement of the vocal cords as a cause of stridor. *Journal of Laryngology and Otology, 92*, 157–158.

Rolak, L. A. (2001). Multiple sclerosis treatment 2001. *Neurology Clinics, 19*, 107–118.

Rontal, E., & Rontal, M. (1986). The immobile cord. In C. Cummings, L. Harker, C. S. Krause, & D. Schuller (Eds.), *Otolaryngology—Head and Neck Surgery* (pp. 2055–2071). St. Louis: CV Mosby.

Rontal, M., Rontal, E., Leuchter, W., & Rolnick, M. (1978). Voice spectrography in the evaluation of myasthenia gravis of the larynx. *Archives of Oto-laryngology, 87,* 722–728.

Rosen, C. A. (1998). Complications of phono-surgery: results of a national survey. *Laryngoscope, 108,* 1697–1703.

Rosen, C. A., & Murry, T. (2000). Voice handicap index in singers. *J Voice, 14,* 370–377.

Rosen, C. A., & Murry, T. (2000). Nomenclature of voice disorders and vocal pathology. *Otolaryngology Clinics of North America, 33,* 1035–1046.

Rosen, D. C., & Sataloff, R. T. (1997). *The psychology of voice.* San Diego: Singular Publishing Group.

Rosenfield, D. B. (1987). Neurolaryngology. *Ear, Nose, and Throat Journal, 66,* 323–326.

Rosenthal, R. S. (1978). Malpractice: cause and its prevention. *Laryngoscope, 88,* 1–11.

Rothenberg, M. (1968). The breath stream dynamics of simple-released plosive production. *Bibliotheca Phonetica, 6.*

Rothenberg, M. (1973). A new inverse filtering technique for deriving the glottal air flow during voicing. *Journal of the Acoustical Society of America, 53,* 1632–1645.

Rothenberg, M. (1977). Measurement of air flow during speech. *Journal of Speech and Hearing Research, 2,* 155–176.

Rothenberg, M. (1981). Some relations between glottal air flow and vocal fold contact area. In C. Ludlow & M. Hart (Eds.), *Proceeding of the Conference on the Assessment of Vocal Pathology* (pp. 88–96). Rockville MD: American Speech-Language-Hearing Association.

Rothenberg, M. (1982). Interpolating subglottal pressure from oral pressure. *Journal of Speech and Hearing Disorders, 47,* 218–224.

Rothenberg, M., & Mahshie, J. J. (1988). Monitoring vocal fold abduction through vocal fold contact area. *Journal of Speech and Hearing Research, 31,* 338–351.

Rothman, H. B., Brown, W. S., Jr., Sapienza, C. M., & Morris, R. J. (2001). Acoustic analyses of trained singers perceptually identified from speaking samples. *Journal of Voice, 15,* 25–35.

Rothman, H. B., Brown, W. S., Jr., & LaFond, J. R. (2002). Spectral changes due to performance environment in singers, nonsingers, and actors. *Journal of Voice, 16,* 323–332.

Rousseau, B., Hirano, S., Wlham, N., Thibeault, S., Bless, D., & Ford, C. (2002). Histological characterization of chronic vocal fold scarring in a rabbit model. 6th International Voice Symposium of Australia. Australia.

Roy, N. (1994). Manual tension reduction: an alternative with functional voice disorders: paper presented at the convention of the American Speech-Language-Hearing Association, New Orleans, LA.

Roy, N. (2004). Psychogenic voice disorders: direct therapy. In R. D. Kent (Ed.), *MIT encyclopedia of communication disorders.* Cambridge, MA: MIT Press.

Roy, N., Gray, S. D., Simon, M., Dove, H., Corbin-Lewis, K., & Stemple, J. C. (2001). An evaluation of the effects of two treatment approaches for teachers with voice disorders: a prospective randomized clinical trial. *Journal of Speech, Language, and Hearing Research, 44,* 286–296.

Roy, N., & Leeper, H. A. (1993). Effects of the manual laryngeal musculoskeletal tension reduction technique as a treatment for functional voice disorders: perceptual and acoustic measures. *Journal of Voice, 7,* 242–249.

Roy, N., Tasko, S. M., & Harvey, S. (1995). Treatment results using the manual laryngeal musculoskeletal tension reduction procedure. Paper presented at the convention of the American Speech-Language-Hearing Association, New Orleans, LA.

Roy, N., Weinrich, B., Gray, S. D., Tanner, K., Toledo, S. W., Dove, H. et al. (2002). Voice amplification versus vocal hygiene instruction for teachers with voice disorders: a treatment outcomes study. *Journal of Speech, Language, and Hearing Research, 45,* 625–638.

Rubin, H. J. (1965). Pitfalls in treatment of dysphonias by intracordal injection of synthetics. *Laryngoscope, 75,* 381–395.

Rubin, H. J., & LeCover, M. (1960). Technique of high speed photography of the larynx. *Annals of Otology, Rhinology and Laryngology, 69,* 1072–1082.

Rubin, J. S., Benjamin, E., Prior, A., Lavy, J., & Ratcliffe, P. (2002). The prevalence of Helicobacter pylori infection in benign laryngeal disorders. *Journal of Voice, 16,* 87–91.

Rullan, A. (1991). Associated laryngeal paralysis. *Archives of Otolaryngology, 64,* 207–212.

Rutala, D. R., Rutala, W. A., Weber, D. J., & Thomann, C. A. (1991). Infection risks associated with spirometry. *Infection Control and Hospital Epidemiology, 12,* 89–92.

Rutala, W. A. (1990). APIC guideline for selection and use of disinfectants. *American Journal of Infection Control, 18,* 99–117.

Rutala, W. A., Clontz, E. P., Weber, D. J., & Hoffmann, K. K. (1991). Disinfection practices for endoscopes and other semicritical items. *Infection Control and Hospital Epidemiology, 12,* 282–288.

Ryan, E. B., & Capadano, H. L. (1978). Age perceptions and evaluative reactions toward adult speakers. *Journal of Gerontology, 33,* 98–102.

Ryan, W. J. (1972). Acoustic aspects of the aging voice. *Journal of Gerontology, 27,* 265–268.

Ryan, W. J., & Burk, K. W. (1974). Perceptual and acoustic correlates of aging in the speech of males. *Journal of Communication Disorders, 7*, 181–192.

Sackner, M. A. (1980). Monitoring of ventilation without physical connection to the airway. In M. A. Sackner (Ed.), *Diagnostic techniques in pulmonary disease* (pp. 503–537). New York N.Y.: Dekker.

Sant'Ambrogio, G., Mathew, O. P., Fisher, J. T., & Sant'Ambrogio, F. B. (1983). Laryngeal receptors responding to transmural pressure, airflow and local muscle activity. *Respiration Physiology, 54*, 317–330.

Salam, M. Z., & Adams, R. D. (1978). The Arnold-Chiari malformation. In P. J. Vinken, G. W. Bruyn, & N. C. Myrianthopoulos (Eds.), *Handbook of clinical neurology* (pp. 99–110). Amsterdam: North Holland.

Salamy, J. N., & Sessions, R. B. (1980). Spastic dysphonia. *Journal of Fluency Disorders, 5*, 281–290.

Sander, E. K. (1989). Arguments against the aggressive pursuit of voice treatment for children. *Language Speech Hearing Services in Schools, 20*, 94–101.

Sapienza, C. M., & Stathopoulos, E. T. (1994). Respiratory and laryngeal measures of children and women with bilateral vocal fold nodules. *Journal of Speech and Hearing Research, 37*, 1229–1243.

Sapienza, C. M., Stathopoulos, E. T., & Brown, W. S., Jr. (1997). Speech breathing during reading in women with vocal nodules. *Journal of Voice, 11*, 195–201.

Sapienza, C. M., Murry, T., & Brown, W. S., Jr. (1998). Variations in adductor spasmodic dysphonia: acoustic evidence. *Journal of Voice, 12*, 214–222.

Sataloff, R. T. (1981). Professional singers: the science and art of clinical care. *American Journal of Otolaryngology, 2*, 251–266.

Sataloff, R. T. (1983). Physical examination of the professional singer. *Journal of Otolaryngology, 12*, 277–281.

Sataloff, R. T. (1986). The professional voice. In C. Cummings, L. Harker, C. S. Krause, & D. Schuller (Eds.), *Otolaryngology-Head Neck Surgery* (pp. 2029–2053). St. Louis: Mosby.

Sataloff, R. T. (1987). Clinical evaluation of the professional singer. *Ear, Nose, and Throat Journal, 66*, 267–277.

Sataloff, R. T. (1987). The professional voice: Part I. Anatomy, function and general health. *Journal of Voice, 1*, 92–104.

Sataloff, R. T. (1987). The professional voice: Part III. Common diagnoses and treatments. *Journal of Voice, 1*, 283–292.

Sataloff, R. T. (1987). The professional voice: Part II. Physical examination. *Journal of Voice, 1*, 191–201.

Sataloff, R. T. (2000). Laryngeal electromyography. *Current Opinion in Otolaryngology & Head & Neck Surgery, 8*, 524–529.

Sataloff, R. T., Hawkshaw, M., Lyons, K. M., & Spiegel, J. R. (1997). Laryngeal granuloma: progression and resolution. *Ear Nose & Throat Journal, 76*, 618.

Sataloff, R. T., & Hawkshaw, M. J. (2000). Teflon granuloma. *Ear Nose & Throat Journal, 79*, 422.

Sataloff, R. T., Ressue, J. C., Portell, M., Harris, R. M., Ossoff, R., Merati, A. L., et al. (2000). Granular cell tumors of the larynx. *Journal of Voice, 14*, 119–134.

Sataloff, R. T., Spiegel, J., Carroll, L., Darby, K., & Rulnick, R. (1987). Objective measures of voice function. *Ear, Nose, and Throat Journal, 66*, 307–312.

Sato, K., & Hirano, M. (1997). Age–related changes of elastic fibers in the superficial layer of the lamina propria of vocal folds. *Annals of Otology, Rhinology, and Laryngology, 106*, 44–48.

Sawashima, M. (1966). Measurements of the phonation time. *Japanese Journal of Logopedics and Phoniatrics, 7*, 23–29.

Sawashima, M., & Hirose, H. (1981). Abduction-adduction of the glottis in speech and voice production. In K. N. Stevens & M. Hirano (Eds.), *Vocal fold physiology* (pp. 329–346). Tokyo Japan: University of Tokyo Press.

Sawashima, M., Sato, M., Funasaka, S., & Totsuk, G. (1958). Electromyographic study of the human larynx and its clinical application. *Journal of Otolaryngology of Japan, 61*, 1357–1364.

Sayani, K., Dodd, C. M., Nedelec, B., Shen, Y. J., Ghahary, A., Tredget, E. E., et al. (2000). Delayed appearance of decorin in healing burn scars. *Histopathology, 36*, 262–272.

Scherer, R. C., & Titze, I. R. (1987). The abduction quotient related to vocal quality. *Journal of Voice, 1*, 246–251.

Scherer, R. C., Brewer, D. W., Colton, R., Rubin, L. S., Raphael, B. N., Miller, R. et al. (1994). The integration of voice science, voice pathology, medicine, public speaking, acting, and singing. *Journal of Voice, 8*, 359–374.

Schiffman, S. S., Reynolds, M. L., & Young, F. W. (1981). *Introduction to multidimensional scaling: theory, methods, application*. New York: Academic Press.

Schilling, R. (1925). Experimentell-phonetische Untersuchunger bei Erkrankunger des extrapyramidalen Systems. *Archives Psychiatrica Nevenkr, 75*, 419–471.

Schultz-Coulon, H. J. (1984). [Clinical course and therapy of congenital malformation of the larynx.] *HNO, 32,* 135–148.

Schutte, H. K., Svec, J. G., & Sram, F. (1998). First results of clinical application of videokymography. *Laryngoscope, 108,* 1206–1210.

Scott, S., & Cairn, F. L. (1983). Speech therapy for Parkinson's disease. *Journal of Neurology, Neurosurgery and Psychiatry, 46,* 140–144.

Segre, R. (1971). Senescence of the voice. *Ear, Nose and Throat Monthly, 50,* 223–233.

Senturia, B. H., & Wilson, F. B. (1968). Otorhinolaryngologic findings in children with voice deviations. *Annals of Otology, Rhinology and Laryngology, 77,* 1027–1042.

Sercarz, J. A., Berke, G. S., Ming, Y., Gerratt, B. R., & Natividad, M. (1992). Videostroboscopy of human vocal fold paralysis. *Annals of Otology, Rhinology and Laryngology, 101,* 567–577.

Sessions, R. B., Dichtel, W. J., & Goepfert, H. (1984). Treatment of recurrent respiratory papillomatosis with interferon. *Ear Nose & Throat Journal, 63,* 488–493.

Sessions, R. B., Miller, S. D., Martin, B. F., Solomon, B. I., Harrison, L. B., & Stackpole, S. (1989). Videolaryngostroboscopic analysis of minimal glottic cancer. *Transactions of the American Laryngological Association, 110,* 56–59.

Shaefer, S. D. (1983). Neuropathology of spasmodic dysphonia. *Laryngoscope, 93,* 1183–1202.

Shaefer, S. D., Freeman, F., Finitzo, T., Close, L., & Cannito, M. (1985). Magnetic resonance imaging findings and correlations in spasmodic dysphonia patients. *Annals of Otology, Rhinology and Laryngology, 94,* 595–601.

Shaefer, S. D., Roark, R. M., Watson, B. C., Kondraske, G. V., Freeman, F. J., Butsch, R. W., & Pohl, J. (1992). Multichannel electromyographic observations in spasmodic dysphonia patients and normal control subjects. *Annals of Otology, Rhinology and Laryngology, 101,* 67–75.

Sharbrough, F. W., Stockard, J. J., & Aronson, A. E. (1975). Brainstem auditory evoked responses in spastic dysphonia. *Transactions of the American Neurological Association, 103,* 198–201.

Shearer, W. (1983). s/z ratio for detection of vocal nodules. *Folia Phoniatrica, 35,* 172.

Shigemori, Y. (1977). Some tests related to the air usage during phonation: Clinical investigations. *Otologia, 23,* 138–166.

Shin, T., Watanabe, H., Oda, M., Umezaki, T., & Nahm, I. (1994). Contact granulomas of the larynx. *European Archives in Otorhinolaryngology, 251,* 67–71.

Shindo, M. L., & Hanson, D. G. (1990). Geriatric voice and laryngeal dysfunction. *Otolaryngologic Clinics of North America, 23,* 1035–1044.

Shindo, M. L., Zaretsky, L. S., & Rice, D. H. (1996). Autologous fat injection for unilateral vocal fold paralysis. *Annals of Otology, Rhinology and Laryngology, 105,* 602–606.

Shipp, T. (1975). Vertical laryngeal position during continuous and discrete vocal frequency change. *Journal of Speech and Hearing Research, 18,* 707–718.

Shipp, T. (1980). Vertical laryngeal position in singing. *Transcripts of the 9th Symposium: Care of the Professional Voice, Part II,* 46–54.

Shipp, T. (1987). Vertical laryngeal position: research findings and application for singers. *Journal of Voice, 1,* 217–219.

Shipp, T., & Huntington, D. (1965). Some acoustic and perceptual factors in acute–laryngitic hoarseness. *Journal of Speech and Hearing Disorders, 30,* 350–359.

Shipp, T., & Hollien, H. (1969). Perception of the aging male voice. *Journal of Speech and Hearing Research, 12,* 703–710.

Shipp, T., Guinn, L., Sundberg, J., & Titze, I. R. (1987). Vertical laryngeal position–research findings and their relationship to singing. *Journal of Voice,* 220–222.

Shipp, T., & Izdebski, K. (1975). Vocal frequency and vertical larynx positioning by singers and nonsingers. *Journal of the Acoustical Society of America, 58,* 1104–1106.

Shipp, T., Izdebski, K., Schutte, H. K., & Morrissey, P. (1988). Subglottal air pressure in spastic dysphonia speech. *Folia Phoniatrica, 40,* 105–110.

Shipp, T., & McGlone, R. (1971). Laryngeal dynamics associated with voice frequency change. *Journal of Speech and Hearing Research, 14,* 761–768.

Shipp, T., Mueller, P., & Zwitman, D. (1980). Intermittent abductory dysphonia. *Journal of Speech and Hearing Disorders, 45,* 283.

Shohet, J. A., Courey, M. S., Scott, M. A., & Ossoff, R. H. (1966). Value of videostroboscopic parameters in differentiating true vocal fold cysts from polyps. *Laryngoscope, 106,* 19–26.

Shvero, J., Koren, R., Hadar, T., Yaniv, E., Sandbank, J., Feinmesser, R. et al. (2000). Clinicopathologic study and classification of vocal cord cysts. *Pathol.Res.Pract., 196,* 95–98.

Silverman, E. M., & Zimmer, C. H. (1975). Incidence of chronic hoarseness among school age children. *Journal of Speech and Hearing Disorders, 40,* 211–215.

Simkin, B. (1964). Corticosteroids in clinical practice. *Eye, Ear, Nose and Throat Monthly, 43* (3), 47–54.

Simpson, G. T., & Strong, M. S. (1983). Recurrent respiratory papillomatosis: the role of the carbon dioxide laser. *Otolaryngology Clinics of North America, 16,* 887–894.

Singh, W., & Ainsworth, W. A. (1992). Computerised measurement of fundamental frequency in Scottish neoglottal patients. *Folia Phoniatrica et Logopedica, 44*, 231–237.

Siribodhi, C., Sundmaker, W., Atkins, J. P., & Bonner, F. L. (1963). Electromyographic studies of laryngeal paralysis and regeneration of laryngeal motor nerve in dogs. *Laryngoscope, 73*, 148–164.

Smith, E., Gray, S. D., Dove, H., Kirchner, L., & Heras, H. (1997). Frequency and effects of teachers' voice problems. *Journal of Voice, 11*, 81–87.

Smith, E., Taylor, M., Mendoza, M., Barkmeier, J., Lemke, J., & Hoffman, H. (1998). Spasmodic dysphonia and vocal fold paralysis: outcomes of voice problems on work-related functioning. *Journal of Voice, 12*, 223–232.

Smith, M. E., Marsh, J. H., Cotton, R. T., & Myer, C. M. III (1993). Voice problems after pediatric laryngotracheal reconstruction: videolaryngostroboscopic, acoustic and perceptual assessment. *International Journal of Pediatric Otorhinolaryngology, 25*, 173–181.

Smith, M. E., & Ramig, L. O. (1995). Neurological disorders and the voice. In J. S. Rubin, R. T. Sataloff, G. S. Korovin, & Gould (Eds.), *Diagnosis and treatment of voice disorders* (pp. 203–224). New York: Igaku-Shoin.

Smith, M. E., Ramig, L. O., Dromey, C., Perez, K. S., & Samandari, R. (1994). Intensive voice treatment in Parkinson's disease: laryngostroboscopic findings. *NCVS Status and Progress Report, 6*, 127–133.

Smith, O. D., Callanan, V., Harcourt, J., & Albert, D. M. (2000). Intracordal cyst in a neonate. *International Journal of Pediatric Otorhinolaryngology, 52*, 277–281.

Smitheran, J. R., & Hixon, T. J. (1981). A clinical method for estimating air way resistance during vowel production. *Journal of Speech and Hearing Disorders, 46*, 138–146.

Snow, J. B., Hirano, M., & Balough, K. (1966). Postintubation granuloma of the larynx. *Anesthesia and Analgesia, 45*, 425.

Södersten, M., & Lindestad, P. A. (1990). Glottal closure and perceived breathiness during phonation in normally speaking subjects. *Journal of Speech and Hearing Research, 33*, 601–611.

Solomon, N. P., McCall, G. N., Trosset, M. W., Gray, W. C. (1989). Laryngeal configuration and constriction during two types of whispering. *Journal of Speech and Hearing Research, 32*, 161–174.

Sondi, M. M. (1975). Measurement of the glottal waveform. *Journal of the Acoustical Society of America, 57*, 228–232.

Sonesson, B. (1959). A method for studying the vibratory movements of the vocal cords. *Journal of Laryngology and Otology, 73*, 732–737.

Sonesson, B. (1960). On the anatomy and vibratory pattern of the human vocal folds. *Acta Oto-Laryngologica.Supplement, 156*, 1–80.

Sorensen, D., & Parker, P. (1993). Response to Mueller, Larson and Summers. *Language Speech Hearing Services in Schools, 24*, 178–179.

Sorin, R., McClean, M. D., Ezerzer, F., & Meissner-Fishbein, B. (1987). Electroglottographic evaluation of the swallow. *Archives of Physical Medicine and Rehabilitation, 68*, 232–235.

Spector, G. J., & Ogura, J. H. (1985). Tumors of the larynx and laryngopharynx. In J. J. Ballenger (Ed.), *Diseases of the nose, throat, ear, head, and neck* (pp. 549–602). Philadelphia PA: Lea and Febiger.

Stark, D. D., Moss, A. A., Gamsu, G., Clark, O. H., & Gooding, G. A. (1984). Magnetic resonance imaging of the neck. Part I: Normal anatomy. *Radiology, 150*, 447–454.

Stathopoulos, E. T., & Sapienza, C. (1993). Respiratory and laryngeal function of women and men during vocal intensity variation. *Journal of Speech and Hearing Research, 36*, 64–75.

Stathopoulos, E. T., & Sapienza, C. M. (1997). Developmental changes in laryngeal and respiratory function with variations in sound pressure level. *Journal of Speech, Language, and Hearing Research, 40*, 595–614.

Stathopoulos, E. T., & Weismer, G. (1985). Oral airflow and air pressure during speech production: a comparative study of children, youths and adults. *Folia Phoniatr. (Basel), 37*, 152–159.

Stemple, J. (2004). Voice therapy: holistic techniques. In R. D. Kent (Ed.), *MIT encyclopedia of communication disorders*. Cambridge, MA: MIT Press.

Stemple, J., Weider, E., Whitehead, W., & Komray, R. (1980). Electromyographic biofeedback training with patients exhibiting a hyperfunctional voice disorder. *Laryngoscope, 90*, 471–475.

Stemple, J. C., Glaze, L., & Gerdeman, B. (1995). *Clinical voice pathology: theory and management* (2nd ed.). San Diego: Singular Publishing Group.

Stevens, K. N., & House, A. (1961). An acoustical theory of vowel production and some of its implications. *Journal of Speech and Hearing Research, 4*, 303–320.

Stoicheff, M. (1981). Speaking fundamental frequency characteristics of nonsmoking female adults. *Journal of Speech and Hearing Research, 24*, 437–441.

Stoicheff, M., Giampi, A., Passi, J., & Fredrickson, J. (1983). The irradiated larynx and voice: a perceptual study. *Journal of Speech and Hearing Research, 26*, 482–485.

Stone, R. E., Jr. (1983). Issues in clinical assessment of laryngeal function: contraindications for subscribing to maximum phonation time and optimum fundamental frequency. In D. M. Bless & J. H. Abbs (Eds.), *Vocal fold physiology: contemporary research and clinical issues* (pp. 410–424). San Diego: College Hill Press.

Strand, E. A., Buder, E. H., Yorkston, K. M., & Ramig, L. O. (1993). Differential phonatory characteristics of women with amyotrophic lateral sclerosis. *NCVS Status and Progress Report, 4,* 151–167.

Stuart, W. D. (1965). The otolaryngologic aspects of myasthenia gravis. *Laryngoscope, 75:*112–121.

Sundberg, J. (1974). Articulatory interpretation of the 'singing formant'. *Journal of the Acoustical Society of America, 55,* 838–844.

Sundberg, J. (1987). *The science of the singing voice.* DeKalb, IL: Northern Illinois University Press.

Sundberg, J., & Askenfelt, A. (1983). Larynx height and voice source: A relationship. In D. M. Bless & J. Abbs (Eds.), *Vocal fold physiology: contemporary research and physiology* (pp. 307–316). College Hill Press: San Diego.

Sundberg, J., Titze, I., & Scherer, R. (1993). Phonatory control in male singing: a study of the effects of subglottal pressure, fundamental frequency, and mode of phonation on the voice source. *Journal of Voice, 7,* 15–29.

Surow, J. B., & Lovetri, J. (2000). "Alternative medical therapy" use among singers: prevalence and implications for the medical care of the singer. *Journal of Voice, 14,* 398–409.

Svec, J. G., & Schutte, H. K. (1996). Videokymography: High-speed line scanning of vocal fold vibration. *Journal of Voice, 10,* 201–205.

Svensson, G., Schalen, L., & Fex, S. (1988). Pathogenesis of idiopathic contact granuloma of the larynx: results of a prospective clinical study. *Acta Otolaryngol.Suppl, 449,* 123–125.

Swenson, M. R., Zwirner, P., Murry, T., & Woodson, G. E. (1992). Medical evaluation of patients with spasmodic dysphonia. *Journal of Voice, 6,* 320–324.

Symington, J. (1881). On the relations of the larynx and trachea to the vertebral column in the fetus and child. *Edinburgh Medical Journal, 26,* 913–916.

Taft, J. M. (1988). Acute inflammatory demyelinating polyradiculoneuropathy: the Landry, Guillain-Barré, Strol syndrome. *American Academy of Physician Assistants, 1,* 219–223.

Tait, N. A., Michel, J. F., & Carpenter, M. A. (1980). Maximum duration of sustained /s/ and /z/ in children. *Journal of Speech and Hearing Disorders, 45,* 239–246.

Takahashi, H., & Koike, Y. (1975). Some perceptual dimensions and acoustical correlates of pathologic voices. *Acta Oto-Laryngologica, 338,* 1–24.

Tanaka, S., & Gould, W. (1985). Vocal efficiency and aerodynamic aspects in voice disorders. *Annales d'Oto-Laryngologie et de Chirurgie Cervico-Faciale, 94,* 29–33.

Tanaka, S., Hirano, M., & Chijiwa, K. (1994). Some aspects of vocal fold bowing. *Annals of Otology, Rhinology and Laryngology, 103,* 357–362.

Tasko, S. M., Roy, N., & Harvey, S. (1994). Using manual laryngeal tension reduction techniques with benign mucosal disorders. Paper presented at the convention of the American Speech-Language-Hearing Association, New Orleans, LA.

Teter, D. L. (1976). Voice disorders. In English, G. M. (Ed.), Otolaryngology: a textbook (pp. 584–599). New York: Harper & Row.

Thack, B. T. (2001). Maturation and transformation of reflexes that protect the laryngeal airway from liquid aspiration from fetal to adult life. *American Journal of Medicine, 111 Suppl. 8A,* 69S–77S.

Thibeault, S. L., Gray, S. D., Li, W., Ford, C. N., Smith, M. E., & Davis, R. K. (2002). Genotypic and phenotypic expression of vocal fold polyps and Reinke's edema: a preliminary study. *Ann. Otol. Rhinol. Laryngol., 111,* 302–309.

Thibeault, S. L., Gray, S. D., Bless, D. M., Chan, R. W., & Ford, C. N. (2002). Histologic and rheologic characterization of vocal fold scarring. *Journal of Voice, 16,* 96–104.

Thomas, J. E., & Schirger, A. (1970). Idiopathic orthostatic hypotension. a study of its natural history in 57 neurologically affected patients. *Archives of Neurology, 22,* 289–293.

Thompson, A. R. (1995). Medications and the voice. In J. S. Rubin, R. T. Sataloff, G. S. Korovin, & W. J. Gould (Eds.), *Diagnosis and treatment of voice disorders* (pp. 237–246). New York: Igaku-Shoin.

Timcke, R., von Leden, H. S., & Moore, G. P. (1958). Laryngeal vibrations: measurements of the glottic wave Part I: The normal vibratory cycle. *Archives of Otolaryngology, 68,* 1–19.

Timcke, R., von Leden, H. S., & Moore, G. P. (1959). Laryngeal vibrations: measurements of the glottic wave Part II: Physiologic variations. *Archives of Otolaryngology, 69,* 438–444.

Titze, I. R. (1981). Heat generation in the vocal folds and its possible effect on vocal endurance. In V. Lawrence (Ed.), *Transcripts of the 10th symposium: care of the professional voice* (pp. 52–59). New York: Voice Foundation.

Titze, I. R. (1984). Parameterization of the glottal area, glottal flow and vocal fold contact area. *Journal of the Acoustical Society of America, 75,* 570–580.

Titze, I. R. (1990). Interpretation of the electroglottographic signal. *Journal of Voice, 4,* 1–9.

Titze, I. R. (1992). Phonation threshold pressure—A missing link in glottal aerodynamics. *Journal of the Acoustical Society of America, 91,* 2926–2935.

Titze, I. R. (1994). *Principles of voice production*. Englewood Cliffs: Prentice-Hall Inc.

Titze, I. R. (1995). Workshop on *Acoustic Voice Analysis—Summary Statement*. Iowa City: National Center for Voice and Speech. Ref Type: Pamphlet.

Titze, I. R. (1996). Regulation of fundamental frequency with a physiologically-based model of the larynx. *National Center for Voice and Speech, 9*, 117–124.

Titze, I. R., & Sundberg, J. (1992). Vocal intensity in speakers and singers. *Journal of the Acoustical Society of America, 91*, 2936–2946.

Titze, I. R., & Talkin, D. (1981). Simulation and interpretation of glottographic waveforms. In C. L. Ludlow & M. Hart (Eds.), *Proceedings of the Conference on the Assessment of Vocal Pathology* (pp. 48–55). Rockville, MD: American Speech-Language-Hearing Association.

Toohill, R. J. (1975). The psychosomatic aspects of children with nodules. *Archives of Otolaryngology, 101*, 591–595.

Trapp, T. K., & Berke, G. S. (1988). Photoelectric measurement of laryngeal paralyses correlated with videostroboscopy. *Laryngoscope, 98*, 486–492.

Tsunoda, K., Soda, Y., Tojima, H., Shinogami, M., Ohta, Y., Nibu, K. et al. (1997). Stroboscopic observation of the larynx after radiation in patients with T1 glottic carcinoma. *Acta Oto-Laryngologica*, 165–166.

Tucker, H. M. (1977). Reinnervation of the unilaterally paralyzed larynx. *Annals of Otology, Rhinology and Laryngology, 86*, 789–794.

Tucker, H. M. (1978). Human laryngeal reinnervation: Long term experience with the nerve-muscle pedicle technique. *Laryngoscope, 88*, 598–604.

Tucker, H. M. (1980). Vocal cord paralysisetiology and management. *Laryngoscope, 90*, 585–590.

Tucker, H. M. (1985). Anterior commissure laryngoplasty for adjustment of vocal fold tension. *Annals of Otology, Rhinology and Laryngology, 94*, 547–549.

Tucker, H. M. (1987). *The larynx*. New York: Thieme Medical Publishers, Inc.

Tucker, H. M. (1989). Laryngeal framework surgery in the management of spasmodic dysphonia: preliminary report. *Annals of Otology, Rhinology and Laryngology, 98*, 52–54.

Tucker, H. M., & Lavertu, P. (1992). Paralysis and paresis of the vocal folds. In A. Blitzer, M. F. Brin, C. T. Sasaki, S. Fahn, & K. S. Harris (Eds.), *Neurologic disorders of the larynx* (pp. 182–189). New York: Thieme.

Tucker, H. M., & Rusnov, M. (1981). Laryngeal reinnervation for unilateral vocal cord paralysis: long term results. *Annals of Otology, Rhinology and Laryngology, 90*, 457–459.

Unal, M. (2004). The successful management of congential laryngeal web with endoscopic lysis and topical mitomycin-C. *International Journal of Pediatric Otorhinolaryngology, 68*, 231–235.

Ungerleider, S. (1986). Athletes in motion: training for the Olympic games with mind and body: two case studies. Paper presented at International Conference on Mental Health and Technology, Winnipeg, Canada.

U.S. Cancer Statistics Working Group (2002). *United States Cancer Statistics: 1999 Incidence*. Atlanta, GA: Department of Health and Human Services, Centers for Disease Control and Prevention and National Cancer Institute.

U.S. Department of Health and Human Services (1985). *The health consequences of smoking: Cancer and chronic diseases in the workplace; A report of the Surgeon General*. Washington DC: U.S. Government Printing Office.

U.S. Department of Health and Human Services (1986). *The health consequences of smoking: A public health service review, 1967–1985*. Washington DC: U. S. Government Printing Office.

Vallancien, B., Gautheron, B., Pasternak, L., Guisez, D., & Paley, B. (1971). Comparaison des signaux microphoniques, diaphanographiques et glottographiques avec application au laryngographe. *Folia Phoniatrica, 23*, 371–380.

van den Berg, J. W. (1956). Physiology and physics of voice production. *Acta Physiologica et Pharmacologica Neerl, 5*, 40–55.

van den Berg, J. W. (1958). Myoelastic–aerodynamic theory of voice production. *Journal of Speech and Hearing Research, 1*, 227–244.

van den Berg, J. W., & Tan, T. S. (1959). Results of experiments with human larynges. *Practica Oto-Rhino-Laryngologica, 21*, 425–450.

Vaughan, C. W. (1982). Diagnosis and treatment of organic voice disorders. *New England Journal of Medicine, 307*, 863–866.

Verdolini, K. (1999). Critical analysis of common terminology in voice therapy: a position paper. *Phonoscope, 2*, 1–8.

Verdolini, K. (2004). Voice therapy for adults. In R. D. Kent (Ed.), *MIT encyclopedia of communication disorders*. Cambridge, MA: MIT Press.

Verdolini, K., Hess, M. M., Titze, I. R., Bierhals, W., & Gross, M. (1999). Investigation of vocal fold impact stress in human subjects. *Journal of Voice, 13*, 184–202.

Verdolini, K., Hoffman, H. T., & McCoy, S. (1994). Nonspecific laryngeal granuloma: a case study of a professional singer. *Journal of Voice, 8*, 352–358.

Verdolini-Marston, K., Titze, I. R., & Druker, D. G. (1990). Changes in phonation threshold pressure with induced conditions of hydration. *Journal of Voice*, *4*, 142–151.

Verdolini-Marston, K., Burke, M. K., Lessac, A., Glaze, L., & Caldwell, E. (1995). Preliminary study of two methods of treatment for laryngeal nodules. *Journal of Voice*, *9*, 74–85.

Verdolini, K., & Titze, I. R. (1995). The application of laboratory formulas to clinical voice management. *American Journal of Speech-Language Pathology*, *4*, 62–69.

Verdolini, K., Titze, I. R., & Fennell, A. (1994). Dependence of phonatory effort on hydration level. *Journal of Speech and Hearing Research*, *37*, 1001–1007.

Von Doersten, P. G., Izdebski, K., Ross, J. C., & Cruz, R. M. (1992). Ventricular dysphonia: a profile of 40 cases. *Laryngoscope*, *102*, 1296–1301.

von Euler, C. (1986). Brain stem mechanisms for generation and control of breathing pattern. In N. S. Cherniack & J. G. Widdicombe (Eds.), *Handbook of physiology, Section 3, The respiratory system* (pp. 1–67). Bethesda: American Physiological Society.

von Leden, H. (1985). Vocal nodules in children. *Ear, Nose and Throat Journal*, *64*, 473–480.

von Leden, H. (1991). The history of phonosurgery. In C. N. Ford & D. M. Bless (Eds.), *Phonosurgery assessment and surgical management of voice disorders* (pp. 3–24). New York: Raven Press.

von Leden, H., & Isshiki, N. (1965). An analysis of cough at the level of the larynx. *Archives of Otolaryngology*, *81*, 616–625.

von Leden, H., & Moore, G. P. (1960). Contact ulcer of the larynx: experimental observations. *Archives of Otolaryngology*, *72*, 746–752.

von Leden, H., Moore, P., & Timcke, R. (1960). Laryngeal vibrations: measurements of the glottic wave. Part III. The pathologic larynx. *Archives of Otolaryngology*, *71*, 26–45.

von Leden, H. S., & Moore, G. P. (1961). Vibratory patterns of the vocal cords in unilateral laryngeal paralysis. *Acta Oto-Laryngologica*, *53*, 493–506.

von Leden, H. S., LeCover, M., Ringel, R. L., & Isshiki, N. (1966). Improvements in laryngeal cinematography. *Archives of Otolaryngology—Head and Neck Surgery*, *83*, 482–487.

Walker, F. O. (1997). Voice fatigue in myasthenia gravis: the sinking pitch sign. *Neurology*, *48*, 1135–1136.

Ward, P. H. (1973). Congenital malformations of the larynx. In M. M. Paparella (Ed.), *Otolaryngology* (pp. 603–608). Philadelphia: Saunders.

Ward, D. (1990). Voice-onset time and electroglottographic dynamics in stutterers' speech: implications for a differential diagnosis. *British Journal of Disorders of Communication*, *25*, 93–104.

Ward, P. H., Cannon, D., & Lindsay, J. R. (1965). The vestibular system in multiple sclerosis. *Laryngoscope*, *75*, 1031–1046.

Ward, P. H., Colton, R., McConnell, F., Malmgren, L., Kashima, H., & Woodson, G. (1989). Aging of the voice and swallowing. *Otolaryngology-Head and Neck Surgery*, *100*, 283–286.

Ward, P. H., Hanson, D., & Berci, G. (1981). Observations on central neurologic etiology for laryngeal dysfunction. *Annals of Otolaryngology*, *90*, 430–441.

Ward, P. D., Thibeault, S. L., & Gray, S. D. (2002). Hyaluronic acid: its role in voice. *Journal of Voice*, *16*, 303–309.

Ward, P. H., Zwitman, D., Hanson, D., & Berci, G. (1980). Contact ulcers and granulomas of the larynx: new insights into their etiology as a basis for a more rational treatment. *Archives of Otolaryngology—Head and Neck Surgery*, *88*, 262–269.

Warr-Leeper, G. A., McShea, R. S., & Leeper, H. (1979). The incidence of voice and speech deviations in a middle school population. *Language Speech Hearing Services in Schools*, *10*, 14–20.

Warner, D. O. (1998). Laryngeal reflexes: exploring terra incognita. *Anesthesiology*, *88*, 1433–1434.

Warren, R. M. (1962). Are 'autophonic' judgments based on loudness? *American Journal of Psychology*, *75*, 452–456.

Warren, W. R., Gutmann, L., & Cody, R. (1977). Stapedius reflex decay in myasthenia gravis. *Archives of Neurology*, *34*, 496–497.

Waters, K. A., Woo, P., Mortelliti, A. J., & Colton, R. (1996). Assessment of the infant airway with video recorded flexible laryngoscopy and the objective analysis of vocal fold abduction. *Otolaryngology—Head and Neck Surgery*, *114*, 554–561.

Watkin, K. L., & Ewanowski, S. J. (1979). The effects of Triamcinolone Acetonide on the voice. *Journal of Speech and Hearing Research*, *22*, 446–455.

Watson, H. (1979). The technology of respiratory inductive plethysmography. *3rd International Symposium on Ambulatory Monitoring*, 1–24.

Watson, P. J., Hixon, T. J., & Maher, M. Z. (1987). To breathe or not to breathe—That is the question: an investigation of speech breathing kinematics in world class Shakespearean actors. *Journals of Voice*, *1*, 269–272.

Watterson, T., Hensen-Magorian, H. J., & McFarlane, S. C. (1988). A demographic description of laryngeal contact ulcers. Paper given at the convention of American Speech Language Hearing Association. Boston: November 1988.

Wechsler, E. (1976). A laryngographic study of voice disorders. *British Journal of Disorders of Communication*, *12*, 9–22.

Weiss, R., Brown, W. S., Jr., & Morris, J. (2001). Singer's formant in sopranos: fact or fiction? *J Voice*, *15*, 457–468.

Weinberg, B., Bosma, J. F., Shanks, J. C., & DeMyer, W. (1968). Myotonic dystrophy initially manifested by speech disability. *Journal of Speech and Hearing Disorders*, *33*, 51–59.

Wendahl, R. W. (1963). Laryngeal analog synthesis of harsh voice quality. *Folia Phoniatrica et Logopedica*, *15*, 241–250.

Wendahl, R. (1966). Some parameters of auditory roughness. *Folia Phoniatrica et Logopedica*, *18*, 26–32.

Wendahl, R. W., & Coleman, R. F. (1967). Vocal cord spectra derived from glottal-area waveforms and subglottal photocell monitoring. *Journal of the Acoustical Society of America*, *41*, 1613A.

Wendahl, R. W., Moore, G. P., & Hollien, H. (1963). Comments on vocal fry. *Folia Phoniatrica et Logopedica*, *15*, 251–255.

Wendler, J., Doherty, E. T., & Hollien, H. (1980). Voice classification by means of long-term speech spectra. *Folia Phoniatrica et Logopedica*, *32*, 51–60.

Wendler, J., Köppen, K., & Fischer, S. (1986). The validity of stroboscopic data in terms of quantitative measures. In S. R. Hibi, D. Bless, & M. Hirano (Eds.), *Proceedings of International Conference on Voice* (pp. 36–43). Kurume, Japan: Kurume University.

Weymuller, E. A. (1988). Laryngeal injury from prolonged endotracheal intubation. *Laryngoscope*, *98*, 1–15.

Wexler, D. B., Jiang, J., Gray, S. D., & Titze, I. R. (1989). Phonosurgical studies: fat-graft reconstruction of injured canine vocal cords. *Annals of Otology, Rhinology and Laryngology*, *98*, 668–673.

Whurr, R., Nye, C., & Lorch, M. (1998). Meta-analysis of botulinum toxin treatment of spasmodic dysphonia: a review of 22 studies. *International Journal of Language and Communication Disorders*, *33 Suppl*, 327–329.

Williams, A. J., Baghat, M. S., DeStableforth, C. R. M., Shenoi, P. M., & Skinner, C. (1983). Dysphonia caused by inhaled steroids: recognition of a characteristic laryngeal abnormality. *Thorax*, *38*, 813–821.

Williams, A. J., Hanson, D., & Calne, D. B. (1979). Vocal cord paralysis in the Shy-Drager syndrome. *Journal of Neurology, Neurosurgery and Psychiatry*, *42*, 151–153.

Williams, R. T., Farquharson, I. M., & Anthony, J. (1975). Fiberoptic laryngoscopy in the assessment of laryngeal disorder. *Journal of Laryngology and Otology*, *89*, 299–306.

Wilson, D. K. (1987). *Voice problems of children*. (3rd ed.) Baltimore: Williams and Wilkins.

Wilson, F. B., & Lamb, M. M. (1973). Comparison of personality characteristics of children with and without vocal nodules on Rorschach protocol interpretation. Paper presented at the convention of the American Speech Language Hearing Association. Atlanta, GA.

Wilson, F. B., & Rice, M. A. (1977). *A programmed approach to voice therapy*. Austin: Learning Concepts.

Wilson, F. B., Wellen, C. J., & Kimbarow, M. L. (1983). Perception of the fundamental frequencies of children's voices by trained and untrained listeners. *Journal of Otolaryngology*, *12*, 341–344.

Wilson, J., Pryde, A., Cecilia, A., & Macintyre, C. (1989). Normal pharyngoesophageal motility: a study of 50 healthy subjects. *Digestive Diseases and Sciences*, *34*, 1590–1599.

Wippold, F. J. (2000). Diagnostic imaging of the larynx. In C. W. Cummings (Ed.), *Otolaryngology head & neck surgery* (3rd ed.), New York: Mosby.

Wirz, S., & Anthony, J. (1979). The use of the Voiscope in improving the speech of profoundly deaf children. *British Journal of Disorders of Communication*, *14*, 137–152.

Wolfe, V. I., & Bacon, M. (1976). Spectrographic comparison of two types of spastic dysphonia. *Journal of Speech and Hearing Disorders*, *41*, 325–332.

Wolfe, V., & Martin, D. (1997). Acoustic correlates of dysphonia: type and severity. *Journal of Communication Disorders*, *30*, 403–415.

Wolfe, V. I., & Ratusnik, D. L. (1988). Acoustic and perceptual measurements of roughness influencing judgments of pitch. *Journal of Speech and Hearing Disorders*, *53*, 15–22.

Wolfe, V. I., & Steinfatt, T. (1987). Prediction of vocal severity within and across voice types. *Journal of Speech and Hearing Research*, *30*, 230–240.

Wolski, W. (1967). Hypernasality as the presenting symptom of myasthenia gravis. *Journal of Speech and Hearing Research*, *32*, 36–38.

Woo, P. (1996). The irritated larynx: edema and inflammation. In W. S. Brown, Jr., B. P. Vinson, & M. A. Crary (Eds.), *Organic Voice Disorders Assessment and treatment* (pp. 193–218). San Diego: Singular Publishing Group, Inc.

Woo, P., & Arandia, H. (1992). Intraoperative laryngeal electromyographic assessment of patients with immobile vocal fold. *Annals of Otology, Rhinology and Laryngology*, *101*, 799–806.

Woo, P., Casper, J., Brewer, D., & Colton, R. H. Long-term voice complications after prolonged intubation. *Archives of Otolaryngology—Head and Neck Surgery*, (in press).

Woo, P., Casper, J., Colton, R., & Brewer, D. (1992). Dysphonia in the aging: Physiology versus disease. *Laryngoscope*, *102*, 139–144.

Woo, P., Casper, J. K., Colton, R. H., & Brewer, D. W. (1994). Aerodynamic and stroboscopic findings before and after microlaryngeal phonosurgery. *Journal of Voice, 8*, 186–194.

Woo, P., Casper, J. K., Colton, R. H., & Brewer, D. W. (1994). Diagnosis and treatment of persistent dysphonia after laryngeal surgery: a retrospective analysis of 62 patients. *Laryngoscope, 104*, 1084–1091.

Woo, P., Casper, J., Griffin, B., Colton, R. H., & Brewer, D. (1995). Endoscopic microsuture repair of vocal fold defects. *Journal of Voice, 9*, 332–339.

Woo, P., Colton, R., Brewer, D., & Casper, J. (1991). Functional staging for vocal cord paralysis. *Otolaryngology—Head and Neck Surgery, 105*, 440–448.

Woo, P., Colton, R. H., Casper, J. K., & Brewer, D. W. (1991). Diagnostic value of stroboscopic examination in hoarse patients. *Journal of Voice, 5*, 231–238.

Woo, P., Colton, R. H., Casper, J. K., & Brewer, D. W. (1992). Analysis of spasmodic dysphonia by aerodynamic and laryngostroboscopic measurements. *Journal of Voice, 6*, 344–351.

Woo, P., Colton, R. H., & Shangold, L. (1987). Phonatory airflow analysis in patients with laryngeal disease. *Annals of Otology, Rhinology and Laryngology, 96*, 549–555.

Woodson, G. E. (1996). The voice care team. In W. S. Brown, Jr., B. P. Vinson, & M. A. Crary (Eds.), *Organic voice disorders assessment and treatment* (pp. 112–118). San Diego: Singular Publishing Group, Inc.

Wright, H. N., & Colton, R. H. (1972). Some parameters of autophonic level. Paper presented at the convention of American Speech Language Hearing Association.

Wright, H. N., & Colton, R. H. (1972). Some parameters of vocal effort. *Journal of the Acoustical Society of America, 51*, 141A.

Wuyts, F. L., Heylen, L., Mertens, F., De Bodt, M., & Van de Heyning, P. H. (2002). Normative voice range profiles of untrained boys and girls. *Journal of Voice, 16*, 460–465.

Wuyts, F. L., Heylen, L., Mertens, F., Du, C. M., Rooman, R., Van de Heyning, P. H., et al. (2003). Effects of age, sex, and disorder on voice range profile characteristics of 230 children. *Annals of Otology, Rhinology and Laryngology, 112*, 540–548.

Wyke, B. (1967). Recent advances in the neurology of phonation: phonatory reflex mechanisms in the larynx. *British Journal of Disorders of Communication, 2*, 2–14.

Wyke, B. (1969). Deus ex machina vocis: An analysis of the laryngeal reflex mechanisms of speech. *British Journal of Disorders of Communication, 4*, 3–25.

Wynder, E. L., Lemon, F. R., & Mantel, N. (1965). Epidemiology of persistent cough. *American Review of Respiratory Diseases., 91*, 679–700.

Wynder, E. L., Covey, L. S., Mabuchi, K., & Muchinski, M. (1976). Environmental factors in cancer of the larynx: a second look. *Cancer, 38*, 1591–1601.

Wynder, E. L., & Stellman, S. D. (1977). Comparative epidemiology of tobacco-related cancers. *Cancer, 37*, 4608–4622.

Yajima, Y., Hayashi, Y., & Yoshii, N. (1982). Ambiguus motoneurons discharging closely associated with ultrasonic vocalization in rats. *Brain Research, 238*, 445–450.

Yamaguchi, H., Yotsukura, Y., Sata, H., Watanabe, Y., Hirose, H., & Kobayashi, N. (1993). Pushing exercise program to correct glottal incompetence. *Journal of Voice, 7*, 250–256.

Yanagihara, N. (1967a). Hoarseness: investigation of the physiological mechanisms. *Annals of Otology, Rhinology and Laryngology, 76*, 472–488.

Yanagihara, N. (1967b). Significance of harmonic changes and noise components in hoarseness. *Journal of Speech and Hearing Research, 10*, 531–541.

Yanagihara, N., & von Leden, H. (1967). Respiration and phonation. *Folia Phoniatrica, 19*, 153–166.

Ylitalo, R., & Hammarberg, B. (2000). Voice characteristics, effects of voice therapy, and long-term follow-up of contact granuloma patients. *Journal of Voice, 14*, 557–566.

Yoshida, Y., Mitsumasu, T., Hirano, M., Morimoto, M., & Kanaseki, T. (1987). Afferent connections to the nucleus ambiguus in the brainstem of the cat—an HRP study. In T. Baer, C. Sasaki, & K. Harris (Eds.), *Laryngeal function in phonation and respiration* (pp. 45–61). San Diego: College Hill Press.

Young, R. R. (1986). Essential-familial tremor. In P. J. Vinken, G. W. Bruyn, & H. L. Klawans (Eds.), Handbook of clinical neurology (pp. 565–582). Amsterdam: Elsevier.

Yumoto, E. (1987). Quantitative assessment of the degree of hoarseness. *Journal of Voice, 1*, 310–313.

Yumoto, E., Gould, W. J., & Baer, T. (1982). Harmonics-to-noise ratio as an index of the degree of hoarseness. *Journal of the Acoustical Society of America, 71*, 1544–1550.

Yumoto, E., Kadota, Y., & Kurokawa, H. (1993). Infraglottic aspect of canine vocal fold vibration: effect of increase of mean airflow rate and lengthening of vocal fold. *Journal of Voice, 7*, 311–318.

Yumoto, E., Sasaki, Y., & Okamura, H. (1984). Harmonics-to-noise ratio and psychological measurement of the degrees of hoarseness. *Journal of Speech and Hearing Research, 27*, 2–6.

Zaretsky, L. S., Shindo, M. L., deTar, M., & Rice, D. H. (1995). Autologous fat injection for vocal fold paralysis: long-term histologic evaluation. *Annals of Otology, Rhinology and Laryngology, 104*, 1–4.

Zeitels, S. M. (1995). Premalignant epithelium and microinvasive cancer of the vocal fold: the evolution of phonomicrosurgical management. *Laryngoscope, 105*, 1–51.

Zeitels, S. M., & Vaughan, C. W. (1991). A submucosal true vocal fold infusion needle. *Otolaryngology—Head and Neck Surgery, 105*, 478–479.

Zeitels, S. M., Hochman, I., & Hillman, R. E. (1998). Adduction arytenopexy: a new procedure for paralytic dysphonia with implications for implant medialization. *Annals of Otology, Rhinology and Laryngology, Suppl, 173*, 2–24.

Zeitels, S. M., Hillman, R. E., Desloge, R. B., & Bunting, G. A. (1999). Cricothyroid subluxation: a new innovation for enhancing the voice with laryngoplastic phonosurgery. *Annals of Otology, Rhinology and Laryngology, 108*, 1126–1131.

Zemlin, W. R. (1962). A comparison of the periodic function of vocal fold vibration in a multiple sclerosis and a normal population. Unpublished doctoral dissertation, University of Minnesota.

Zemlin, W. R. (1988). *Speech and Hearing Science: Anatomy and physiology.* Englewood Cliffs NJ: Prentice Hall.

Zhang, S. P., Davis, P. J., Carrive, P., & Bandler, R. (1992). Vocalization and marked pressor effect evoked from the region of the nucleus retroambigualis in the caudal ventrolateral medulla of the cat. *Neuroscience Letters, 140*, 103–107.

Zhang, S. P., Davis, P. J., Bandler, R., & Carrive, P. (1994). Brain stem integration of vocalization: role of the midbrain periaqueductal gray. *Journal of Neurophysiology, 72*, 1337–1356.

Zwirner, P., Murry, T., Swenson, M., & Woodson, G. E. (1991). Acoustic changes in spasmodic dysphonia after botulinum toxin injection. *Journal of Voice, 5*, 78–84.

Zwitman, D. (1979). Bilateral cord dysfunctions: abductor type spastic dysphonia. *Journal of Speech and Hearing Disorders, 44*, 373–378.

Figure and Table Credits

Figures

Figure 2.3. Coleman, R. F., Mabis, J. H., & Hinson, J. K. (1977). Fundamental frequency-sound pressure level profiles of adult male and female voices. *Journal of Speech and Hearing Research, 20,* 197–204.

Figures 4.1–4.7. Cornut, G., & Bouchayer, M. (2004). *Assessing dysphonia: the role of videostroboscopy.* KayPentax: Lincoln Park, NJ.

Figure 5.3. Colton, R. H., & Brewer, D. W. (1985). Fiberoptic/vibratory relationships in patients with voice disorders. In V. Lawrence (Ed.), *Transcripts of the 14th symposium: care of the professional voice* (pp. 271–275). New York: Voice Foundation.

Figure 5.4. Aronson, A. E., Brown, J. R., Litin, E. M., & Pearson, J. S. (1968). Spastic dysphonia II. Comparison with essential (voice) tremor and other neurologic and psychogenic dysphonias. *Journal of Speech and Hearing Disorders, 33,* 219–231.

Figure 5.5. Smith, M. E., Ramig, L. O., Dromey, C., Perez, K. S., & Samandari, R. (1994). Intensive voice treatment in Parkinson's disease: Laryngostroboscopic findings. *NCVS Status and Progress Report, 6,* 127–133.

Figures 5.6–5.7. Perez, K. S., Ramig, L. O., Smith, M. E., & Dromey, C. (1994). The Parkinson larynx: tremor and videostroboscopic findings. *NCVS Status and Progress Report, 7,* 33–39.

Figure 5.8. Hanson, D. G., Ludlow, C., & Bassich, C. (1983). Vocal fold paresis in Shy-Drager syndrome. *Annals of Otology, Rhinology, and Laryngology, 92,* 85–90.

Figure 5.9. A. Terris, D. J., Arnstein, D. P., & Nguyen, H. H. (1992). Contemporary evaluation of unilateral vocal cord paralysis [review]. *Otolaryngology—Head and Neck Surgery, 107,* 84–90. **B.** Tucker, H. M. (1980). Vocal cord paralysis—etiology and management. *Laryngoscope, 90,* 585–590.

Figures 5.11–5.12. Hanson, D. G., Gerratt, B. R., Karin, R. R., & Berke, G. S. (1988). Glottographic measures of vocal fold vibration: an examination of laryngeal paralysis. *Laryngoscope, 98,* 541–549.

Figure 5.13. Casper, J. K., Colton, R. H., & Brewer, D. W. (1985). Selected therapy techniques and laryngeal physiological changes in patients with vocal fold immobility. In V. Lawrence (Ed.), *Transcripts of the 14th symposium: care of the professional voice* (pp. 318–323). New York: Voice Foundation.

Figure 5.14. Aronson, A. E., Brown, J. R., Litin, E. M., & Pearson, J. S. (1968). Spastic dysphonia, I. Voice, neurologic, and psychiatric aspects. *Journal of Speech and Hearing Disorders, 33,* 203–218.

Figure 5.15. Izdebski, K. (1984). Overpressure and breathiness in spastic dysphonia. *Acta Otolaryngologica (Stockholm), 97,* 373–378.

Figure 5.16. Wolfe, V. I., & Bacon, M. (1976). Spectrographic comparison of two types of spastic dysphonia. *Journal of Speech and Hearing Disorders, 41,* 325–332.

Figure 5.17. Aronson, A. E., Brown, J. R., Litin, E. M., & Pearson, J. S. (1968). Spastic dysphonia II. Comparison with essential (voice) tremor and other neurologic and psychogenic dysphonias. *Journal of Speech and Hearing Disorders, 33,* 219–231.

Figures 5.19. Aronson, A. E., Brown, J. R., Litin, E. M., & Pearson, J. S. (1968). Spastic dysphonia II. Comparison with essential (voice) tremor and other neurologic and psychogenic dysphonias. *Journal of Speech and Hearing Disorders, 33,* 219–231.

Figures 5.20. Aronson, A. E., Brown, J. R., Litin, E. M., & Pearson, J. S. (1968). Spastic dysphonia II. Comparison with essential (voice) tremor and other neurologic and psychogenic dysphonias. *Journal of Speech and Hearing Disorders, 33,* 219–231.

Figure 5.21. Aronson, A. E., Brown, J. R., Litin, E. M., & Pearson, J. S. (1968). Spastic dysphonia II. Comparison with essential (voice) tremor and other neurologic and psychogenic dysphonias. *Journal of Speech and Hearing Disorders, 33,* 219–231.

Figures 5.24. Aronson, A. E., Brown, J. R., Litin, E. M., & Pearson, J. S. (1968). Spastic dysphonia II. Comparison with essential (voice) tremor and other neurologic and psychogenic dysphonias. *Journal of Speech and Hearing Disorders, 33,* 219–231.

Figures 6.1, 6.3, & 6.5. Color photographs by Eijii Yanagisawa, M.D.

Figures 6.8–6.10. Colton, R. H., Reed, G., Sagerman, R., & Chung, C. (1982). An investigation of voice change after radiotherapy. In *Final Report, National Cancer Institute,* NIH. Bethesda, MD: National Institutes of Health.

Figure 8.1. Conture, E. G., Schwartz, H., & Brewer, D. (1985). Laryngeal behavior during stuttering: a further study. *Journal of Speech and Hearing Research, 28,* 233–240.

Figure 8.4. Redrawn from Kitzing, P. (1985). Stroboscopy—a pertinent laryngological examination. *Journal of Otolaryngology, 14,* 151–157.

Figure 8.5. Hirano, M., & Bless, D. M. (1993). *Videostroboscopic examination of the larynx.* San Diego: Singular Publishing Group.

Figure 8.6. Metz, D. E., Whitehead, R. L., Peterson, D. H. (1980). An optical illumination system for high speed laryngeal cinematography. *Journal of the Acoustical Society of America, 67,* 719–720.

Figures 8.9–8.10. Drawn from data of Colton, R. H., Reed, G., Sagerman, R., & Chung, C. (1982). An investigation of voice change after radiotherapy.

In *Final Report, National Cancer Institute*, NIH. Bethesda, MD: National Institutes of Health.

Figure 8.12. *Application notes: acoustic measurement of vocal function.* Courtesy of Kay Elemetrics Co., Pine Brook, NJ.

Figure 8.18. Data drawn from Tait, N. A., Michel, J. F., & Carpenter, M. A. (1980). Maximum duration of sustained /s/ and /z/ in children. *Journal of Speech and Hearing Disorders, 45,* 239–246.

Figure 8.19. Based on data reported by Wright, H. N., & Colton, R. H. (1972a). Some parameters of vocal effort. *Journal of the Acoustical Society of America, 51,* 141A.

Figure 9.1. From Zeitels. S. M. (2000). Phonomicrosurgery I: principles and equipment. *Otolaryngol Clin North Am, 33,* 1047–1062.

Figure 9.2. From Zeitels, S. M. (2000). Phonomicrosurgery I: principles and equipment. *Otolaryngol Clin North Am, 33,* 1047–1062.

Figure 9.3. From Kleinsasser, O. (1990). *Microlaryngoscopy and endolaryngeal microsurgery.* (Third ed.) Philadelphia: Hanley & Belfus, Inc.

Figure 9.4–9.6. From Dyce, O. H., Tufano, R. P., & Flint, P. W. (2003). Powered instrumentation in laryngeal surgery. *Operative Techniques in Otolaryngology—Head and Neck Surgery, 14,* 12–17.

Figures 9.7, 9.8, 9.11, 9.12, 9.13. Hirano, M. (1988). Endolaryngeal microsurgery. In G. M. English (Ed.), *Otolaryngology* (Vol. 3, pp. 1–22). Philadelphia: JB Lippincott.

Figure 9.10. Pontes, P., & Behlau, M. (1993). Treatment of sulcus vocalis: auditory perceptual and acoustical analysis of the slicing mucosa surgical technique. *Journal of Voice, 7,* 365–376.

Figures 9.17–9.18. Reproduced by permission from Hirano, M. (1989). Surgical alteration of voice quality. In C. W. Cummings, J. M. Fredrickson, L. A. Harker, C. J. Krause, D. E. Schuller (Eds.), *Otolaryngology—Head and Neck Surgery, Update I.* St. Louis: CV Mosby.

Figure 10.1. Hixon, T. J. (1973). Respiratory function in speech. In F. D. Minifie, T. J. Hixon, & W. Williams (Eds.), *Normal aspects of speech, hearing and language* (p. 107). Englewood Cliffs, NJ: Prentice-Hall.

Figure 10.3. Data obtained from Holmberg, E. B., Hillman, R. E., & Perkell, J. S. (1988). Glottal airflow and transglottal air pressure measurements for male and female speakers in soft, normal and loud voice. *Journal of the Acoustical Society of America, 84,* 511–529.

Figure 11.5. Hirano, M. (1981). *Clinical examination of voice.* Vienna: Springer-Verlag.

Figure 11.6. Dickson, D. R., & Dickson, W. M. (1982). *Anatomical and physiological bases of speech.* Boston: Little, Brown.

Figure 12.2. Titze, I. R. (1994). *Principles of voice production.* Englewood Cliffs, NJ: Prentice-Hall, p. 101.

Figure 12.3. Based on data from Hollien, H., & Moore, G. P. (1960). Measurements of the vocal folds during changes in pitch. *Journal of Speech and Hearing Research, 3,* 157–165.

Figure 12.4. Based on data from Hollien, H., & Colton, R. H. (1969). Four laminagraphic studies of vocal fold thickness. *Folia Phoniatrica, 21,* 179–198.

Figure 12.5. Based on data from van den Berg, J. W., & Tan, T. S. (1959). Results of experiments with human larynges. *Practica Otology Rhinology Laryngology, 21,* 425–450.

Figures 12.6–12.7. Data obtained from Holmberg, E. B., Hillman, R. E., & Perkell, J. S. (1988). Glottal airflow and transglottal air pressure measurements for male and female speakers in soft, normal and loud voice. *Journal of the Acoustical Society of America, 84,* 511–529 (Tables AI–AVI).

Figure 12.9. Based on data from Colton, R. H., Estill, J., & Gerstman, L. (1981). *Identification of four selected voice qualities by spectral analysis.* Paper presented at the Vocal Fold Physiology Conference, Madison, WI.

Figure 13.1. McClean, M. D. (1988). Neuromotor aspects of speech production and dysarthria. In K. M. Yorkston, D. R. T. Beukelman, & K. R. Bell (Eds.), *Clinical management of dysarthric speakers* (pp. 19–58). Boston: College Hill Press.

Figure 13.2. Based on data from Penfield, W., & Roberts, L. (1959). *Speech and brain mechanisms.* Princeton, NJ: Princeton University Press.

Figures 13.3–13.4. Riklan, M., & Levita, E. (1969). *Subcortical correlates of human behavior.* Baltimore: Williams & Wilkins.

Figure 13.5. Based on data from Penfield, W., & Roberts, L. (1959). *Speech and brain mechanisms.* Princeton, NJ: Princeton University Press.

Figures 13.6–13.7. Eccles, J. C. (1977). *The understanding of the brain.* New York: McGraw-Hill.

Figure 13.8. House, E. L., & Pansky, B. (1967). *A functional approach to neuroanatomy.* New York: McGraw-Hill.

Tables

Table 5.2. Adapted from Hoehn, M. M., & Yahr, M. D. (1967). Parkinsonism: onset, progression and mortality. *Neurology, 17,* 427–442.

Table 5.4. Adapted from Ballenger, J. J. (1985). Neurologic diseases of the larynx. In J. J. Ballenger (Ed.), *Diseases of the nose, throat, ear, head, and neck* (pp. 513–548). Philadelphia: Lea & Febiger.

Table 5.5. Adapted from Ballenger, J. J. (1985). Neurologic diseases of the larynx. In J. J. Ballenger (Ed.), *Diseases of the nose, throat, ear, head, and neck* (pp. 513–548). Philadelphia: Lea & Febiger.

Table 5.6. Adapted from Hirano, M., Feder, R., & Bless, D. M. (1983). Clinical evaluation of patients with voice disorders: stroboscopic evaluation. Paper presented at the convention of the American Speech-Language-Hearing Association, Cincinnati, OH.

Table 5.7. Adapted from Carpenter, R. J., McDonald, T. J., & Howard, F. M. (1988). The otolaryngologic presentation of amyotrophic lateral sclerosis. *Otolaryngology, 86*, 479–484.

Table 5.8. Adapted from Carrow, E., Mauldin, M., & Shamblin, L. (1974). Deviant speech characteristics in motor neuron disease. *Archives of Otolaryngology, 100*, 212–218.

Table 5.10. Adapted from Jarema, A. D., Kennedy, J. L., & Shoulson, I. (1985). *Acoustic and aerodynamic measurements of hyperkinetic dysarthria in Huntington's disease.* Paper presented at the convention of the American Speech-Language-Hearing Association, Washington, DC.

Tables 5.11–5.12. Adapted from Darley, F. L., Brown, J. R., & Goldstein, N. P. (1972). Dysarthria in multiple sclerosis. *Journal of Speech and Hearing Research, 15*, 229–245.

Table 6.1. Based on American Joint Committee for Cancer Staging and End Results Reporting. (1983). Philadelphia: JB Lippincott.

Table 14.2. Data from Brown, W. S., Jr., Morris, R. J., Hollien, H., & Howell, E. (1991). Speaking fundamental frequency characteristics as a function of age and professional singing. *Journal of Voice, 5*, 310–315.

Table 14.3. Data from Casper, J. K. (1983). *Frequency perturbation in normal speakers: a descriptive and methodological study.* Unpublished doctoral dissertation, Syracuse University, Syracuse, NY.

Table 14.6. Adapted from Baken, R. J. (1987). *Clinical measurement of speech and voice.* San Diego: College Hill Press, p. 117.

Table 14.9. Adapted from Table 2 in Kent, R. D., Kent, J., & Rosenbek, J. (1987). Maximum performance tests of speech production. *Journal of Speech and Hearing Research, 52*, 367–387.

Index

Page numbers followed by an "f" denote figures; those followed by a "t" denote tables.

Abuse, 86–90, 86t
  breathy phonation for, 339–340
  coughing, 86t, 87–88
  elimination of habitual, 327, 329
  excessive, prolonged loudness,
    86–87, 86t
  identification and reduction of,
    355–356
  misuse versus, 85–86
  of screamer and noise maker, 86t,
    88–89
  sigh, aspirate, easy initiation of
    phonation for, 341
  by sports/exercise enthusiast, 86t,
    89–90
  strained, excessive use during
    swelling/inflammation, 86t,
    87
  throat clearing, 86t, 87–88
Acoustic signs, 21–29, 22t
  amplitude, 25–26, 26f
  frequency breaks, 29
  fundamental frequency, 22–24,
    22t, 23f, 25f
  normal acoustics, 29
  phonation time, 27–29
  signal-to-noise ratio, 26–27
  tremor, 27, 28f
  vocal rise or fall time, 27
  voice stoppages, 29
Acoustic spectrum
  definition of, 256
  one-third octave analysis of, 256
  spectrum analysis and software
    for, 256
Acoustic studies, 248–257
  acoustic spectrum analysis in, 256,
    257f
  of fundamental frequency,
    248–250
  of perturbation, 253–255
  of phonational range, 250–251
  spectrograms in, 255–256
  of vocal intensity, 251–253
Acoustics
  in aging voice, 5
  normal, 29
Actors, voice, 2
Adam's apple, 377–378
Age and gender differences, in lamina
  propria, 69–71
Aged voice (see Geriatric voice)
Aging (see also Geriatric voice)
  acoustics in, 5
  essential tremor and, 163
  theories of, 215–217
  voice in, 5
Air pressure (see also Subglottal (lung)
  air pressure)
  and airflow, 416, 417t

normal versus pathologic, 30
in spasmodic dysphonia, 149–150
Air volumes and capacities, 263
Airflow
  air pressure and, 418, 418t
  average rates of, 416, 417t
  drugs affecting, 94–95
  maximum flow declination rate of,
    418, 419t
  with nodules, 102–103
  normal versus pathologic, 30
  normative data for, 416–419
  in spasmodic dysphonia, 149–150
  in unilateral vocal fold paralysis,
    141–142, 141f
  vibratory, 416, 417t, 418
Airflow waveforms (see also Inverse
  filtering)
  inverse filtering of, 260
Alcohol
  carcinoma from, 193
  voice quality and, 4
Allergic reaction
  effect on voice, 317
  medical management of,
    317–318
ALS (see Amyotrophic lateral sclerosis
  [ALS])
Alternative therapies, herbal
  preparations and, 97–98, 98t
American Medical Association (AMA),
  284
Amino glycoside antibiotics,
  ototoxicity of, 97
Amplitude, 25–26, 26f
  dynamic range of, 25–26, 26f
  sound pressure level in, 23f, 25,
    26f
  variability of, 25
Amplitude perturbation, 26, 413, 414t
  in amyotrophic lateral sclerosis,
    161, 161t
  measurement of, 255
  with nodules, 102
  in Parkinson's disease, 129–130,
    130t
  in vocal fold paralysis, 139
Amyotrophic lateral sclerosis (ALS),
  159–162
  acoustic signs in, 160–161, 161t
  description and etiology of, 159,
    160t
  pathophysiology of, 162
  perceptual voice signs and
    symptoms in, 159–160, 160f
  physiological signs of, 161–162
  speech signs in, 159, 160f
  symptoms of, 159–160, 160f
Anatomical malformations,
  laryngoscopic view of, 35

Anatomy
  of larynx, 373–382
  of vocal folds, 382, 383f, 384–385,
    385f
Androgen-containing hormones,
  adverse effect of, 335
Androgens, effect on vocal structure,
  96–97
Ankylosis of the cricoarytenoid joint,
  185–186
  versus vocal fold paralysis,
    185–186
Ansa cervicalis nerve, 407
Anterior commissure advancement,
  312–313, 312f, 313f
Anterior commissure pushback, for
  vocal fold slackening, 313, 313f
Anterior glottal web
  cause of, 315
  endolaryngeal surgery for,
    315–316, 315f
  thyrotomy for, 315, 315f
Antidepressants, mucosal drying from,
  96
Antihistamines
  effect on voice, 317
  mucosal drying from, 96
Antihypertensives, mucosal drying
  from, 96
Antipsychotics, mucosal drying from,
  96
Antitussives, mucosal drying from, 96
Aphonia
  in differential diagnosis, 16
    case study of, 51–53, 52t,
      60t–62t
    consistent, 21
    episodic, 21
    as perceptual sign, 17t
    psychological, 84–85
    signs associated with, 52t
Apraxia, phonatory, 36
Arnold-Chiari malformation
  description of, 173
  types of, 173–174
  vocal fold paralysis in, 174, 206
Articular cartilages, aging of, 217
Articulation error, in Parkinson's
  disease, 129
Aryepiglottic folds, function of, 1, 384
Arytenoid adduction (see Arytenoid
  cartilages, rotation of)
Arytenoid cartilages, 331, 377f,
  378–379, 379f
  excision (arytenoidectomy), 310,
    311f
  in medialization surgery, 309–310,
    309f
    cricoarytenoid fixation, 310
    rotation of, 309–310, 309f